a LANGE medical book

Vaughan & Asbury's
General Ophthalmology

BMA

. . . Now do you not see that the eye embraces the beauty of the whole world? It is the lord of astronomy and the maker of cosmography; it counsels and corrects all the arts of mankind; it leads men to the different parts of the world; it is the prince of mathematics, and the sciences founded on it are absolutely certain. It has measured the distances and sizes of the stars; it has found the elements and their locations; it . . . has given birth to architecture, and to perspective, and to the divine art of painting. Oh excellent thing, superior to all others created by God! . . . What peoples, what tongues will fully describe your true function? The eye is the window of the human body through which it feels its way and enjoys the beauty of the world. Owing to the eye the soul is content to stay in its bodily prison, for without it such bodily prison is torture.

Leonardo da Vinci (1452–1519)

Vaughan & Asbury's
General Ophthalmology

EIGHTEENTH EDITION

Edited by

Paul Riordan-Eva, FRCOphth
Consultant Ophthalmologist
King's College Hospital, London, United Kingdom
Honorary Senior Lecturer (Teaching)
King's College London School of Medicine at Guy's, King's College and St. Thomas' Hospitals,
London, United Kingdom

Emmett T. Cunningham, Jr., MD, PhD, MPH
Director, The Uveitis Service
Department of Ophthalmology
California Pacific Medical Center
San Francisco, California
Adjunct Clinical Professor of Ophthalmology
Stanford University School of Medicine
Stanford, California

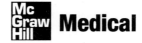
Medical

New York   Chicago   San Francisco   Lisbon   London   Madrid   Mexico
Milan   New Delhi   San Juan   Seoul   Singapore   Sydney   Toronto

Vaughan & Asbury's General Ophthalmology, Eighteenth Edition

1 2 3 4 5 6 7 8 9 0   DOC/DOC   15 14 13 12 11

ISBN 978-0-07-163420-5
MHID 0-07-163420-7
ISSN 1550-0004

Notice

Medicine is an ever-changing science. As new research and clinical experience broaden our knowledge, changes in treatment and drug therapy are required. The authors and the publisher of this work have checked with sources believed to be reliable in their efforts to provide information that is complete and generally in accord with the standards accepted at the time of publication. However, in view of the possibility of human error or changes in medical sciences, neither the authors nor the publisher nor any other party who has been involved in the preparation or publication of this work warrants that the information contained herein is in every respect accurate or complete, and they disclaim all responsibility for any errors or omissions or for the results obtained from use of the information contained in this work. Readers are encouraged to confirm the information contained herein with other sources. For example and in particular, readers are advised to check the product information sheet included in the package of each drug they plan to administer to be certain that the information contained in this work is accurate and that changes have not been made in the recommended dose or in the contraindications for administration. This recommendation is of particular importance in connection with new or infrequently used drugs.

This book was set in Minion by Glyph International.
The editors were Brian Belval and Peter J. Boyle.
The production supervisor was Sherri Souffrance.
Project management was provided by Rajni Pisharody, Glyph International.
The text was designed by Alan Barnett Design.
RR Donnelley was printer and binder.

This book is printed on acid-free paper.

International Edition ISBN 978-0-07-176729-3; MHID 0-07-176729-0. Copyright © 2011. Exclusive rights by The McGraw-Hill Companies, Inc., for manufacture and export. This book cannot be re-exported from the country to which it is consigned by McGraw-Hill. The International Edition is not available in North America.

This edition of
General Ophthalmology
is dedicated with gratitude to
John ("Jack") P. Whitcher, MD, MPH
who was a title page editor for the seventeenth edition,
as well as having contributed to many previous editions.

Contents

Color plates follow page 466

Authors

Taylor Asbury, MD
Vice Chair for Development, Department of
  Ophthalmology, University of Cincinnati;
  Department of Ophthalmology, University of
  Cincinnati College of Medicine, Cincinnati, Ohio
Strabismus

James J. Augsburger, MD
Professor and Chairman, Department of
  Ophthalmology, University of Cincinnati College of
  Medicine, Cincinnati, Ohio
*Lids & Lacrimal Apparatus; Conjunctiva & Tears; Uveal Tract
  & Sclera; Retina; Ophthalmic Genetics; Ophthalmic Trauma*

Roderick Biswell, MD
Associate Professor of Ophthalmology, University of
  California, San Francisco; University of California,
  San Francisco Hospital; O'Connor Hospital, San Jose,
  California
Cornea

Toby Y.B. Chan, MD, BSc
Ophthalmology Resident, Department of Ophthalmology,
  Ivey Eye Institute, University of Western Ontario,
  London, Ontario, Canada
Immunologic Diseases of the Eye

David F. Chang, MD
Clinical Professor, University of California,
  San Francisco
Ophthalmologic Examination

Steve Charles, MD
Clinical Professor of Ophthalmology, Department of
  Ophthalmology, University of Tennessee
  Memphis, Tennessee
Vitreous

N. H. Victor Chong, MPhil, DO, FRCS, FRCOphth
Consultant Ophthalmic Surgeon, Oxford Eye Hospital,
  University of Oxford, Oxford United Kingdom
Retina; Lasers in Ophthalmology

August Colenbrander, MD
Affiliate Senior Scientist, Rehabilitation Engineering Center,
  Smith-Kettlewell Eye Research Institute, San Francisco,
  California
Vision Rehabilitation; Appendix: Functional Vision Score

Zélia M. Corrêa MD, PhD
Associate Professor, Department of Ophthalmology,
  University of Cincinnati College of Medicine, Cincinnati,
  Ohio
*Lids & Lacrimal Apparatus; Conjunctiva & Tears; Uveal Tract
  & Sclera, Retina; Ophthalmic Genetics; Ophthalmic
  Trauma*

Emmett T. Cunningham, Jr., MD, PhD, MPH
Director, The Uveitis Service, Department of
  Ophthalmology, California Pacific Medical Center,
  San Francisco, California
Uveal Tract & Sclera

Eleanor E. Faye, MD, FACS
Associate Professor Retired, Department of Ophthalmology,
  New York University, New York, New York
Low Vision

Allan J. Flach, PharmD, MD
Professor of Ophthalmology, University of California,
  San Francisco
Ophthalmic Therapeutics

Emily C. Fletcher, MBChB, MRCOphth
Specialist Registrar, Department of Ophthalmology, Oxford
  Eye Hospital, John Radcliffe Hospital, Oxford, United
  Kingdom
Retina

Frederick W. Fraunfelder, MD
Assistant Professor of Ophthalmology, Casey Eye
  Institute at Oregon Health and Science University,
  Portland, Oregon
Ophthalmic Therapeutics

Douglas R. Fredrick, MD, FACS
Clinical Professor of Ophthalmology and Pediatrics,
  Department of Ophthalmology, Stanford University,
  Stanford, California
Special Subjects of Pediatric Interest

Francisco J. Garcia-Ferrer, MD
Associate Professor, Department of Ophthalmology and
  Vision Science, Univerisity of California, Davis, School of
  Medicine, Sacramento, California
Conjunctiva &Tears

Elizabeth M. Graham, FRCP, FRCOphth
Consultant Medical Ophthalmologist, St. Thomas' Hospital and National Hospital for Neurology and Neurosurgery, London, United Kingdom
Ocular Disorders Associated with Systemic Diseases

Richard A. Harper, MD
Professor, Department of Ophthalmology, University of Arkansas for Medical Sciences Little Rock, Arkansas
Lens

William G. Hodge, MD, MPH, PhD, FRCSC
University of Ottawa Eye Institute; The Ottawa Hospital, Ottawa, Ontario, Canada
Immunologic Diseases of the Eye; Causes and Prevention of Vision Loss

William F. Hoyt, MD
Professor Emeritus, University of California, San Francisco
Neuro-Ophthalmology

Shefalee Shukla Kent, MD, FRCSC
Fellow, Department of Neuro-Ophthalmology, University of Toronto, Toronto, Canada
Causes and Prevention of Vision Loss

W. Walker Motley, MS, MD
Clinical Assistant Professor of Ophthalmology, Department of Ophthalmology, University of Cincinnati, Cincinnati, Ohio
Strabismus

Lisa M. Nijm, MD, JD
Volunteer Clinical Assistant Professor of Ophthalmology, Department of Surgery, Southern Illinois University School of Medicine, Springfield, Illinois
Conjunctiva & Tears

Carlos Pavesio, MD, FRCOphth
Consultant Ophthalmologist, Medical Retina, Moorfields Eey Hospital, London, United Kingdom
Uveal Tract & Sclera

Adnan Pirbhai, MD, FRCS(C)
Resident, Ivey Eye Institute, Department of Ophthalmology, University of Western Ontario, London, Ontario, Canada
Causes and Prevention of Vision Loss

Edward Pringle MA, MRCP, MRCOphth
Specialist Registrar, Medical Eye Unit, St Thomas' Hospital, London, United Kingdom
Ocular Disorders Associated with Systemic Diseases

Paul Riordan-Eva, FRCOphth
Consultant Ophthalmologist, King's College Hospital, London, United Kingdom; Honorary Senior Lecturer (Teaching), King's College London School of Medicine at Guy's, King's College and St. Thomas' Hospitals, London, United Kingdom
Anatomy & Embryology of the Eye; Ophthalmic Emergencies; Neuro-Ophthalmology; Optics & Refraction

John F. Salmon, MD, FRCS
Consultant Ophthalmologist, Department of Ophthalmology, University of Oxford, Oxford, United Kingdom
Glaucoma

Ivan R. Schwab, MD, FACS
Professor, Department of Ophthalmology, University of California, Davis, Sacramento, California
Conjunctiva & Tears

John P. Shock, MD
Executive Vice Chancellor, Professor and Chairman, Department of Ophthalmology, University of Arkansas for Medical Sciences, Little Rock, Arkansas
Lens

Gwen K. Sterns, MD
Clinical Professor of Ophthalmology, Department of Ophthalmology, University of Rochester School of Medicine and Dentistry, Rochester, New York
Low Vision

John H. Sullivan, MD
Clinical Professor, Department of Ophthalmology, University of California, San Francisco, California
Lids & Lacrimal Apparatus; Orbit

M. Reza Vagefi, MD
Assistant Professor of Ophthalmology, Department of Ophthalmology, Scheie Eye Institute, University of Pennsylvania, Philadelphia, Pennsylvania
Lids & Lacrimal Apparatus

Preface

For five decades, *General Ophthalmology* has served as the most concise, current, and authoritative review of the subject for medical students, ophthalmology residents, practicing ophthalmologists, nurses, optometrists, and colleagues in other fields of medicine and surgery, as well as health-related professionals. The eighteenth edition has been revised and updated in keeping with that goal. It contains the following changes from the seventeenth edition:

- Increased number of color illustrations, more available in the online version at accessmedicine.com
- New chapters on Ophthalmic Emergencies (3), Vision Rehabilitation (25), and Functional Vision Score (Appendix)
- Major revision of the tumors sections of Chapters 4 (Lids and Lacrimal Apparatus), 5 (Conjunctiva & Tears), 7 (Uveal Tract & Sclera), and 10 (Retina), of the sclera section of Chapter 7, and of Chapters 12 (Strabismus), 18 (Ophthalmic Genetics), 19 (Ophthalmic Trauma) and 24 (Low Vision)
- Reorganization of causes and prevention of vision loss into a single chapter (20).

As in past revisions, we have relied on the assistance of many authorities in special fields who have given us the benefit of their advice. We particularly thank David Albiani, Robert Campbell, William Edward, Debra Shetlar, Dhanes Thomas, Constance West and Jack Whitcher for their contributions to previous editions. We warmly welcome our new authors, Toby Chan, August Colenbrander, Zélia Corrêa, Walker Motley, Lisa Nijm, Carlos Pavesio, Adnan Pirbhai, Edward Pringle, Shefalee Shukla Kent, Gwen Sterns, and Reza Vagefi.

Paul Riordan-Eva, FRCOphth
Emmett T. Cunningham, Jr., MD, PhD, MPH
May 2011

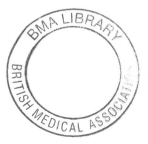

Acknowledgments

Margot Riordan-Eva

Elliott Riordan-Eva

Natasha Riordan-Eva

Anastasia Riordan-Eva

Mary Elaine Armacost

Arthur Asbury

Laurie Campbell

Patricia Cunnane

Harry Hind

Lionel Sorenson

Sharon Shaw

Aidan Cunningham

Ava Cunningham

Jack Whitcher

Heinrich König

Charles Leiter

Barbara Miller

Patricia Pascoe

Geraldine Hruby

Vicente Jocson

Anatomy & Embryology of the Eye

Paul Riordan-Eva, FRCOphth

A thorough understanding of the anatomy of the eye, orbit, visual pathways, upper cranial nerves, and central pathways for the control of eye movements is a prerequisite for proper interpretation of diseases having ocular manifestations. Furthermore, such anatomic knowledge is essential to the proper planning and safe execution of ocular and orbital surgery. Whereas most knowledge of these matters is based on anatomic dissections, either postmortem or during surgery, noninvasive techniques—particularly magnetic resonance imaging (MRI), ultrasonography, and optical coherence tomography (OCT)—are increasingly providing additional information. Investigating the embryology of the eye is clearly a more difficult area because of the relative scarcity of suitable human material, and thus there is still great reliance on animal studies, with the inherent difficulties in inferring parallels in human development. Nevertheless, a great deal is known about the embryology of the human eye, and—together with the recent expansion in molecular genetics—this has led to a much deeper understanding of developmental anomalies of the eye.

▼ I. NORMAL ANATOMY

THE ORBIT (FIGURES 1–1 AND 1–2)

The orbital cavity is schematically represented as a pyramid of four walls that converge posteriorly. The medial walls of the right and left orbit are parallel and are separated by the nose. In each orbit, the lateral and medial walls form an angle of 45°, which results in a right angle between the two lateral walls. The orbit is compared to the shape of a pear, with the optic nerve representing its stem. The anterior circumference is somewhat smaller in diameter than the region just within the rim, which makes a sturdy protective margin.

The volume of the adult orbit is approximately 30 mL, and the eyeball occupies only about one-fifth of the space. Fat and muscle account for the bulk of the remainder.

The anterior limit of the orbital cavity is the **orbital septum**, which acts as a barrier between the eyelids and orbit (see Eyelids later in this chapter).

The orbits are related to the frontal sinus above, the maxillary sinus below, and the ethmoid and sphenoid sinuses medially. The thin orbital floor is easily damaged by direct trauma to the globe, resulting in a "blowout" fracture with herniation of orbital contents into the maxillary antrum. Infection within the sphenoid and ethmoid sinuses can erode the paper-thin medial wall (lamina papyracea) and involve the contents of the orbit. Defects in the roof (eg, neurofibromatosis) may result in visible pulsations of the globe transmitted from the brain.

▶ Orbital Walls

The roof of the orbit is composed principally of the orbital plate of the **frontal bone**. The lacrimal gland is located in the lacrimal fossa in the anterior lateral aspect of the roof. Posteriorly, the lesser wing of the **sphenoid bone** containing the optic canal completes the roof.

The lateral wall is separated from the roof by the superior orbital fissure, which divides the lesser from the greater wing of the sphenoid bone. The anterior portion of the lateral wall is formed by the orbital surface of the **zygomatic (malar) bone**. This is the strongest part of the bony orbit. Suspensory ligaments, the lateral palpebral tendon, and check ligaments have connective tissue attachments to the lateral orbital tubercle.

The orbital floor is separated from the lateral wall by the inferior orbital fissure. The orbital plate of the maxilla forms the large central area of the floor and is the region where blowout fractures most frequently occur. The frontal process of the **maxilla** medially and the zygomatic bone laterally complete the inferior orbital rim. The orbital process of the **palatine** bone forms a small triangular area in the posterior floor.

The boundaries of the medial wall are less distinct. The **ethmoid bone** is paper-thin but thickens anteriorly as it meets

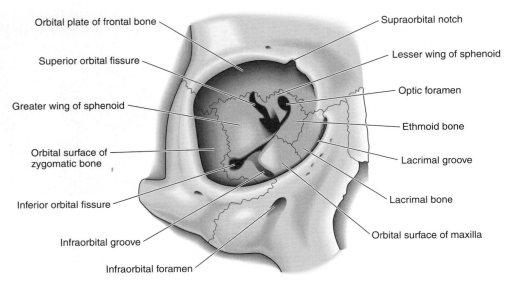

▲ Figure 1–1. Anterior view of bones of right orbit.

Orbital plate of frontal bone

Superior orbital fissure

Greater wing of sphenoid

Orbital surface of zygomatic bone

Inferior orbital fissure

Infraorbital groove

Infraorbital foramen

Supraorbital notch

Lesser wing of sphenoid

Optic foramen

Ethmoid bone

Lacrimal groove

Lacrimal bone

Orbital surface of maxilla

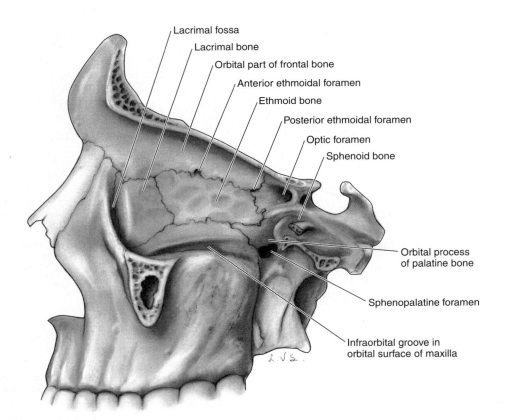

▲ Figure 1–2. Medial view of bony wall of left orbit.

Lacrimal fossa

Lacrimal bone

Orbital part of frontal bone

Anterior ethmoidal foramen

Ethmoid bone

Posterior ethmoidal foramen

Optic foramen

Sphenoid bone

Orbital process of palatine bone

Sphenopalatine foramen

Infraorbital groove in orbital surface of maxilla

the **lacrimal bone**. The body of the sphenoid forms the most posterior aspect of the medial wall, and the angular process of the frontal bone forms the upper part of the posterior lacrimal crest. The lower portion of the posterior lacrimal crest is made up of the lacrimal bone. The anterior lacrimal crest is easily palpated through the lid and is composed of the frontal process of the maxilla. The lacrimal groove lies between the two crests and contains the lacrimal sac.

▶ Orbital Apex (Figure 1–3)

The apex of the orbit is the main portal for all nerves and vessels to the eye and the site of origin of all extraocular muscles

except the inferior oblique. The **superior orbital fissure** lies between the body and the greater and lesser wings of the sphenoid bone. The superior ophthalmic vein and the lacrimal, frontal, and trochlear nerves pass through the lateral portion of the fissure that lies outside the annulus of Zinn. The superior and inferior divisions of the oculomotor nerve and the abducens and nasociliary nerves pass through the medial portion of the fissure within the annulus of Zinn. The optic nerve and ophthalmic artery pass through the optic canal, which also lies within the annulus of Zinn. The inferior ophthalmic vein frequently joins the superior ophthalmic vein before exiting the orbit. Otherwise, it may pass through any part of the superior orbital fissure, including the portion adjacent to the body

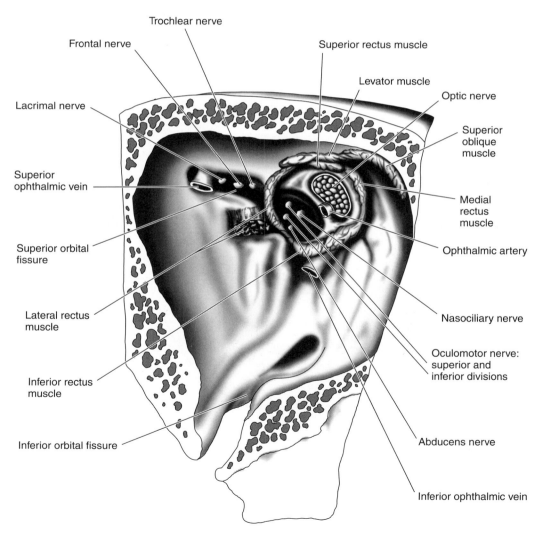

▲ **Figure 1–3.** Anterior view of apex of right orbit.

of the sphenoid that lies inferomedial to the annulus of Zinn, or through the inferior orbital fissure.

▶ Blood Supply (Figures 1-4, 1-5, and 1-6)

The principal arterial supply of the orbit and its structures derives from the ophthalmic artery, the first major branch of the intracranial portion of the internal carotid artery. This branch passes beneath the optic nerve and accompanies it through the optic canal into the orbit. The first intraorbital branch is the central retinal artery, which enters the optic nerve about 8–15 mm behind the globe. Other branches of the ophthalmic artery include the lacrimal artery, supplying the lacrimal gland and upper eyelid; muscular branches to the various muscles of the orbit; long and short posterior ciliary arteries; medial palpebral arteries to both eyelids; and

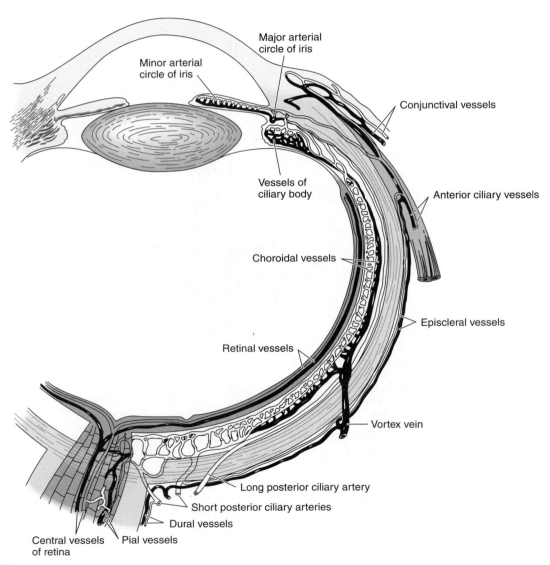

Major arterial circle of iris

Minor arterial circle of iris

Conjunctival vessels

Vessels of ciliary body

Anterior ciliary vessels

Choroidal vessels

Episcleral vessels

Retinal vessels

Vortex vein

Long posterior ciliary artery

Short posterior ciliary arteries

Dural vessels

Central vessels of retina   Pial vessels

▲ **Figure 1-4.** Vascular supply to the eye. All arterial branches originate with the ophthalmic artery. Venous drainage is through the cavernous sinus and the pterygoid plexus.

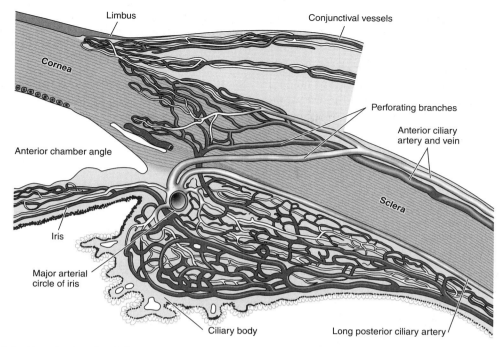

▲ Figure 1–5. Vascular supply of the anterior segment.

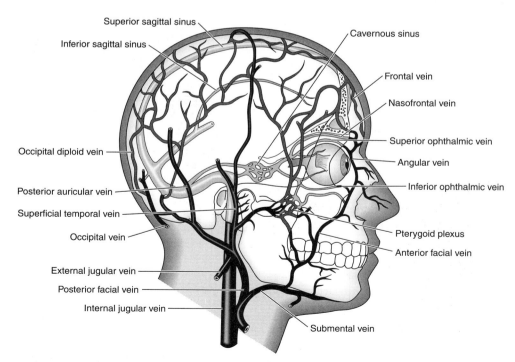

▲ Figure 1–6. Venous drainage system of the eye.

the supraorbital and supratrochlear arteries. The short posterior ciliary arteries supply the choroid and parts of the optic nerve. The two long posterior ciliary arteries supply the ciliary body and anastomose with each other and with the anterior ciliary arteries to form the major arterial circle of the iris. The anterior ciliary arteries are derived from the muscular branches to the rectus muscles. They supply the anterior sclera, episclera, limbus, and conjunctiva and contribute to the major arterial circle of the iris. The most anterior branches of the ophthalmic artery contribute to the formation of the arterial arcades of the eyelids, which make an anastomosis with the external carotid circulation via the facial artery.

The venous drainage of the orbit is primarily through the superior and inferior ophthalmic veins, into which drain the vortex veins, the anterior ciliary veins, and the central retinal vein. The ophthalmic veins communicate with the cavernous sinus via the superior orbital fissure and the pterygoid venous plexus via the inferior orbital fissure. The superior ophthalmic vein is initially formed from the supraorbital and supratrochlear veins and from a branch of the angular vein, all of which drain the skin of the periorbital region. This provides a direct communication between the skin of the face and the cavernous sinus, thus forming the basis of the potentially lethal cavernous sinus thrombosis, secondary to superficial infection of the periorbital skin.

THE EYEBALL

The normal adult globe is approximately spherical, with an anteroposterior diameter averaging 24 mm.

THE CONJUNCTIVA

The conjunctiva is the thin, transparent mucous membrane that covers the posterior surface of the lids (the palpebral conjunctiva) and the anterior surface of the sclera (the bulbar conjunctiva). It is continuous with the skin at the lid margin (a mucocutaneous junction) and with the corneal epithelium at the limbus.

The **palpebral conjunctiva** lines the posterior surface of the lids and is firmly adherent to the tarsus. At the superior and inferior margins of the tarsus, the conjunctiva is reflected posteriorly (at the superior and inferior fornices) and covers the episcleral tissue to become the bulbar conjunctiva.

The **bulbar conjunctiva** is loosely attached to the orbital septum in the fornices and is folded many times. This allows the eye to move and enlarges the secretory conjunctival surface. (The ducts of the lacrimal gland open into the superior temporal fornix.) Except at the limbus (where Tenon's capsule and the conjunctiva are fused for about 3 mm), the bulbar conjunctiva is loosely attached to Tenon's capsule and the underlying sclera.

A soft, movable, thickened fold of bulbar conjunctiva (the **semilunar fold**) is located at the inner canthus and corresponds to the nictitating membrane of some lower animals.

A small, fleshy, epidermoid structure (the caruncle) is attached superficially to the inner portion of the semilunar fold and is a transition zone containing both cutaneous and mucous membrane elements.

▶ Histology

The **conjunctival epithelium** consists of two to five layers of stratified columnar epithelial cells—superficial and basal. Conjunctival epithelium near the limbus, over the caruncle, and near the mucocutaneous junctions at the lid margins consists of stratified squamous epithelial cells. The **superficial epithelial cells** contain round or oval mucus-secreting goblet cells. The mucus, as it forms, pushes aside the goblet cell nucleus and is necessary for proper dispersion of the precorneal tear film. The **basal epithelial cells** stain more deeply than the superficial cells and may contain pigment near the limbus.

The **conjunctival stroma** is divided into an adenoid (superficial) layer and a fibrous (deep) layer. The **adenoid layer** contains lymphoid tissue and in some areas may contain "follicle-like" structures without germinal centers. The adenoid layer does not develop until after the first 2 or 3 months of life. This explains why inclusion conjunctivitis of the newborn is papillary in nature rather than follicular and why it later becomes follicular. The **fibrous layer** is composed of connective tissue that attaches to the tarsal plate. This explains the appearance of the papillary reaction in inflammations of the conjunctiva. The fibrous layer is loosely arranged over the globe.

The **accessory lacrimal glands** (glands of Krause and Wolfring), which resemble the lacrimal gland in structure and function, are located in the stroma. Most of the glands of Krause are in the upper fornix, and the remaining few are in the lower fornix. The glands of Wolfring lie at the superior margin of the upper tarsus.

▶ Blood Supply, Lymphatics, & Nerve Supply

The conjunctival arteries are derived from the anterior ciliary and palpebral arteries. The two arteries anastomose freely and—along with the numerous conjunctival veins that generally follow the arterial pattern—form a considerable conjunctival vascular network. The conjunctival lymphatics are arranged in superficial and deep layers and join with the lymphatics of the eyelids to form a rich lymphatic plexus. The conjunctiva receives its nerve supply from the first (ophthalmic) division of the fifth nerve. It possesses a relatively small number of pain fibers.

TENON'S CAPSULE (FASCIA BULBI)

Tenon's capsule is a fibrous membrane that envelops the globe from the limbus to the optic nerve (Figure 1–19). Adjacent to the limbus, the conjunctiva, Tenon's capsule, and episclera are fused together. More posteriorly, the inner surface of Tenon's capsule lies against the sclera, and its outer aspect is in contact with orbital fat and other structures within the extraocular muscle cone. At the point where Tenon's capsule is pierced by tendons of the extraocular muscles in their passage to their attachments to the globe, it sends a tubular reflection around each of these muscles. These fascial reflections become continuous with the fascia of the muscles, the fused fasciae sending expansions to the surrounding structures and to the orbital bones. The fascial expansions are quite tough and limit the action of the extraocular muscles, and are therefore known as **check ligaments** (Figure 1–20). They regulate the direction of action of the extraocular muscles and may act as their functional mechanical origins, possibly with active neuronal control (active pulley hypothesis). The lower segment of Tenon's capsule is thick and fuses with the fascia of the inferior rectus and the inferior oblique muscles to form the suspensory ligament of the eyeball (Lockwood's ligament), upon which the globe rests.

THE SCLERA & EPISCLERA

The **sclera** is the fibrous outer protective coating of the eye, consisting almost entirely of collagen (Figure 1–7). It is dense and white, and continuous with the cornea anteriorly and the dural sheath of the optic nerve posteriorly. Across the posterior scleral foramen are bands of collagen and elastic tissue, forming the **lamina cribrosa**, between which pass the axon bundles of the optic nerve. The outer surface of the anterior sclera is covered by a thin layer of fine elastic tissue, the **episclera**, which contains numerous blood vessels that

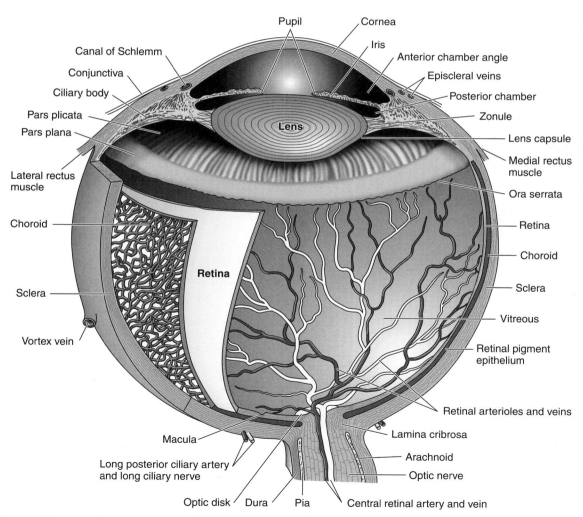

▲ **Figure 1–7.** Internal structures of the human eye.

nourish the sclera. The brown pigment layer on the inner surface of the sclera is the lamina fusca, which forms the outer layer of the suprachoroidal space.

At the insertion of the rectus muscles, the sclera is about 0.3 mm thick; elsewhere it is about 0.6 mm thick. Around the optic nerve, the sclera is penetrated by the long and short posterior ciliary arteries and the long and short ciliary nerves (Figure 1–8). The long posterior ciliary arteries and long ciliary nerves pass from the optic nerve to the ciliary body in a shallow groove on the inner surface of the sclera at the 3 and 9 o'clock meridians. Slightly posterior to the equator, the four vortex veins draining the choroid exit through the sclera, usually one in each quadrant. About 4 mm posterior to the limbus, slightly anterior to the insertion of the respective rectus muscle, the four anterior ciliary arteries and veins penetrate the sclera. The nerve supply to the sclera is from the ciliary nerves.

Histologically, the sclera consists of many dense bands of parallel and interlacing collagen bundles, each of which is 10–16 μm thick and 100–140 μm wide. The histologic structure of the sclera is remarkably similar to that of the corneal stroma (see the next section) but it is opaque rather than transparent because of irregularity of the collagen lamellae, higher water content, and less proteoglycans.

THE CORNEA

The cornea is a transparent tissue comparable in size and structure to the crystal of a small wristwatch (Figure 1–9). It is

inserted into the sclera at the limbus, the circumferential depression at this junction being known as the scleral sulcus. The average adult cornea is 550 μm thick in the center, although there are racial variations, and about 11.7 mm in diameter horizontally and 10.6 mm vertically. From anterior to posterior, it has five distinct layers (Figure 1–10): the epithelium (which is continuous with the epithelium of the bulbar conjunctiva), Bowman's layer, the stroma, Descemet's membrane, and the endothelium. The epithelium has five or six layers of cells. Bowman's layer is a clear acellular layer, a modified portion of the stroma. The corneal stroma accounts for about 90% of the corneal thickness. It is composed of intertwining lamellae of collagen fibrils 10–250 μm in width and 1–2 μm in height that run almost the full diameter of the cornea. They run parallel to the surface of the cornea and by virtue of their regularity, are optically clear. The lamellae lie within a ground substance of hydrated proteoglycans in association with the keratocytes that produce the collagen and ground substance. Descemet's membrane, constituting the basal lamina of the corneal endothelium, has a homogeneous appearance on light microscopy but a laminated appearance on electron microscopy due to structural differences between its prenasal and postnatal portions. It is about 3 μm thick at birth but increases in thickness throughout life, reaching 10–12 μm in adulthood. The endothelium has only one layer of cells, but this is responsible for maintaining the essential deturgescence of the corneal stroma. The endothelium is quite susceptible to injury as well as undergoing loss of cells with age: the normal density reducing from 23,000 cells/mm^2 at birth to

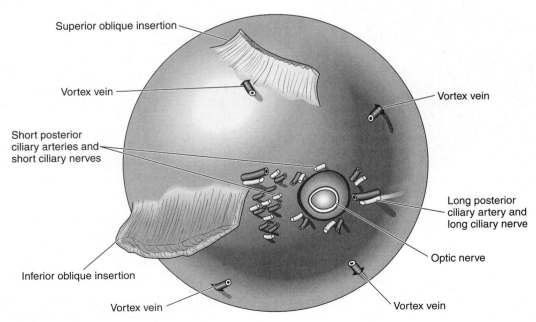

▲ **Figure 1–8.** Posterior view of left eye.

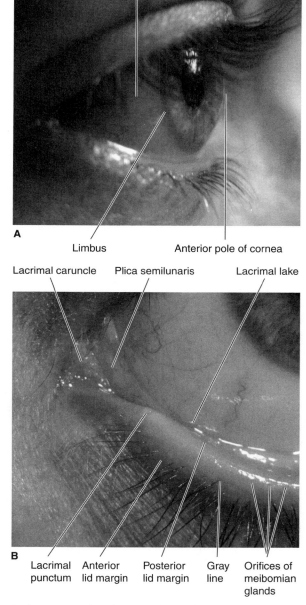

Sclera

Limbus   Anterior pole of cornea

A

Lacrimal caruncle   Plica semilunaris   Lacrimal lake

Lacrimal   Anterior   Posterior   Gray   Orifices of
punctum   lid margin   lid margin   line   meibomian
                                              glands

B

▲ **Figure 1–9. (A, B)** External landmarks of the eye. The sclera is covered by transparent conjunctiva.

2000 cells/mm² in old age. Endothelial repair is limited to enlargement and sliding of existing cells, with little capacity for cell division. Failure of endothelial function leads to corneal edema.

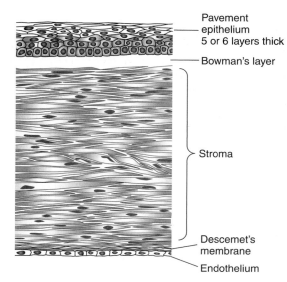

Pavement epithelium 5 or 6 layers thick

Bowman's layer

Stroma

Descemet's membrane

Endothelium

▲ **Figure 1–10.** Transverse section of cornea.

Sources of nutrition for the cornea are the vessels of the limbus, the aqueous, and the tears. The superficial cornea also gets most of its oxygen from the atmosphere. The sensory nerves of the cornea are supplied by the first (ophthalmic) division of the fifth (trigeminal) cranial nerve.

The transparency of the cornea is due to its uniform structure, avascularity, and deturgescence.

THE UVEAL TRACT

The uveal tract is composed from anterior to posterior of the iris, the ciliary body, and the choroid (Figure 1–7). It is the middle vascular layer of the eye and is protected by the cornea and sclera. It contributes blood supply to the retina.

▶ Iris

The **iris** is a shallow cone pointing anteriorly with a centrally situated round aperture, the **pupil**. It is positioned in front of the lens, dividing the **anterior chamber** from the **posterior chamber**, each of which contains aqueous humor that passes through the pupil. There are no epithelial cells covering the anterior stroma. The sphincter and dilator muscles develop from the anterior epithelium, which covers the posterior surface of the stroma and represents an anterior extension of the retinal pigment epithelium. The heavily pigmented posterior epithelium represents an anterior extension of the neuroretina.

The arterial blood supply to the iris is from the major circle of the iris (Figure 1–4). Iris capillaries have a non-fenestrated endothelium, and hence do not normally leak intravenously injected fluorescein. Sensory nerve supply to the iris is via fibers in the ciliary nerves.

The iris controls the amount of light entering the eye. Pupillary size is principally determined by a balance between constriction due to parasympathetic activity transmitted via the third cranial nerve and dilation due to sympathetic activity (see Chapter 14).

▶ The Ciliary Body

The **ciliary body**, roughly triangular in cross section, extends forward from the anterior end of the choroid to the root of the iris (about 6 mm). It consists of a corrugated anterior zone, the pars plicata (2 mm), and a flattened posterior zone, the pars plana (4 mm). The ciliary processes arise from the pars plicata (Figure 1–11). They are composed mainly of capillaries and veins that drain through the vortex veins. The capillaries are large and fenestrated, and hence leak intravenously injected fluorescein. There are two layers of ciliary epithelium: an internal nonpigmented layer, representing the anterior extension of the neuroretina, and an external pigmented layer, representing an extension of the retinal pigment epithelium. The ciliary processes and their covering ciliary epithelium are responsible for the formation of aqueous.

The **ciliary muscle** is composed of a combination of longitudinal, radial, and circular fibers. The function of the circular fibers is to contract and relax the zonular fibers, which originate in the valleys between the ciliary processes (Figure 1–12). This alters the tension on the capsule of the lens, giving the lens a variable focus for both near and distant objects in the visual field. The longitudinal fibers of the ciliary muscle insert into the trabecular meshwork to influence its pore size.

The arterial blood supply to the ciliary body is derived from the major circle of the iris. The nerve supply is via the short ciliary nerves.

▶ The Choroid

The choroid is the posterior segment of the uveal tract, between the retina and the sclera. It is composed of three layers of choroidal blood vessels: large, medium, and small. The deeper the vessels are placed in the choroid, the wider their lumens (Figure 1–13). The internal portion of the choroid vessels is known as the choriocapillaris. Blood from the choroidal vessels drains via the four vortex veins, one in each of the four posterior quadrants. The choroid is bounded internally by Bruch's membrane and externally by the sclera. The suprachoroidal space lies between the choroid and the sclera. The choroid is firmly attached posteriorly to the margins of the optic nerve. Anteriorly, the choroid joins with the ciliary body.

The aggregate of choroidal blood vessels serves to nourish the outer portion of the retina (Figure 1–4). The nerve supply to the choroid is via the ciliary nerves.

THE LENS

The lens is a biconvex, avascular, colorless, and almost completely transparent structure, about 4 mm thick and 9 mm in diameter. It is suspended behind the iris by the zonule, which connects it with the ciliary body. Anterior to the lens is the aqueous; posterior to it, the vitreous.

The lens capsule (see The Vitreous later in the chapter) is a semipermeable membrane (slightly more permeable than a capillary wall) that will admit water and electrolytes. A subcapsular epithelium is present anteriorly (Figure 1–14). With age, subepithelial lamellar fibers are continuously produced, so that the lens gradually becomes larger and less elastic throughout life. The nucleus and cortex are made up of long concentric lamellae, the lens nucleus being harder than the cortex. The suture lines formed by the end-to-end joining of these lamellar fibers are Y-shaped when viewed with the slit-lamp (Figure 1–15). The Y is upright anteriorly and inverted posteriorly.

Each lamellar fiber contains a flattened nucleus. These nuclei are evident microscopically in the peripheral portion of the lens near the equator and are continuous with the subcapsular epithelium.

The lens is held in place by a suspensory ligament known as the zonule (zonule of Zinn), which is composed of numerous fibrils that arise from the surface of the ciliary body and insert into the lens equator.

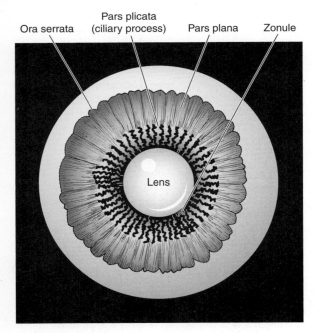

Ora serrata   Pars plicata (ciliary process)   Pars plana   Zonule

Lens

▲ **Figure 1–11.** Posterior view of ciliary body, zonule, lens, and ora serrata.

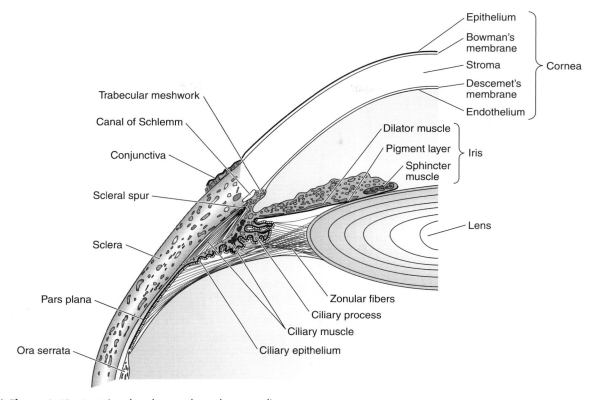

▲ **Figure 1–12.** Anterior chamber angle and surrounding structures.

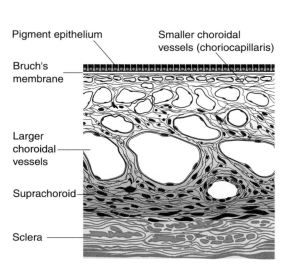

▲ **Figure 1–13.** Cross section of choroid.

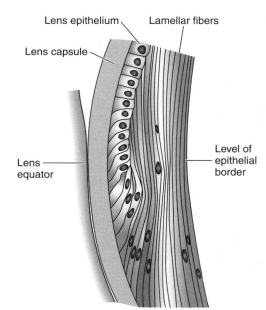

▲ **Figure 1–14.** Magnified view of lens showing termination of subcapsular epithelium (vertical section).

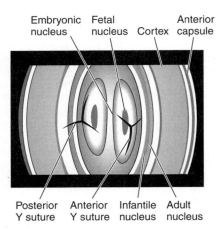

▲ Figure 1–15. Zones of lens showing Y sutures.

The lens consists of about 65% water, about 35% protein (the highest protein content of any tissue of the body), and a trace of minerals common to other body tissues. Potassium is more concentrated in the lens than in most tissues. Ascorbic acid and glutathione are present in both oxidized and reduced forms.

There are no pain fibers, blood vessels, or nerves in the lens.

THE AQUEOUS

Aqueous humor is produced by the ciliary body. Entering the posterior chamber, it passes through the pupil into the anterior chamber (Figure 1–7) and then peripherally toward the anterior chamber angle. The physiology of the aqueous is discussed in Chapter 11.

THE ANTERIOR CHAMBER ANGLE

The anterior chamber (iridocorneal) angle lies at the junction of the peripheral cornea and the root of the iris (Figures 1–12 and 1–16). Its main anatomic features are Schwalbe's line, the trabecular meshwork (which overlies Schlemm's canal), and the scleral spur.

Schwalbe's line marks the termination of the corneal endothelium. The trabecular meshwork is triangular in cross section, with its base directed toward the ciliary body. It is composed of perforated sheets of collagen and elastic tissue, forming a filter with decreasing pore size as the canal of Schlemm is approached. The internal portion of the meshwork, facing the anterior chamber, is known as the uveal meshwork; the external portion, adjacent to the canal of Schlemm, is called the corneoscleral meshwork. The longitudinal fibers of the ciliary muscle insert into the trabecular meshwork. The scleral spur is an inward extension of the

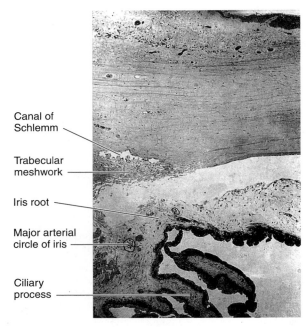

▲ Figure 1–16. Photomicrograph of anterior chamber angle and related structures. (Courtesy of I Wood and L Garron.)

sclera between the ciliary body and Schlemm's canal, to which the iris and ciliary body are attached. Efferent channels from Schlemm's canal (about 30 collector channels and up to 12 aqueous veins) communicate with the episcleral venous system.

THE RETINA

The retina is a thin, semitransparent, multilayered sheet of neural tissue that lines the inner aspect of the posterior two-thirds of the wall of the globe. It extends almost as far anteriorly as the ciliary body, ending at that point in a ragged edge, the ora serrata (Figure 1–12). In adults the ora serrata is about 6.5 mm behind Schwalbe's line on the temporal side and 5.7 mm behind it nasally. The outer surface of the sensory retina is apposed to the retinal pigment epithelium, and thus related to Bruch's membrane, the choroid, and the sclera. In most areas, the retina and retinal pigment epithelium are easily separated to form the subretinal space, such as occurs in retinal detachment. But at the optic disk and the ora serrata, the retina and retinal pigment epithelium are firmly bound together, thus limiting the spread of subretinal fluid in retinal detachment. This contrasts with the potential suprachoroidal space between the choroid and sclera, which extends to the scleral spur. Choroidal detachments thus extend beyond the ora serrata, under the pars plana and pars plicata. The epithelial layers of the inner surface of the ciliary body and the posterior surface of the iris represent anterior extensions of the retina and retinal pigment epithelium. The inner surface of the retina is apposed to the vitreous.

The layers of the retina, starting from its inner aspect, are: (1) internal limiting membrane; (2) nerve fiber layer, containing the ganglion cell axons passing to the optic nerve; (3) ganglion cell layer; (4) inner plexiform layer, containing the connections of the ganglion cells with the amacrine and bipolar cells; (5) inner nuclear layer of bipolar, amacrine, and horizontal cell bodies; (6) outer plexiform layer, containing the connections of the bipolar and horizontal cells with the photoreceptors; (7) outer nuclear layer of photoreceptor cell nuclei; (8) external limiting membrane; (9) photoreceptor layer of rod and cone inner and outer segments; and (10) retinal pigment epithelium (Figure 1–17). The inner layer of Bruch's membrane is actually the basement membrane of the retinal pigment epithelium.

The retina is 0.1 mm thick at the ora serrata and 0.56 mm thick in parts of the posterior pole. In the center of the posterior retina is the 5.5- to 6.0-mm-diameter macula, defined clinically as the area bounded by the temporal retinal vascular arcades. It is known to anatomists as the area centralis, being defined histologically as that part of the retina in which the ganglion cell layer is more than one cell thick. The macula lutea is defined anatomically as the 3-mm-diameter area containing the yellow luteal pigment xanthophyll. The

1.5-mm-diameter fovea is characterized histologically by thinning of the outer nuclear layer and absence of the other parenchymal layers as a result of the oblique course of the photoreceptor cell axons (Henle fiber layer) and the centrifugal displacement of the retinal layers that are closer to the inner retinal surface. In the center of the macula, 4 mm lateral to the optic disk, is the 0.3-mm-diameter foveola, clinically apparent as a depression that creates a particular reflection when viewed ophthalmoscopically. It is the thinnest part of area of the retina (0.25 mm), containing only cone photoreceptors, and corresponds to the retinal avascular zone on fluorescein angiography. The histologic features of the fovea and foveola provide for fine visual discrimination, the foveola providing optimal visual acuity. The normally empty extracellular space of the retina is potentially greatest at the macula. Diseases that lead to accumulation of extracellular material particularly cause thickening of this area (macular edema).

The retina receives its blood supply from two sources: the choriocapillaris immediately outside Bruch's membrane, which supplies the outer third of the retina, including the outer plexiform and outer nuclear layers, the photoreceptors, and the retinal pigment epithelium; and branches of the central retinal artery, which supply the inner two-thirds (Figure 1–4). The foveola is supplied entirely by the choriocapillaris and is susceptible to irreparable damage when the retina is detached. The retinal blood vessels have a nonfenestrated endothelium, which forms the inner blood-retinal barrier, whereas the endothelium of choroidal vessels is fenestrated. The outer blood-retinal barrier lies at the level of the retinal pigment epithelium.

THE VITREOUS

The vitreous is a clear, avascular, gelatinous body that comprises two-thirds of the volume and weight of the eye. It fills the space bounded by the lens, retina, and optic disk (Figure 1–7). The outer surface of the vitreous—the hyaloid membrane—is normally in contact with the following structures: the posterior lens capsule, the zonular fibers, the pars plana epithelium, the retina, and the optic nerve head. The base of the vitreous maintains a firm attachment throughout life to the pars plana epithelium and the retina immediately behind the ora serrata. The attachment to the lens capsule and the optic nerve head is firm only in early life.

The vitreous is about 99% water. The remaining 1% includes two components, collagen and hyaluronan, which give the vitreous a gel-like form and consistency because of their ability to bind large volumes of water.

THE EXTERNAL ANATOMIC LANDMARKS

Accurate localization of the position of internal structures with reference to the external surface of the globe is important in many surgical procedures. The distance of structures from the limbus as measured externally is less than their

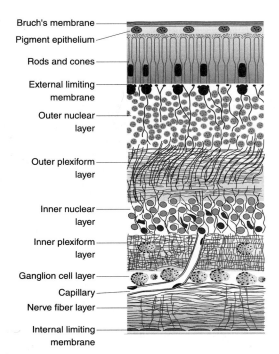

Bruch's membrane
Pigment epithelium
Rods and cones
External limiting membrane
Outer nuclear layer
Outer plexiform layer
Inner nuclear layer
Inner plexiform layer
Ganglion cell layer
Capillary
Nerve fiber layer
Internal limiting membrane

▲ **Figure 1–17.** Layers of the retina.

actual length. Externally, the ora serrata is situated approximately 5.5 mm from the limbus on the medial side and 7 mm on the temporal side of the globe. This corresponds to the level of insertion of the rectus muscles. Injections into the vitreous cavity through the pars plana should be given 3.5–4.0 mm from the limbus in the phakic eye and 3–3.5 mm from the limbus in the pseudophakic or aphakic eye. The pars plicata, which is the target for cyclodestructive procedures in the treatment of intractable glaucoma, occupies the 2–3 mm directly posterior to the limbus.

THE EXTRAOCULAR MUSCLES

Six extraocular muscles control the movement of each eye: four rectus and two oblique muscles.

Rectus Muscles

The four rectus muscles originate at a common ring tendon (annulus of Zinn) surrounding the optic nerve at the posterior apex of the orbit (Figure 1–3). They are named according to their insertion into the sclera on the medial, lateral, inferior, and superior surfaces of the eye. The principal action of the respective muscles is thus to adduct, abduct, depress, and elevate the globe (see Chapter 12). The muscles are about 40 mm long, becoming tendinous 4–8 mm from the point of insertion, where they are about 10 mm wide. The approximate distances of the points of insertion from the corneal limbus are: medial rectus, 5.5 mm; inferior rectus, 6.5 mm; lateral rectus, 7 mm; superior rectus, 7.5 mm (Figure 1–18). With the eye in the primary position, the vertical rectus muscles make an angle of about 23° with the optic axis.

Oblique Muscles

The two oblique muscles primarily control torsional movement and, to a lesser extent, upward and downward movements of the globe (see Chapter 12).

The **superior oblique** is the longest and thinnest of the ocular muscles. It originates above and medial to the optic foramen and partially overlaps the origin of the levator palpebrae superioris muscle. The superior oblique has a thin, fusiform belly (30-mm long) and passes anteriorly in the form of a tendon (10-mm long) to its trochlea, or pulley. It is then reflected backwards and downwards as a further length of tendon to attach in a fan shape to the sclera beneath the superior rectus. The trochlea is a cartilaginous structure attached to the frontal bone 3 mm behind the orbital rim. The superior oblique tendon is enclosed in a synovial sheath as it passes through the trochlea.

The **inferior oblique** muscle originates from the nasal side of the orbital wall just behind the inferior orbital rim and lateral to the nasolacrimal duct. It passes beneath the inferior rectus and then under the lateral rectus muscle to insert onto the sclera with a short tendon. The insertion is

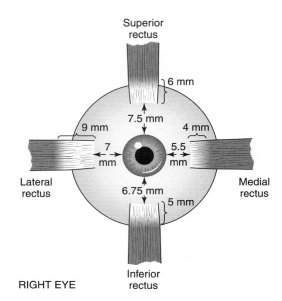

▲ **Figure 1–18.** Approximate distances of the rectus muscles from the limbus, and the approximate lengths of tendons.

into the posterotemporal segment of the globe and just over the macular area. The muscle is about 35-mm long.

In the primary position, the muscle plane of the superior and inferior oblique muscles forms an angle of 51–54° with the optic axis.

Fascia

All the extraocular muscles are ensheathed by fascia. Near the points of insertion of these muscles, the fascia is continuous with Tenon's capsule, and fascial condensations to adjacent orbital structures (check ligaments) act as the functional origins of the extraocular muscles (Figures 1–19 and 1–20).

Nerve Supply

The oculomotor nerve (III) innervates the medial, inferior, and superior rectus muscles and the inferior oblique muscle. The abducens nerve (VI) innervates the lateral rectus muscle; the trochlear nerve (IV) innervates the superior oblique muscle.

Blood Supply

The blood supply to the extraocular muscles is derived from the muscular branches of the ophthalmic artery. The lateral rectus and inferior oblique muscles are also supplied by branches from the lacrimal artery and the infraorbital artery, respectively.

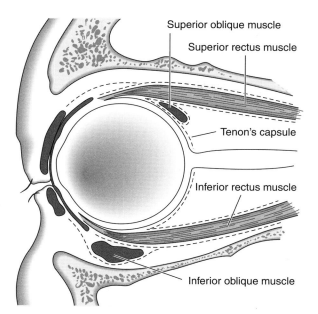

▲ **Figure 1–19.** Fascia about muscles and eyeball (Tenon's capsule).

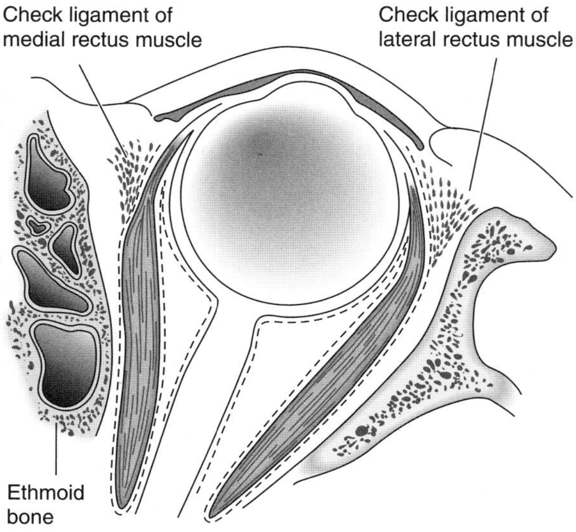

THE OCULAR ADNEXA

1. EYEBROWS

The eyebrows are folds of thickened skin covered with hair. The skin fold is supported by underlying muscle fibers. The glabella is the hairless prominence between the eyebrows.

2. EYELIDS

The upper and lower eyelids (palpebrae) are modified folds of skin that can close to protect the anterior eyeball (Figure 1–21). Blinking helps spread the tear film, which protects the cornea and conjunctiva from dehydration. The upper lid ends at the eyebrows; the lower lid merges into the cheek.

The eyelids consist of five principal planes of tissues. From superficial to deep, they are the skin layer, a layer of striated muscle (orbicularis oculi), areolar tissue, fibrous tissue (tarsal plates), and a layer of mucous membrane (palpebral conjunctiva) (Figure 1–22).

▶ **Structures of the Eyelids**

A. Skin Layer

The skin of the eyelids differs from skin on most other areas of the body in that it is thin, loose, and elastic and possesses few hair follicles and no subcutaneous fat.

B. Orbicularis Oculi Muscle

The function of the orbicularis oculi muscle is to close the lids. Its muscle fibers surround the palpebral fissure in

▲ **Figure 1–20.** Check ligaments of medial and lateral rectus muscles, right eye (diagrammatic).

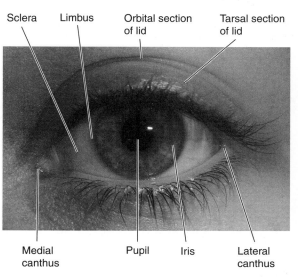

▲ **Figure 1–21.** External landmarks of the eye.

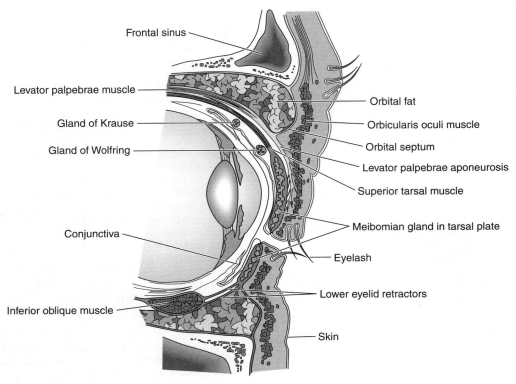

Frontal sinus

Levator palpebrae muscle

Gland of Krause

Gland of Wolfring

Conjunctiva

Inferior oblique muscle

Orbital fat

Orbicularis oculi muscle

Orbital septum

Levator palpebrae aponeurosis

Superior tarsal muscle

Meibomian gland in tarsal plate

Eyelash

Lower eyelid retractors

Skin

▲ **Figure 1–22.** Cross section of the eyelids. (Courtesy of C Beard.)

concentric fashion and spread for a short distance around the orbital margin. Some fibers run onto the cheek and the forehead. The portion of the muscle that is in the lids is known as its pretarsal portion; the portion over the orbital septum is the preseptal portion. The segment outside the lid is called the orbital portion. The orbicularis oculi is supplied by the facial nerve.

C. Areolar Tissue

The submuscular loose areolar tissue that lies deep to the orbicularis oculi muscle communicates with the subaponeurotic layer of the scalp.

D. Tarsal Plates

The main supporting structure of the eyelids is a dense fibrous tissue layer that—along with a small amount of elastic tissue—is called the tarsal plate. The lateral and medial angles and extensions of the tarsal plates are attached to the orbital margin by the lateral and medial palpebral ligaments. The upper and lower tarsal plates are also attached by a condensed, thin fascia to the upper and lower orbital margins. This thin fascia forms the orbital septum.

E. Palpebral Conjunctiva

The lids are lined posteriorly by a layer of mucous membrane, the palpebral conjunctiva, which adheres firmly to the tarsal plates. A surgical incision through the gray line of the lid margin (see the next section) splits the lid into an anterior lamella (margin) of the skin and the orbicularis muscle and a posterior lamella (margin) of the tarsal plate and the palpebral conjunctiva.

▶ Lid Margins

The free lid margin is 25–30-mm long and about 2-mm wide. It is divided by the gray line (mucocutaneous junction) into anterior and posterior margins.

A. Anterior Margin

1. **Eyelashes**—The eyelashes project from the margins of the eyelids and are arranged irregularly. The upper lashes are longer and more numerous than the lower lashes and turn upward; the lower lashes turn downward.

2. **Glands of Zeis**—These are small, modified sebaceous glands that open into the hair follicles at the base of the eyelashes.

3. **Glands of Moll**—These are modified sweat glands that open in a row near the base of the eyelashes.

B. Posterior Margin

The posterior lid margin is in close contact with the globe, and along this margin are the small orifices of modified sebaceous glands (meibomian, or tarsal, glands).

C. Lacrimal Punctum

At the medial end of the posterior margin of the lid, a small elevation with a central small opening can be seen on the upper and lower lids. The puncta serve to carry the tears down through the corresponding canaliculus to the lacrimal sac.

Palpebral Fissure

The palpebral fissure is the elliptic space between the two open lids. The fissure terminates at the medial and lateral canthi. The lateral canthus is about 0.5 cm from the lateral orbital rim and forms an acute angle. The medial canthus is more elliptic than the lateral canthus and surrounds the lacrimal lake (Figure 1–21).

Two structures are identified in the lacrimal lake: the **lacrimal caruncle**, a yellowish elevation of modified skin containing large modified sweat glands and sebaceous glands that open into follicles that contain fine hair (Figure 1–9), and the **plica semilunaris**, a vestigial remnant of the third eyelid of lower animal species.

In the Asian population, a skin fold known as **epicanthus** passes from the medial termination of the upper lid to the medial termination of the lower lid, hiding the caruncle.

Epicanthus may be present normally in young infants of all races and disappears with the development of the nasal bridge but persists throughout life in Asians.

Orbital Septum

The orbital septum is the fascia behind that portion of the orbicularis muscle that lies between the orbital rim and the tarsus and serves as a barrier between the lid and the orbit.

The orbital septum is pierced by the lacrimal vessels and nerves, the supratrochlear artery and nerve, the supraorbital vessels and nerves, the infratrochlear nerve (Figure 1–23), the anastomosis between the angular and ophthalmic veins, and the levator palpebrae superioris muscle.

The superior orbital septum blends with the tendon of the levator palpebrae superioris and the superior tarsus; the inferior orbital septum blends with the inferior tarsus.

Lid Retractors

The lid retractors are responsible for opening the eyelids. They are formed by a musculofascial complex, with both striated and smooth muscle components, known as the levator complex in the upper lid and the capsulopalpebral fascia in the lower lid.

In the upper lid, the striated muscle portion is the **levator palpebrae superioris**, which arises from the apex of the orbit and passes forward to divide into an aponeurosis and a deeper portion that contains the smooth muscle fibers of **Müller's (superior tarsal) muscle** (Figure 1–22). The aponeurosis elevates the anterior lamella of the lid, inserting into the posterior surface of the orbicularis oculi and through this into the overlying skin to form the upper lid skin crease. Müller's muscle inserts into the upper border of the tarsal plate and the superior fornix of the conjunctiva, thus elevating the posterior lamella.

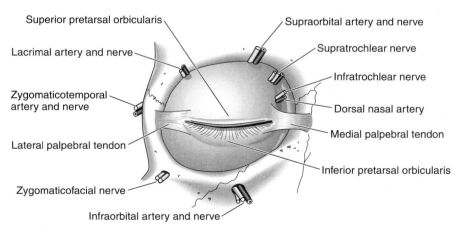

▲ Figure 1–23. Vessels and nerves to extraocular structures.

In the lower lid, the main retractor is the inferior rectus muscle, from which fibrous tissue extends to enclose the inferior oblique muscle and insert into the lower border of the tarsal plate and the orbicularis oculi. Associated with this aponeurosis are the smooth muscle fibers of the inferior tarsal muscle.

The smooth muscle components of the lid retractors are innervated by sympathetic nerves. The levator and inferior rectus muscles are supplied by the third cranial (oculomotor) nerve. Ptosis is thus a feature of both Horner's syndrome and third nerve palsy.

▶ Levator Palpebrae Superioris Muscle

The levator palpebrae muscle arises with a short tendon from the undersurface of the lesser wing of the sphenoid above and ahead of the optic foramen. The tendon blends with the underlying origin of the superior rectus muscle. The levator belly passes forward, forms an aponeurosis, and spreads like a fan. The muscle, including its smooth muscle component (Müller's muscle), and its aponeurosis form an important part of the upper lid retractor (see previous section). The palpebral segment of the orbicularis oculi muscle acts as its antagonist.

The two extremities of the levator aponeurosis are called its medial and lateral horns. The medial horn is thin and is attached below the frontolacrimal suture and into the medial palpebral ligament. The lateral horn passes between the orbital and palpebral portions of the lacrimal gland and inserts into the orbital tubercle and the lateral palpebral ligament.

The sheath of the levator palpebrae superioris is attached to the superior rectus muscle inferiorly. The superior surface, at the junction of the muscle belly and the aponeurosis, forms a thickened band (Whitnall's ligament) that is attached medially to the trochlea and laterally to the lateral orbital wall, the band forming the check ligaments of the muscle.

The levator is supplied by the superior branch of the oculomotor nerve (III). Blood supply to the levator palpebrae superioris is derived from the lateral muscular branch of the ophthalmic artery.

▶ Sensory Nerve Supply

The sensory nerve supply to the eyelids is derived from the first and second divisions of the trigeminal nerve (V). The lacrimal, supraorbital, supratrochlear, infratrochlear, and external nasal nerves are branches of the ophthalmic division of the fifth nerve. The infraorbital, zygomaticofacial, and zygomaticotemporal nerves are branches of the maxillary (second) division of the trigeminal nerve.

▶ Blood Supply & Lymphatics

The blood supply to the lids is derived from the lacrimal and ophthalmic arteries by their lateral and medial palpebral branches. Anastomoses between the lateral and medial palpebral arteries form the tarsal arcades that lie in the submuscular areolar tissue.

Venous drainage from the lids empties into the ophthalmic vein and the veins that drain the forehead and temple (Figure 1–6). The veins are arranged in pretarsal and posttarsal plexuses.

Lymphatics from the lateral segment of the lids run into the preauricular and parotid nodes. Lymphatics draining the medial side of the lids empty into the submandibular lymph nodes.

3. THE LACRIMAL APPARATUS

The lacrimal complex consists of the lacrimal gland, accessory lacrimal glands, lacrimal puncta, lacrimal canaliculi, lacrimal sac, and nasolacrimal duct (Figure 1–24).

The lacrimal gland consists of the following structures:

1. The almond-shaped **orbital portion**, located in the lacrimal fossa in the anterior upper temporal segment of the orbit, is separated from the palpebral portion by the lateral horn of the levator palpebrae muscle. To reach this portion of the gland surgically, one must incise the skin, the orbicularis oculi muscle, and the orbital septum.

2. The smaller **palpebral portion** is located just above the temporal segment of the superior conjunctival fornix. Lacrimal secretory ducts, which open by approximately 10 fine orifices, connect the orbital and palpebral portions of the lacrimal gland to the superior conjunctival fornix. Removal of the palpebral portion of the gland cuts off all of the connecting ducts, and thus prevents secretion by the entire gland.

The accessory lacrimal glands (glands of Krause and Wolfring) are located in the substantia propria of the palpebral conjunctiva.

Tears drain from the lacrimal lake via the upper and lower puncta and canaliculi to the lacrimal sac, which lies in the lacrimal fossa. The nasolacrimal duct continues downward from the sac and opens into the inferior meatus of the nasal cavity, lateral to the inferior turbinate. Tears are directed into the puncta by capillary attraction and gravity and by the blinking action of the eyelids. The combined forces of capillary attraction in the canaliculi, gravity, and the pumping action of Horner's muscle, which is an extension of the orbicularis oculi muscle to a point behind the lacrimal sac, all tend to continue the flow of tears down the nasolacrimal duct into the nose.

▶ Blood Supply & Lymphatics

The blood supply of the lacrimal gland is derived from the lacrimal artery. The vein that drains the gland joins the ophthalmic vein. The lymphatic drainage joins with the conjunctival lymphatics to drain into the preauricular lymph nodes.

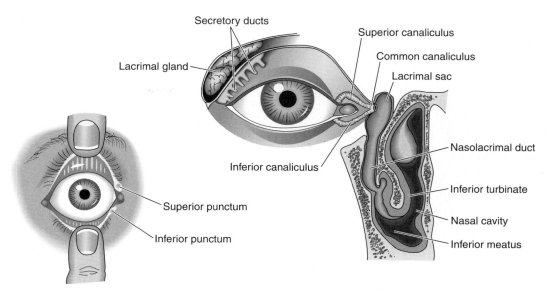

▲ **Figure 1-24.** The lacrimal drainage system.

▶ Nerve Supply

The nerve supply to the lacrimal gland is by (1) the lacrimal nerve (sensory), a branch of the trigeminal first division; (2) the great petrosal nerve (parasympathetic secretory), which comes from the superior salivary nucleus and is a branch of the facial nerve; and (3) sympathetic nerves in the deep petrosal nerve and accompanying the lacrimal artery and the lacrimal nerve. The greater and deep petrosal nerves form the nerve of the pterygoid canal (Vidian nerve).

▶ Related Structures

The **medial palpebral ligament** connects the upper and lower tarsal plates to the frontal process at the inner canthus anterior to the lacrimal sac. The portion of the lacrimal sac below the ligament is covered by a few fibers of the orbicularis oculi muscle. These fibers offer little resistance to swelling and distention of the lacrimal sac. The area below the medial palpebral ligament becomes swollen in acute dacryocystitis, and fistulas commonly open in the area.

The angular vein and artery lie just deep to the skin, 8 mm to the nasal side of the inner canthus. Skin incisions made in surgical procedures on the lacrimal sac should always be placed 2–3 mm to the nasal side of the inner canthus to avoid these vessels.

THE OPTIC NERVE

The trunk of the optic nerve consists of about 1 million axons that arise from the ganglion cells of the retina (nerve fiber layer). The optic nerve emerges from the posterior surface of the globe through the posterior scleral foramen, a short, circular opening in the sclera about 1 mm below and 3 mm nasal to the posterior pole of the eye (Figure 1–8). The nerve fibers become myelinated on leaving the eye, increasing the diameter from 1.5 mm (within the sclera) to 3 mm (within the orbit). The orbital segment of the nerve is 25–30 mm long; it travels within the optic muscle cone, via the bony optic canal, and thus gains access to the cranial cavity. The intracanalicular portion measures 4–9 mm. After a 10 mm intracranial course, the nerve joins the opposite optic nerve to form the optic chiasm.

Eighty percent of the optic nerve consists of visual fibers that synapse in the lateral geniculate body on neurons whose axons terminate in the primary visual cortex of the occipital lobes. Twenty percent of the fibers are pupillary and bypass the geniculate body en route to the pretectal area. Since the ganglion cells of the retina and their axons are part of the central nervous system, they will not regenerate if severed.

▶ Sheaths of the Optic Nerve (Figure 1-25)

The fibrous wrappings that ensheathe the optic nerve are continuous with the meninges. The pia mater is loosely attached to the nerve near the chiasm and only for a short distance within the cranium, but it is closely attached around most of the intracanalicular and all of the intraorbital portions. The pia consists of some fibrous tissue with numerous small blood vessels (Figure 1–26). It divides the nerve fibers into bundles by sending numerous septa into the nerve

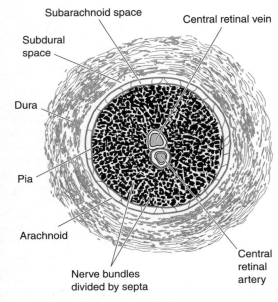

▲ Figure 1–25. Cross section of the optic nerve.

nerve to the globe, where it ends in the sclera and overlying dura. This sheath is a diaphanous connective tissue membrane with many septate connections with the pia mater, which it closely resembles. It is more intimately associated with pia than with dura.

The dura mater lining the inner surface of the cranial vault comes in contact with the optic nerve as it leaves the optic canal. As the nerve enters the orbit from the optic canal, the dura splits, one layer (the periorbita) lining the orbital cavity and the other forming the outer dural covering of the optic nerve. The dura becomes continuous with the outer two-thirds of the sclera. The dura consists of tough, fibrous, relatively avascular tissue lined by endothelium on the inner surface.

The subdural space is between the dura and the arachnoid; the subarachnoid space is between the pia and the arachnoid. Both are more potential than actual spaces under normal conditions but are direct continuations of their corresponding intracranial spaces. Increased cerebrospinal fluid pressure results in dilatation of the subarachnoid component of the optic nerve sheaths. The meningeal layers are adherent to each other and to the optic nerve and the surrounding bone within the optic foramen, making the optic nerve resistant to traction from either end.

substance. The pia continues to the sclera, with a few fibers running into the choroid and lamina cribrosa.

The arachnoid comes in contact with the optic nerve at the intracranial end of the optic canal and accompanies the

▶ Blood Supply (Figure 1–26)

The surface layer of the optic disk receives blood from branches of the retinal arterioles. In the region of the lamina

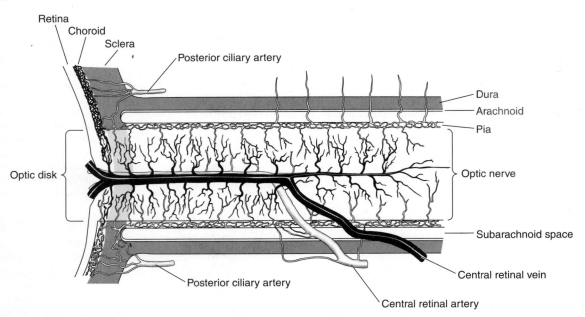

▲ Figure 1–26. Blood supply of the optic nerve. (Redrawn from: Hayreh SS: Trans. Am. Acad. Ophthalmol. Otolaryngol. 1974;78:240.)

cribrosa, comprising the prelaminar, laminar, and retrolaminar segments of the optic nerve, the arterial supply is from the short posterior ciliary arteries. The anterior intraorbital optic nerve receives some blood from branches of the central retinal artery. The remainder of the intraorbital nerve, as well as the intracanalicular and intracranial portions, are supplied by a pial network of vessels derived from the various branches of the ophthalmic artery and other branches of the internal carotid.

THE OPTIC CHIASM

The optic chiasm is located at the junction of the floor and anterior wall (lamina terminalis) of the third ventricle. It is variably situated near the top of the diaphragm of the sella turcica, most often posteriorly, lying 1 cm above it and continuing the 45° upward angulation of the optic nerves after their emergence from the optic canals (Figure 1–27). The internal carotid arteries lie just laterally, adjacent to the cavernous sinuses. The chiasm is made up of the junction of the two optic nerves and provides for crossing of the nasal fibers to the opposite optic tract and passage of temporal fibers to the ipsilateral optic tract. The macular fibers are arranged similarly to the rest of the fibers except that their decussation

is farther posteriorly and superiorly. The chiasm receives many small blood vessels from the neighboring circle of Willis.

THE RETROCHIASMATIC VISUAL PATHWAYS

Each optic tract begins at the posterolateral angle of the chiasm and sweeps around the upper part of the cerebral peduncle to end in the lateral geniculate nucleus. Afferent pupillary fibers leave the tract just anterior to the nucleus and pass via the brachium of the superior colliculus to the midbrain. (The pupillary pathway is diagrammed in Figure 14–2.) Afferent visual fibers terminate on cells in the lateral geniculate nucleus that give rise to the geniculocalcarine tract. This tract traverses the posterior limb of the internal capsule and then fans out into a broad bundle called the optic radiation. The fibers in this bundle curve backward around the anterior aspect of the temporal horn of the lateral ventricle and then medially to reach the calcarine cortex of the occipital lobe, where they terminate. The most inferior fibers, which carry projections from the superior aspect of the contralateral half of the visual field, course anteriorly into the temporal lobe in a configuration known as Meyer's loop. Lesions of the temporal lobe that extend 5 cm back

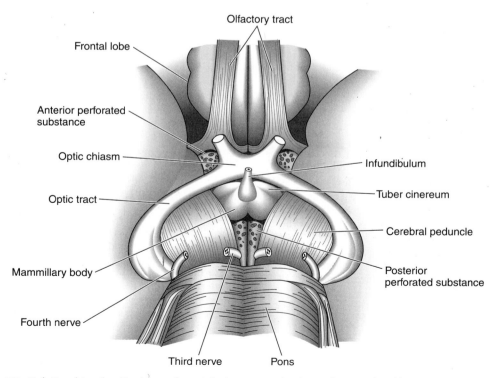

▲ **Figure 1–27.** Relationship of optic chiasm from inferior aspect. (Redrawn from: Duke-Elder WS: System of Ophthalmology, vol 2. Mosby, 1961.)

from the anterior tip involve these fibers and can produce superior quadrantanopic field defects.

The primary visual cortex (area V1) occupies the upper and lower lips and the depths of the calcarine fissure on the medial aspect of the occipital lobe. Each lobe receives input from the two ipsilateral half-retinas, representing the contralateral half of the binocular visual field. Projection of the visual field onto the visual cortex occurs in a precise retinotopic pattern. The macula is represented at the medial posterior pole, and the peripheral parts of the retina project to the most anterior part of the calcarine cortex. On either side of area V1 lies area V2, and then area V3. V2 appears to function in a manner very similar to V1. Area V4, situated on the medial surface of the cerebral hemisphere but more anterior and inferior than V1 in the region of the fusiform gyrus, is primarily concerned with color processing. Motion detection localizes to area V5 at the junction of the occipital and temporal lobes, lateral to area V1.

THE OCULOMOTOR NERVE (III)

The oculomotor nerve leaves the brainstem between the cerebral peduncles and passes near the posterior communicating artery of the circle of Willis. Lateral to the pituitary gland, it is closely approximated to the optic tract, and here it pierces the dura to course in the lateral wall of the cavernous sinus. As the nerve leaves the cavernous sinus, it divides into superior and inferior divisions. The superior division enters the orbit within the annulus of Zinn at its highest point and adjacent to the trochlear nerve (Figure 1–3). The inferior division enters the annulus of Zinn low and passes below the optic nerve to supply the medial and inferior rectus muscles. A large branch from the inferior division extends forward to supply the inferior oblique. A small twig from the proximal end of the nerve to the inferior oblique carries parasympathetic fibers to the ciliary ganglion.

THE TROCHLEAR NERVE (IV)

The thinnest of the cranial nerves, the trochlear nerve (Figure 1–3) is the only nerve to originate on the dorsal surface of the brain stem. The fibers decussate before they emerge from the brainstem just below the inferior colliculi, where they are subject to injury from the tentorium. The nerve pierces the dura behind the sella turcica and travels within the lateral walls of the cavernous sinus to enter the superior orbital fissure medial to the frontal nerve. From this point it travels within the periorbita of the roof over the levator muscle to the upper surface of the superior oblique muscle.

THE TRIGEMINAL NERVE (V) (FIGURE 1–3)

The trigeminal nerve originates from the pons, and its sensory roots form the trigeminal ganglion. The first (ophthalmic) of the three divisions passes through the lateral wall of the cavernous sinus and divides into the lacrimal, frontal, and nasociliary nerves. The **lacrimal nerve** passes through the upper lateral aspect of the superior orbital fissure, outside the annulus of Zinn, and continues its lateral course in the orbit to terminate in the lacrimal gland, providing its sensory innervation. Slightly medial to the lacrimal nerve within the superior orbital fissure is the frontal nerve, which is the largest of the first division of branches of the trigeminal nerve. It also crosses over the annulus of Zinn and follows a course over the levator to the medial aspect of the orbit, where it divides into the supraorbital and supratrochlear nerves. These provide sensation to the brow and forehead. The nasociliary nerve is the sensory nerve of the eye. After entering through the medial portion of the annulus of Zinn, it lies between the superior rectus and the optic nerve. Branches to the ciliary ganglion and those forming the ciliary nerves provide sensory supply to the cornea, iris, and ciliary body. The terminal branches are the infratrochlear nerve, which supplies the medial portion of the conjunctiva and eyelids, and the anterior ethmoidal nerve, which provides sensation to the tip of the nose. Thus, the skin on the tip of the nose may be affected with vesicular lesions prior to the onset of herpes zoster ophthalmicus.

The second (maxillary) division of the trigeminal nerve passes through the foramen rotundum and enters the orbit through the inferior orbital fissure. It passes through the infraorbital canal, becoming the **infraorbital nerve**, and exits via the infraorbital foramen, supplying sensation to the lower lid and adjacent cheek. It is frequently damaged in fractures of the orbital floor.

THE ABDUCENS NERVE (VI)

The abducens nerve (Figure 1–3) originates between the pons and medulla and pursues an extended course, having the longest intracranial course of any cranial nerve, up the clivus to the posterior clinoid, penetrates the dura, and passes within the cavernous sinus. (All other nerves course through the lateral wall of the cavernous sinus.) After passing through the superior orbital fissure within the annulus of Zinn, the nerve continues laterally to innervate the lateral rectus muscle.

THE FACIAL NERVE (VII)

The facial nerve exits the brainstem at the lower border of the pons, the greater petrosal nerve forming part of the separate portion known as the nervus intermeidus, and passes through the internal acoustic meatus with the vestibulocochlear (VII) nerve into the facial canal. At the geniculate ganglion the greater petrosal nerve, which contains parasympathetic secretomotor fibers, joins the lesser petrosal nerve to form the nerve of the pterygoid canal (Vidian nerve) and pass through the pterygopalatine ganglion, where the parasympathetic fibers synapse, to reach the lacrimal gland. The facial nerve exits the facial canal at the stylomastoid foramen, passes through the parotid gland and then branches out across the face to supply the muscles of facial expression, including orbicularis oculi.

II. EMBRYOLOGY OF THE EYE

The eye is derived from three of the primitive embryonic layers: surface ectoderm, including its derivative—the neural crest; neural ectoderm; and mesoderm. Endoderm does not enter into the formation of the eye. Mesenchyme, derived from mesoderm or the neural crest, is the term for embryonic connective tissue. Most of the mesenchyme of the head and neck is derived from the neural crest.

The **surface ectoderm** gives rise to the lens, the lacrimal gland, the epithelium of the cornea, conjunctiva and adnexal glands, and the epidermis of the eyelids.

The **neural crest**, which arises from the surface ectoderm in the region immediately adjacent to the neural folds of neural ectoderm, is responsible for the formation of the corneal keratocytes, the endothelium of the cornea and the trabecular meshwork, the stroma of the iris and choroid, the ciliary muscle, the fibroblasts of the sclera, the vitreous, and the optic nerve meninges. It is also involved in the formation of the orbital cartilage and bone, the orbital connective tissues and nerves, the extraocular muscles, and the subepidermal layers of the eyelids.

The **neural ectoderm** gives rise to the optic vesicle and optic cup, and is thus responsible for the formation of the retina and retinal pigment epithelium, the pigmented and nonpigmented layers of ciliary epithelium, the posterior epithelium, the dilator and sphincter muscles of the iris, and the optic nerve fibers and glia.

The **mesoderm** contributes to the vitreous, extraocular and lid muscles, and the orbital and ocular vascular endothelium.

Optic Vesicle Stage

The embryonic plate is the earliest stage in fetal development during which ocular structures can be differentiated. At 2 weeks, the edges of the neural groove thicken to form the neural folds. The folds then fuse to form the neural tube, which sinks into the underlying mesoderm and detaches itself from the surface epithelium. The site of the optic groove or optic sulcus is in the cephalic neural folds on either side of and parallel to the neural groove, which forms when the neural folds begin to close at 3 weeks (Figure 1–28).

At 4 weeks, just before the anterior portion of the neural tube closes completely, neural ectoderm grows outward and toward the surface ectoderm on either side to form the spherical optic vesicles. The optic vesicles are connected to the forebrain by the optic stalks. At this stage also, a thickening of the surface ectoderm (lens plate) begins to form opposite the ends of the optic vesicles.

Optic Cup Stage

As the optic vesicle invaginates to produce the optic cup, the original outer wall of the vesicle approaches its inner wall. The invagination of the ventral surface of the optic stalk and of the optic vesicle occurs simultaneously and creates a groove, the optic (embryonic) fissure. The margins of the optic cup then grow around the optic fissure. At the same time, the lens plate invaginates to form first a cup and then a hollow sphere known as the lens vesicle. By 6 weeks, the lens vesicle separates from the surface ectoderm and lies free in the rim of the optic cup.

The optic fissure allows mesodermal mesenchyme to enter the optic stalk and eventually to form the hyaloid system of the vitreous cavity. As invagination is completed, the optic fissure narrows and closes, leaving one small permanent opening at the anterior end of the optic stalk through which the hyaloid artery passes. At 4 months, the retinal artery and vein pass through this opening.

Once the optic fissure has closed, the ultimate general structure of the eye has been determined. Further development consists in differentiation of the individual optic structures. In general, differentiation of the optic structures occurs more rapidly in the posterior than in the anterior segment of the eye during the early stages and more rapidly in the anterior segment during the later stages of gestation.

EMBRYOLOGY OF SPECIFIC STRUCTURES

Lids & Lacrimal Apparatus

The lids develop from mesenchyme except for the epidermis of the skin and the epithelium of the conjunctiva, which are derivatives of surface ectoderm. The lid buds are first seen at 6 weeks growing in front of the eye, where they meet and fuse by 8 weeks. They separate during the fifth month. The lashes and meibomian and other lid glands develop as downgrowths from the epidermis.

The lacrimal and accessory lacrimal glands develop from the conjunctival epithelium. The lacrimal drainage system (canaliculi, lacrimal sac, and nasolacrimal duct) are also surface ectodermal derivatives, which develop from a solid epithelial cord that becomes buried between the maxillary and nasal processes of the developing facial structures. This cord canalizes just before birth.

Sclera & Extraocular Muscles

The sclera and extraocular muscles are formed from condensations of mesenchyme encircling the optic cup and are identifiable by 7 weeks. Development of these structures is well advanced by the fourth month. Tenon's capsule appears about the insertions of the rectus muscles at 12 weeks and is complete at 5 months.

Anterior Segment

The anterior segment of the globe is formed by the invasion of the neural crest mesenchymal cells into the space between the surface ectoderm, which develops into the corneal epithelium, and the lens vesicle, which has become separated from it. The invasion occurs in three stages: the first is responsible for formation of the corneal endothelium, the

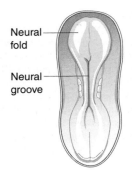

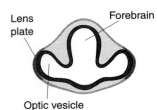

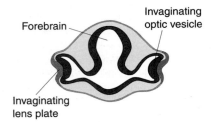

3 weeks. Dorsal view. Neural folds beginning to close.

4 weeks. Transverse section. Formation of optic vesicles and lens plates.

4½ weeks. Transverse section. Invagination of optic vesicles and lens plates.

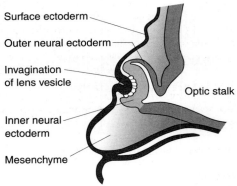

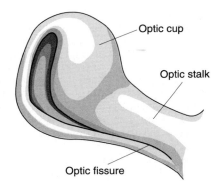

5 weeks. Cross section. Development of optic cup and lens vesicle.

6 weeks. External view. Closure of optic fissure through which hyaloid vessels enter the optic cup.

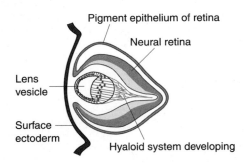

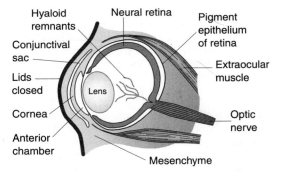

7 weeks. Cross section. Differentiation of layers of neural ectoderm into pigment epithelium and neural retina and expansion of lens vesicle.

8 weeks. Cross section. Fusion of lids and development of extraocular muscles from mesenchyme.

▲ **Figure 1–28.** Embryologic development of ocular structures.

second for formation of the iris stroma, and the third for formation of the corneal stroma. The anterior chamber angle is formed from a residual condensation of mesenchyme at the anterior rim of the optic cup. The mechanism of formation of the anterior chamber itself—and hence the angle structures—is still debated but seems to involve patterns of migration of neural crest cells and subsequent changes in their structure rather than cleavage of mesodermal tissue, as previously thought.

The corneal epithelium and endothelium are first apparent at 6 weeks, when the lens vesicle has separated from the surface ectoderm. Descemet's membrane is secreted by the flattened endothelial cells by 11 weeks. The stroma slowly thickens and forms an anterior condensation just under the epithelium that is recognizable at 4 months as Bowman's layer. A definite corneoscleral junction is present at 4 months.

The double row of iris epithelium is a forward extension of the anterior rim of the optic cup. This grows forward during the third month to lie posterior to the neural crest cells that form the iris stroma. These two epithelial layers become pigmented in the iris, whereas only the outer layer is pigmented in the ciliary body. By the fifth month, the sphincter muscle of the pupil is developing from the anterior epithelial layer of the iris near the pupillary margin. Soon after the sixth month, the dilator muscle appears in the anterior epithelial layer near the ciliary body.

The anterior chamber of the eye first appears at 7 weeks and remains very shallow until birth. At 10 weeks, Schlemm's canal appears as a vascular channel at the level of the recess of the angle and gradually assumes a relatively more anterior location as the angle recess develops. The iris, which in the early stages of development is quite anterior, gradually lies relatively more posteriorly as the chamber angle recess develops, most likely because of the difference in the rate of growth of the anterior segment structures. The trabecular meshwork develops from the loose mesenchymal tissue lying originally at the margin of the optic cup. The aqueous drainage system is ready to function before birth.

Lens

Soon after the lens vesicle lies free in the rim of the optic cup (6 weeks), the cells of its posterior wall elongate, encroach on the empty cavity, and finally fill it in (7 weeks). At about 6 weeks, a hyaline capsule is secreted by the lens cells. Secondary lens fibers elongate from the equatorial region and grow forward under the subcapsular epithelium, which remains as a single layer of cuboidal epithelial cells, and backward under the lens capsule. These fibers meet to form the lens sutures (upright Y anteriorly and inverted Y posteriorly), which are complete by the seventh month. (This growth and proliferation of secondary lens fibers continues at a decreasing rate throughout life; the lens therefore continues to enlarge slowly, causing compression of the lens fibers.)

Ciliary Body & Choroid

The ciliary epithelium is formed from the same anterior extension of the optic cup that is responsible for the iris epithelium. Only the outer layer becomes pigmented. The ciliary muscle and blood vessels are derived from mesenchyme.

At 3½ weeks, a network of capillaries encircles the optic cup and develops into the choroid. By the third month, the intermediate and large venous channels of the choroid are developed and drain into the vortex veins to exit from the eye.

Retina

The outer layer of the optic cup remains as a single layer and becomes the pigment epithelium of the retina. Pigmentation begins at 5 weeks. Secretion of the inner layer of Bruch's membrane occurs by 6 weeks. The inner layer of the optic cup undergoes a complicated differentiation into the other nine layers of the retina. This occurs slowly throughout gestation. By the seventh month, the outermost cell layer (consisting of the nuclei of the rods and cones) is present as well as the bipolar, amacrine, and ganglion cells and nerve fibers. The macular region is thicker than the rest of the retina until the eighth month, when the macular depression begins to develop. Macular development is not complete in anatomic terms until 6 months after birth.

Vitreous

A. First Stage

(Primary vitreous, 3–6 weeks.) At about 3 weeks, cells and fibroblasts derived from mesenchyme at the rim of the optic cup or associated with the hyaloid vascular system, together with minor contributions from the embryonic lens and the inner layer of the optic vesicle, form the vitreous fibrils of the primary vitreous. Ultimately, the primary vitreous comes to lie just behind the posterior pole of the lens in association with remnants of the hyaloid vessels (Cloquet's canal).

B. Second Stage

(Secondary vitreous, 6–10 weeks.) The fibrils and cells (hyalocytes) of the secondary vitreous are thought to originate from the vascular primary vitreous. Anteriorly, the firm attachment of the secondary vitreous to the internal limiting membrane of the retina constitutes the early stages of formation of the vitreous base. The hyaloid system develops a set of vitreous vessels as well as vessels on the lens capsule surface (tunica vasculosa lentis). The hyaloid system is at its height at 2 months and then atrophies from posterior to anterior.

C. Third Stage

(Tertiary vitreous, 10 weeks on.) During the third month, the marginal bundle of Drualt is forming. This consists of vitreous fibrillar condensations extending from the future ciliary epithelium of the optic cup to the equator of the lens. Condensations then form the suspensory ligament of the lens, which is well developed by 4 months. The hyaloid system atrophies complete during this stage.

▶ Optic Nerve

The axons of the ganglion cells of the retina form the nerve fiber layer. The fibers slowly form the optic stalk (7 weeks) and then the optic nerve. Mesenchymal elements enter the surrounding tissue to form the vascular septa of the nerve. Myelination extends from the brain peripherally down the optic nerve and at birth has reached the lamina cribrosa. Myelination is completed by age 3 months.

▶ Blood Vessels

Long ciliary arteries bud off from the hyaloid system at 6 weeks and anastomose around the optic cup margin with the major circle of the iris by 7 weeks. The hyaloid artery gives rise to the central retinal artery and its branches (4 months). Buds arise in the region of the optic disc and gradually extend to the peripheral retina, reaching the ora serrata at 8 months. The branches of the central retinal vein develop simultaneously. The hyaloid system (see Vitreous, earlier in this section) has atrophied completely by the eighth month.

▼ III. GROWTH & DEVELOPMENT OF THE EYE

▶ Eyeball

At birth, the eye is larger in relation to the rest of the body than is the case in children and adults, but in relation to its ultimate size (reached at 7–8 years), it is comparatively short, averaging 16.6 mm in anteroposterior diameter. This would make the eye markedly rather than the usual mildly hyperopic if it were not for the greater refractive power due to steeper corneal curvature and more spherical lens.

▶ Cornea

The newborn infant has a relatively large cornea that reaches adult size by the age of 2 years. It is steeper than the adult cornea, and its curvature is greater at the periphery than in the center. (The reverse is true in adults.)

▶ Lens

At birth, the lens is more nearly spherical in shape than later in life, producing a greater refractive power that helps to compensate for the short anteroposterior diameter of the eye. The lens grows throughout life as new fibers are added to the periphery, making it flatter.

The consistency of the lens material changes throughout life. At birth, it may be compared with soft plastic; in old age, the lens is of a glass-like consistency. This accounts for the greater resistance to change of shape in accommodation with age.

▶ Iris

At birth, there is little or no pigment in the stroma of the anterior iris but the epithelium, particularly the posterior layer, is heavily pigmented. Nevertheless, reflection of light by the stroma gives the eyes of most infants a bluish color. Iris color is subsequently determined by pigmentation and thickness of the stroma, the latter influencing visibility of the epithelial pigment.

Ophthalmologic Examination

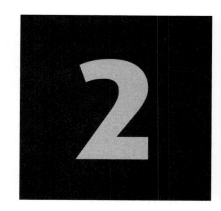

David F. Chang, MD

Of all the organs of the body, the eye is most accessible to direct examination. Visual function can be quantified by simple subjective testing. The external anatomy of the eye is visible to inspection with the unaided eye and with fairly simple instruments. With more complicated instruments, the interior of the eye is visible through the clear cornea. The eye is the only part of the body where blood vessels and central nervous system tissue (retina and optic nerve) can be viewed directly. Important systemic effects of infectious, autoimmune, neoplastic, and vascular diseases may be identified from ocular examination.

The purpose of sections I and II of this chapter is to provide an overview of the ocular history and basic complete eye examination as performed by an ophthalmologist. In section III, more specialized examination techniques will be presented.

▼ I. OCULAR HISTORY

The **chief complaint** is characterized according to its duration, frequency, intermittency, and rapidity of onset. The location, the severity, and the circumstances surrounding onset are important, as well as any associated symptoms. Current eye medications being used and all other current and past ocular disorders are recorded, and a review of other pertinent ocular symptoms is performed.

The **past medical history** centers on the patient's general state of health and principal systemic illnesses, if any. Vascular disorders commonly associated with ocular manifestations—such as diabetes and hypertension—should be asked about specifically. Just as a general medical history should include ocular medications being used, the eye history should list the patient's systemic medications. This provides a general indication of health status and may include medications that affect ocular health, such as corticosteroids. Finally, any drug allergies should be recorded.

The **family history** is pertinent for ocular disorders, such as strabismus, amblyopia, glaucoma, or cataracts, and retinal problems, such as retinal detachment or macular degeneration. Medical diseases such as diabetes may be relevant as well.

COMMON OCULAR SYMPTOMS

A basic understanding of ocular symptomatology is necessary for performing a proper ophthalmic examination. Ocular symptoms can be divided into three basic categories: abnormalities of vision, abnormalities of ocular appearance, and abnormalities of ocular sensation—pain and discomfort.

Symptoms and complaints should always be fully characterized. Was the **onset** gradual, rapid, or asymptomatic? (For example, was blurred vision in one eye not discovered until the opposite eye was inadvertently covered?) Was the **duration** brief, or has the symptom continued until the present visit? If the symptom was intermittent, what was the frequency? Is the **location** focal or diffuse, and is involvement unilateral or bilateral? Finally, does the patient characterize the **degree** as mild, moderate, or severe?

One should also determine what therapeutic measures have been tried and to what extent they have helped. Has the patient identified circumstances that trigger or worsen the symptom? Have similar instances occurred before, and are there any other associated symptoms?

The following is a brief overview of ocular complaints. Representative examples of some causes are given here and discussed more fully elsewhere in this book.

ABNORMALITIES OF VISION

▶ Visual Loss

Loss of visual acuity may be due to abnormalities anywhere along the optical and neurologic visual pathway. One must therefore consider refractive (focusing) error, lid ptosis, clouding or interference from the ocular media (eg, corneal edema, cataract, or hemorrhage in the vitreous or aqueous space), and malfunction of the retina (macula), optic nerve, or intracranial visual pathway.

A distinction should be made between decreased central acuity and peripheral vision. The latter may be focal, such as a scotoma, or more expansive, as with hemianopia. Abnormalities of the intracranial visual pathway usually disturb the visual field more than central visual acuity.

Transient loss of central or peripheral vision is frequently due to circulatory changes anywhere along the neurologic visual pathway from the retina to the occipital cortex, for example amaurosis fugax and migrainous scotoma.

The degree of visual impairment may vary under different circumstances. For example, uncorrected nearsighted refractive error may seem worse in dark environments. This is because pupillary dilation allows more misfocused rays to reach the retina, increasing the blur. A central focal cataract may seem worse in sunlight. In this case, pupillary constriction prevents more rays from entering and passing around the lens opacity. Blurred vision from corneal edema may improve as the day progresses owing to corneal dehydration from surface evaporation.

▶ Visual Aberrations

Glare or **halos** may result from uncorrected refractive error, scratches on spectacle lenses, excessive pupillary dilation, and hazy ocular media, such as corneal edema or cataract. **Visual distortion** (apart from blurring) may be manifested as an irregular pattern of dimness, wavy or jagged lines, and image magnification or minification. Causes may include the aura of migraine, optical distortion from strong corrective lenses, or lesions involving the macula and optic nerve. **Flashing** or **flickering** lights may indicate retinal traction (if instantaneous) or migrainous scintillations that last for several seconds or minutes. **Floating spots** may represent normal vitreous strands due to vitreous "syneresis" or separation (see Chapter 9) or the pathologic presence of pigment, blood, or inflammatory cells. **Oscillopsia** is a shaking field of vision due to ocular instability.

It must be determined whether **double vision** is monocular or binocular (ie, disappears if one eye is covered). **Monocular diplopia** is often a split shadow or ghost image. Causes include uncorrected refractive error, such as astigmatism, or focal media abnormalities, such as cataracts or corneal irregularities (eg, scars, keratoconus). **Binocular diplopia** (see Chapters 12 and 14) can be vertical, horizontal, diagonal, or torsional. If the deviation occurs or increases in one gaze direction as opposed to others, it is called "incomitant." Neuromuscular dysfunction or mechanical restriction of globe rotation is suspected. "Comitant" deviation is one that remains constant regardless of the direction of gaze. It is usually due to childhood or long-standing strabismus.

ABNORMALITIES OF APPEARANCE

Complaints of "red eye" call for differentiation between redness of the lids and periocular area versus redness of the globe. The latter can be caused by subconjunctival hemorrhage or by vascular congestion of the conjunctiva, sclera, or episclera (connective tissue between the sclera and conjunctiva). Causes of such congestion may be either external surface inflammation, such as conjunctivitis and keratitis, or intraocular inflammation, such as iritis and acute glaucoma (see Inside Front Cover). Color abnormalities other than redness may include jaundice and hyperpigmented spots on the iris or outer ocular surface.

Other changes in appearance of the **globe** that may be noticeable to the patient include focal lesions of the ocular surface, such as a pterygium, and asymmetry of pupil size (anisocoria). The **lids** and **periocular tissues** may be the source of visible signs, such as edema, redness, focal growths, and lesions, and abnormal position or contour, such as ptosis. Finally, the patient may notice bulging or displacement of the globe, such as with exophthalmos.

PAIN & DISCOMFORT

"Eye pain" may be periocular, ocular, retrobulbar (behind the globe), or poorly localized. Examples of **periocular** pain are tenderness of the lid, tear sac, sinuses, or temporal artery. **Retrobulbar** pain can be due to orbital inflammation of any kind. Certain locations of inflammation, such as optic neuritis or orbital myositis, may produce pain on eye movement. Many **nonspecific** complaints such, as "eyestrain," "pulling," "pressure," "fullness," and certain kinds of "headaches," are poorly localized. Causes may include fatigue from ocular accommodation or binocular fusion or referred discomfort from nonocular muscle tension or fatigue.

Ocular pain itself may seem to emanate from the surface or from deeper within the globe. Corneal epithelial damage typically produces a superficial sharp pain or foreign body sensation exacerbated by blinking. Topical anesthesia will immediately relieve this pain. Deeper internal aching pain occurs with acute glaucoma, iritis, endophthalmitis, and scleritis. The globe is often tender to palpation in these situations. Reflex spasm of the ciliary muscle and iris sphincter can occur with iritis or keratitis, producing brow ache and painful "photophobia" (light sensitivity). This discomfort is markedly improved by instillation of cycloplegic/mydriatic agents (see Chapter 22).

▶ Eye Irritation

Superficial ocular discomfort usually results from surface abnormalities. **Itching**, as a primary symptom, is often a sign of allergic sensitivity. Symptoms of **dryness**, burning, grittiness, and mild foreign body sensation can occur with dry eyes or other types of mild corneal irritation. **Tearing** may be of two general types. Sudden reflex tearing is usually due to irritation of the ocular surface. In contrast, chronic watering and "epiphora" (tears rolling down the cheek) may indicate abnormal lacrimal drainage (see Chapter 4).

Ocular **secretions** are often diagnostically nonspecific. Severe amounts of discharge that cause the lids to be glued shut upon awakening usually indicate viral or bacterial conjunctivitis. More scant amounts of mucoid discharge can also be seen with allergic and noninfectious irritations. Dried matter and crusts on the lashes may occur acutely with conjunctivitis or chronically with blepharitis (lid margin inflammation).

II. BASIC OPHTHALMOLOGIC EXAMINATION

The purpose of the ophthalmologic physical examination is to evaluate both the function and the anatomy of the two eyes. Function includes vision and nonvisual functions, such as eye movements and alignment. Anatomically, ocular problems can be subdivided into three areas: those of the adnexa (lids and periocular tissue), the globe, and the orbit.

VISION

Just as assessment of vital signs is a part of every physical examination, any ocular examination must include assessment of vision, regardless of whether vision is mentioned as part of the chief complaint. Good vision results from a combination of an intact neurologic visual pathway, a structurally healthy eye, and proper focus of the eye. An analogy might be made to a video camera, requiring a functioning cable connection to the monitor, a mechanically intact camera body, and a proper focus setting. Vision can be divided broadly into central and peripheral, quantified by visual acuity and visual field testing, respectively. Clinical assessment of visual acuity and visual field is subjective rather than objective, since it requires responses on the part of the patient.

▶ Visual Acuity Testing

Visual acuity can be tested either for distance or near, conventionally at 20 feet (6 meters) and 14 inches (33 cms) away, respectively, but distance acuity is the general standard for comparison. For diagnostic purposes visual acuity is always tested separately for each eye, whereas binocular visual acuity is useful for assessing functional vision (see Chapter 25), such as for assessing the eligibility to drive.

Visual acuity is measured with a display of different-sized optotypes shown at the appropriate distance from the eye. The familiar "Snellen chart" is composed of rows of progressively smaller letters, each row designated by a number corresponding to the distance in feet (or meters) from which a normal eye can read the letters of the row. For example, the letters in the "40" row are large enough for the normal eye to see from 40 feet away. Whereas wall-mounted illuminated charts, or projection systems are commonly used, wall-mounted LCD screens provide better standardization and calibration (Figure 2–1). Mainly for clinical trials but increasingly for specific clinical situations, LogMAR charts are being used (see Chapter 24).

Visual acuity is scored as a fraction (eg, "20/40"). The first number represents the testing distance between the chart and the patient, and the second number represents the smallest row of letters that the patient's eye can read. Hence normal

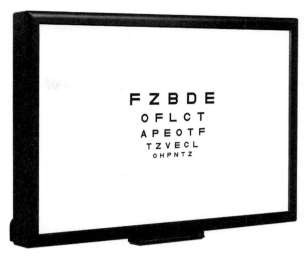

▲ **Figure 2–1.** LCD screen displaying Snellen visual acuity chart with 20/40 letters at the top (Photo courtesy of M&S Technologies).

vision is 20/20 and 20/60 acuity indicates that the patient's eye can only read from 20 feet letters large enough for a normal eye to read from 60 feet.

Charts containing numerals can be used for patients not familiar with the English alphabet. The "illiterate E" chart is used to test small children or if there is a language barrier. "E" figures are randomly rotated in each of four different orientations throughout the chart. For each target, the patient is asked to point in the same direction as the three "bars" of the E (Figure 2–2). Most children can be tested in this manner beginning at about age 3½ years.

Uncorrected visual acuity is measured without glasses or contact lenses. **Corrected** acuity means that these aids were worn. Since poor uncorrected distance acuity may simply be due to refractive error, corrected visual acuity is a more relevant assessment of ocular health.

▶ Pinhole Test

If the patient needs glasses or if his or her glasses are unavailable, the corrected acuity can be estimated by testing vision through a "pinhole." Refractive blur (eg, myopia, hyperopia, astigmatism) is caused by multiple misfocused rays entering through the pupil and reaching the retina. This prevents formation of a sharply focused image.

Viewing the Snellen chart through a placard of multiple tiny pinhole-sized openings prevents most of the misfocused rays from entering the eye. Only a few centrally aligned focused rays will reach the retina, resulting in a sharper image. In this manner, the patient may be able to read within one or two lines of what would be possible if proper corrective glasses were being used.

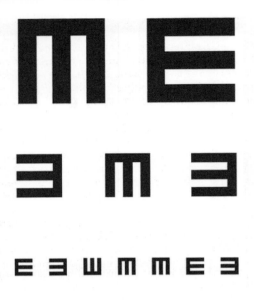

▲ **Figure 2–2.** "Illiterate E" chart.

▶ Refraction

The unaided distant focal point of the eye varies among normal individuals depending on the shape of the globe and the cornea (Figure 2–3). An **emmetropic** eye is naturally in optimal focus for distance vision. An **ametropic** eye (ie, one with myopia, hyperopia, or astigmatism) needs corrective lenses to be in proper focus for distance. This optical abnormality is called **refractive error.**

Refraction is the procedure by which any refractive error is characterized and quantified (Figure 2–4) (see Chapter 21), allowing the best measure of corrected visual acuity. In addition, it is the most reliable means to distinguish between blurred vision caused by refractive error or by other abnormalities of the visual system. Thus, in addition to being the basis for prescription of corrective glasses or contact lenses, refraction serves a crucial diagnostic function.

▶ Testing Poor Vision

The patient unable to read the largest ("20/200") letter on a Snellen chart should be moved closer to the chart until that letter can be read. The distance from the chart is then recorded as the first number. Visual acuity of "5/200" means that the patient can identify correctly the largest letter from a distance of 5 feet but not further away. An eye unable to read any letters is tested by the ability to count fingers. "CF at 2 ft" indicates that the eye was able to count fingers held 2 feet

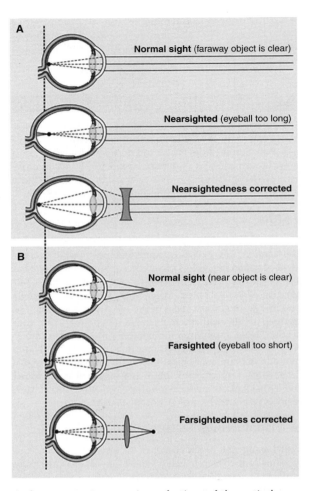

▲ **Figure 2–3.** Common imperfections of the optical system of the eye **(refractive errors)**. Ideally, light rays from a distant target should automatically arrive in focus on the retina if the retina is situated precisely at the eye's natural focal point. Such an eye is called **emmetropic**. In **hyperopia** ("farsightedness"), the light rays from a distant target instead come to a focus behind the retina, causing the retinal image to be blurred. A biconvex (+) lens corrects this by increasing the refractive power of the eye and shifting the focal point forward. In **myopia** ("nearsightedness"), the light rays come to a focus in front of the retina, as though the eyeball is too long. Placing a biconcave (–) lens in front of the eye diverges the incoming light rays; this effectively weakens the optical power of the eye enough so that the focus is shifted backward and onto the retina. (Modified and reproduced, with permission, from Ganong WF: Review of Medical Physiology, 15th ed. McGraw-Hill, 1991.)

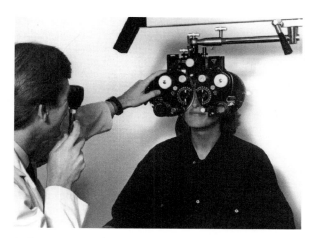

▲ **Figure 2–4.** Refraction being performed using a "phoropter." This device contains the complete range of corrective lens powers, which can quickly be changed back and forth, allowing the patient to subjectively compare various combinations while viewing the eye chart at a distance. (Photo by M Narahara.)

away but not farther away. If counting fingers is not possible, the eye may be able to detect a hand moving vertically or horizontally ("HM," or "hand motions" vision). The next lower level of vision would be the ability to perceive light ("LP," or "light perception"). An eye that is totally blind is recorded as having no light perception ("NLP").

▶ Visual Field Testing

Visual field testing should be included in every complete ophthalmologic examination because even dense visual field abnormalities may not be apparent to the patient. Since the visual fields of the two eyes overlap, for diagnostic purposes each eye must be tested separately. Binocular visual field testing is useful in assessment of functional vision (see Chapter 25).

Assessment of visual fields can be quickly achieved using **confrontation testing**. The patient is seated facing the examiner with one eye covered while the examiner closes the opposite eye (eg, the patient's left eye is covered and the examiner's right eye is closed so that the patient's right eye looks into the examiner's left eye). Presentation of targets at a distance halfway between the patient and the examiner allows direct comparison of the field of vision of each eye of the patient and the examiner. Since the patient and examiner are staring eye to eye, any loss of fixation by the patient will be noticed.

For gross assessment, the examiner briefly shows a number of fingers of one hand (usually one, two, or four fingers) peripherally in each of the four quadrants. The patient must identify the number of fingers flashed while maintaining straight-ahead fixation. The upper and lower temporal and

the upper and lower nasal quadrants are all tested in this fashion for each eye.

A 5-mm-diameter red sphere or disk attached to a handle as the target allows detection and quantification of more subtle visual field defects, particularly if areas of abnormal reduction in color (desaturation) are sought.

In disease of the right cerebral hemisphere, particularly involving the parietal lobe, there may be **visual neglect** (visual inattention) in which there is no comparable visual field loss on testing of each eye separately, but objects are not identified in the left hemifield of either eye if objects are simultaneously presented in the right hemifield. The patient functions as if there is a left homonymous hemianopia. Visual neglect is detected by **simultaneous confrontation testing**. The examiner holds both hands out peripherally, one on each side. The patient, with both eyes open, is asked to signify on which side (right, left, or both) the examiner is intermittently wiggling his or her fingers. The patient will still be able to detect the fingers in the left hemifield when wiggled alone but not when the fingers in the right hemifield are wiggled simultaneously.

More sophisticated means of visual field testing, important for detection of subtle visual field loss, such as in the diagnosis of early glaucoma and for quantification of any visual field defect, are discussed later in this chapter.

PUPILS

▶ Basic Examination

The pupils should be symmetric, and each one should be examined for size, shape (circular or irregular), and reactivity to both light and accommodation. Pupillary abnormalities may be due to (1) neurologic disease, (2) intraocular inflammation causing either spasm of the pupillary sphincter or adhesions of the iris to the lens (posterior synechiae), (3) markedly elevated intraocular pressure causing atony of the pupillary sphincter, (4) prior surgical alteration, (5) the effect of systemic or eye medications, and (6) benign variations of normal.

To avoid accommodation, the patient is asked to fixate on a distant target as a penlight is directed toward each eye. Dim lighting conditions help to accentuate the pupillary response and may best demonstrate an abnormally small pupil. Likewise, an abnormally large pupil may be more apparent in brighter background illumination. The **direct response** to light refers to constriction of the illuminated pupil. The reaction may be graded as either brisk or sluggish. The **consensual response** is the normal simultaneous constriction of the opposite nonilluminated pupil. The neuroanatomy of the pupillary pathway is discussed in Chapter 14.

▶ Swinging Penlight Test for Marcus Gunn Pupil

As a light is swung back and forth in front of the two pupils, one can compare the reactions to stimulation of each eye, which should be equal. If the neural response to stimulation of the left eye is impaired, the pupil response in *both eyes* will be reduced on stimulation of the left eye compared to stimulation of the right eye. As the light is swung from the right to the left eye, both pupils will begin to dilate normally as the light is moved away from the right eye and then not constrict or paradoxically *widen* as the light is shone into the left eye (since the direct response in the left eye and the consensual response in the right eye are reduced compared to the consensual response in the left eye and direct response in the right eye from stimulation of the right eye). When the light is swung back to the right eye, both pupils will begin to dilate as the light is moved away from the left eye and then constrict normally as the light is shone into the right eye. This phenomenon is called a relative afferent pupillary defect (RAPD). It is usually a sign of optic nerve disease but may occur in retinal disease. Importantly, it does not occur in media opacities such as corneal disease, cataract, and vitreous hemorrhage. Because the pupils are normal in size and may appear to react normally when each is stimulated alone, the swinging flashlight test is the only means of demonstrating a relative afferent pupillary defect. Also, because the pupils react equally, detection of a relative afferent pupillary defect requires inspection of only one pupil and can still be achieved when one pupil is structurally damaged or cannot be visualized, as in dense corneal opacity. Relative afferent pupillary defect is further discussed and illustrated in Chapter 14.

OCULAR MOTILITY

The objective of ocular motility testing is to evaluate the alignment of the eyes and their movements, both individually ("ductions") and in tandem ("versions"). A more complete discussion of ocular motility testing and eye movement abnormalities is presented in Chapters 12 and 14.

▶ Testing Alignment

Normal patients have binocular vision. Since each eye generates a visual image separate from and independent of that of the other eye, the brain must be able to fuse the two images in order to avoid "double vision." This is achieved by having each eye positioned so that both foveas are simultaneously fixating on the object of regard.

A simple test of binocular alignment is performed by having the patient look toward a penlight held several feet away. A pinpoint light reflection, or "reflex," should appear on each cornea and should be centered over each pupil if the two eyes are straight in their alignment. If the eye positions are convergent, such that one eye points inward ("esotropia"), the light reflex will appear temporal to the pupil in that eye. If the eyes are divergent, such that one eye points outward ("exotropia"), the light reflex will be located more nasally in that eye. This test can be used with infants.

The **cover test** (see Chapter 12) is a more accurate method of verifying normal ocular alignment. The test requires good vision in both eyes. The patient is asked to gaze at a distant target with both eyes open. If both eyes are fixating together on the target, covering one eye should not affect the position or continued fixation of the other eye.

To perform the test, the examiner suddenly covers one eye and carefully watches to see that the second eye does not move (indicating that it was fixating on the same target already). If the second eye was not identically aligned but was instead turned abnormally inward or outward, it could not have been simultaneously fixating on the target. Thus, it will have to quickly move to find the target once the previously fixating eye is covered. Fixation of each eye is tested in turn.

An abnormal cover test is expected in patients with diplopia. However, diplopia is not always present in many patients with long-standing ocular misalignment. When the test is abnormal, prism lenses of different power can be used to neutralize the refixation movement of the misaligned eye (prism cover test). In this way, the amount of eye deviation can be quantified based on the amount of prism power needed.

▶ Testing Extraocular Movements

The patient is asked to follow a target with both eyes as it is moved in each of the four cardinal directions of gaze. The examiner notes the speed, smoothness, range, and symmetry of movements and observes for unsteadiness of fixation (eg, nystagmus).

Impairment of eye movements can be due to neurologic problems (eg, cranial nerve palsy), primary extraocular muscular weakness (eg, myasthenia gravis), or mechanical constraints within the orbit limiting rotation of the globe (eg, orbital floor fracture with entrapment of the inferior rectus muscle). Deviation of ocular alignment that is the same amount in all directions of gaze is called "comitant." It is "incomitant" if the amount of deviation varies with the direction of gaze.

EXTERNAL EXAMINATION

Before studying the eye under magnification, a general external examination of the ocular adnexa (eyelids and periocular area) is performed. Skin lesions, growths, and inflammatory signs such as swelling, erythema, warmth, and tenderness are evaluated by gross inspection and palpation.

The positions of the eyelids are checked for abnormalities, such as ptosis or lid retraction. Asymmetry can be quantified by measuring the central width (in millimeters) of the "palpebral fissure"—the space between the upper and lower lid margins. Abnormal motor function of the lids, such as impairment of upper lid elevation or forceful lid closure, may be due to either neurologic or primary muscular abnormalities.

Malposition of the globe, such as proptosis, may occur in orbital disease. Palpation of the bony orbital rim and periocular soft tissue should always be done in instances of

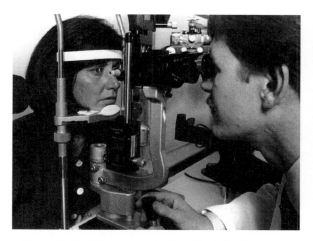

▲ **Figure 2–5.** Slitlamp examination. (Photo by M Narahara. Courtesy of the American Academy of Ophthalmology.)

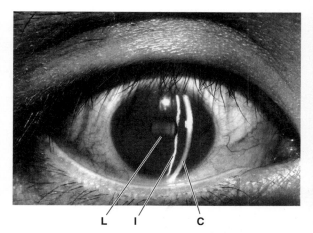

▲ **Figure 2–6.** Slitlamp photograph of a normal right eye. The curved slit of light to the right is reflected off of the cornea (C), while the slit to the left is reflected off of the iris (I). As the latter slit passes through the pupil, the anterior lens (L) is faintly illuminated in cross section. (Photo by M Narahara.)

suspected orbital trauma, infection, or neoplasm. The general facial examination may contribute other pertinent information as well. Depending on the circumstances, checking for enlarged preauricular lymph nodes, sinus tenderness, temporal artery prominence, or skin or mucous membrane abnormalities may be diagnostically relevant.

SLITLAMP EXAMINATION

▶ Basic Slitlamp Biomicroscopy

The slitlamp (Figure 2–5) is a table-mounted binocular microscope with a special adjustable illumination source attached. A linear slit beam of incandescent light is projected onto the globe, illuminating an optical cross section of the eye (Figure 2–6). The angle of illumination can be varied along with the width, length, and intensity of the light beam. The magnification can be adjusted as well (normally 10× to 16× power). Since the slitlamp is a binocular microscope, the view is "stereoscopic," or three-dimensional.

　　The patient is seated while being examined, and the head is stabilized by an adjustable chin rest and forehead strap. Using the slitlamp alone, the anterior half of the globe—the "anterior segment"—can be visualized. Details of the lid margins and lashes, the palpebral and bulbar conjunctival surfaces, the tear film and cornea, the iris, and the aqueous can be studied. Through a dilated pupil, the crystalline lens and the anterior vitreous can be examined as well.

　　Because the slit beam of light provides an optical cross section of the eye, the precise anteroposterior location of abnormalities can be determined within each of the clear ocular structures (eg, cornea, lens, vitreous body). The highest magnification setting is sufficient to show the abnormal presence of cells within the aqueous, such as red or white blood cells or pigment granules. Aqueous turbidity, called "flare," resulting from increased protein concentration can be detected in the presence of intraocular inflammation. Normal aqueous is optically clear, without cells or flare.

▶ Adjunctive Slitlamp Techniques

The eye examination with the slitlamp is supplemented by the use of various techniques. Tonometry is discussed separately in a subsequent section.

A. Lid Eversion

Lid eversion, to examine the undersurface of the upper lid, can be performed either at the slitlamp or without the aid of that instrument. It should always be done if the presence of a superficial foreign body is suspected but not already identified (see Chapter 19). A semirigid plate of cartilage called the tarsus gives each lid its contour and shape. In the upper lid, the superior edge of the tarsus lies centrally about 8–9 mm above the lashes. On the undersurface of the lid, it is covered by the tarsal palpebral conjunctiva.

　　Following topical anesthesia, the patient is positioned at the slitlamp and instructed to look down. The examiner gently grasps the upper lashes with the thumb and index finger of one hand while using the other hand to position an applicator handle just above the superior edge of the tarsus (Figure 2–7). The lid is everted by applying slight downward pressure with the applicator as the lash margin is simultaneously lifted. The patient continues to look down, and the lashes are held pinned to the skin overlying the superior orbital rim as the applicator is withdrawn. The tarsal conjunctiva is then examined under magnification. To undo

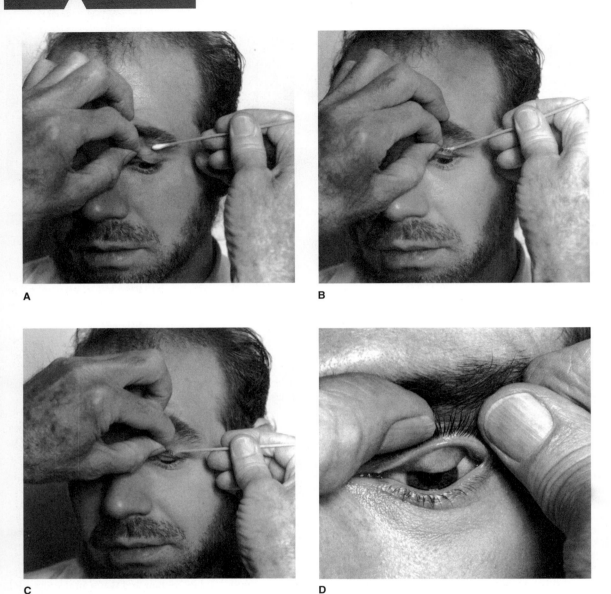

▲ **Figure 2–7.** Technique of lid eversion. **A:** With the patient looking down, the upper lashes are grasped with one hand as an applicator stick is positioned at the superior edge of the upper tarsus (at the upper lid crease). **B** and **C:** As the lashes are lifted, slight downward pressure is simultaneously applied with the applicator stick. **D:** The thumb pins the lashes against the superior orbital rim, allowing examination of the undersurface of the tarsus. (Photos by M Narahara.)

eversion, the lid margin is gently stroked downward as the patient looks up.

B. Fluorescein Staining

Fluorescein is a specialized dye that stains the cornea and highlights any irregularities of its epithelial surface. Sterile paper strips containing fluorescein are wetted with sterile saline or local anesthetic and touched against the inner surface of the lower lid, instilling the yellowish dye into the tear film. The illuminating light of the slitlamp is made blue with a filter, causing the dye to fluoresce.

A uniform film of dye should cover the normal cornea. If the corneal surface is abnormal, excessive amounts of dye will absorb into or collect within the affected area. Abnormalities can range from tiny punctate dots, such as those resulting from excessive dryness or ultraviolet light damage, to large geographic defects in the epithelium, such as those seen in corneal abrasions or infectious ulcers.

C. Special Lenses

Special examining lenses can expand and further magnify the slitlamp examination of the eye's interior. A goniolens (Figure 2–8) provides visualization of the anterior chamber "angle" formed by the iridocorneal junction. Other lenses placed on or in front of the eye allow slitlamp evaluation of the posterior half of the globe's interior—the "posterior segment." Since the slitlamp is a binocular microscope, these lenses provide a magnified three-dimensional view of the posterior vitreous, the fundus, and the disk. Examples are the Goldmann-style three-mirror lens (Figure 2–8) and the Volk-style range of lenses.

D. Special Attachments

Special attachments to the slitlamp allow it to be used with several techniques requiring microscopic visualization. Special camera bodies can be attached for photographic documentation and for special applications such as corneal endothelial cell studies. Special instruments for the study of visual potential require attachment to the slitlamp. Finally, laser sources are attached to a slitlamp to allow microscopic visualization and control of eye treatment.

TONOMETRY

The globe can be thought of as an enclosed compartment through which there is a constant circulation of aqueous humor. This fluid maintains the shape and a relatively uniform pressure within the globe. Tonometry is the method of measuring intraocular pressure using calibrated instruments. The normal range is 10 to 21 mm Hg.

In **applanation tonometry**, intraocular pressure is determined by the force required to flatten the cornea by a standard amount. The force required increases with intraocular pressures. The **Schiotz tonometer**, now rarely used, measures the amount of corneal indentation produced by preset weights. Less corneal indentation is produced as intraocular pressure rises. Since both methods employ devices that touch the patient's cornea, they require topical anesthetic and disinfection of the instrument tip prior to use. (Tonometer disinfection techniques are discussed in Chapter 21.) With any method of tonometry, care must be taken to avoid pressing on the globe and artificially increasing its pressure.

▶ Applanation Tonometry

The Goldmann applanation tonometer (Figure 2–9) is attached to the slitlamp and measures the amount of force

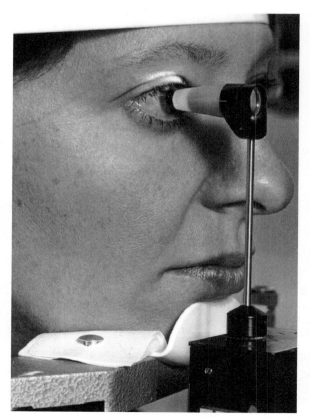

▲ **Figure 2–9.** Applanation tonometry, using the Goldmann tonometer attached to the slit lamp. (Photo by M Narahara. Courtesy of the American Academy of Ophthalmology.)

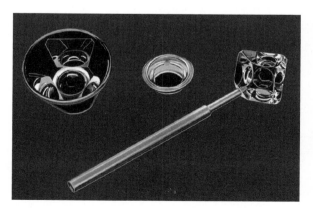

▲ **Figure 2–8.** Three types of goniolenses. **Left:** Goldmann three-mirror lens. Besides the goniomirror, there are also two peripheral retinal mirrors and a central fourth mirror for examining the central retina. **Center:** Koeppe lens. **Right:** Posner/Zeiss-type lens. (Photo by M Narahara.)

required to flatten the corneal apex by a standard amount. The higher the intraocular pressure, the greater the force required. Since Goldmann applanation tonometer is a more accurate method than Schiotz tonometry, it is preferred by ophthalmologists.

Following topical anesthesia and instillation of fluorescein, the patient is positioned at the slitlamp and the tonometer is swung into place. To visualize the fluorescein, the cobalt blue filter is used with the brightest illumination setting. After grossly aligning the tonometer in front of the cornea, the examiner looks through the slitlamp ocular just as the tip contacts the cornea. A manually controlled counterbalanced spring varies the force applied by the tonometer tip.

Upon contact, the tonometer tip flattens the central cornea and produces a thin circular outline of fluorescein. A prism in the tip visually splits this circle into two semicircles that appear green while viewed through the slitlamp oculars. The tonometer force is adjusted manually until the two semicircles just overlap, as shown in Figure 2–10. This visual end point indicates that the cornea has been flattened by the set standard amount. The amount of force required to do this is translated by the scale into a pressure reading in millimeters of mercury.

Accuracy of intraocular pressure measurement is affected by central corneal thickness. The thinner the cornea, the more easily it is indented, but the calibration of tonometers generally assumes a cornea of standard thickness. If the cornea is relatively thin, the actual intraocular pressure is higher than the measured value, and if the cornea is relatively thick, the actual intraocular pressure is lower than the measured value. Thus ultrasonic measurement of corneal thickness (pachymetry) may be helpful in assessment of intraocular pressure. The **Pascal dynamic contour tonometer**, a contact but non-applanating technique, measures intraocular pressure independent of corneal thickness.

Other applanation tonometers are the **Perkins tonometer**, a portable mechanical device with a mechanism similar to the Goldmann tonometer, the **Tono-Pen**, a portable electronic applanation tonometer that is reasonably accurate but requires daily recalibration, and the **pneumatotonometer**, which is particularly useful when the cornea has an irregular surface. The Perkins tonometer and Tono-Pen are commonly used when examination at the slitlamp is not feasible, for example, in emergency rooms in cases of orbital trauma with retrobulbar hemorrhage and in operating rooms during examinations under anesthesia.

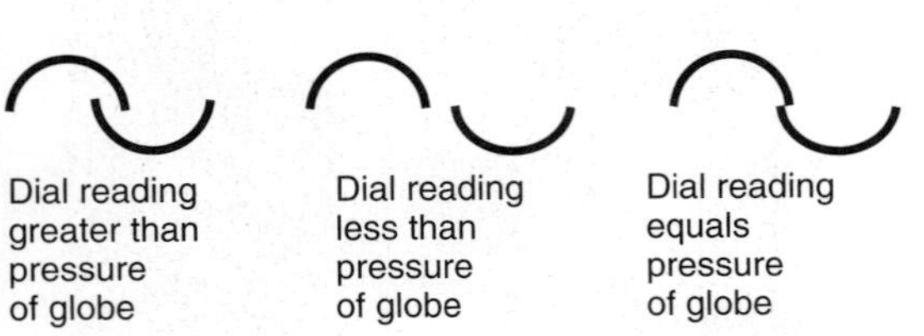

▶ Schiotz Tonometry

The advantage of this method is that it is simple, requiring only a relatively inexpensive, easily portable hand-held instrument. It can be used in any clinic or emergency room setting, at the hospital bedside, or in the operating room, but it requires greater expertise and has generally been superseded by applanation tonometers.

▶ Noncontact Tonometry

The **noncontact ("air-puff") tonometer** is not as accurate as applanation tonometers. A small puff of air is blown against the cornea. The air rebounding from the corneal surface hits a pressure-sensing membrane in the instrument. This method does not require anesthetic drops, since no instrument touches the eye. Thus, it can be more easily used by optometrists or technicians and is useful in screening programs.

DIAGNOSTIC MEDICATIONS

▶ Topical Anesthetics

Eye drops such as proparacaine, tetracaine, and benoxinate provide rapid onset, short-acting topical anesthesia of the cornea, and conjunctiva. They are used prior to ocular contact with diagnostic lenses and instruments such as the tonometer. Other diagnostic manipulations utilizing topical anesthetics will be discussed later. These include corneal and conjunctival scrapings, lacrimal canalicular and punctal probing, and scleral depression.

▶ Mydriatic (Dilating) Drops

The pupil can be pharmacologically dilated by either stimulating the iris dilator muscle with a sympathomimetic agent (eg, 2.5% phenylephrine) or by inhibiting the sphincter muscle with an anticholinergic eye drop (eg, 0.5% or 1% tropicamide) (see Chapter 22). Anticholinergic medications also inhibit accommodation (cycloplegic). This may aid the process of refraction but causes further inconvenience for the patient. Therefore, drops with the shortest duration of action (usually several hours) are used for diagnostic applications. Combining drops from both pharmacologic classes produces the fastest onset (15–20 minutes) and widest dilation.

Because dilation can cause a small rise in intraocular pressure, tonometry should always be performed before these drops are instilled. There is also a small risk of precipitating an attack of acute angle-closure glaucoma if the patient has preexisting narrow anterior chamber angles (between the iris and cornea). Such an eye can be identified using the technique illustrated in Figure 11–4. Finally, excessive instillation of these drops should be avoided because of the systemic

| Dial reading greater than pressure of globe | Dial reading less than pressure of globe | Dial reading equals pressure of globe |

▲ **Figure 2–10.** Appearance of fluorescein semicircles, or "mires," through the slitlamp ocular, showing the end point for applanation tonometry.

absorption that can occur through the nasopharyngeal mucous membranes following lacrimal drainage.

A more complete discussion of diagnostic drops is found in Chapter 22.

DIRECT OPHTHALMOSCOPY

▶ Instrumentation

The hand-held direct ophthalmoscope provides a monocular image, including a 15× magnified view of the fundus. Because of its portability and the detailed view of the disk and retinal vasculature it provides, direct ophthalmoscopy is a standard part of the general medical examination. The intensity, color, and spot size of the illuminating light can be adjusted, as well as the ophthalmoscope's point of focus. The latter is changed using a wheel of progressively higher-power lenses that the examiner dials into place. These lenses are sequentially arranged and numbered according to their power in diopters. Usually the (+) converging lenses are designated by black numbers and the (−) divergent lenses are designated by red numbers.

▶ Anterior Segment Examination

Using the high plus lenses, the direct ophthalmoscope can be focused to provide a magnified view of the conjunctiva, cornea, and iris. The slitlamp allows a far superior and more magnified examination of these areas, but it is not portable and may be unavailable.

▶ Red Reflex Examination

If the illuminating light is aligned directly along the visual axis, more obviously when the pupil is dilated, the pupillary aperture normally is filled by a homogeneous bright reddish-orange color. This **red reflex,** equivalent to the "red eye"

effect of flash photography, is formed by reflection of the illuminating light by the fundus through the clear ocular media—the vitreous, lens, aqueous, and cornea. It is best observed by holding the ophthalmoscope at arm's length from the patient as he looks toward the illuminating light and dialing the lens wheel to focus the ophthalmoscope in the plane of the pupil.

Any opacity located along the central optical pathway will block all or part of the red reflex and appear as a dark spot or shadow. If a focal opacity is seen, have the patient look momentarily away and then back toward the light. If the opacity is still moving or floating, it is located within the vitreous (eg, small hemorrhage). If it is stationary, it is probably in the lens (eg, focal cataract) or on the cornea (eg, scar).

▶ Fundus Examination

The primary value of the direct ophthalmoscope is in examination of the fundus (Figure 2–11). The view may be impaired by cloudy ocular media, such as a cataract, or by a small pupil. Darkening the room usually causes enough natural pupillary dilation to allow evaluation of the central fundus, including the disk, the macula, and the proximal retinal vasculature. Pharmacologically dilating the pupil greatly enhances the view and permits a more extensive examination of the peripheral retina.

Examination of the fundus is also optimized by holding the ophthalmoscope as close to the patient's pupil as possible (approximately 1–2 inches), just as one can see more through a keyhole by getting as close to it as possible. This requires using the examiner's right eye and hand to examine the patient's right eye and the left eye and hand to examine the patient's left eye (Figure 2–12).

The spot size and color of the illuminating light can be varied. If the pupil is well dilated, the large spot size of light

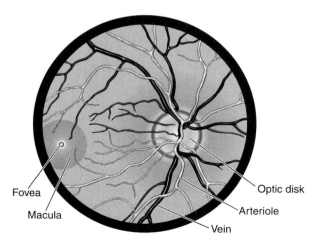 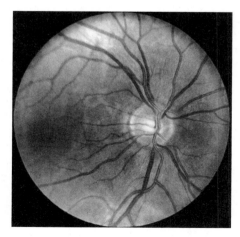

Fovea

Macula

Optic disk

Arteriole

Vein

▲ **Figure 2–11.** Photo and corresponding diagram of a normal fundus. Note that the retinal vessels all stop short of and do not cross the fovea. (Photo by Diane Beeston.)

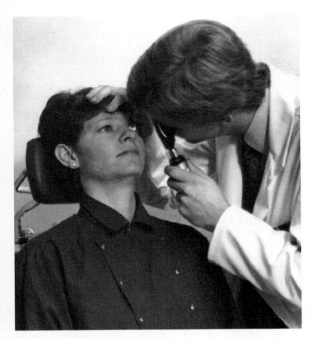

▲ **Figure 2–12.** Direct ophthalmoscopy. The examiner uses the left eye to evaluate the patient's left eye.
(Photo by M Narahara. Courtesy of the American Academy of Ophthalmology.)

affords the widest area of illumination. With an undilated pupil, however, much of this light would be reflected back toward the examiner's eye by the patient's iris, interfering with the view, and the pupil will constrict. For this reason, the smaller spot size of light is usually better for undilated pupils.

The refractive error of the patient's and the examiner's eyes will determine the lens power needed to bring the fundus into optimal focus. If the examiner wears spectacles, they can be left either on or off. The patient's spectacles are usually left off, but it may be helpful to leave them on if there is high refractive error.

As the patient fixates on a distant target with the opposite eye, the examiner first brings retinal details into sharp focus. Since the retinal vessels all arise from the disk, the latter is located by following any major vascular branch back to this common origin. At this point, the ophthalmoscope beam will be aimed slightly nasal to the patient's line of vision, or "visual axis." One should study the shape, size, and color of the disk, the distinctness of its margins, and the size of the pale central "physiologic cup." The ratio of cup size to disk size is of diagnostic importance in glaucoma (Figures 2–13 and 2–14).

The macular area (Figure 2–11) is located approximately two "disk diameters" temporal to the edge of the disk. A small pinpoint white reflection or "reflex" marks the central fovea. This is surrounded by a more darkly pigmented and poorly circumscribed area called the macula. The retinal vascular branches approach from all sides but stop short of the fovea. Thus, its location can be confirmed by the focal absence of

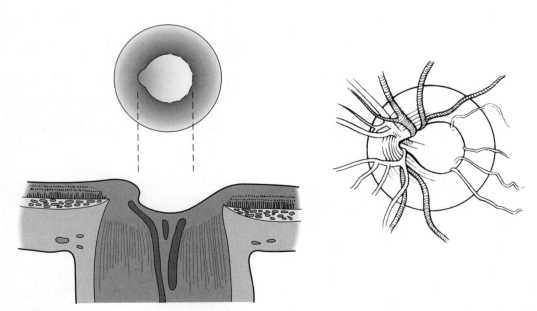

▲ **Figure 2–13.** Diagram of a moderately cupped disk viewed on end and in profile, with an accompanying sketch for the patient's record. The width of the central cup divided by the width of the disk is the "cup-to-disk ratio." The cup-to-disk ratio of this disk is approximately 0.5.

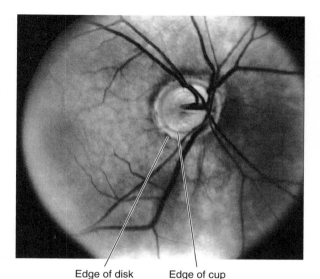

Edge of disk   Edge of cup

▲ **Figure 2–14.** Cup-to-disk ratio of 0.9 in a patient with end-stage glaucoma. The normal disk tissue is compressed into a peripheral thin rim surrounding a huge pale cup.

retinal vessels or by asking the patient to stare directly into the light.

The major retinal vessels are then examined and followed as far distally as possible in each of the four quadrants (superior, inferior, temporal, and nasal). The veins are darker and wider than their paired arteries. The vessels are examined for color, tortuosity, and caliber, as well as for associated abnormalities, such as aneurysms, hemorrhages, or exudates. Sizes and distances within the fundus are often measured in "disk diameters" (DD). (The typical optic disk is generally 1.5–2 mm in diameter.) Thus, one might describe a "1 DD area of hemorrhage located 2.5 DD inferotemporal to the fovea." The green "red-free" filter assists in the examination of the retinal vasculature and the subtle striations of the nerve fiber layer as they course toward the disk (see Chapter 14).

To examine the retinal periphery, which is greatly enhanced by dilating the pupil, the patient is asked to look in the direction of the quadrant to be examined. Thus, the temporal retina of the right eye is seen when the patient looks to the right, while the superior retina is seen when the patient looks up. When the globe rotates, the retina and the cornea move in opposite directions. As the patient looks up, the superior retina rotates downward into the examiner's line of vision.

INDIRECT OPHTHALMOSCOPY

▶ Instrumentation

The binocular indirect ophthalmoscope (Figure 2–15) complements and supplements the direct ophthalmoscopic

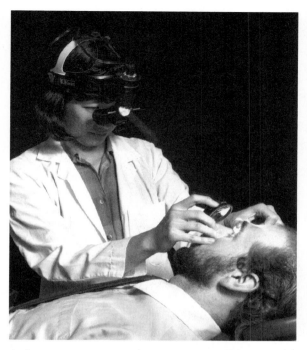

▲ **Figure 2–15.** Examination with head-mounted binocular indirect ophthalmoscope. A 20-diopter hand-held condensing lens is used. (Photo by M Narahara.)

examination. Since it requires wide pupillary dilation and is difficult to learn, this technique is used primarily by ophthalmologists. The patient can be examined while seated, but the supine position is preferable.

The indirect ophthalmoscope is worn on the examiner's head and allows binocular viewing through a set of lenses of fixed power. A bright adjustable light source attached to the headband is directed toward the patient's eye. As with direct ophthalmoscopy, the patient is told to look in the direction of the quadrant being examined. A convex lens is hand-held several inches from the patient's eye in precise orientation so as to simultaneously focus light onto the retina and an image of the retina in midair between the patient and the examiner. Using the preset head-mounted ophthalmoscope lenses, the examiner can then "focus on" and visualize this midair image of the retina.

▶ Comparison of Indirect & Direct Ophthalmoscopy

Indirect ophthalmoscopy is so called because one is viewing an "image" of the retina formed by a hand-held "condensing lens." In contrast, direct ophthalmoscopy allows one to focus on the retina itself. Compared with the direct ophthalmoscope (15× magnification), indirect ophthalmoscopy provides a much wider field of view (Figure 2–16) with less overall magnification (approximately 3.5× using a standard

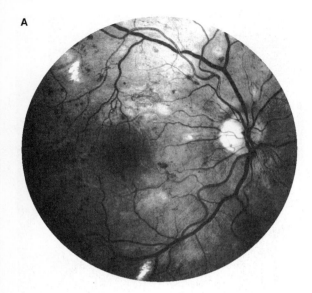

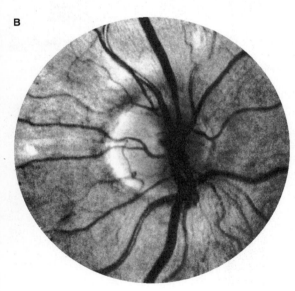

▲ **Figure 2–16.** Comparison of view within the same fundus using the indirect ophthalmoscope **(A)** and the direct ophthalmoscope **(B)**. The field of view with the latter is approximately 10°, compared with approximately 37° using the indirect ophthalmoscope. In this patient with diabetic retinopathy, an important overview is first seen with the indirect ophthalmoscope. The direct ophthalmoscope can then provide magnified details of a specific area. (Photos by M Narahara.)

20-diopter hand-held condensing lens). Thus, it presents a wide panoramic fundus view from which specific areas can be selectively studied under higher magnification using either the direct ophthalmoscope or the slitlamp with special auxiliary lenses.

Indirect ophthalmoscopy has three distinct advantages over direct ophthalmoscopy. One is the brighter light source that permits much better visualization through cloudy media. A second advantage is that by using both eyes, the examiner enjoys a stereoscopic view, allowing visualization of elevated masses or retinal detachment in three dimensions. Finally, indirect ophthalmoscopy can be used to examine the entire retina, even out to its extreme periphery, the ora serrata. This is possible for two reasons. Optical distortions caused by looking through the peripheral lens and cornea interfere very little with the indirect ophthalmoscopic examination compared with the direct ophthalmoscope. In addition, the adjunct technique of scleral depression can be used.

Scleral depression (Figure 2–17) is performed as the peripheral retina is being examined with the indirect ophthalmoscope. A smooth, thin metal probe is used to gently indent the globe externally through the lids at a point just behind the corneoscleral junction (limbus). As this is done, the ora serrata and peripheral retina are pushed internally into the examiner's line of view. By depressing around the entire circumference, the peripheral retina can be viewed in its entirety.

Because of all of these advantages, indirect ophthalmoscopy is used preoperatively and intraoperatively in the evaluation and surgical repair of retinal detachments. A disadvantage of indirect ophthalmoscopy, which also applies to the Volk-style of lenses for examination of the posterior segment with a slitlamp, is that it provides an inverted image of the fundus, which requires a mental adjustment on the examiner's part. Its brighter light source can also be more uncomfortable for the patient.

EYE EXAMINATION BY THE NONOPHTHALMOLOGIST

The preceding sequence of tests would comprise a complete routine or diagnostic ophthalmologic evaluation. A general medical examination would often include many of these same testing techniques.

Assessment of pupils, extraocular movements, and confrontation visual fields is part of any complete neurologic assessment. Direct ophthalmoscopy should always be performed to assess the appearance of the disk and retinal vessels. Separately testing the visual acuity of each eye (particularly with children) may uncover either a refractive or a medical cause of decreased vision. The three most common preventable causes of permanent visual loss in developed nations are amblyopia, diabetic retinopathy, and glaucoma. All can remain asymptomatic while the opportunity for preventive measures is gradually lost. During this time, the pediatrician

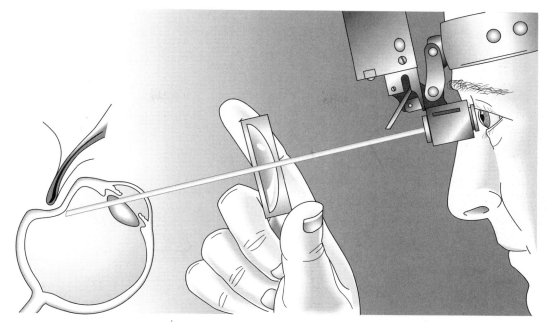

▲ **Figure 2–17.** Diagrammatic representation of indirect ophthalmoscopy with scleral depression to examine the far peripheral retina. Indentation of the sclera through the lids brings the peripheral edge of the retina into visual alignment with the dilated pupil, the hand-held condensing lens, and the head-mounted ophthalmoscope.

or general medical practitioner may be the only physician the patient visits.

By testing children for visual acuity in each eye, examining and referring diabetics for regular dilated fundus ophthalmoscopy, and referring patients with suspicious discs to the ophthalmologist, the nonophthalmologist may indeed be the one who truly "saves" that patient's eyesight. This represents both an important opportunity and responsibility for every primary care physician.

▼ III. SPECIALIZED OPHTHALMOLOGIC EXAMINATIONS

This section will discuss ophthalmologic examination techniques with more specific indications that would not be performed on a routine basis. They will be grouped according to the function or anatomic area of primary interest.

DIAGNOSIS OF VISUAL ABNORMALITIES

1. PERIMETRY

Perimetry is used to examine the central and peripheral visual fields. Usually performed separately for each eye, it assesses the combined function of the retina, the optic nerve, and the intracranial visual pathway. It is used clinically to detect or monitor field loss due to disease at any of these locations. Damage to specific parts of the neurologic visual pathway may produce characteristic patterns of change on serial field examinations.

The visual field of the eye is measured and plotted in degrees of arc. Measurement of degrees of arc remains constant regardless of the distance from the eye that the field is checked. The sensitivity of vision is greatest in the center of the field (corresponding to the fovea) and least in the periphery. Perimetry relies on subjective patient responses, and the results will depend on the patient's psychomotor as well as visual status. Perimetry must always be performed and interpreted with this in mind.

▶ The Principles of Testing

Although perimetry is subjective, the methods discussed below have been standardized to maximize reproducibility and permit subsequent comparison. Perimetry requires (1) steady fixation and attention by the patient; (2) a set distance from the eye to the screen or testing device; (3) a uniform, standard amount of background illumination and contrast; (4) test targets of standard size and brightness; and (5) a universal protocol for administration of the test by examiners.

As the patient's eye fixates on a central target, test objects are randomly presented at different locations throughout the field. If they are seen, the patient responds either verbally or with a hand-held signaling device. Varying the target's size or brightness permits quantification of visual sensitivity of different areas in the field. The smaller or dimmer the target seen, the higher the sensitivity of that location.

There are two basic methods of target presentation—static and kinetic—that can be used alone or in combination during an examination. In **static perimetry**, different locations throughout the field are tested one at a time. A dim stimulus, usually a white light, is first presented at a particular location. If it is not seen, the size or intensity is incrementally increased until it is just large enough or bright enough to be detected. This is called the "threshold" sensitivity level of that location. This sequence is repeated at a series of other locations, so that the sensitivity of multiple points in the field can be evaluated and combined to form a profile of the visual field.

In **kinetic perimetry,** the sensitivity of the entire field to one single test object (of fixed size and brightness) is first tested. The object is slowly moved toward the center from a peripheral area until it is first spotted. By moving the same object inward from multiple directions, a boundary called an "**isopter**" can be mapped out that is specific for that target. The isopter outlines the area within which the target can be seen and beyond which it cannot be seen. Thus, the larger the isopter, the better the visual field of that eye. The boundaries of the isopter are measured and plotted in degrees of arc. By repeating the test using objects of different size or brightness, multiple isopters can then be plotted for a given eye. The smaller or dimmer test objects will produce smaller isopters.

▶ Methods of Perimetry

The **tangent screen** is the simplest apparatus for standardized perimetry. It utilizes different-sized pins on a black wand presented against a black screen and is used primarily to test the central 30° of visual field. The advantages of this method are its simplicity and rapidity, the possibility of changing the subject's distance from the screen, and the option of using any assortment of fixation and test objects, including different colors.

The more sophisticated **Goldmann perimeter** (Figure 2–18) is a hollow white spherical bowl positioned a set distance in front of the patient. A light of variable size and intensity can be presented by the examiner (seated behind the perimeter) in either static or kinetic fashion. This method can test the full limit of peripheral vision and was for years the primary method for plotting fields in glaucoma patients.

Computerized automated perimeters (Figure 2–19) now constitute the most sophisticated and sensitive equipment available for visual field testing. Using a bowl similar to the Goldmann perimeter, these instruments display test lights of varying brightness and size but use a quantitative static threshold testing format that is more precise and comprehensive than other methods. Numerical scores (Figure 2–20)

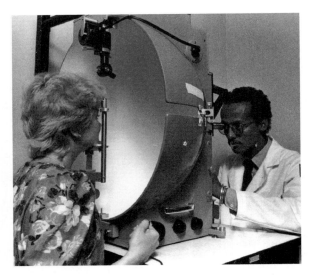

▲ **Figure 2–18.** Goldmann perimeter. (Photo by M Narahara.)

corresponding to the threshold sensitivity of each test location can be stored in the computer memory and compared statistically with results from previous examinations or from other normal patients. The higher the numerical score, the better the visual sensitivity of that location in the field.

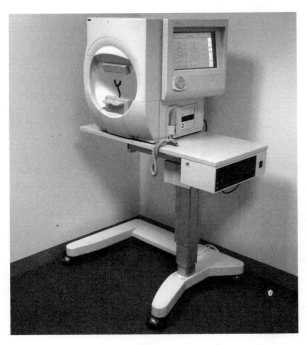

▲ **Figure 2–19.** Computerized automated perimeter.

A

RIGHT

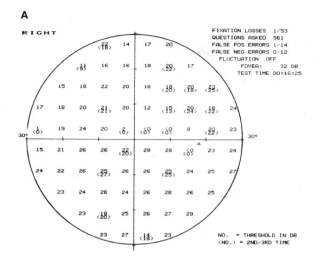

B

RIGHT

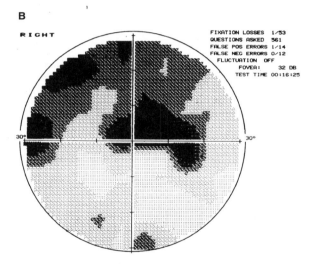

FIXATION LOSSES   1/53
QUESTIONS ASKED   561
FALSE POS ERRORS 1/14
FALSE NEG ERRORS 0/12
FLUCTUATION OFF
FOVEA: 32 DB
TEST TIME 00:16:25

▲ **Figure 2–20.** **A:** Numerical printout of threshold sensitivity scores derived by using the static method of computerized perimetry. This is the 30° field of a patient's right eye with glaucoma. The higher the numbers, the better the visual sensitivity. The computer retests many of the points (bracketed numbers) to assess consistency of the patient's responses. **B:** Diagrammatic "gray scale" display of these same numerical scores. The darker the area, the poorer the visual sensitivity at that location.

Another important advantage is that the test presentation is programmed and automated, eliminating any variability on the part of the examiner. Analysis of the results provides information on whether visual field loss is diffuse or focal and on the patient's ability to perform the test reliably.

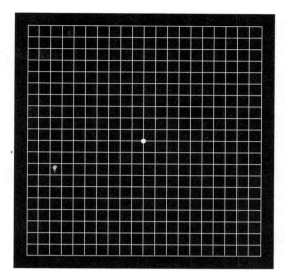

▲ **Figure 2–21.** Amsler grid.

2. AMSLER GRID

The Amsler grid is used to test the central 20° of the visual field. The grid (Figure 2–21) is viewed by each eye separately at normal reading distance and with reading glasses on if the patient uses them. It is most commonly used to test macular function.

While fixating on the central dot, the patient checks to see that the lines are all straight, without distortion, and that no spots or portions of the grid are missing. One eye is compared with the other. A scotoma or blank area—either central or paracentral—can indicate disease of the macula or optic nerve. Wavy distortion of the lines (metamorphopsia) can indicate macular edema or submacular fluid.

The grid can be used by patients at home to test their own central vision. For example, patients with age-related macular degeneration (see Chapter 10) can use the grid to monitor for sudden metamorphopsia. This often is the earliest symptom of acute fluid accumulation beneath the macula arising from leaking sub-retinal neovascularization. Since these abnormal vessels may respond to prompt treatment, early detection is important.

3. BRIGHTNESS ACUITY TESTING

The visual abilities of patients with media opacities may vary depending on conditions of lighting. For example, when dim illumination makes the pupil larger, one may be able to "see around" a central focal cataract, whereas bright illumination causing pupillary constriction would have the contrary effect. Bright lights may also cause disabling glare in patients with corneal edema or diffuse clouding of the crystalline lens due to light scattering.

Because the darkened examining room may not accurately elicit the patient's functional difficulties in real life, instruments have been developed to test the effect of varying levels of brightness or glare on visual acuity. Distance acuity with the Snellen chart is usually tested under standard levels of incrementally increasing illumination, and the information may be helpful in making therapeutic or surgical decisions. Asking cataract patients specific questions about how their vision is affected by various lighting conditions is even more important.

4. COLOR VISION TESTING

Normal color vision requires healthy function of the macula and optic nerve. The most common abnormality is red-green "color blindness," which is present in approximately 8% of the male population. This is due to an X-linked congenital deficiency of one specific type of retinal photoreceptor. Depressed color vision may also be a sensitive indicator of certain kinds of acquired macular or optic nerve disease. For example, in optic neuritis or optic nerve compression (eg, by a mass), abnormal color vision is often an earlier indication of disease than visual acuity, which may still be 20/20.

The most common testing technique utilizes a series of polychromatic plates, such as those of Ishihara or Hardy-Rand-Rittler (Figure 2–22). The plates are made up of dots of the primary colors printed on a background mosaic of similar dots in a confusing variety of secondary colors. The primary dots are arranged in simple patterns (numbers or geometric shapes) that cannot be recognized by patients with deficient color perception.

5. CONTRAST-SENSITIVITY TESTING

Contrast sensitivity is the ability of the eye to discern subtle degrees of contrast. Retinal and optic nerve disease and clouding of the ocular media (eg, cataracts) can impair this ability. Like color vision, contrast sensitivity may become depressed before Snellen visual acuity is affected in many situations.

Contrast sensitivity is best tested by using standard preprinted charts with a series of test targets (Figure 2–23). Since illumination greatly affects contrast, it must be standardized and checked with a light meter. Each separate target consists of a series of dark parallel lines in one of three different orientations. They are displayed against a lighter, contrasting gray background. As the contrast between the lines and their background is progressively reduced from one target to the next, it becomes more difficult for the patient to judge the orientation of the lines. The patient can be scored according to the lowest level of contrast at which the pattern of lines can still be discerned.

6. ASSESSING POTENTIAL VISION

When opacities of the cornea or lens coexist with disease of the macula or optic nerve, the visual potential of the eye is often in doubt. The benefit of corneal transplantation or cataract extraction will depend on the severity of coexisting retinal or optic nerve impairment. Several methods are available for assessing central visual potential under these circumstances.

Even with a totally opaque cataract that completely prevents a view of the fundus, the patient should still be able to

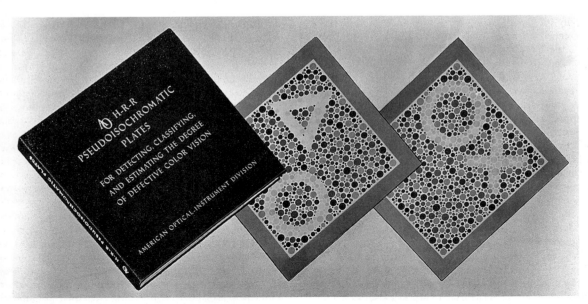

▲ **Figure 2–22.** Hardy-Rand-Rittler (H-R-R) pseudoisochromatic plates for testing color vision.

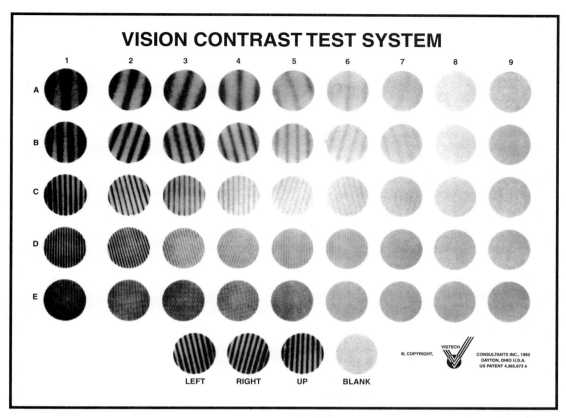

▲ **Figure 2–23.** Contrast-sensitivity test chart. (Courtesy of Vistech Consultants, Inc.)

identify the direction of a light directed into the eye from different quadrants. When a red lens is held in front of the light, the patient should be able to differentiate between white and red light. The presence of a relative afferent pupillary defect indicates significant disease of the retina or optic nerve, and thus a poor visual prognosis.

A gross test of macular function involves the patient's ability to perceive so-called **entoptic phenomena.** For example, as the eyeball is massaged with a rapidly moving penlight through the closed lids, the patient should be able to visualize an image of the paramacular vascular branches if the macula is healthy. These may be described as looking like "the veins of a leaf." Because this test is highly subjective and subject to interpretation, it is only helpful if the patient is able to recognize the vascular pattern in at least one eye. Absence of the pattern in the opposite eye then suggests macular impairment.

In addition to these gross methods, sophisticated quantitative instruments have been developed for more direct determination of visual potential in eyes with media opacities. These instruments project a narrow beam of light containing a pattern of images through any relatively clear portion of the media (eg, through a less-dense region of a cataract) and onto the retina. The patient's vision is then graded according to the size of the smallest patterns that can be seen.

Two different types of patterns are used. **Laser interferometry** employs laser light to generate interference fringes or gratings, which the patient sees as a series of parallel lines. Progressively narrowing the width and spacing of the lines causes an end point to be reached where the patient can no longer discern the orientation of the lines. The narrowest image width the patient can resolve is then correlated with a Snellen acuity measurement to determine the visual potential of that eye. The **potential acuity meter** projects a standard Snellen acuity chart onto the retina. The patient is then graded in the usual fashion, according to the smallest line of letters read.

Although both instruments appear useful in measuring potential visual acuity, false-positive and false-negative results do occur, with a frequency dependent on the type of disease present. Thus, these methods are helpful but not completely reliable in determining the visual prognosis of eyes with cloudy media.

7. TESTS FOR FUNCTIONAL VISUAL LOSS

The measurement of vision is subjective, requiring responses on the part of the patient. The validity of the test may therefore be limited by the alertness or cooperation of the patient. "Functional" visual loss is a subjective complaint of impaired vision without any demonstrated organic or objective basis. Examples include hysterical blindness and malingering.

Recognition of functional visual loss or malingering depends on the use of testing variations in order to elicit inconsistent or contradictory responses. An example would be eliciting "tunnel" visual fields using the tangent screen. A patient claiming "poor vision" and tested at the standard distance of 1 meter may map out a narrow central zone of intact vision beyond which even large objects—such as a hand—allegedly cannot be seen. The borders ("isopter") of this apparently small area are then marked. The patient is then moved back to a position 2 meters from the tangent screen. From this position, the field should be twice as large as the area plotted from 1 meter away. If the patient outlines an area of the same size from both testing distances, this raises a strong suspicion of functional visual loss, but a number of conditions, such as advanced glaucoma, severe retinitis pigmentosa, and cortical blindness, would need to be excluded.

A variety of other different tests can be chosen to assess the validity of different degrees of visual loss that may be in question.

DIAGNOSIS OF OCULAR ABNORMALITIES

1. MICROBIOLOGY & CYTOLOGY

Like any mucous membrane, the conjunctiva can be cultured with swabs for the identification of bacterial infection. Specimens for cytologic examination are obtained by lightly scraping the palpebral conjunctiva (ie, lining the inner aspect of the lid), such as with a small platinum spatula, following topical anesthesia. For the cytologic evaluation of conjunctivitis, Giemsa's stain is used to identify the types of inflammatory cells present, while Gram's stain may demonstrate the presence (and type) of bacteria. These applications are discussed at length in Chapter 5.

The cornea is normally sterile. The base of any suspected infectious corneal ulcer should be scraped with the platinum spatula or other device for Gram staining and culture. This procedure is performed at the slitlamp. Because in many cases only trace quantities of bacteria are recoverable, the scrapings should be transferred directly onto culture plates without the intervening use of transport media. Any amount of culture growth, no matter how scant, is considered significant, but many cases of infection may still be "culture-negative."

Culture of intraocular fluids is the standard method of diagnosing or ruling out bacterial endophthalmitis. Aqueous can be tapped by inserting a short 25-gauge needle on a tuberculin syringe through the limbus parallel to the iris. Care must be taken not to traumatize the lens. The diagnostic yield is better if vitreous is cultured. Vitreous specimens can be obtained by a needle tap through the pars plana or by doing a surgical vitrectomy. Polymerase chain reaction of vitreous samples has become the standard method of diagnosing viral retinitis. In the evaluation of noninfectious intraocular inflammation, cytology specimens are occasionally obtained using similar techniques.

2. TECHNIQUES FOR CORNEAL EXAMINATION

Several additional techniques are available for more specialized evaluation of the cornea. The **keratometer** is a calibrated instrument that measures the radius of curvature of the cornea in two meridians 90° apart. If the cornea is not perfectly spherical, the two radii will be different. This results in **corneal astigmatism**, which is quantified by the difference between the two radii of curvature. Keratometer measurements are used in contact lens fitting and for intraocular lens power calculations prior to cataract surgery.

Many corneal diseases result in distortion of the otherwise smooth surface of the cornea, which impairs its optical quality. The **photokeratoscope** is an instrument that assesses the uniformity and evenness of the surface by reflecting a pattern of concentric circles onto it. This pattern, which can be visualized and photographed through the instrument, should normally appear perfectly regular and uniform. Focal corneal irregularities will instead distort the circular patterns reflected from that particular area.

Computerized corneal topography is an advanced technique of mapping the anterior corneal surface. Whereas keratometry provides only a single corneal curvature measurement and photokeratoscopy provides only qualitative information, these computer systems combine and improve on the features of both. A real-time video camera records the concentric keratoscopic rings reflected from the cornea. A computer digitizes the data from thousands of locations across the corneal surface and displays the measurements in a color-coded map (Figure 2–24). This enables one to quantify and analyze minute changes in shape and refractive power across the entire cornea induced by disease or surgery. Wavefront aberrometry measures the quality of the eye's optics, and may be combined together with corneal topography in a single instrument (Figure 2–24). By recording the path of diagnostic laser beams bouncing off of the retina, these devices can diagnose optical distortions called higher-order aberrations that are caused either by the cornea or the lens. Higher-order aberrations can result in blurred vision, halos, glare, and starbursts that are most symptomatic at night due to larger pupil size. These optical distortions are not corrected by eyeglasses.

The endothelium is a monolayer of cells lining the posterior corneal surface, which function as fluid pumps and are responsible for keeping the cornea thin and dehydrated, thereby maintaining its optical clarity. If these cells become

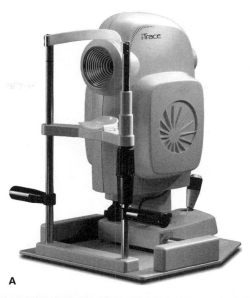

A

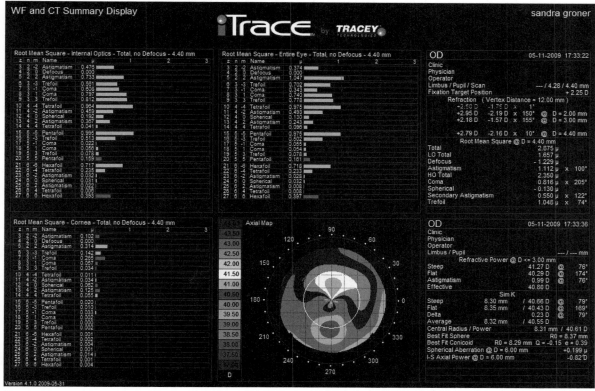

B

▲ **Figure 2–24. A:** Computerized corneal topography and wavefront aberrometry system. **B:** Color-coded corneal topographic display of curvature across the entire corneal surface, combined with quantitative measurements of higher order aberrations from the total eye (top right), lens (top left), and cornea (bottom left). See color insert. (Photos courtesy of Tracey Technologies, Inc.)

impaired or depleted, corneal edema and thickening result, ultimately decreasing vision. The endothelial cells themselves can be photographed with a special slitlamp camera, enabling one to study cell morphology and perform cell counts. Central corneal thickness can be accurately measured with an ultrasonic pachymeter. These measurements are useful for monitoring increasing corneal thickness due to edema caused by progressive endothelial cell loss and, as discussed earlier, in determining the validity of intraocular pressure measurements obtained by applanation tonometry.

3. GONIOSCOPY

The anterior chamber—the space between the iris and the cornea—is filled with liquid aqueous humor, which is produced behind the iris by the ciliary body and exits the eye through the sieve-like drainage system of the trabecular meshwork. The meshwork is arranged as a thin circumferential band of tissue just anterior to the base of the iris and within the angle formed by the iridocorneal junction (Figure 11–3). This angle recess can vary in its anatomy, pigmentation, and width of opening—all of which may affect aqueous drainage and be of diagnostic relevance for glaucoma.

Gonioscopy is the method of examination of the anterior chamber angle anatomy using binocular magnification and a special **goniolens.** The Goldmann and Posner–Zeiss types of goniolenses (Figure 2–8) have special mirrors angled so as to provide a line of view parallel with the iris surface and directed peripherally toward the angle recess, the anterior chamber angle not being amenable to direct visualization (see Chapter 21). After topical anesthesia, the patient is seated at the slitlamp and the goniolens is placed on the eye (Figure 2–25). Magnified details of the anterior chamber angle are viewed stereoscopically. By rotating the mirror, the entire 360° circumference of the angle can be examined. The same lens can be used to direct laser treatment toward the angle as therapy for glaucoma.

A third type of goniolens, the Koeppe lens, requires a special illuminator and a separate hand-held binocular microscope. It is used with the patient lying supine and can thus be used either in the office or in the operating room (either diagnostically or for surgery).

4. GOLDMANN THREE-MIRROR LENS

The Goldmann lens is a versatile adjunct to the slitlamp examination (Figure 2–8). Three separate mirrors, all with different angles of orientation, allow the examiner's line of sight to be directed peripherally at three different angles while using the standard slitlamp. The most anterior and acute angle of view is achieved with the goniolens, discussed above.

Through a dilated pupil, the other two mirrored lenses angle the examiner's view toward the retinal mid periphery and far periphery, respectively. As with gonioscopy, each lens can be rotated 360° circumferentially and can be used to aim

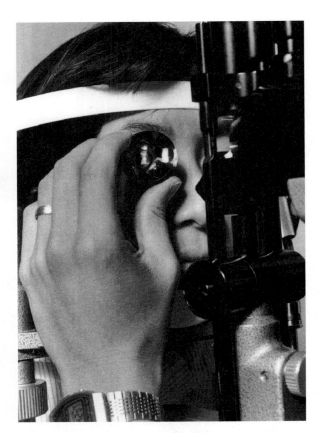

▲ **Figure 2–25.** Gonioscopy with slitlamp and Goldmann-type lens. (Photo by M Narahara.)

laser treatment. A fourth central lens (no mirror) is used to examine the posterior vitreous and the central-most area of the retina. The stereoscopic magnification of this method provides the greatest three-dimensional detail of the macula and disk.

The patient's side of the lens has a concavity designed to fit directly over the topically anesthetized cornea. A clear, viscous solution of methylcellulose is placed in the concavity of the lens prior to insertion onto the patient's eye. This eliminates interference from optical interfaces, such as bubbles, and provides mild adhesion of the lens to the eye for stabilization.

5. FUNDUS PHOTOGRAPHY

Special retinal cameras are used to document details of the fundus for study and future comparison. In the past, standard film was used for 35-mm color slides. Digital photography is now more common. As with any form of ophthalmoscopy, a dilated pupil and clear ocular media provide the most optimal view. All of the fundus photographs in this textbook were taken with such a camera.

One of the most common applications is disk photography, used in the evaluation for glaucoma. Since the slow progression of glaucomatous optic nerve damage may be evident only by subtle alteration of the disk's appearance over time (see Chapter 11), precise documentation of its morphology is needed. By slightly shifting the camera angle on two consecutive shots, a "stereo" pair of slides can be produced that will provide a three-dimensional image when studied through a stereoscopic slide viewer. Stereo disk photography thus provides the most sensitive means of detecting increases in glaucomatous cupping.

6. FLUORESCEIN ANGIOGRAPHY

The capabilities of fundus photographic imaging can be tremendously enhanced by fluorescein, a dye whose molecules emit green light when stimulated by blue light. When photographed, the dye highlights vascular and anatomic details of the fundus. Fluorescein angiography is invaluable in the diagnosis and evaluation of many retinal conditions. Because it can so precisely delineate areas of abnormality, it is an essential guide for planning laser treatment of retinal vascular disease.

▶ Technique

The patient is seated in front of the retinal camera following pupillary dilation. After a small amount of fluorescein is injected into a vein in the arm, it circulates throughout the body before eventually being excreted by the kidneys. As the dye passes through the retinal and choroidal circulation, it can be visualized and photographed because of its properties of fluorescence. Two special filters within the camera produce this effect. A blue **"excitatory"** filter bombards the fluorescein molecules with blue light from the camera flash, causing them to emit a green light. The **"barrier"** filter allows only this emitted green light to reach the photographic film, blocking out all other wavelengths of light. A digital black and white photograph results, in which only the fluorescein image is seen.

Because the fluorescein molecules do not diffuse out of normal retinal vessels, the latter are highlighted photographically by the dye (Figure 2–26). The diffuse, background "ground glass" appearance results from fluorescein filling of the separate underlying choroidal circulation. The choroidal and retinal circulations are anatomically separated by a thin, homogeneous monolayer of pigmented cells—the "retinal pigment epithelium." Denser pigmentation located in the macula obscures more of this background choroidal fluorescence (Figure 2–26), causing the darker central zone on the photograph. In contrast, focal atrophy of the pigment epithelium causes an abnormal increase in visibility of the background fluorescence (Figure 2–27).

▶ Applications

A high-speed motorized frame advance allows for rapid sequence photography of the dye's transit through the

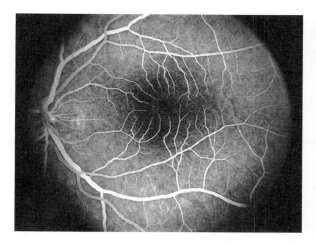

▲ **Figure 2–26.** Normal angiogram of the central retina. The photo has been taken after the dye (appearing white) has already sequentially filled the choroidal circulation (seen as a diffuse, mottled whitish background), the arterioles, and the veins. The macula appears dark due to heavier pigmentation, which obscures the underlying choroidal fluorescence that is visible everywhere else. (Photo courtesy of R Griffith and T King.)

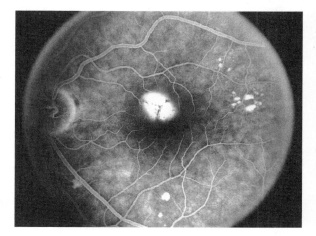

▲ **Figure 2–27.** Abnormal angiogram in which dye-stained fluid originating from the choroid has pooled beneath the macula. This is one type of abnormality associated with age-related macular degeneration (see Chapter 10). Secondary atrophy of the overlying retinal pigment epithelium in this area causes heightened, un-obscured visibility of this increased fluorescence. (Photo courtesy of R Griffith and T King.)

retinal and choroidal circulations over time. A fluorescein study or "angiogram" therefore consists of multiple sequential black and white photos of the fundi taken at different times following dye injection (Figure 2–28). Early-phase photos document the dye's initial rapid, sequential perfusion of the choroid, the retinal arteries, and the retinal veins. Later-phase photos may, for example, demonstrate the gradual, delayed leakage of dye from abnormal vessels. This extravascular dye-stained edema fluid will persist long after the intravascular fluorescein has exited the eye.

Figure 2–28 illustrates several of the retinal vascular abnormalities that are well demonstrated by fluorescein angiography. The dye delineates structural vascular alterations, such as aneurysms or neovascularization. Changes in blood flow such as ischemia and vascular occlusion are seen as an interruption of the normal perfusion pattern. Abnormal vascular permeability is seen as a leaking cloud of dye-stained edema fluid increasing over time. Hemorrhage does not stain with dye but rather appears as a dark, sharply demarcated void. This is due to blockage and obscuration of the underlying background fluorescence.

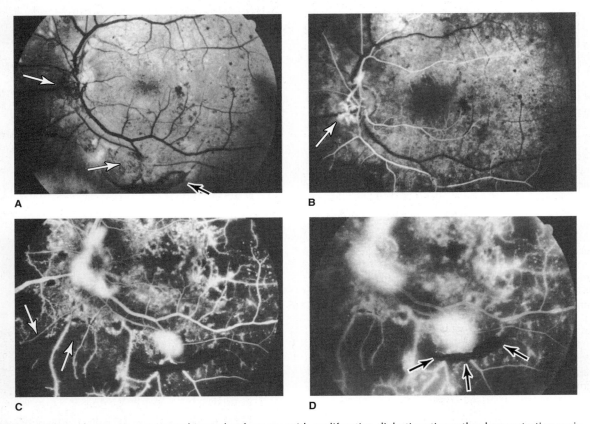

▲ **Figure 2–28.** Fluorescein angiographic study of an eye with proliferative diabetic retinopathy demonstrating variations in the dye pattern over several minutes' time. **A:** Fundus photograph of left eye (before fluorescein) showing neovascularization (abnormal new vessels) on the disk and inferior to the macula **(arrows)**. This latter area has bled, producing the arcuate preretinal hemorrhage at the bottom of the photo **(open arrow)**. **B:** Early-phase angiogram of the same eye, in which fluorescein has initially filled the arterioles and highlighted the area of the disk neovascularization. **C:** Midphase angiogram of the same eye, in which dye has begun to leak out of the hyperpermeable areas of neovascularization. In addition to the irregular venous caliber and the microaneurysms (white dots), extensive areas of ischemia are apparent by virtue of the gross absence of vessels (and therefore dye) in many areas **(see arrows)**. **D:** Late-phase photo demonstrating increasing amounts of dye leakage over time. Although the preretinal hemorrhage does not stain with dye, it is detectable as a solid black area since it obscures all underlying fluorescence **(arrows)**. (Photos courtesy of University of California, San Francisco.)

7. INDOCYANINE GREEN ANGIOGRAPHY

The principal use for fluorescein angiography in age-related macular degeneration (Chapter 10) is in locating subretinal choroidal neovascularization for possible laser photocoagulation. The angiogram may show a well-demarcated neovascular membrane. Frequently, however, the area of choroidal neovascularization is poorly defined ("occult") because of surrounding or overlying blood, exudate, or serous fluid.

Indocyanine green angiography is a separate technique that is superior for imaging the choroidal circulation. Fluorescein diffuses out of the choriocapillaris, creating a diffuse background fluorescence. As opposed to fluorescein, indocyanine green is a larger molecule that binds completely to plasma proteins, causing it to remain in the choroidal vessels. Thus, larger choroidal vessels can be imaged. Unique photochemical properties allow the dye to be transmitted better through melanin (eg, in the retinal pigment epithelium), blood, exudate, and serous fluid. This technique therefore serves as an important adjunct to fluorescein angiography for imaging occult choroidal neovascularization and other choroidal vascular abnormalities.

Following dye injection, angiography is performed using special digital video cameras. The digital images can be further enhanced and analyzed by computer.

8. OPTICAL COHERENCE TOMOGRAPHY

Optical Coherence Tomography (OCT) is a computerized, cross sectional tomographic imaging modality used to examine and measure intraocular structures in three dimensions. The operational principle of OCT is analogous to ultrasound, except that it uses 840-nm-wavelength light instead of sound. Because the speed of light is nearly one million times faster than the speed of sound, OCT can image and measure structures on a 5-μm scale, compared to the 100-μm image resolution for ultrasound. OCT can be performed through an undilated pupil and, unlike ultrasound, does not require contact with the tissue examined. The instrumentation is similar to a fundus camera and is used in the office.

The OCT interferometer measures the echo delay time of light that is projected from a superluminescent diode and then reflected from different structures within the eye. Posterior segment OCT enables detailed analysis of the optic disk, retinal nerve fiber layer, and macula. Microscopic changes in the macula, such as edema (Figure 2–29), can be imaged and measured. For the anterior segment, a different OCT instrument projecting a longer-wavelength infrared light beam (1300 nm) is used. This can provide high-resolution images and measurements of the cornea, iris, and intraocular devices and lenses.

9. LASER IMAGING TECHNOLOGIES (FOR DISK & RETINA)

In early glaucoma, morphologic changes of the disk and retinal nerve fiber layer (RNFL) usually precede the appearance of visual field abnormalities. Newer technologies such as scanning laser polarimetry, scanning laser tomography (SLT), and OCT are able to image and quantify the microscopic details of the optic disk and the surrounding RNFL.

In confocal SLT reflections from a scanning laser beam are recorded at different tissue depths so as to provide a series of 64 tomographic coronal sections perpendicular to the optical axis—like a series of computed tomography (CT) scans. Software programs display this data as three-dimensional topographic images (Figure 2–30), similar analyses also being obtainable from OCT images (Figure 2-31). Comparing the thickness of the RNFL and the volume of the cup to data from normal individuals and repeated examinations facilitates early detection and monitoring of glaucoma.

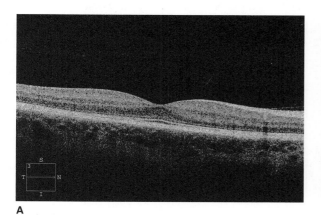

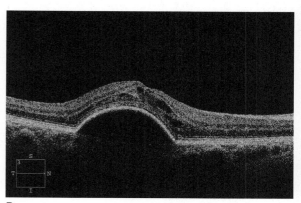

A   **B**

▲ **Figure 2–29.** Optical coherence tomography cross section image of a normal macula **(A)** and a macula with pigment epithelial detachment showing fluid beneath the retinal pigment epithelium **(B)**. (Images taken with Cirrus Spectral Domain OCT, Carl Zeiss Meditec, Inc.)

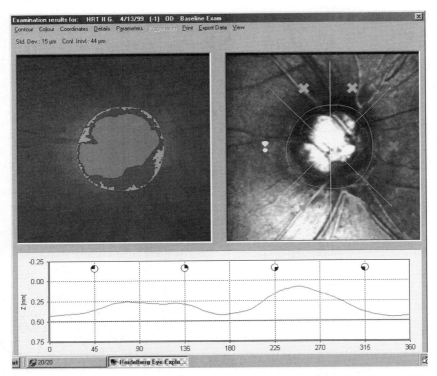

▲ Figure 2–30. Confocal scanning laser topographic image generated by the Heidelberg Retinal Tomograph II. Upper left image color codes areas according to height, the central area being the depression of the cup. Upper right image statistically analyzes cup-disk proportions in six sectors. "X" indicates abnormal sectors. Bottom graph plots retinal nerve fiber layer thickness. (Photo courtesy of Heidelberg Engineering.)

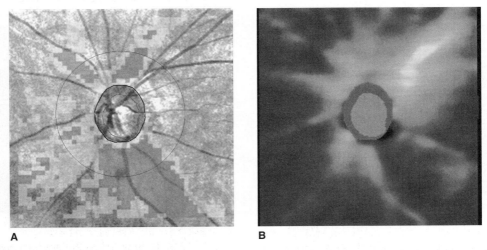

A   B

▲ Figure 2–31. OCT-derived color-coded maps of retinal nerve fiber layer thickness, with disc and cup masked **(A)** and indicating deviation from normal with cup and disc edges outlined **(B)**. See color insert.

10. ELECTROPHYSIOLOGIC TESTING

Physiologically, "vision" results from a series of electrical signals initiated in the retina and ending in the occipital cortex. Electroretinography, electro-oculography, and visual evoked response testing are methods of evaluating the integrity to the neural circuitry.

▶ Electroretinography & Electro-Oculography

Electroretinography (ERG) measures the electrical response of the retina to flashes of light, **the flash electroretinogram,** or to a reversing checkerboard stimulus, the **pattern ERG (PERG)**. The recording electrode is placed on the surface of the eye, and a reference electrode is placed on the skin of the face. The amplitude of the electrical signal is less than 1 mV, and amplification of the signal and computer averaging of the response to repeated trials are thus necessary to achieve reliable results.

The flash ERG has two major components: the "a wave" and the "b wave." An early receptor potential preceding the "a wave" and oscillatory potentials superimposed on the "b wave" may be recorded under certain circumstances. The early part of the flash ERG reflects photoreceptor function, whereas the later response particularly reflects the function of the Müller cells, which are glial cells within the retina. Varying the intensity, wavelength, and frequency of the light stimulus and recording under conditions of light or dark adaptation modulates the waveform of the flash ERG and allows examination of rod and cone photoreceptor function. The flash ERG is a diffuse response from the whole retina and is thus sensitive only to widespread, generalized diseases of the retina, eg, inherited retinal degenerations (retinitis pigmentosa), in which flash ERG abnormalities precede visual loss; congenital retinal dystrophies, in which flash ERG abnormalities may precede ophthalmoscopic abnormalities; and toxic retinopathies from drugs or chemicals (eg, iron intraocular foreign bodies). It is not sensitive to focal retinal disease, even when the macula is affected, and is not sensitive to abnormalities of the retinal ganglion cell layer, such as in optic nerve disease.

The PERG also has two major components: a positive wave at about 50 ms (P50) and a negative wave at about 95 ms (N95) from the time of the pattern reversal. The P50 reflects macular retinal function, whereas the N95 appears to reflect ganglion cell function. Thus, the PERG is useful in distinguishing retinal and optic nerve dysfunction and in diagnosing macular disease.

Electro-oculography (EOG) measures the standing corneoretinal potential. Electrodes are placed at the medial and lateral canthi to record the changes in electrical potential while the patient performs horizontal eye movements. The amplitude of the corneoretinal potential is least in the dark and maximal in the light. The ratio of the maximum potential in the light to the minimum in the dark is known as the

Arden index. Abnormalities of the EOG principally occur in diseases diffusely affecting the retinal pigment epithelium and the photoreceptors and often parallel abnormalities of the flash ERG. Certain diseases, such as Best's vitelli-form dystrophy, produce a normal ERG but a characteristically abnormal EOG. EOG is also used to record eye movements.

▶ Visual Evoked Response

Like electroretinography, the visual evoked response (VER) measures the electrical potential resulting from a visual stimulus. However, because it is measured by scalp electrodes placed over the occipital cortex, the entire visual pathway from retina to cortex must be intact in order to produce a normal electrical waveform reading. Like the ERG wave, the VER pattern is plotted on a scale displaying both amplitude and latency (Figure 2–32).

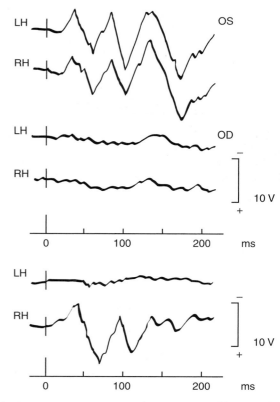

▲ **Figure 2–32. Top:** Normal VER generated by stimulating the left eye (OS) is contrasted with the absent response from the right eye (OD), which has a severe optic nerve lesion. LH and RH signify recordings from electrodes over the left and right hemispheres of the occipital lobe. **Bottom:** VER with right homonymous hemianopia. No response is recorded from over the left hemisphere. (Courtesy of M Feinsod.)

Interruption of neuronal conduction by a lesion will result in reduced amplitude of the VER. Reduced speed of conduction, such as with demyelination, abnormally prolongs the latency of the VER. Unilateral prechiasmatic (retinal or optic nerve) disease can be diagnosed by stimulating each eye separately and comparing the responses. Postchiasmatic disease (eg, homonymous hemianopia) can be identified by comparing the electrode responses measured separately over each hemisphere.

Proportionately, the majority of the occipital lobe area is devoted to the macula. This large cortical area representing the macula is also in close proximity to the scalp electrode, so that the clinically measured VER is primarily a response generated by the macula and optic nerve. Thus the VER can be used to assess visual acuity, making it a valuable objective test in situations where subjective testing is unreliable, such as in infants, unresponsive individuals, and suspected malingerers.

11. DARK ADAPTATION

In going from conditions of bright light to darkness, a certain period of time must pass before the retina regains its maximal sensitivity to low amounts of light. This phenomenon is called dark adaptation. It can be quantified by measuring the recovery of retinal sensitivity to low-light levels over time following a standard period of bright-light exposure. Dark adaptation is often abnormal in retinal diseases characterized by rod photoreceptor dysfunction and impaired night vision.

DIAGNOSIS OF EXTRAOCULAR ABNORMALITIES

1. LACRIMAL SYSTEM EVALUATION

▶ Evaluation of Tear Production

Tears and their components are produced by the lacrimal gland and accessory glands in the lid and conjunctiva (see Chapter 5). The **Schirmer test** is a simple method for assessing gross tear production. Schirmer strips are disposable 35-mm-length dry strips of filter paper. The tip of one end is folded at the preexisting notch so that it can drape over the lower lid margin just lateral to the cornea.

Tears in the conjunctival sac will cause progressive wetting of the paper strip. The distance between the leading edge of wetness and the initial fold can be measured after 5 minutes using a millimeter ruler. The ranges of normal measurements vary depending on whether topical anesthetic is used. Without anesthesia, irritation from the Schirmer strip itself will cause reflex tearing, thereby increasing the measurement. With anesthesia, less than 5 mm of wetting after 5 minutes is considered abnormal.

Significant degrees of chronic dryness cause surface changes in the exposed areas of the cornea and conjunctiva. **Fluorescein** will stain punctate areas of epithelial loss on the cornea. Another dye, **rose bengal**, is able to stain devitalized cells of the conjunctiva and cornea before they actually degenerate and drop off.

▶ Evaluation of Lacrimal Drainage

The anatomy of the lacrimal drainage system is discussed in Chapters 1 and 4. The pumping action of the lids draws tears nasally into the upper and lower canalicular channels through the medially located "punctal" openings in each lid margin. After collecting in the lacrimal sac, the tears then drain into the nasopharynx via the nasolacrimal duct. Symptoms of watering are frequently due to increased tear production as a reflex response to some type of ocular irritation. However, the patency and function of the lacrimal drainage system must be checked in the evaluation of otherwise unexplained tearing.

The **Jones I** test evaluates whether the entire drainage system as a whole is functioning. Concentrated fluorescein dye is instilled into the conjunctival sac on the side of the suspected obstruction. After 5 minutes, a cotton Calgiswab is used to attempt to recover dye from beneath the inferior nasal turbinate. Alternatively, the patient blows his or her nose into a tissue, which is checked for the presence of dye. Recovery of any dye indicates that the drainage system is functioning.

The **Jones II** test is performed if no dye is recovered, indicating some abnormality of the system. Following topical anesthesia, a smooth-tipped metal probe is used to gently dilate one of the puncta (usually lower). A 3-mL syringe with sterile water or saline is prepared and attached to a special lacrimal irrigating cannula. This blunt-tipped cannula is used to gently intubate the lower canaliculus, and fluid is injected as the patient leans forward. With a patent drainage system, fluid should easily flow into the patient's nasopharynx without resistance.

If fluorescein can now be recovered from the nose following irrigation, a partial obstruction might have been present. Recovery of clear fluid without fluorescein, however, may indicate inability of the lids to initially pump dye into the lacrimal sac with an otherwise patent drainage apparatus. If no fluid can be irrigated through to the nasopharynx using the syringe, total occlusion is present. Finally, some drainage problems may be due to stenosis of the punctal lid opening, in which case the preparatory dilation may be therapeutic.

2. METHODS OF ORBITAL EVALUATION

▶ Exophthalmometry

A method is needed to measure the anteroposterior location of the globe with respect to the bony orbital rim. The lateral orbital rim is a discrete, easily palpable landmark and is used as the reference point.

The exophthalmometer (Figure 2–33) is a hand-held instrument with two identical measuring devices (one for each eye), connected by a horizontal bar. The distance

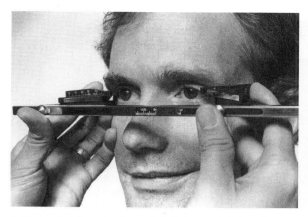

▲ **Figure 2–33.** Hertel exophthalmometer. (Photo by M Narahara.)

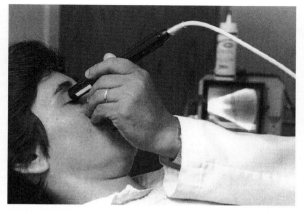

▲ **Figure 2–34.** Ultrasonography using B-scan probe. The image will appear on the oscilloscope screen, visible in the background. (Photo by M Narahara.)

between the two devices can be varied by sliding one toward or away from the other, and each has a notch that fits over the edge of the corresponding lateral orbital rim. When properly aligned, an attached set of mirrors reflects a side image of each eye profiled alongside a measuring scale, calibrated in millimeters. The tip of the corneal image aligns with a scale reading representing its distance from the orbital rim.

The patient is seated facing the examiner. The distance between the two measuring devices is adjusted so that each aligns with and abuts against its corresponding orbital rim. To allow reproducibility for repeat measurements in the future, the distance between the two devices is recorded from an additional scale on the horizontal bar. Using the first mirror scale, the patient's right eye position is measured as it fixates on the examiner's left eye. The patient's left eye is measured while fixating on the examiner's right eye.

The distance from the cornea to the orbital rim typically ranges from 12 to 20 mm, and the two eye measurements are normally within 2 mm of each other. A greater distance is seen in exophthalmos, which can be unilateral or bilateral. This abnormal forward protrusion of the eye can be produced by any significant increase in orbital mass, because of the fixed size of the bony orbital cavity. Causes might include orbital hemorrhage, neoplasm, inflammation, or edema.

▶ Ultrasonography

Ultrasonography utilizes the principle of sonar to study structures that may not be directly visible. It can be used to evaluate either the globe or the orbit. High-frequency sound waves are emitted from a special transmitter toward the target tissue. As the sound waves bounce back off the various tissue components, they are collected by a receiver that amplifies and displays them on an oscilloscope screen.

A single probe that contains both the transmitter and receiver is placed against the eye and used to aim the beam of sound (Figure 2–34). Various structures in its path will reflect separate echoes (which arrive at different times) back toward the probe. Those derived from the most distal structures arrive last, having traveled the farthest.

There are two methods of clinical ultrasonography: A scan and B scan. In **A- scan ultrasonography**, the sound beam is aimed in a straight line. Each returning echo is displayed as a spike whose amplitude is dependent on the density of the reflecting tissue. The spikes are arranged in temporal sequence, with the latency of each signal's arrival correlating with that structure's distance from the probe (Figure 2–35). If the same probe is now swept across the eye, a continuous series of individual A scans is obtained. From spatial summation of these multiple linear scans, a two-dimensional image, or **B scan**, can be constructed.

Both A and B scans can be used to image and differentiate orbital disease or intraocular anatomy concealed by opaque media. In addition to defining the size and location of intraocular and orbital masses, A and B scans can provide clues to the tissue characteristics of a lesion (eg, solid, cystic, vascular, calcified).

For purposes of measurement, the A scan is the most accurate method. Sound echoes reflected from two separate locations will reach the probe at different times. This temporal separation can be used to calculate the distance between the points, based on the speed of sound in the tissue medium. The most commonly used ocular measurement is the axial length (cornea to retina). This is important in cataract surgery in order to calculate the power for an intraocular lens implant. A scan can also be used to quantify tumor size and monitor growth over time.

The application of pulsed ultrasound and spectral Doppler techniques to orbital ultrasonography provides information on the orbital vasculature. It is certainly possible to determine the direction of flow in the ophthalmic artery and the ophthalmic veins and reversal of flow in these vessels

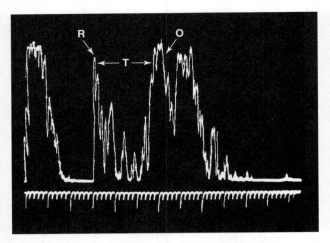 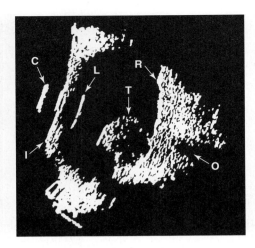

▲ **Figure 2–35.** A scan **(left)** and B scan **(right)** of an intraocular tumor (melanoma). C = cornea; I = iris; L = posterior lens surface; O = optic nerve; R = retina; T = tumor. (Courtesy of RD Stone).

occurring in internal carotid artery occlusion and carotid-cavernous fistula, respectively. As yet, the value of measuring flow velocities in various vessels, including the posterior ciliary arteries, without being able to measure blood vessel diameter is not fully established.

3. OPHTHALMIC RADIOLOGY (x-RAY, CT SCAN)

Plain x-rays and CT scans (Figures 13–1 and 13–2) are useful in the evaluation of **orbital** and **intracranial** conditions. CT scan in particular has become the most widely used method for localizing and characterizing structural disease in the extraocular visual pathway. Common orbital abnormalities demonstrated by CT scan include neoplasms, inflammatory masses, fractures, and extraocular muscle enlargement associated with Graves' disease (Figure 13–4).

The **intraocular** applications of radiology are primarily in the detection of foreign bodies following trauma and the demonstration of intraocular calcium in tumors such as retinoblastoma. CT scan is useful for foreign body localization because of its multidimensional reformatting capabilities and its ability to image the ocular walls.

4. MAGNETIC RESONANCE IMAGING

The technique of magnetic resonance imaging (MRI) has many applications in orbital and intracranial diagnosis. Improvements such as surface receiver coils and thin section techniques have improved the anatomic resolution in the eye and orbit.

Unlike CT, the MRI technique does not expose the patient to ionizing radiation. Since MRI might cause movement of metal, it should not be used if a metallic foreign body is suspected.

Because it can better differentiate between tissues of different water content, MRI is superior to CT in its ability to image edema, areas of demyelination, and vascular lesions. Bone generates a weak MRI signal, allowing improved resolution of intraosseous disease and a clearer view of the intracranial posterior fossa. Examples of MRI scans are presented in Chapters 13 and 14.

REFERENCES

Agarwal A: *Fundus Fluorescein and Indocyanine Green Angiography: A Textbook and Atlas.* Slack, 2008.

Alward W: *Color Atlas of Gonioscopy.* American Academy of Ophthalmology, 2000.

Broadway D et al: *Ophthalmology Examination Techniques: Questions and Answers.* Butterworth Heinemann, 1999.

Byrne SF, Green RL: *Ultrasound of the Eye and Orbit,* 2nd ed. Mosby, 2001.

Chauhan BC et al: Optic disc and visual field changes in a prospective longitudinal study of patients with glaucoma. Comparison of scanning laser tomography with conventional perimetry and optic disc photography. Arch Ophthalmol 2001;119:1492. [PMID: 11594950]

Choplin NT, Edwards RP: *Visual Field Testing with the Humphrey Field Analyzer: A Text and Clinical Atlas,* 2nd ed. Slack, 1999.

Cohen EJ et al: Corneal endothelial photography. A report by the American Academy of Ophthalmology. Ophthalmology 1997;104:1360–1365.

Cohen EJ et al: Corneal topography. A report by the American Academy of Ophthalmology. Ophthalmology 1999;106: 1628–1638.

Delgado MF et al: Automated perimetry: A report by the American Academy of Ophthalmology. Ophthalmology 2002;109:2362–2374.

Drake M: *A Primer on Automated Perimetry.* Vol 11, No. 8, in: *Focal Points 1993: Clinical Modules for Ophthalmologists.* American Academy of Ophthalmology, 1993.

Ellis BD, Hogg JP: *Neuroimaging for the General Ophthalmologist.* Vol 16, No. 8, in: *Focal Points 1998: Clinical Modules for Ophthalmologists.* American Academy of Ophthalmology, 1998.

Faulkner W: *Macular Function Testing Through Opacities.* Vol 4, Module 2, in: *Focal Points 1986: Clinical Modules for Ophthalmologists.* American Academy of Ophthalmology, 1986.

Fishman GA et al: *Electrophysiologic Testing in Disorders of the Retina, Optic Nerve, and Visual Pathway,* 2nd ed. American Academy of Ophthalmology, 2001.

Garcia-Ferrer FJ et al: *New Laboratory Diagnostic Techniques for Corneal and External Diseases.* Vol 20, Module 9, in: *Focal Points 2002: Clinical Modules for Ophthalmologists.* American Academy of Ophthalmology, 2002.

Goins KM, Wagoner MD: *Imaging the Anterior Segment.* Vol 27, No. 11, in: *Focal Points 2009. Clinical Modules for Ophthalmologists.* American Academy of Ophthalmology, 2009.

Gundogan FC, Sobaci, G, Bayer A: Pattern visual evoked potentials in the assessment of visual acuity in malingering. Ophthalmology 2007;114:2332. [PMID: 17618689]

Holder GE, Gale RP, Acheson JF, Robson AG: Electrodiagnostic assessment in optic nerve disease. Curr Opin Neurol 2009;22:3. [PMID: 19155758]

Holder GE: The pattern electroretinogram in anterior visual pathway dysfunction and its relationship to the pattern visual evoked potential: A personal clinical review of 743 eyes. Eye 1997;11:924.

Hosten N, Bornfeld N: *Imaging of the Globe and Orbit.* Thieme, 1998.

Hoyt CS, Paks MM: *How to Examine the Eye of the Neonate.* Vol 7, Module 1, in: *Focal Points 1989: Clinical Modules for Ophthalmologists.* American Academy of Ophthalmology, 1989.

Huang D, Kaiser P, Lowder C, Traboulsi E: *Retinal Imaging.* Mosby, 2006.

Ip MS, Duker JS: *Advances in Posterior Segment Imaging Techniques.* Vol 17, Module 7, in: *Focal Points 1999: Clinical Modules for Ophthalmologists.* American Academy of Ophthalmology, 1999.

James CB, Benjamin L: *Ophthalmology: Investigation and Examination Techniques.* Mosby, 2006.

Johnson CA, Spry P: *Automated Perimetry.* Vol 20, No. 10, in: *Focal Points 2002: Clinical Modules for Ophthalmologists.* American Academy of Ophthalmology, 2002.

Laquis SJ et al: *Orbital Imaging.* Vol 22, Module 12, in: *Focal Points 2004: Clinical Modules for Ophthalmologists.* American Academy of Ophthalmology, 2004.

Ledford JK: *The Complete Guide to Ocular History Taking.* Slack, 1999.

Lee MS: *Diplopia: Diagnosis and Management.* Vol 25, No. 12, in: *Focal Points 2007. Clinical Modules for Ophthalmologists.* American Academy of Ophthalmology, 2007.

Lin SC, et al. Optic nerve head and retinal nerve fiber layer analysis: A report by the American Academy of Ophthalmology. Ophthalmology 2007;114:1937–49.

Maguire LJ: *Computerized Corneal Analysis.* Vol 14, No. 5, in: *Focal Points 1996: Clinical Modules for Ophthalmologists.* American Academy of Ophthalmology, 1996.

Masters BR: *Noninvasive Diagnostic Techniques in Ophthalmology.* Springer, 1990.

McBain VA, Robson AG, Hogg CR, Holder GE: Assessment of patients with suspected non-organic visual loss using pattern appearance visual evoked potentials. Graefes Arch Clin Exp Ophthalmol 2007;245:502. [PMID: 17111152]

Miller BW: A review of practical tests for ocular malingering and hysteria. Surv Ophthalmol 1973;17:241.

Newman SA: *Automated Perimetry in Neuro-Ophthalmology.* Vol 13, No. 6, in: *Focal Points 1995: Clinical Modules for Ophthalmologists.* American Academy of Ophthalmology, 1995.

Parmar H, Trobe JD: A "first cut" at interpreting brain MRI signal intensities: What's white, what's black, and what's gray. J Neuro-Ophthalmol 2010;30:91. [PMID: 20182216]

Rosenthal ML, Fradin S: The technique of binocular indirect ophthalmoscopy. Highlights Ophthalmol 1966;9:179. (Reprinted as Appendix in: Hilton GF et al: *Retinal Detachment,* 2nd ed. American Academy of Ophthalmology, 1995.)

Salinas Van Orman E et al: *Nerve Fiber Layer and Optic Disk Imaging in Glaucoma.* Vol 24, Module 8, in: *Focal Points 2006: Clinical Modules for Ophthalmologists.* American Academy of Ophthalmology, 2006.

Savage JA: *Gonioscopy in the Management of Glaucoma.* Vol 24, Module 3, in: *Focal Points 2006: Clinical Modules for Ophthalmologists.* American Academy of Ophthalmology, 2006.

Schuman JS, Puliafito CA, Fujimoto JG: *Optical Coherence Tomography of Ocular Diseases,* 2nd ed. Slack, 2004.

Schwartz B: *Optic Disc Evaluation in Glaucoma.* Vol 8, Module 12, in: *Focal Points 1990: Clinical Modules for Ophthalmologists.* American Academy of Ophthalmology, 1990.

Schwartz GS: *The Eye Exam: A Complete Guide.* Slack, 2006.

Slavin ML: *Functional Visual Loss.* Vol 9, Module 2, in: *Focal Points 1991: Clinical Modules for Ophthalmologists.* American Academy of Ophthalmology, 1991.

Spry PGD et al: *Advances in Automated Perimetry.* Vol 20, Module 10, in: *Focal Points 2002: Clinical Modules for Ophthalmologists.* American Academy of Ophthalmology, 2002.

Stein HA et al: *The Ophthalmic Assistant: A Guide for Ophthalmic Medical Personnel,* 7th ed. Mosby, 2000.

Steinert RF, Huang D. *Anterior Segment Optical Coherence Tomography.* Slack, 2008.

Sunness JS: *Clinical Retinal Function Testing.* Vol 9, Module 1, in: *Focal Points 1991: Clinical Modules for Ophthalmologists.* American Academy of Ophthalmology, 1991.

Thompson HS, Kardon RH: *Clinical Importance of Pupillary Inequality.* Vol 10, No. 10, in: *Focal Points 1992: Clinical Modules for Ophthalmologists.* American Academy of Ophthalmology, 1992.

Tomsak RL: *Magnetic Resonance Imaging in Neuro-ophthalmology.* Vol 4, Module 10, in: *Focal Points 1986: Clinical Modules for Ophthalmologists.* American Academy of Ophthalmology, 1986.

von Noorden GK, Campos EC: *Binocular Vision and Ocular Motility: Theory and Management of Strabismus,* 6th ed. Mosby, 2002.

Walsh TJ: *Visual Fields: Examination and Interpretation,* 2nd ed. American Academy of Ophthalmology, 1996.

Wang M: *Corneal Topography in the Wavefront Era: A Guide for Clinical Application.* Slack, 2006.

Williams GA et al: Single-field fundus photography for diabetic retinopathy screening. A report by the American Academy of Ophthalmology. Ophthalmology 2004; 111:1055–1062.

Wilson FM: *Practical Ophthalmology: A Manual for Beginning Residents,* 5th ed. American Academy of Ophthalmology, 2005.

Wirtschafter JD et al: *Magnetic Resonance Imaging and Computed Tomography: Clinical Neuro-Orbital Anatomy.* American Academy of Ophthalmology, 1992.

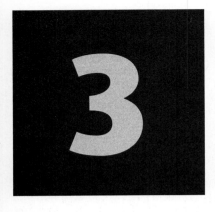

Ophthalmic Emergencies

Paul Riordan-Eva, FRCOphth

INTRODUCTION

Prompt recognition and treatment of ophthalmic emergencies are crucial to prevention of unnecessary visual impairment. Although specific diagnosis may require specialist ophthalmic expertise, using simple guidelines non-ophthalmologists as well as ophthalmologists can identify patients requiring emergency or urgent evaluation. Intensity and duration of pain, rapidity of onset and severity of visual loss (primarily assessed by visual acuity, which should be measured for each eye in all patients presenting with ophthalmic emergencies), gross appearance of the globe, and abnormalities on ophthalmoscopy are particularly important parameters.

Excluding ocular and orbital trauma, which is covered in Chapter 19, this chapter reviews the common ophthalmic emergencies, for the most part grouped according to the predominant symptom. For each group, the section on triage highlight the features that are crucial during initial assessment by a non-ophthalmologist, for instance on presentation to an emergency department. The section on clinical assessment emphasizes what is important during ophthalmological evaluation. The management of the more common or important entities is then briefly discussed, principally to provide reference to discussion in other chapters.

ACUTE RED EYE

The majority of patients with acute red eye have a relatively benign condition, such as bacterial, viral, or allergic conjunctivitis, subconjunctival hemorrhage, or blepharitis, which poses little or no threat to vision. Conversely a few are at risk of rapid progression within a few hours or days to severe visual impairment, even blindness, such as from acute angle closure glaucoma, intraocular infection (endophthalmitis), bacterial, viral, amebic, or fungal corneal infection, acute uveitis, or scleritis.

▶ Triage

(See Differential Diagnosis of Common Causes of the Inflamed Eye on Inside Front Cover)

Emergency or urgent ophthalmic evaluation should be arranged for any patient with acute red eye and a history within the past few weeks of intraocular surgery, which predisposes to endophthalmitis; contact lens wear, which predisposes to corneal infection (see Figure 6–3); recent or distant history of corneal transplantation because of the possibility of graft rejection; previous episodes of acute uveitis or scleritis; or systemic diseases predisposing to uveitis or scleritis, such as ankylosing spondylitis and rheumatoid arthritis. In acutely ill patients, particularly those with sepsis or requiring prolonged intravenous cannulation such as in intensive therapy units or for parenteral nutrition, an acute red eye may be due to bacterial or fungal endophthalmitis (see Figure 15–32). Ocular involvement in toxic epidermal necrolysis, Stevens-Johnson syndrome, or erythema multiforme requires urgent ophthalmic assessment.

Pain, rather than discomfort, should be regarded as inconsistent with conjunctivitis, episcleritis, or blepharitis. It is suggestive of keratitis, intraocular or scleral inflammation, or elevated intraocular pressure, with the likelihood of a serious cause increasing with increasing severity. Associated nausea and vomiting are particularly suggestive of markedly elevated intraocular pressure. Deep, boring pain, typically waking the patient at night, is characteristic of scleritis. Photophobia characteristically occurs in keratitis and anterior uveitis.

Reduced vision, whether reported by the patient or identified by measurement of visual acuity, in the absence of a pre-existing explanation, should also be regarded as inconsistent with conjunctivitis, episcleritis, or blepharitis and, as with pain, the greater the severity the greater the likelihood of a serious cause.

Severity of redness is not necessarily a guide to the seriousness of the underlying condition, for instance subconjunctival hemorrhage with its bright red appearance being a benign entity (see Figure 5–34). Distribution of redness can be helpful, with predominance around the limbus (circumcorneal) being indicative of intraocular disease, whereas diffuse redness involving the tarsal and bulbar conjunctiva

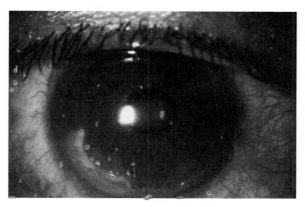

▲ **Figure 3-1.** Acute red eye with peripheral corneal ulceration.

being indicative of conjunctivitis (see Figure 16–1); focal or diffuse redness of the globe being consistent with episcleritis; and redness of the eyelid margins being indicative of blepharitis. Bluish redness (violaceous discoloration) of the globe (see Figure 7–28), best identified in natural rather than artificial light, is characteristic of scleritis. Vesicles or ulceration of the lids or periocular skin are typical of ophthalmic zoster (shingles) (see Figure 5–13) and less commonly varicella or primary herpes simplex virus infection.

Conjunctivitis usually causes purulent, mucoid, or watery discharge, and allergic conjunctivitis typically causes itching. Profuse purulent discharge is characteristic of gonococcal conjunctivitis, which requires emergency treatment (see later in the chapter).

Any abnormality of the cornea apparent on gross examination, such as ulceration (Figure 3–1) or focal opacity (Figure 3–2), which may be due to infection, or diffuse cloudiness, which may be due to markedly elevated intraocular pressure when it is usually associated with a semi-dilated unreactive pupil, warrants emergency ophthalmic assessment unless it is known to be longstanding, for example

pterygium (see Figure 5–32). Instillation of fluorescein facilitates identification of an epithelial defect (Figure 3–3), including dendritic ulceration due to herpes simplex virus keratitis (see Figure 5–10). A constricted pupil is suggestive of intraocular inflammation, typically due to anterior uveitis. Hypopyon (pus within the anterior chamber), a feature of corneal infection, intraocular infection, or acute anterior uveitis (iritis) (see Figures 3–4 and 16–5), necessitates emergency ophthalmic assessment.

▶ **Clinical Assessment**

Slitlamp examination (see Figure 2–6) facilitates assessment of distribution of redness; identification of conjunctival abnormalities, including examination of the superior tarsal conjunctiva following eversion of the upper eyelid (see Figure 2–7); diagnosis of episcleritis and scleritis (see Figures 7–26 to 7–29); characterization of corneal lesions; and detection of corneal keratic precipitates (see Figure 7–3), anterior chamber flare and cells, and possibly hypopyon indicative of anterior chamber inflammation due to anterior uveitis, intraocular infection, or secondary to corneal inflammation,

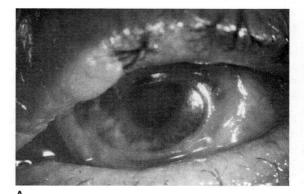

A

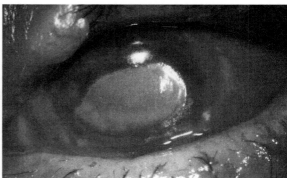

B

▲ **Figure 3-3.** Large corneal epithelial defect. **A:** Before instillation of fluorescein. **B:** After instillation of fluorescein. See color insert.

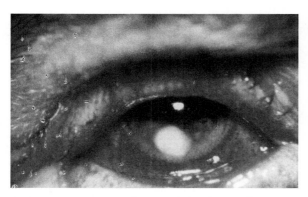

▲ **Figure 3-2.** Acute red eye with focal corneal opacity.

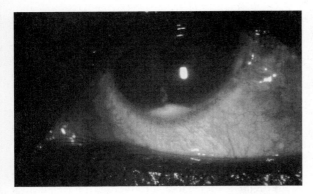

▲ **Figure 3–4.** Hypopyon in acute anterior uveitis (iritis).

including infection. In cases of intraocular inflammation, dilated fundal examination is essential to determine whether there is involvement of the vitreous, retina (see Figures 7–8, 15–30, 15–31 and 15–33) or choroid (see Figures 15–25 and 15–27), which is important to diagnosis as well as assessment of severity.

▶ Management

There are many causes of acute conjunctivitis (see Table 5–1), which in most case is a benign, often self-limiting, condition (see Chapter 5). However care needs to be exercised in neonates (**ophthalmia neonatorum**) (see Chapter 17) because of the possibility of infection with **chlamydia**, which may be associated with non-ocular disease and needs systemic therapy, **gonococcus**, or **herpes simplex virus**, which may be associated with encephalitis and requires hospitalization and parenteral antiviral therapy. Gonococcal conjunctivitis in neonates or adults, characteristically causing profuse purulent discharge (see Figure 5–1) as well as severe conjunctival inflammation, necessitates emergency investigation by microscopy and culture of the discharge and parenteral antibiotic therapy with ceftriaxone to avoid progression to severe corneal damage (see Table 6–1). Treatment with parenteral antiviral therapy within 72 hours of the appearance of the rash reduces the likelihood of ocular complications in ophthalmic zoster (shingles) (see Chapters 5 and 6). Skin lesions on the tip of the nose (Hutchinson's sign) or the eyelid margins are predictive of ocular complications.

Management of acute **keratitis** primarily revolves around identification and treatment of infection, for which contact lens wear and pre-existing ocular surface disease, including corneal anesthesia or exposure, are the common predisposing factors (see Chapter 6). Occasionally it is apparent straightaway that there is a non-infectious inflammatory process, requiring other therapy, possibly topical or systemic steroids but steroid therapy should not be started without ophthalmic assessment.

Management of acute intraocular inflammation (**uveitis**) also primarily revolves around identification and treatment of infection, particularly if there is posterior segment involvement (vitritis, retinitis, or choroiditis) or recent history of intraocular surgery, but a non-infectious inflammatory process is more common than in acute keratitis. Topical or systemic steroid therapy should not be started without ophthalmic assessment. Scleritis is infrequently caused by infection, autoimmune disease being more commonly responsible (see Table 7–7), and can often be managed in the first instance by oral nonsteroidal anti-inflammatory agents (NSAIDS) but ophthalmic assessment is necessary to make the diagnosis and exclude other entities.

In **acute angle closure glaucoma** prompt recognition and treatment are required if severe visual loss is to be avoided (see Chapter 11). The mainstay of initial treatment is intravenous and oral acetazolamide, as well as topical agents, to reduce intraocular pressure, supplemented by topical steroids to reduce inflammation, and topical pilocarpine to constrict the pupil. Definitive treatment is usually laser peripheral iridotomy with prophylactic treatment to the fellow eye. Emergency ophthalmic assessment is essential to establish the diagnosis, including exclusion of other causes of markedly raised intraocular pressure that may require distinctly different treatment.

ACUTE ORBITAL DISEASE

Acute orbital disease is uncommon but a few entities need to be recognized promptly to avoid the severe visual loss, or even non-ocular morbidity and possibly mortality that may result from delay in treatment (see Chapter 13).

▶ Triage

Orbital cellulitis is usually a disease of childhood and due to spread of infection from the ethmoid sinuses. It is characterized by fever, pain, eyelid swelling and erythema, proptosis, limitation of extraocular movements, and systemic upset with leukocytosis. **Pre-septal cellulitis**, in which there is no proptosis or limitation of eye movement, may be due to a localized infection in the anterior (pre-septal) portion of the eyelid or may be the early manifestation of orbital cellulitis. In adolescents and young adults orbital signs may be indicative of extension of infection from the fronto-ethmoidal sinus complex. In diabetics and the immunocompromised, acute orbital disease may be due to fungal infection (**mucormycosis**), with a high risk of death even with early treatment.

Usually occurring in patients with autoimmune hyperthyroidism (Grave's disease), which may or may not have been diagnosed previously, acute Graves' ophthalmopathy may lead to marked proptosis (see Figures 5–30, 13–3 and 15–23), with the possibility of corneal exposure or optic nerve compression, and limitation of eye movements. Pseudotumor, another inflammatory orbital disease, and carotid artery-cavernous sinus fistula, due to dural shunts that typically occur in patients with diabetes and/or systemic hypertension, or due to spontaneous rupture of an intracavernous internal carotid artery aneurysm, may present in a similar manner.

▶ Clinical Assessment

Reduced vision unexplained by corneal exposure, especially if associated with impaired color vision and/or a relative afferent pupillary defect, indicates optic nerve dysfunction. In orbital cellulitis non-axial proptosis implies abscess formation. Other complications include cavernous sinus thrombosis and intracranial infection, the latter being more likely if there is infection in the frontal sinus.

▶ Management

Orbital cellulitis is a clinical diagnosis and requires hospitalization and immediate institution of antibiotic therapy, usually intravenously, together with early ophthalmic and otolaryngologic assessments. Orbital imaging may be undertaken in all cases or reserved for those in whom orbital abscess or another complication is suspected.

Orbital imaging, usually CT but possibly MRI, is generally sufficient to differentiate between Graves' ophthalmopathy, orbital pseudotumor, and carotid artery-cavernous sinus fistula, but orbital ultrasound blood flow studies are particularly helpful in diagnosing the third.

ACUTE PAINLESS VISUAL LOSS

Sudden onset painless visual loss is a very important symptom, because it may be due to ophthalmic disease that requires emergency or urgent treatment; ocular vascular disease with immediate or early threat to the patient's life or remaining vision; or acute intracranial disease.

▶ Triage

It is essential to determine from the outset whether the reported visual loss involves one or both eyes, including clearly distinguishing monocular visual loss from loss of vision to one side in both eyes, ie, homonymous hemianopia. Patients often will not have checked, by closing one eye and then the other, and if necessary they should be asked to carry out this simple test. Monocular visual loss indicates disease of the globe or optic nerve, whereas bilateral visual loss, including homonymous hemianopia, indicates a lesion at or posterior to the optic chiasm.

Also it is essential to determine whether the visual loss that has been noticed is definitely of recent onset, or whether it may have been longstanding and only recently identified. This requires establishing when the patient was last aware that vision in the affected eye(s) was unaffected, such as when last tested by an optometrist.

History of recent onset of black spots or shapes ("floaters") with flashing lights (photopsia) followed by a field defect progressing upwards from below in one eye is characteristic of retinal detachment (see Chapter 9). Preservation of good central vision, implying that the central retina (macula) has not yet detached, warrants emergency ophthalmic referral. Sudden onset of floaters may also be caused by vitreous hemorrhage, of which the main causes are retinal tear and proliferative retinopathy due to diabetes or retinal vein occlusion. Any patient with sudden onset floaters and/or flashes, even with otherwise normal vision, requires urgent ophthalmic assessment. Unless another cause is apparent, patients aged 55 or older with acute or subacute unilateral central visual loss, particularly if associated with distortion of images, should be assumed to have neovascular age-related macular degeneration and urgent ophthalmic referral arranged.

A reliable account of the rapidity of progression of visual loss can be a very helpful clue to diagnosis, an abrupt onset being very suggestive of an arterial vascular event. Whether there has been any recovery of vision is important, full recovery after a short period of impairment being suggestive of an embolic arterial event. All patients with possible ocular vascular disease should be asked about vascular risk factors, such as diabetes mellitus, systemic hypertension, and hyperlipidemia. Patients aged 55 or older with suspected arterial disease must be questioned about symptoms of giant cell arteritis, as well as their erythrocyte sedimentation rate (ESR) and/or C-reactive protein (CRP) being checked.

Ophthalmoscopy (see Chapter 2) often provides the diagnosis in acute painless visual loss. Lack of a red reflex with abnormal or absent view of the retina is suggestive of vitreous hemorrhage or retinal detachment, for which urgent or emergency ophthalmic referral is required (see Chapter 10). Widespread or sectoral retinal hemorrhages indicate central or branch retinal vein occlusion (see Figures 10–14, 10–15, and 15–8) for which urgent ophthalmic assessment is indicated. Widespread retinal whitening with a cherry-red spot (see Figures 10–16 and 15–4) indicates central retinal artery occlusion for which emergency ophthalmic assessment must be arranged, and giant cell arteritis and embolic disease need to be excluded. Sectoral retinal whitening indicates branch retinal artery occlusion, for which urgent ophthalmic assessment is important to confirm the diagnosis but prompt investigations for embolic disease need to be undertaken. Optic disk swelling in an eye with recent acute or subacute visual loss is commonly due to anterior ischemic optic neuropathy (see Figure 14–13), for which giant cell arteritis must be excluded in patients aged 55 or over.

▶ Clinical Assessment

The ophthalmologist must clarify whether the visual loss is monocular or binocular, not only by reviewing the history but by assessment of visual acuity and visual field in each eye, the latter initially by confrontation testing but if necessary by perimetry. Detection of bilateral visual field loss, including abnormality in a subjectively unaffected fellow eye, may establish that the disease process involves the optic chiasm, when there is a bitemporal hemianopia or a temporal hemianopia in the subjectively unaffected fellow eye, or the retrochiasmal visual pathways, when there is homonymous hemianopia. Assessment of color vision and pupillary reactions to light, particularly looking for a relative afferent pupillary defect (see Figure 14–32) are important in detection of optic nerve disease.

Fundal examination following pupillary dilation provides the best means of diagnosing retinal tears with or without retinal detachment; vitreous hemorrhage and its cause if the hemorrhage is not too dense, otherwise ultrasound examination is necessary; age-related macular degeneration, including whether it has features of the neovascular stage; retinal vein or artery occlusion; and anterior ischemic optic neuropathy. In giant cell arteritis fundal examination may be normal when visual loss is due to choroidal ischemia or posterior ischemic optic neuropathy.

▶ **Management**

Retinal detachment is usually treated surgically, with urgency primarily being determined by whether the macula is detached but also the underlying cause (see Chapter 10). Management of vitreous hemorrhage is determined by the underlying cause (see Chapters 9 and 10). Repeated intravitreal injection of inhibitors of vascular endothelial growth factor (VEGF) has become the standard treatment for neovascular age-related macular degeneration (see Chapter 10).

There is debate about the role of carotid endarterectomy in patients with ocular transient ischemia attacks (TIAs) due to carotid artery stenosis, but all patients with transient monocular visual loss ("amaurosis fugax") likely to be due to retinal emboli should undergo investigations for carotid and cardiac sources (see Chapters 14 and 15). Transient visual loss can also be due to giant cell arteritis or optic disk swelling due to raised intracranial pressure (see later in the chapter).

No treatment in the acute stage is established to alter visual outcome in central or branch retinal vein occlusion but various treatments, including intravitreal injections of VEGF inhibitors or triamcinolone, retinal laser photocoagulation, and various surgical techniques are effective for the long term complications (see Chapter 10). Various treatments, including intra-arterial thrombolytic therapy, are advocated in the acute stage of central retinal artery occlusion but evidence for their usefulness is lacking, particularly in view of the risk of adverse events in the case of intra-arterial thrombolysis (see Chapters 10 and 14). No treatment in the acute stage is established to alter visual outcome in anterior ischemic optic neuropathy (see Chapters 14 and 15). Failure to treat promptly giant cell arteritis causing anterior ischemic optic neuropathy or central retinal artery occlusion is likely to lead rapidly to complete bilateral blindness (see Chapters 14 and 15).

Sudden visual loss due to optic chiasmal or retrochiasmal disease necessitates emergency imaging and appropriate management thereafter, which may involve neurology or neurosurgery referral.

ACUTE PAINFUL VISUAL LOSS WITHOUT A RED EYE

A number of relatively uncommon but important conditions present with painful visual loss without a red eye because for the most part they are retrobulbar in location.

▶ **Triage**

There are many causes of optic nerve inflammation ("**optic neuritis**") (see Table 14–1). The most common is the acute demyelinative optic neuropathy associated with multiple sclerosis, occurring as the initial manifestation or part of a subsequent relapse. It characteristically presents as subacute monocular visual loss with peri- or retro-ocular discomfort exacerbated by eye movements (see Chapter 14).

Pituitary apoplexy, usually due to hemorrhagic infarction of a pituitary tumor, is rare but requires prompt recognition and treatment to reduce the risk of severe morbidity, possibly death, as well severe visual loss, possibly complete blindness. Characteristically it presents with sudden onset headache, unilateral or bilateral visual loss, sometimes impaired eye movements, and metabolic and circulatory derangement due to pituitary failure, particularly resulting in adrenal insufficiency. **Sphenoid sinusitis** also presents with headache, typically localized to the vertex, and acute unilateral or bilateral visual loss. Diagnosis of **posterior scleritis** is often delayed because of the frequent lack of specific diagnostic features, including the absence of apparent inflammation of the globe to suggest an inflammatory condition (see Chapter 7).

▶ **Clinical Assessment**

In acute demyelinative optic neuropathy there are features of optic nerve dysfunction (impaired color vision, visual field loss, and a relative afferent pupillary defect), with progression of visual loss over a few days, and usually no ophthalmoscopic abnormality but mild optic disk swelling is present in one third of cases (see Figure 14–8).

The ophthalmic manifestations of pituitary apoplexy are unilateral or bilateral often severe visual loss with impaired pupillary light reactions, sometimes impaired eye movements (external ophthalmoplegia) due to ocular motor cranial nerve palsies, and normal or pale optic disks depending upon whether the pituitary tumor previously has caused anterior visual pathway compression.

In sphenoid sinusitis the visual loss also has features of optic nerve dysfunction, with normal or pale optic disks depending upon whether there has been chronic optic nerve compression from a pre-existing sphenoid sinus mucocele (see Chapter 13). The clinical signs in posterior scleritis include proptosis, limitation of eye movements, induced refractive error, choroidal folds, fundal mass, serous retinal detachment, and optic disk swelling (see Chapter 7). Ultrasound is the best diagnostic test (see Figure 7–35).

Management

In most cases of acute demyelinative optic neuropathy the vision recovers spontaneously, and management centers on investigation of the likelihood of multiple sclerosis and the need for disease modifying therapy, but the crucial issue in the acute management is excluding other entities that require urgent treatment. Pituitary apoplexy is an endocrine and neurosurgical emergency. The patient may require emergency resuscitation. Intravenous hydrocortisone should be given to all patients prior to investigation with MRI, or CT if the patient's condition is unstable. Urgent neurosurgery is frequently required, particularly in patients with visual loss. Sphenoid sinusitis causing visual loss requires surgical drainage as well as antibiotic therapy. Posterior scleritis may respond to oral NSAIDS but oral steroid therapy may be required.

DOUBLE VISION AND EYE MOVEMENT ABNORMALITIES

Double vision has many causes ranging from the benign entity of an incorrect spectacle prescription to the life-threatening expansion of a posterior communicating artery aneurysm. Ocular, orbital, intracranial, generalized neurological, and systemic diseases can all present with double vision.

▶ Triage

Assessment of double vision is complex and can cause non-ophthalmologists, as well as ophthalmologists, great difficulty. In oculomotor (third cranial) nerve palsy there may be clues from associated ptosis or pupillary abnormality. Otherwise, unless the pattern of double vision reported by the patient or the examination of the range of eye movements quickly leads to identification of a specific entity, such as an abducens (sixth cranial) nerve (lateral rectus) palsy (see Figures 12–2 and 12–10), the non-ophthalmologist will derive more useful guidance to the clinical urgency from eliciting information about other features, such as whether there is also impairment of vision, orbital signs such as lid swelling or proptosis, periocular pain or headache, non-ocular neurologic abnormalities, or systemic illness. In general, patients with multiple cranial nerve palsies or other neurologic features, severe headache, associated systemic illness, or age under 50 with single or multiple cranial nerve palsy are most likely to have a serious underlying condition.

▶ Clinical Assessment

Double vision is usually due to ocular misalignment, but the first step in its evaluation is to determine whether it is monocular or binocular. If double vision, or even more than two images, is present when the patient is viewing with only one eye (monocular), whether it is just with one eye or with each eye alone, the visual disturbance is not due to ocular misalignment. Instead it is likely to be due to refractive error, lens opacity, or possibly macular disease. Unless there are other features to clearly implicate cerebral disease, multiple images on monocular viewing can be assumed not to be due to intracranial disease.

Effectively every episode of double vision has an acute onset, because double vision is either present or not. What needs to be established is for how long double vision has been noticed and whether, during the one or many episodes that have occurred, there has been change in the pattern, as judged by the direction of separation of images and the directions of gaze in which double vision has been present, or severity, as judged by the distance separating the two images. It is also helpful to establish whether the double vision can be overcome with voluntary effort, because this implies a longstanding abnormality that has become more difficult to overcome (decompensated).

Whenever an ocular motor cranial nerve palsy is diagnosed, it is essential to determine whether it is isolated or part of multiple cranial nerve dysfunction, including assessment of trigeminal nerve as well optic nerve function, not only to provide anatomical localization of the disease process but as a guide to the likelihood of a serious underlying condition.

In oculomotor nerve palsy the presence of pupillary dysfunction, either anisocoria or particularly an impaired response to light, provides an important clue to the possibility of a compressive lesion such as a posterior communicating artery aneurysm (see Chapter 14). Severe pain is another important clue to the presence of an aneurysm, but also may occur in pituitary apoplexy (see earlier in the chapter).

In all cases of double vision, careful attention needs to be paid to identification of any orbital signs, not least to avoid unnecessary investigation for a possible intracranial lesion. Specific eye movement abnormalities provide precise anatomical localization. Internuclear ophthalmoplegia, in which there is impairment of adduction of one or both eyes (see Figure 14–12), localizes to the medial longitudinal fasciculus within the brainstem (see Chapter 14). Horizontal gaze palsy, in which there is loss of conjugate horizontal gaze to one or both sides, localizes to the pons, whereas vertical gaze palsy localizes to the midbrain (see Chapter 14). Variability of double vision, during or between episodes, typically with increasing severity with fatigue that may also manifest as increasing ptosis, is suggestive of myasthenia gravis (see Chapter 14).

▶ Management

Investigation of patients with binocular double vision depends upon the clinical assessment. Many cases of isolated ocular motor cranial nerve palsy in patients over 50 are due to ischemic (microvascular) disease, which requires little investigation apart from exclusion of giant cell arteritis and review of vascular risk factors, and in which spontaneous recovery is the rule. In contrast, in isolated oculomotor nerve palsy suspicion of posterior communicating artery aneurysm due to pupillary involvement, severity of pain, or age under 50, necessitates emergency imaging, outcome being much better if treatment can be undertaken prior to subarachnoid hemorrhage due to aneurysm rupture. Similarly, multiple cranial nerve dysfunction requires urgent investigation, usually guided primarily by a neurologist, who will also guide investigations when the disease process localizes to the brainstem. Management of orbital disease usually depends upon the outcome of imaging with CT or MRI. When clinical evaluation suggests decompensation of a longstanding abnormality, such as a congenital superior oblique (trochlear) palsy, further investigation may not be required and initial treatment will be with prisms (see Chapter 14).

In any patient with suspected myasthenia gravis it is important to establish whether there is non-ocular weakness suggesting generalized disease, especially impairment of breathing or swallowing for which emergency neurologic assessment is essential.

PUPIL ABNORMALITIES

Abnormalities of pupil size and/or reactions result from a wide variety of causes, including structural abnormalities of the iris usually also causing pupillary distortion, miosis in intraocular inflammation, mydriasis in markedly elevated intraocular pressure, tonic pupil, oculomotor nerve palsy, Horner's syndrome, and midbrain dysfunction.

▶ Triage

Acute isolated dilated, unreactive pupil in an otherwise well individual is rarely due to a serious underlying condition, the likely possibilities being the benign entity of tonic pupil (see Chapter 14) or pharmacological mydriasis, such as from accidental ocular inoculation with the anticholinergic agent in travel sickness mediation. In contrast, isolated dilated, unreactive pupil in a patient with depressed conscious level due to head injury or other acute intracranial disease is an ominous sign, being suggestive of tentorial herniation. As discussed above, pupil involvement in oculomotor nerve palsy is an important clue to the possibility of a compressive lesion, including posterior communicating artery aneurysm. Miosis with ptosis is characteristic of Horner's syndrome (see Chapter 14). Acute painful Horner's syndrome, possibly following neck trauma, requires urgent exclusion of carotid dissection. Pupillary light-near dissociation (impaired pupillary constriction to light with better constriction to near) is traditionally associated with central nervous system syphilis (Argyll Robertson pupils), but can be due to midbrain dysfunction, typically compression from a pineal tumor or dilated third ventricle in hydrocephalus, when usually there is also impairment of vertical eye movements.

▶ Clinical Assessment

Besides confirming a suspected diagnosis of oculomotor nerve palsy or Horner's syndrome, the ophthalmologist's

particular role in assessment of acute pupil abnormalities is the identification of benign entities, such as tonic pupil and pharmacological mydriasis, to avoid unnecessary investigation, and ophthalmic entities, such as acute angle closure glaucoma, to direct management. In all 3 instances, there will be no related ptosis or impairment of eye movements. Tonic pupil may be identified by the delayed dilation following a near response from which it derives its name; abnormal spiralling ("vermiform") movements of the iris when constricting to a light stimulus, best seen on slitlamp examination; or constriction to dilute (0.125%) pilocarpine eye drops. Pharmacological mydriasis is characterized by lack of pupil constriction to bright light and standard strength (2%) pilocarpine eye drops.

BILATERAL OPTIC DISK SWELLING

There are many causes of optic disk swelling, including inflammatory (see Figure 14–8) or ischemic (see Figure 14–13) optic neuropathy, central retinal vein occlusion (see Figures 10–14 and 15–8), uveitis (see Figure 15–38), posterior scleritis (see Figure 7–34), and intra-orbital optic nerve compression, of which all are usually unilateral. Bilateral optic disk swelling is a characteristic feature of raised intracranial pressure (see Figures 14–9, 14–14, 14–15, and 14–16) and malignant (accelerated) systemic hypertension (see Figure 15–11), both requiring emergency or urgent investigation and treatment.

▶ Triage

Papilledema (optic disk swelling due to raised intracranial pressure) is usually identified as part of the examination of a patient with neurological symptoms, particularly headache. It may be indentified incidentally, such as during routine optometric examination, but even then still requires urgent head imaging to exclude an intracranial mass lesion. Blood pressure should be checked in every patient with bilateral optic disk swelling, even a child.

▶ Clinical Assessment

When the abnormalities are florid (see Figure 14–14 A), recognition of optic disk swelling is straightforward. When the abnormalities are less marked (see Figure 14–9), ophthalmological assessment may be crucial particularly to identify other entities such as myelinated nerve fibers (see Figure 14–17), optic nerve head drusen (see Figure 14–25), or congenitally small and crowded optic disks (pseudopapilledena) (Figure 3–5) that mimic optic disk swelling, so that unnecessary investigations and anxiety can be avoided. In individuals with papilledema, particularly when it is acute with retinal exudates (see Figure 14–4 B) or atrophic (see Figure 14–16), assessment of vision by an ophthalmologist, including visual fields, is a crucial guide to urgency of treatment. In malignant hypertension, optic disk swelling is usually accompanied by retinal and choroidal abnormalities and is an indication for urgent reduction in blood pressure, although

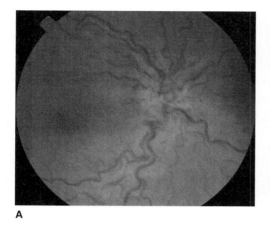 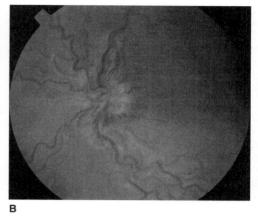

A   B

▲ **Figure 3–5.** Congenitally small and crowded optic disks (pseudopapilledema). **A:** Right eye. **B:** Left eye.

precipitous reduction should be avoided to reduce the risk of optic nerve infarction.

REFERENCES

Akagi T, Miyamoto K, Kashii S, Yoshimura N: Cause and prognosis of neurologically isolated third, fourth, or sixth cranial nerve dysfunction in cases of oculomotor palsy. Jpn J Ophthalmol 2008;52:32. [PMID: 18369697]

Amraoui F, van Montfrans GA, van den Born BJ: Value of retinal examination in hypertensive encephalopathy. J Hum Hypertens 2010;24:274. [PMID: 19865107]

Arashvand K: Images in clinical medicine. Central retinal artery occlusion. N Engl J Med 2007;356:841. [PMID: 17314343]

Atkins EJ, Bruce BB, Newman NJ, Biousse V: Treatment of nonarteritic anterior ischemic optic neuropathy. Surv Ophthalmol 2010;55:47. [PMID: 20006051]

Babineau MR, Sanchez LD: Ophthalmologic procedures in the emergency department. Emerg Med Clin North Am 2008;26:17. [PMID: 18249255]

Beran DI, Murphy-Lavoie H: Acute, painless vision loss. J La State Med Soc 2009;161:214. [PMID: 19785313]

Bielory L, Friedlaender MH: Allergic conjunctivitis. Immunol Allergy Clin North Am 2008;28:43. [PMID: 18282545]

Brazis PW: Isolated palsies of cranial nerves III, IV, and VI. Semin Neurol 2009;29:14. [PMID: 19214929]

Bruce BB, Biousse V, Newman NJ: Third nerve palsies. Semin Neurol 2007;27:257. [PMID: 17577867]

Chen CS, Lee AW: Management of acute central retinal artery occlusion. Nat Clin Pract Neurol 2008;4:376. [PMID: 18542123]

Chew SS, Kerr NM, Danesh-Meyer HV: Giant cell arteritis. J Clin Neurosci 2009;16:1263. [PMID: 19586772]

Coffee RE, Westfall AC, Davis GH, Mieler WF, Holz ER: Symptomatic posterior vitreous detachment and the incidence of delayed retinal breaks: case series and meta-analysis. Am J Ophthalmol 2007;144:409. [PMID: 17583667]

Coluciello M: Images in clinical medicine. Retinal arteriolar cholesterol emboli. N Engl J Med 2008;358:826. [PMID: 18287605]

Cronau H, Kankanala RR, Mauger T: Diagnosis and management of red eye in primary care. Am Fam Physician 2010;81:137. [PMID: 20082509]

D'Amico DJ: Clinical practice. Primary retinal detachment. N Engl J Med 2008;359:2346. [PMID: 19038880]

Dargin JM, Lowenstein RA: The painful eye. Emerg Med Clin North Am 2008;26:199. [PMID: 18249263]

Fraser JA, Weyand CM, Newman NJ, Biousse V: The treatment of giant cell arteritis. Rev Neurol Dis 2008;5:140. [PMID: 18838954]

Fraser SG, Adams W: Interventions for acute non-arteritic central retinal artery occlusion. Cochrane Database Syst Rev 2009;1:CD001989. [PMID: 19160204]

Galor A, Jeng BH: Red eye for the internist: when to treat, when to refer. Cleve Clin J Med 2008;75:137. [PMID: 18290357]

Germann CA, Baumann MR, Hamzavi S: Ophthalmic diagnoses in the ED: optic neuritis. Am J Emerg Med 2007;25:834. [PMID: 17870491]

Goff MJ, McDonald HR, Johnson RN, et al: Causes and treatment of vitreous hemorrhage. Compr Ophthalmol Update 2006;7:97. [PMID: 16882398]

Grosser S: Red eyes, red flags: answers to frequently asked questions about the eye. Minn Med 2009;92:31. [PMID: 19653469]

Hall JK: Giant-cell arteritis. Curr Opin Ophthalmol 2008;19:454. [PMID: 18854689]

Hazin R, Dixon JA, Bhatti MT: Thrombolytic therapy in central retinal artery occlusion: cutting edge therapy, standard of care therapy, or impractical therapy? Curr Opin Ophthalmol 2009;20:210. [PMID: 19367164]

He L, Zhang D, Zhou M, Zhu C: Corticosteroids for preventing postherpetic neuralgia. Cochrane Datbase Syst Rev 2008;1:CD005582. [PMID: 18254083]

Hodge C, Lawless M: Ocular emergencies. Aust Fam Physician 2008;37:506. [PMID: 18592066]

Hollands H, Johnson D, Brox AC et al: Acute-onset floaters and flashes: is this patient at risk for retinal detachment? JAMA 2009;302:2243. [PMID: 19934426]

Kang HK, Luff AJ: Management of retinal detachment: a guide for non-ophthalmologists. BMJ 2008;336:1235. [PMID: 18511798]

Kawasaki A, Purvin V: Giant cell arteritis: an updated review. Acta Ophthalmol 2009;87:13. [PMID: 18937808]

Kerr NM, Chew SS, Danesh-Meyer HV: Non-arteritic anterior ischaemic optic neuropathy: a review and update. J Clin Neurosci 2009;16:994. [PMID: 19596112]

Koch J, Sikes K: Getting the red out: primary angle-closure glaucoma. Nurse Pract 2009;34:6. [PMID: 19390391]

Lam DS, Tham CC, Lai JS, Leung DY: Current approaches to the management of acute primary angle closure. Curr Opin Ophthalmol 2007;18:146. [PMID: 17301617]

Li Q, Chen N, Yang J: Antiviral treatment for preventing postherpetic neuralgia. Cochrane Database Syst Rev 2009;2:CD006866. [PMID: 19370655]

Luneau K, Newman NJ, Biousse V: Ischemic optic neuropathies. Neurologist 2008;14:341. [PMID: 19008740]

Magauran B: Conditions requiring emergency ophthalmologic consultation. Emerg Med Clin North Am 2008;26:233. [PMID: 18249265]

Mahmood AR, Narang AT: Diagnosis and management of the acute red eye. Emerg Med Clinic North Am 2008;26:35. [PMID: 18249256]

Margo CE, Harman LE: Posterior vitreous detachment. How to approach sudden-onset floaters and flashing lights. Postgrad Med 2005;117:37. [PMID: 15782672]

Mathys KC, Garg S: Images in clinical medicine. Central hemiretinal arterial occlusion. N Engl J Med 2008;358:2716. [PMID: 18565864]

Moeller JJ, Maxner CE: The dilated pupil: an update. Curr Neurol Neurosci Rep 2007;7:417. [PMID: 17764632]

Mueller JB, McStay CM: Ocular infection and inflammation. Emerg Med Clin North Am 2008;26:57. [PMID: 18249257]

Opstelten W, Eekhof J, Neven AK, Verheij T: Treatment of herpes zoster. Can Fam Physician 2008;54:373. [PMID: 18337531]

Patel A, Hammersmith K: Contact lens-related microbial keratitis: recent outbreaks. Curr Opin Ophthalmol 2008;19:302. [PMID: 18545011]

Pavan-Langston D: Herpes zoster antivirals and pain management. Ophthalmology 2008;115:S13. [PMID: 18243927]

Pokhrel PK, Loftus SA: Ocular emergencies. Am Fam Physician 2007;76:829. [PMID: 17910297]

Prentiss KA, Dorfman DH: Pediatric ophthalmology in the emergency department. Emerg Med Clin North Am 2008;26:181. [PMID: 18249262]

Reich SG: Teaching video is it III alone, or III and IV? Neurology 2007;68:E34. [PMID: 17515533]

Roufail ED, Polkinghorne P: Vitreous floaters. Compr Ophthalmol Update 2006;7:171. [PMID: 17007730]

Rudkin AK, Lee AW, Aldrich E, Miller NR, Chen CS: Clinical characteristics and outcome of current standard management of central retinal artery occlusion. Clin Experiment Ophthalmol 2010;38:496. [PMID: 20584027]

Saligan LN, Yeh S: Seeing red: guiding the management of ocular hyperemia. Nurs Pract 2008;33:14. [PMID: 18528197]

Schumacher M, Schmidt D, Jurklies B, et al: Central retinal artery occlusion: local intra-arterial fibrinolysis versus conservative treatment, a multicenter randomized trial. Ophthalmology 2010;117:1367. [PMID: 20609991]

Tarabishy AB, Jeng BH: Bacterial conjunctivitis: a review for internists. Cleve Clin J Med 2008;75:507. [PMID: 18646586]

Vortmann M, Schneider JI: Acute monocular visual loss. Emerg Med Clin North Am 2008;26:73. [PMID: 18249258]

Weizblit N, Noble J: Ophthaproblem. Central retinal artery occlusion. Can Fam Physician 2009;55:167. [PMID: 19221078]

Woodruff MM, Edlow JA: Evaluation of third nerve palsy in the Emergency Department. J Emerg Med 2008;35:239. [PMID: 17976817]

Yang M, Quah BL, Seah LL, Looi A: Orbital cellulitis in children—medical treatment versus surgical management. Orbit 2009;28;124. [PMID: 19839897]

Yau JW, Lee P, Wong TY, Best J, Jenkins A: Retinal vein occlusion: an approach to diagnosis, systemic risk factors and management. Intern Med 2008;38:904. [PMID: 19120547]

Zhang X, Ji X, Luo Y, et al: Intra-arterial thrombolysis for acute central retinal artery occlusion. Neurol Res 2009;31:385. [PMID: 19508824]

Lids & Lacrimal Apparatus

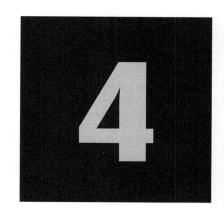

M. Reza Vagefi, MD, John H. Sullivan, MD,
Zélia M. Corrêa MD, PhD, and James J. Augsburger, MD

4.1. Lids

M. Reza Vagefi, MD, and John H. Sullivan, MD

▼ ANATOMY OF THE LIDS (FIGURE 1–22)

The eyelids are thin structures comprised of skin, muscle, and fibrous tissue that serve to protect the eye. The great mobility of the lids is possible because the skin is among the thinnest of the body. Beneath the skin lies a very thin fibroadipose layer through which septa pass and closely adhere to the orbicularis oculi muscle. The orbicularis oculi muscle consists of striated muscle innervated on its deep surface by the facial nerve (cranial nerve VII). The muscle functions to close the lids and is divided into orbital, preseptal, and pretarsal divisions. The orbital portion, which functions primarily in forcible closure, is a circular muscle with no temporal insertion. The preseptal and pretarsal muscles are more involved in involuntary lid movements (blink). They have superficial and deep medial heads that participate in lacrimal pump function (see Section II. Lacrimal Apparatus).

The lid margins are supported by the tarsi, rigid fibrous plates connected to the orbital rim by the medial and lateral canthal tendons. The lateral canthus lies 1–2 mm higher than the medial. The orbital septum originates from the orbital rim and functions as an important barrier between the eyelids and the orbit. In the upper lid, the septum attaches to the levator aponeurosis which then joins the tarsus. Behind the septum lies the medial and the central or preaponeurotic fat pad, a helpful surgical landmark. In the lower lid, the septum joins the inferior border of the tarsus. The lower lid has three anatomically distinct fat pads beneath the orbital septum.

Deep to the fat lies the levator muscle complex—the principal retractor of the upper eyelid—and its equivalent, the capsulopalpebral fascia in the lower lid. The levator muscle originates in the apex of the orbit and is innervated by the oculomotor nerve (cranial nerve III). As it enters the eyelid, it forms an aponeurosis that attaches to the lower third of the superior tarsus. In the lower lid, the capsulopalpebral fascia originates from the inferior rectus muscle and inserts on the inferior border of the tarsus. It serves to retract the lower lid in downgaze. The superior (Müller's muscle) and inferior tarsal muscle form the next layer, which is adherent to the conjunctiva. These sympathetically innervated muscles are also lid retractors. Conjunctiva lines the inner surface of the lids. It is continuous with that of the eyeball and contains glands essential for lubrication of the ocular surface.

The upper lid is larger and more mobile than the lower. A deep crease usually present in the mid position of the upper lid in Caucasian populations represents an attachment of levator muscle fibers. The crease is much lower or is absent in the Asian eyelid. With age, the thin skin of the upper lid tends to hang over the lid crease and may touch the eyelashes. Aging also thins the orbital septum and reveals the underlying fat pads.

▼ INFECTIONS & INFLAMMATIONS OF THE LIDS

HORDEOLUM

A hordeolum is an infection of one or more glands of the eyelid. When the meibomian glands are involved, it is called an internal hordeolum. An external hordeolum (sty) is an infection of a gland of Zeis or Moll.

Pain, redness, and swelling are the principal symptoms. The intensity of the pain is a function of the amount of lid swelling. An internal hordeolum may point to the skin or to the conjunctival surface. An external hordeolum always points to the skin.

Most hordeola are caused by staphylococcal infections, usually *Staphylococcus aureus.* Culture is seldom required. Treatment consists of warm compresses three or four times a day for 10–15 minutes. If the process does not begin to resolve within 48 hours, incision and drainage of the purulent material is indicated. A vertical incision should be made on the conjunctival surface to avoid cutting across the meibomian glands. The incision should not be squeezed to express residual pus. If the hordeolum is pointing externally, a horizontal incision should be made on the skin to minimize scar formation.

Antibiotic ointment is routinely applied to the conjunctival sac 4 times daily. Systemic antibiotics are indicated if cellulitis develops.

CHALAZION

A chalazion (Figure 4–1) is a sterile, focal, chronic inflammation of the eyelid that results from obstruction of a meibomian gland. It is commonly associated with rosacea and posterior blepharitis. Symptoms begin with mild inflammation and tenderness that persists over a period of weeks to months. It is differentiated from a hordeolum by the absence of acute inflammatory signs. Most chalazia point toward the conjunctival surface, which may be slightly reddened or elevated. If sufficiently large, a chalazion may press on the globe and cause astigmatism. Excision is indicated if the lesion distorts vision or is cosmetically unacceptable.

Laboratory studies are seldom indicated, but on histologic examination, there is proliferation of the endothelium of the acinus and a granulomatous inflammatory response that includes Langerhans-type giant cells. Biopsy is indicated for recurrent chalazion, since sebaceous gland carcinoma may mimic the appearance of chalazion.

Surgical excision is performed via a vertical incision into the tarsal gland from the conjunctival surface followed by careful curettement of the gelatinous material and glandular epithelium. Intralesional steroid injections alone may be useful for small lesions, and in combination with surgery in difficult cases.

ANTERIOR BLEPHARITIS

Anterior blepharitis (Figure 4–2) is a common, chronic bilateral inflammation of the lid margins. There are two main types: staphylococcal and seborrheic. Staphylococcal blepharitis may be due to infection with *S aureus, Staphylococcus epidermidis* or coagulase-negative staphylococci. Seborrheic blepharitis is usually associated with the presence of *Pityrosporum ovale,* although this organism has not been shown to be causative. Often, both types are present (mixed).

The chief symptoms are irritation, burning, and itching of the lid margins. The eyes are "red-rimmed." Many scales or scurf can be seen clinging to the lashes of both the upper and lower lids. In the staphylococcal type, the scales are dry, the lids are erythematous, the lid margins are ulcerated, and the lashes tend to fall out. In the seborrheic type, the scales are greasy, ulceration does not occur, and the lid margins are less inflamed. Seborrhea of the scalp, brows, and ears is also frequently found. In the more common mixed type, both dry and greasy scales are present with lid margin inflammation and possible ulceration. Staphylococcal species and *P ovale* can be seen together or singly in stained material scraped from the lid margins.

Staphylococcal blepharitis may be complicated by hordeola, chalazia, epithelial keratitis of the lower third of the cornea, and marginal corneal infiltrates (see Chapter 6). Both forms of anterior blepharitis predispose to recurrent conjunctivitis.

Treatment consists of eyelid hygiene particularly in the seborrheic type of blepharitis. Scales must be removed daily from the lid margins by gentle mechanical scrubbing with a damp cotton applicator and baby shampoo.

Staphylococcal blepharitis is treated with antistaphylococcal antibiotic or sulfacetamide ointment applied on a cotton applicator once daily to the lid margins.

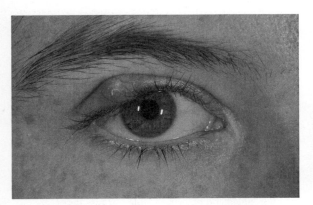

▲ **Figure 4-1.** Chalazion of right upper eyelid.

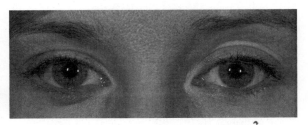

▲ **Figure 4-2.** Severe anterior blepharitis. See color insert.

Both types may run a chronic course over a period of months or years if not treated adequately. Associated staphylococcal conjunctivitis or keratitis usually disappears promptly following local antistaphylococcal medication.

POSTERIOR BLEPHARITIS

Posterior blepharitis (Figure 4–3) is inflammation of the eyelids secondary to dysfunction of the meibomian glands. Like anterior blepharitis, it is a bilateral, chronic condition. Anterior and posterior blepharitis may coexist. Seborrheic dermatitis is commonly associated with meibomian gland dysfunction. Colonization or frank infection with strains of staphylococci is frequently associated with meibomian gland disease and may represent one reason for the disturbance of meibomian gland function. Bacterial lipases may cause inflammation of the meibomian glands and conjunctiva and disruption of the tear film.

Posterior blepharitis is manifested by a broad spectrum of symptoms involving the lids, tears, conjunctiva, and cornea. Meibomian gland changes include inflammation of the meibomian orifices (meibomianitis), plugging of the orifices with inspissated secretions, dilatation of the meibomian glands in the tarsal plates, and production of abnormal soft, cheesy secretion upon pressure over the glands. Hordeola and chalazia may also occur. The lid margin shows hyperemia and telangiectasia, and may become rounded and rolled inward as a result of scarring of the tarsal conjunctiva, causing an abnormal relationship between the precorneal tear film and the meibomian gland orifices. The tears may be frothy or abnormally greasy. Hypersensitivity to staphylococci may produce a secondary keratopathy. The cornea may also develop peripheral vascularization and thinning, particularly inferiorly, sometimes with frank marginal infiltrates. Posterior blepharitis is often associated with rosacea (see Chapter 15).

Regardless of disease severity, the primary therapy is application of warm compresses to the eyelids, with periodic meibomian gland expression. Further treatment is determined by the associated conjunctival and corneal changes. Topical therapy with antibiotics is guided by results of bacterial cultures from the lid margins. Frank inflammation of the lids calls for anti-inflammatory treatment, including long-term therapy with topical metrogel (0.75% twice daily) and/or systemic doxycycline (50–100 mg twice daily). Short-term treatment with weak topical steroids (eg, prednisolone acetate, 0.125% twice daily) can be considered. Tear film dysfunction may necessitate artificial tears, but toxic reactions to preservatives need to be identified. Hordeola and chalazia should be treated appropriately.

ANATOMIC DEFORMITIES OF THE LIDS

ENTROPION

Entropion is an inward turning of the lid margin (Figure 4–4). It may be involutional, spastic, cicatricial, or congenital. Involutional entropion is the most common and by definition occurs as a result of aging. It always affects the lower lid and is the result of a combination of horizontal eyelid laxity, disinsertion of the lower lid retractors, and upward migration of the preseptal orbicularis muscle.

Cicatricial entropion may involve the upper or lower lid and is the result of conjunctival and tarsal scar formation. It is most often found with chronic inflammatory diseases such as trachoma or pemphigoid.

Congenital entropion is rare and should not be confused with congenital **epiblepharon**, which usually afflicts Asians. In congenital entropion, the lid margin is rotated toward the cornea, whereas in epiblepharon, the pretarsal skin and muscle cause the lashes to rotate around the tarsal border.

Trichiasis is misdirection of eyelashes toward the cornea and may be due to entropion, epiblepharon, or simply

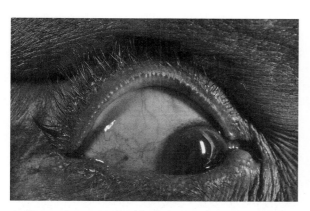

▲ **Figure 4–3.** Posterior blepharitis with inspissated meibomian glands.

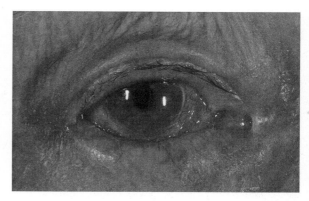

▲ **Figure 4–4.** Involutional entropion of right lower eyelid.

misdirected growth. It causes corneal irritation and encourages ulceration. Chronic inflammatory lid diseases such as blepharitis may cause scarring of the lash follicles and subsequent misdirected growth.

Distichiasis is a condition manifested by accessory eyelashes, often growing from the orifices of the meibomian glands. It may be congenital or the result of inflammatory metaplastic changes in the glands of the eyelid margin.

Surgery to evert the lid is effective in all kinds of entropion. Useful temporary measures in involutional entropion are to tape the lower lid to the cheek with tension exerted temporally and inferiorly or to inject botulinum toxin. Trichiasis without entropion can be temporarily relieved by epilating the offending eyelashes. Permanent relief may be achieved with electrolysis, laser, cryotherapy or lid surgery.

ECTROPION

Ectropion is an outward turning of the lid margin (Figure 4–5). It may be involutional, paralytic, cicatricial, mechanical or congenital. Involutional ectropion is the result of horizontal eyelid laxity from aging. Paralytic ectropion follows facial nerve palsy. Cicatricial ectropion is caused by contracture of the skin of the lid from trauma or inflammation. Mechanical ectropion usually occurs because of bulky tumors of the lid. Symptoms of tearing and irritation with exposure keratitis may occur with any type.

Involutional and paralytic ectropion can be treated surgically by horizontal shortening of the lid. Treatment of cicatricial ectropion requires surgical revision of the scar and often skin grafting. Correction of mechanical ectropion requires removal of the neoplasm followed by eyelid reconstruction.

COLOBOMA

Congenital coloboma is the result of incomplete fusion of fetal maxillary processes. The consequence is a lid margin cleft of variable size. The medial aspect of the upper lid is most often involved, and there is often an associated dermoid tumor. Surgical reconstruction can usually be delayed for years but should be done immediately if the cornea is at risk. A full-thickness eyelid defect from any cause is sometimes referred to as a coloboma.

EPICANTHUS

Epicanthus is characterized by vertical folds of skin over the medial canthi. It is typical of Asians and is present to some degree in most children of all races. The skinfold is often large enough to cover part of the nasal sclera and cause "pseudoesotropia." The eye appears to be crossed when the medial aspect of the sclera is not visible. The most frequent type is **epicanthus tarsalis,** in which the superior lid fold is continuous medially with the epicanthal fold. In **epicanthus inversus,** the skinfold blends into the lower lid. Other types are less common. Epicanthal skinfolds may also be acquired after surgery or trauma to the medial eyelid and nose. The cause of epicanthus is vertical shortening of the skin between the canthus and the nose. Surgical correction is directed at vertical lengthening and horizontal shortening. Epicanthal folds in normal children, however, diminish gradually by puberty and seldom require surgery.

TELECANTHUS

The normal distance between the medial canthus of each eye, the intercanthal distance, is equal to the length of each palpebral fissure (approximately 30 mm in adults). A wide intercanthal distance may be the result of traumatic disinsertion or congenital craniofacial dysgenesis. Minor degrees of telecanthus (eg, blepharophimosis syndrome) can be corrected with skin and soft-tissue surgery. Major craniofacial reconstruction, however, is required when the orbits are widely separated, as in Crouzon's disease (see Chapter 17).

▼ BLEPHAROCHALASIS

Blepharochalasis (Figure 4–6) is a rare condition of unknown cause, sometimes familial, which resembles angioneurotic edema. Repeated attacks begin near puberty, diminish during

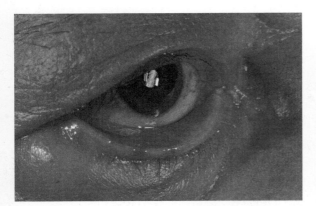

▲ **Figure 4–5.** Involutional ectropion of right lower eyelid.

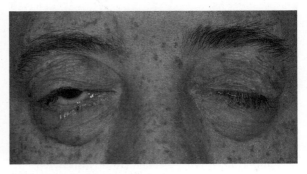

▲ **Figure 4–6.** Blepharochalasis.

adulthood, and cause atrophy of periorbital structures. Eyelid skin appears thin, wrinkled, and redundant and is described as resembling cigarette paper. A sunken appearance is the result of fat atrophy. Involvement of the levator aponeurosis produces moderate to severe ptosis. Medical management is limited to symptomatic treatment of edema. Surgical repair of levator dehiscence and excision of redundant skin is most likely to be successful after attacks have abated.

DERMATOCHALASIS

Dermatochalasis (Figure 4–7) is eyelid skin redundancy and loss of elasticity, usually as a result of aging. In the upper lid, the preseptal skin and orbicularis muscle, which normally forms a crease near the upper tarsal border in Caucasians, hangs over the pretarsal portion of the lid. When dermatochalasis is severe, the superior visual field is obstructed. Weakness of the orbital septum causes the medial and preaponeurotic fat pads to bulge. "Bags" in the preseptal region of the lower lid represent herniated orbital fat.

Blepharoplasty may be indicated for visual or cosmetic reasons. In the upper lid, superfluous eyelid skin is removed as well as muscle and fat for optimum aesthetics. Lower lid blepharoplasty is considered cosmetic surgery unless extreme redundancy contributes to ectropion of the lid margin.

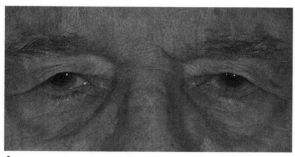

A

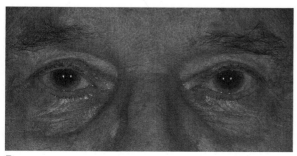

B

▲ **Figure 4–7.** Blepharoplasty. **(A)** Dermatochalasis of upper lids. **(B)** Upper eyelid blepharoplasty surgery results in removal of excess skin and improved peripheral vision.

Pulsed CO_2 and erbium lasers, while effective for facial aesthetic surgery, must be used with extreme caution in the periocular area.

BLEPHAROSPASM

Benign essential blepharospasm is an uncommon type of involuntary muscle contraction characterized by bilateral, synchronous, involuntary, spasms of the eyelids with onset typically during adulthood. The spasms tend to progress in force and frequency, resulting in a grimacing expression and involuntary closure of the eyes. Patients are incapacitated and often only able to experience only brief intervals of vision between spasms. When the entire face and neck are involved, the condition is known as Meige syndrome. Diagnosis is frequently delayed.

The cause of blepharospasm is not known, but studies have implicated dysfunction of the basal ganglia and a number of cortical and subcortical centers that control blinking. Emotional stress and fatigue sometimes make the condition worse.

It is important to differentiate benign essential blepharospasm from hemifacial spasm. The latter condition tends to be unilateral and to involve the upper and lower face. Hemifacial spasm can result from compression of the facial nerve by an artery or posterior fossa tumor. Jenetta's neurosurgical decompression is the definitive mode of treatment; however, temporary neuromuscular blockade (see below) is less invasive and more frequently employed.

Other types of involuntary facial movements include **tardive dyskinesia,** which results from prolonged phenothiazine therapy and seldom affects the orbicularis muscle selectively; and **facial tics,** common in children, which are thought to be psychogenic.

The primary treatment of blepharospasm is repeated injections of botulinum toxin to produce temporary neuromuscular paralysis of the orbicularis oculi muscle. Rarely, unusual instances of psychoneurotic behavior may be identified that benefit from psychotherapy, neuroleptic drug treatment, biofeedback training, and hypnosis. If intolerance or unresponsiveness to botulinum toxin develops, selective extirpation of the orbicularis muscles or surgical ablation of the facial nerve can be performed.

BLEPHAROPTOSIS

The upper lid normally rests approximately midway between the superior limbus and the pupillary margin. Considerable variation may exist as long as symmetry is maintained. Blepharoptosis, or "ptosis," as it is more commonly called, is the condition in which one or both upper eyelids assume an abnormally low position.

▶ Classification

Blepharoptosis may be congenital or acquired (Table 4–1). Classification is important for selection of appropriate treatment.

Table 4–1. Classification of Blepharoptosis

Congenital ptosis
  Myogenic
    Simple
    With superior rectus weakness
    Blepharophimosis syndrome
  Neurogenic
    Congenital oculomotor nerve palsy
    Congenital Horner's syndrome
    Marcus Gunn Jaw-Winking syndrome
    Congenital fibrosis of the extraocular muscles
  Mechanical
    Eyelid mass (eg. capillary hemangioma)

Acquired ptosis
  Aponeurotic
    Senescent (Involutional)
    Trauma
    Blepharochalasis
    Pregnancy
    Graves' disease
  Myogenic
    Chronic progressive external ophthalmoplegia
    Oculopharyngeal dystrophy
    Myotonic dystrophy
    Myasthenia gravis
  Neurogenic
    Acquired oculomotor nerve palsy
      Ischemia (microvascular disease)
      Trauma
      Compression
    Acquired Horner's syndrome
    Levator muscle botulinum toxin injection
  Mechanical

Pseudo-ptosis
  Dermatochalasis
  Contralateral upper lid retraction
  Hypotropia
  Reduced orbital volume
    Enophthalmos
    Microphthalmos
    Phthisis Bulbi

CONGENITAL PTOSIS

A. Congenital Myogenic Ptosis

Congenital myogenic ptosis is the result of an isolated dystrophy of the levator muscle affecting both contraction and relaxation of the fibers. Ptosis is present in the primary position of gaze, and there is reduced movement of the lid in upgaze and impaired closure on downgaze. Lid lag on downgaze is an important clue to diagnosis of levator maldevelopment. Other ocular abnormalities, such as strabismus, may be present. In 25% of cases, the superior rectus muscle shares the same dystrophic changes as the levator, resulting in weakness

of upgaze. Successful surgical outcome in the presence of superior rectus weakness requires the resection of an additional length of levator.

Blepharophimosis syndrome accounts for 5% of cases of congenital ptosis. Severe ptosis with poor levator function is accompanied by telecanthus, epicanthus inversus, and sometimes ectropion of the lower lids. It can also be associated with premature ovarian failure in females. The condition is autosomal dominant and caused by a mutation in the FOXL2 gene on chromosome 3.

B. Congenital Neurogenic Ptosis

Congenital oculomotor nerve palsy may be partial or complete and manifests as blepharoptosis associated with the inability to elevate, depress, or adduct the globe. Mydriasis may also be observed. If the lid is completely closed deprivational amblyopia will develop unless the ptosis is corrected.

Congenital Horner's syndrome manifests as mild ptosis, miosis with decreased pigmentation of the iris resulting in heterochromia, and anhidrosis of the ipsilateral face. In most cases no etiology is identified and failure of development of the sympathetic nervous chain may be responsible. Birth trauma is the most commonly identified etiology but neuroblastoma is responsible in a few cases and urine testing for catecholamines may be required. Unexplained acquired Horner's in infants necessitates imaging for neuroblastoma.

In **Marcus Gunn jaw-winking syndrome**, aberrant innervation of the levator muscle by the motor division of the trigeminal nerve (cranial nerve V) results in a synkinesis, manifesting as elevation of the ptotic eyelid with movement of the mandible.

Congenital fibrosis of the extraocular muscles (CFEOM) is a rare genetic disorder manifesting as ptosis and restrictive ophthalmoplegia. The name of the disease is a misnomer as recent studies support a defect in neuronal differentiation. Several types exist and are classified according to genotype and phenotype. Inherited is usually autosomal dominant pattern. Mutations of KIF21A (chromosome 12) and PHOX2A (chromosome 11) genes have been identified.

ACQUIRED PTOSIS

A. Aponeurotic Ptosis

Senescent or involutional ptosis is the most common type of acquired ptosis. It results from partial disinsertion or dehiscence of the levator aponeurosis from the tarsal plate with age. Typically, there are sufficient residual attachments to the tarsus to maintain full excursion of the lid with upgaze. Upward displacement or loss of insertion of the levator fibers into the skin and orbicularis muscle results in an unusually high lid crease. Thinning of the lid may also occur. Ptosis due to trauma (including ocular surgery or birth trauma), and blepharochalasis, or associated with pregnancy, is also usually due to disinsertion of the levator aponeurosis. Ptosis in Graves' disease may be aponeurotic but myasthenia gravis should also be considered (see later in the chapter).

B. Acquired Myogenic Ptosis

Chronic progressive external ophthalmoplegia (CPEO), one form of mitochondrial cytopathy, is a slowly progressive neuromuscular disease that usually begins in mid life. Although it is associated with deletions in mitochondrial DNA, the disease is usually sporadic because of new mutations rather than inherited. All extraocular muscles, including the levator, and the muscles of facial expression gradually become affected. A wide range of other neuro-degenerative disorders may be present. In **Kearns-Sayre syndrome,** ophthalmoplegia, pigmentary retinopathy, and heart block manifest before age 15.

Oculopharyngeal dystrophy, an autosomal-dominant disease affecting individuals of French-Canadian descent, predominantly manifests as dysphagia but also as facial weakness, ptosis, and usually mild ophthalmoplegia. Ptosis and facial weakness occur in **myotonic dystrophy.** Other findings include cataract, pupillary abnormalities, frontal baldness, testicular atrophy, and diabetes.

Myasthenia gravis (see Chapter 14) is an autoimmune disorder in which circulating antibodies impair binding of acetylcholine at the post-synaptic neuromuscular junction and thus muscle contraction. Ptosis and/or diplopia are commonly the initial manifestation of both the ocular and generalized forms. Lid fatigue with increasing ptosis on prolonged upgaze is a consistent sign. Ptosis may be reversed by rest or the local application of ice. The orbicularis oculi muscles are also frequently involved. Cogan's lid twitch, in which the upper lid twitches upward on rapid movements of the eyes from downward gaze to primary position, is sometimes present but is not specific. Circulating antibodies to acetylcholine receptors (AChR), which can be divided into binding, blocking and modulating, or muscle-specific kinase (MuSK), or electromyography (EMG), particularly single-fiber studies of orbicularis oculi in ocular myasthenia, may be diagnostic. The diagnosis can also be confirmed by the reversal of muscle weakness following administration of intravenous edrophonium or intramuscular neostigmine, which prevents the breakdown of acetylcholine by inhibiting cholinesterase. Medical management with anti-cholinesterase agents, systemic steroids, or other immunosuppressants is usually effective. Thymectomy may be helpful in selected cases.

C. Acquired Neurogenic Ptosis

Although the majority of **acquired oculomotor nerve palsies** are caused by ischemia (microvascular disease), usually secondary to arteriosclerosis, some are due to serious intracranial disease such as aneurysm or tumor (see Chapter 14). Typically there is lid ptosis and impairment of adduction, depression, and elevation of the globe, but the severity of each component varies. Pupillary abnormalities are common in traumatic palsies and compressive lesions. Acute painful isolated oculomotor nerve palsy with pupil involvement should be considered to be due to aneurysmal compression until proven otherwise. Oculomotor palsy due to trauma, acute aneurysmal compression, or chronic compression, typically cavernous sinus lesions, may be complicated by oculomotor synkinesis (aberrant regeneration), resulting in inappropriate movements of the globe, eyelid, or pupil (e.g. lid elevation on downgaze).

Acquired Horner's syndrome results from disruption of sympathetic innervation. It results in mild ptosis, due to paralysis of Müller's muscle in the upper eyelid, and mild elevation of the lower eyelid, due to paralysis of the smooth muscle component of the inferior tarsal muscle, the combination giving a false impression of enophthalmos, and miosis. If the lesion of the sympathetic pathway is proximal to the superior cervical ganglion, there is absence of sweating (anhidrosis) of the ipsilateral face and neck (see Chapter 14).

Temporary neurogenic ptosis, such as for the treatment of corneal disease, can be induced by injection of botulinum toxin into the levator muscle.

D. Mechanical Ptosis

The upper lid may be prevented from opening completely because of the mass effect of a neoplasm, or the tethering effect of scar formation. Excessive horizontal shortening of the upper lid is a common cause of mechanical ptosis. Another form is seen following enucleation, absence of support from the globe allowing the lid to drop.

PSEUDO-PTOSIS

In severe dermatochalasis, excess skin of the upper lid may conceal the lid margin and give the appearance of ptosis. Alternatively, contralateral upper lid retraction may be mistakenly interpreted as ipsilateral ptosis. Hypotropia may also give the appearance of ptosis. When the eye looks down, the upper lid drops more than the lower lid. The narrowed palpebral fissure and the ptotic upper lid are much more apparent than the hypotropic globe. Occlusion of the contralateral eye, causing the ipsilateral eye to take up fixation, clarifies the situation. Conditions in which orbital volume is reduced such as enophthalmos, microphthalmos, and phthisis bulbi, can create the appearance of ptosis.

▶ Treatment

With the exception of myasthenia gravis, all types of ptosis are treated surgically. In children, surgery can be performed once accurate evaluation can be obtained and the child is able to cooperate postoperatively. Astigmatism and myopia may be associated with childhood ptosis. Early surgery might be helpful in preventing anisometropic amblyopia, but this has not been proved. Deprivational amblyopia probably occurs only with complete ptosis, as in congenital oculomotor nerve palsy.

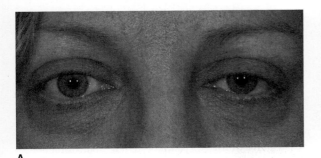
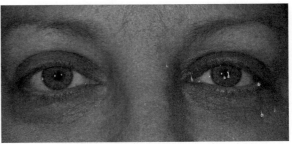

A   B

▲ **Figure 4–8.** Blepharoptosis correction. **(A)** Blepharoptosis of the left upper lid. **(B)** External levator resection on left side results in improvement of upper eyelid height.

Symmetry is the goal of surgery, and symmetry in all positions of gaze is possible only if levator function is unimpaired. In most cases, the best result that can be achieved is to balance the lids in the primary position. With unilateral ptosis, achievement of symmetry in other positions of gaze is proportionate to levator function.

Most ptosis operations involve resection of the levator aponeurosis or superior tarsal muscle (or both). The superior portion of the tarsus is often resected for additional elevation. Many approaches, from both skin and conjunctiva, are currently in use. In recent years, emphasis has been placed on the advantages of confining the operation to advancement and resection of the levator aponeurosis, especially in acquired ptosis (Figure 4–8).

Patients with little or no levator function, as in severe neurogenic or myogenic ptosis, require an alternative elevating source. Suspension of the lids to the brow allows the patient to elevate the lids with the natural movement of the frontalis muscle. Autogenous fascia lata is usually considered the best means of suspension, but other materials such as Mersilene mesh or silicone rod may be used. When lid closure, Bell's phenomenon, and other extraocular movements are impaired, ptosis surgery must be undertaken with caution because of the risk of exposure keratitis.

4.2. Eyelid Tumors
Zélia M. Corrêa, MD, PhD, and James J. Augsburger, MD

This section presents an overview of the most common and most important neoplasms, choristomas, and hamartomas of the eyelid. Simulating lesions of inflammatory, infectious, or degenerative natures (eg, chalazion, hordeolum, molluscum contagiosum, and xanthelasma) are discussed in other sections of this chapter.

▼ BENIGN TUMORS OF THE EYELIDS

Benign neoplasms are acquired cellular tumors of cells that are atypical but not sufficient to be classified as malignant. They may enlarge slowly but have little or no invasive potential and no metastatic capability. **Hamartomas** are congenital tumors composed of normal or near-normal cells and tissues for the anatomic site but in excessive amounts. **Choristomas** are congenital tumors consisting of normal cells and tissue elements but not occurring normally at the anatomic site.

▶ Benign Epidermal Neoplasms

The epidermis and dermis of the eyelid may be affected by many acquired neoplasms that range from completely benign to pre-cancerous. Each type of epithelial tumor exhibits some variation in its clinical features, such that clinical diagnosis may not be reliable and definitive diagnosis requires histopathological examination.

Squamous papilloma (Figure 4–9) of the skin (skin tag) is a focal hyperplasia of the stratified squamous epithelium of the epidermis. Single or multiple, with a fleshy color and irregular surface, squamous papillomas may be sessile or pedunculated. Treatment is surgical excision.

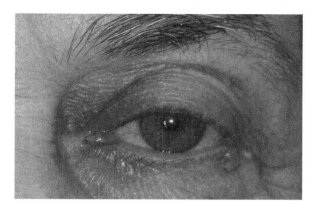

▲ **Figure 4–9.** Squamous papillomas (skin tags)—two fleshy pedunculated lesions by the external canthus—of left lower eyelid. (Courtesy of Tiana G. Burmann)

Seborrheic keratosis (Figure 4–10) predominantly occurs in middle aged and older adults. It manifests as a dome-shaped to verrucoid (wart-like) adherent papule that is fleshy to gray-brown in color, with a crusty surface due to hyperkeratosis. Treatment of cosmetically bothersome lesions is surgical excision.

Keratoacanthoma is often mistaken for a low-grade squamous cell carcinoma. It usually manifests as a rapidly growing single nodule in a middle-aged individual. Umbilicated, with a distinctive crater filled with a keratin plug, the lesion develops over a few weeks but typically undergoes spontaneous involution

within 6 months leaving an atrophic scar. It is a common feature of the Muir-Torre syndrome. Treatment of an actively enlarging keratoacanthoma is surgical excision.

Actinic keratosis (solar or senile keratosis) manifests as an erythematous, scaly flat lesion, developing in a middle-aged or older person. The frequency of malignant transformation to squamous cell carcinoma has been estimated to be as high as 20%. Treatment is surgical excision.

▶ Benign Melanocytic Neoplasms (Figure 4–11)

Melanocytic skin lesions may arise from epidermal (dendritic) melanocytes, nevus cells in the epidermis, or dermal (fusiform) melanocytes. Most benign melanocytic neoplasms are melanocytic nevi, of which the three principal subtypes are termed junctional, compound, and intradermal. A junctional nevus typically appear as a small, flat tan macule that first becomes apparent in childhood and gradually increases in size but only to a limited extent. It represents nests of melanocytes within the epidermis at the dermal-epidermal junction. As the lesion stops growing, some of the nests of melanocytes migrate into the dermis forming a compound nevus, which clinically is slightly elevated and melanotic. Further evolution of the lesion, with the remaining epidermal nests migrating into the dermis, produces an intradermal nevus, which, may be dome-shaped, pedunculated, or papillomatous. Intradermal nevi are commonly present in adults and usually are hypomelanotic or amelanotic. Diagnosis of melanocytic nevi is based on clinical appearance. Although malignant transformation is rare, it may occur in the junctional or compound stages. Suspicious looking lesions that demonstrate significant growth should be excised.

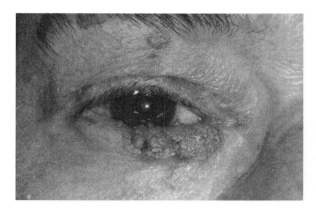

▲ **Figure 4–10.** Seborrheic keratosis (gray-brown verrucoid (wart-like) adherent papule with irregular crusty surface due to hyperkeratosis) of the lower and actinic keratoses (multiple erythematous, flat, scaly lesions of sun-exposed skin) of the upper right eyelids. (Courtesy of Tiana G. Burmann)

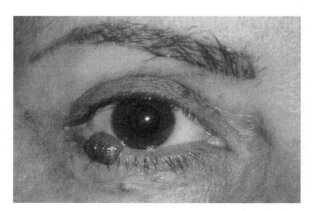

▲ **Figure 4–11.** Nevus (papillomataous melanocytic lesion with eyelashes) of lateral right lower eyelid margin. (Courtesy of Tiana G. Burmann)

Adnexal Neoplasms

Adnexal tumors of the eyelid are benign neoplasms arising from tissues such as hair follicle epithelium, sweat glands (glands of Moll), and sebaceous glands (Meibomian glands in the tarsus and glands of Zeiss in the eyelashes). Two noteworthy categories are **sebaceous adenoma,** which arises from Meibomian glands of the tarsus and therefore develops close to or contiguous with a hair follicle, and the **trichoepithelioma,** which arises from the hair follicle epithelium and therefore develops adjacent to hair shafts, including the eyelashes. These tumors typically appear as solitary, well-circumscribed, superficial nodules. Treatment is surgical excision.

Hamartomas

Vascular hamartomas of the eyelid comprise a spectrum of benign blood vessel tumors that includes **nevus flammeus** (congenital teleangiectatic hemangioma), the classic cutaneous feature of the Sturge-Webber syndrome, and **capillary hemangioma** (strawberry nevus) as the principal variants, as well as **cavernous hemangioma** (Figure 4–12). Capillary hemangioma is composed of a hamartomatous proliferation of vascular endothelial cells. It is sometimes evident at birth but usually becomes apparent during the first few months of life, then progressively enlarges for several months. Becoming stable around age 1 year, it usually involutes by the age of 3 years. Almost all cases will have regressed by the age of 7 years. Clinically, the usual superficial lesion typically manifests as a red vascular macule that may become large enough to cause ptosis, indentational astigmatism, and amblyopia. A deeper lesion has a blue-gray color, is soft to palpation, and becomes more evident when the child cries or strains. It may cause proptosis and/or strabismus. Since most capillary hemangiomas regress spontaneously, the principal indication for treatment is amblyopia or another complication. Surgical excision is appropriate for large lesions, whereas treatments that hasten tumor regression, such as intralesional injection of corticosteroid or interferon alfa, are frequently employed for small to medium-sized lesions.

Lymphangioma of the eyelid is a congenital overgrowth of lymph channels. More than half are evident at birth and approximately 90% are clinically apparent by age 2. It usually lies deep to the epidermis and manifests as a dark blue, soft, fluctuant mass. There may also be conjunctival or orbital involvement. Spontaneous or post-traumatic bleeding may occur. Management options include observation of small lesions, surgical resection of cosmetically bothersome circumscribed lesions, and surgical debulking of diffuse lesions.

Choristomas

Choristomas of the eyelid are rare. Present at birth, they slowly enlarge. Several types are recognized, including phakomatous choristoma (Zimmerman tumor) consisting of lens material; odontogenic choristoma consisting of dental tissue; osseous choristoma consisting of bone tissue;, **epidermoid cyst** consisting of a wall of stratified squamous epithelium and a central cavity filled with desquamated keratinized cells; and **dermoid cyst** that consists of mature skin complete with hair follicles and sweat glands, hair, and often pockets of sebum, blood, fat, bone, nails, teeth, eyes, cartilage, and thyroid tissue. Eyelid choristomas can develop in the superficial or deep tissues of the lid and orbit and are found in almost any location. Clinically, they manifest as a solitary, firm, slowly enlarging, nontender masses, most commonly in the lateral upper eyelid and brow. Treatment is complete surgical removal.

MALIGNANT TUMORS OF THE EYELIDS

Primary Malignant Epidermal Neoplasms

Basal cell carcinoma (Figure 4–13) arises from pluripotent stem cells within the basal layers of the epidermis and external root sheaths of hair follicles. It does not appear to arise from

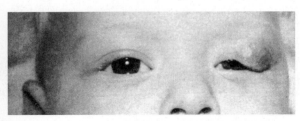

▲ **Figure 4–12.** Cavernous hemangioma of the left upper eyelid in an infant, causing ptosis and indentation of the globe.

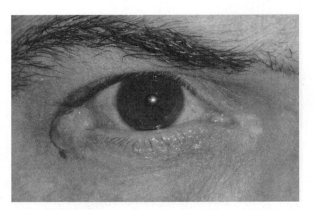

▲ **Figure 4–13.** Basal cell carcinoma, with a pearly surface, lid notching, loss of eyelashes, and teleangiectatic surface vessels, at the lateral canthus of the right lower eyelid. (Courtesy of Tiana G. Burmann)

mature differentiated basal cells. It comprises about 90% of all eyelid malignancies. The incidence of basal cell carcinoma of the eyelid skin increases with age and there is a slight male preponderance (3:2 male to female ratio). Clinically, it typically manifests as a firm painless indurated nodule with a pearly, rolled border and fine (small) telangiectatic surface vessels. 65% of cases occur in the lower eyelid. Treatment consists of complete surgical excision. Incisional punch biopsy of larger tumors is frequently recommended to confirm the diagnosis, prior to wide surgical excision that may require complex plastic surgery to reconstruct the eyelid.

Squamous cell carcinoma (Figure 4–14) arises from the stratified squamous epithelium. It tends to be locally invasive but rarely metastasizes. It comprises 5–10% of all eyelid malignancies, being much less common than basal cell carcinoma. Risk factors for eyelid squamous cell carcinoma of the skin include ultraviolet light/actinic damage, chronic exposure to arsenic, hydrocarbons, radiation, or immunosuppressive drugs, genetic disorders such as albinism and xeroderma pigmentosum, and chronic skin lesions. Although typically observed in elderly patients, squamous cell carcinoma may be seen in younger patients with a history of radiotherapy or in patients infected with HIV. Clinically, eyelid squamous cell carcinoma typically appears as a slow growing, painless, hyperkeratotic nodule that eventually becomes ulcerated. Subsequently there is shallow ulceration with a granular, red base surrounded by an elevated, hard border. Treatment is surgical excision of the entire lesion whenever possible, either by conventional methods or Mohs micrographic surgery, followed by reconstruction of the defect. Focal radiation therapy is used occasionally to treat perineural invasion into bone or the orbit, and exenteration is generally performed in cases with extensive eyelid destruction or massive

orbital invasion. All patients with squamous cell carcinoma of the eyelid should be advised of the risk of residual or recurrent tumor post-treatment and encouraged to adhere to recommended follow up.

Sebaceous gland carcinoma of the eyelid arises from sebaceous glands in the skin. Clinically, it appears as a painless subcutaneous nodularity extending into the tarsal conjunctiva. Lash loss in involved areas is common. Initially, sebaceous carcinoma of the eyelid is frequently misdiagnosed as a benign condition such as recurrent chalazia and chronic blepharitis leading to delay in effective treatment. Histopathologically, the tumor exhibits a disordered invasion of the dermis by lobules of poorly defined sebaceous cells or basaloid/squamoid cells. Tumor cells tend to have multivacuolated clear cytoplasm, causing the nucleus to be scalloped from the lipid invasion. Moderate-to-severe atypia can be found, as well as a high nuclear/cytoplasm ratio and a perinuclear halo. Tumor cells are frequently found in the adjacent epithelia separate from the main tumor, a feature known as pagetoid spread. This typically occurs within the conjunctiva, but it can also occur in the skin or cornea. Special stains to confirm the histologic diagnosis are oil red-O and Sudan black (specific for cytoplasmic fat) and epithelial membrane antigen (EMA) immunoperoxidase staining (specific for sebaceous differentiation). Sebaceous gland carcinoma exhibits an aggressive clinical course, with a significant tendency for both local recurrence after excision and distant metastasis. Delay in diagnosis contributes to poor outcome, potentially avoidable by a high degree of clinical awareness and readiness to biopsy suspicious lesions. Definitive treatment is wide surgical excision. Radiation therapy has traditionally been considered palliative but not curative.

Cutaneous **melanoma** accounts for only 1% of all eyelid tumors but is associated with relatively high frequencies of metastasis and tumor-related death. It generally affects Caucasians and occurs preferentially in areas of skin exposed excessively to ultra-violet light. There are four types of primary cutaneous melanoma: lentigo maligna, superficial spreading melanoma, nodular melanoma, and acral lentigious melanoma. The typical clinical appearance of an eyelid melanomas is a variably melanotic mass that can bleed or ulcerate. Metastasis from eyelid melanomas usually first manifests in the regional lymph nodes of the head and neck, emphasizing the importance of examination for preauricular and submandibular lymphadenopathy. Treatment is wide surgical excision followed by reconstructive surgery. Exenteration of the orbit is performed for some patients with massive orbital invasion, although there is little evidence that such surgery improves survival. The prognosis in eyelid melanoma is related to size of the tumor, depth of invasion, atypicality of tumor cells, and completeness of initial excision.

▶ Other Malignant Tumors

Eyelid metastasis, due to occasional hematogenous spread from non-ophthalmic primary cancer, typically manifests as

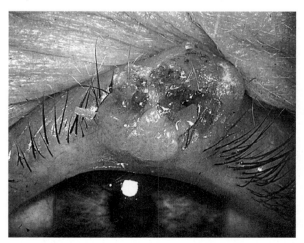

▲ **Figure 4–14.** Squamous cell carcinoma, with a typical nodular shape and ulcerated center, of the upper eyelid. (Courtesy of A. Rosenberg)

an abruptly enlarging subepidermal mass, metastases at various other anatomic sites also usually being detectable. The survival prognosis of a patient with an eyelid metastasis is poor. Recommended treatment is radiotherapy if the tumor becomes large and/or painful.

✳ **Kaposi sarcoma** is a malignant mesenchymal neoplasm first reported by Kaposi in 1872 as an idiopathic multiple-pigmented sarcoma. Previously relatively rare and encountered mainly in southern Europe in persons 40 years of age or older, recently the vast majority of affected patients have been younger persons with AIDS. The extremities are involved most frequently, but any region of the skin can be affected. Eyelid Kaposi sarcoma manifests as a red to purple subcutaneous lesion that can be circumscribed, diffuse, nodular, or pedunculated. Histopathologically, Kaposi sarcoma comprises a network of proliferating endothelial cells that form a channel-like structure filled with blood. Treatment for Kaposi sarcoma of the eyelid consists of intravenous chemotherapy (especially if the patient has multiple skin lesions in various anatomic sites) or focal palliative radiotherapy.

Eyelid **lymphoma**, in which there is infiltration by malignant lymphocytic cells, tends to cause thickening and lumpiness of the involved eyelid. Usually it is not tender or painful, but severe recurrent itchiness is common. Unlike conjunctival, intraocular, and orbital lymphomas, which are almost always disorders of B-cell derived lymphocytes, a relatively high proportion of eyelid lymphomas are classified immunopathologically as T-cell lymphomas. The classic primary T-cell lymphoma of the skin occurs in **mycosis fungoides**. Diagnosis is usually based on pathologic analysis of a biopsy specimen. Despite usually having an indolent course, **extranodal marginal zone B-cell lymphomas** are renowned for recurrence in extranodal sites, including other ocular adnexal sites. Management of patients with ocular adnexal lymphomas generally begins with a thorough baseline systemic staging examination. Treatment of disseminated cutaneous lymphoma is usually intravenous chemotherapy. However, radiation therapy can be used for treatment of limited disease, including eyelid involvement. Prognostic factors for survival in patients with cutaneous lymphoma include the lymphoma subtype, as determined using the REAL classification, the clinical course, responsiveness to treatment, and the age and general health of the patient at the time of diagnosis.

4.3. Lacrimal Apparatus

M. Reza Vagefi, MD, and John H. Sullivan, MD

The lacrimal apparatus comprises structures involved in the production and drainage of tears (also see Chapter 5). The secretory system consists of the glands that produce the various components of the tear film, which is distributed over the surface of the eye by the action of blinking. The lacrimal puncta, canaliculi, and sac, and the nasolacrimal duct form the drainage system, ultimately draining into the nose.

LACRIMAL SECRETORY SYSTEM

The tear film is composed of three layers. Unicellular goblet cells, which are scattered throughout the conjunctiva, secrete glycoprotein in the form of mucin that comprises the innermost layer of the tear film. The intermediate aqueous layer is provided by the main and accessory lacrimal glands. The lipid layer is the final layer of the tear film that is produced by the meibomian glands of the tarsus.

The largest volume of the aqueous layer is produced by the lacrimal gland located in the lacrimal fossa in the superior temporal quadrant of the orbit. This almond-shaped gland is divided by the lateral horn of the levator aponeurosis into a larger orbital lobe and a smaller palpebral lobe.

Ducts from the orbital lobe join those of the palpebral lobe and empty into the superior temporal fornix (see Chapter 1). The normal palpebral lobe can sometimes be visualized by everting the upper lid. The accessory lacrimal glands, although only one-tenth of the mass of the major gland, have an essential role and are known as the "basal secretors." Their secretions are normally sufficient to maintain the health of the cornea. They are comprised of the glands of Krause and Wolfring, which are identical in structure to the lacrimal gland, but lack ductules. These glands are located in the conjunctiva mainly in the superior fornix and superior tarsal border.

Secretions from the lacrimal gland are triggered by emotion or physical irritation and cause tears to flow copiously over the lid margin (epiphora). The afferent pathway of the reflex arc is the ophthalmic branch of the trigeminal nerve. The efferent pathway is comprised of parasympathetic and sympathetic contributions. Parasympathetic innervation, originating from the pontine lacrimal (superior salivary) nucleus, is conveyed by the greater petrosal nerve, which is contained in the separate part of the facial nerve known as the nervus intermedius, the nerve of the pterygoid canal (Vidian nerve), synapsing in the pterygopalatine ganglion, and then via an uncertain route to the lacrimal gland. The sympathetic pathway is less well characterized.

DISORDERS OF THE SECRETORY SYSTEM

▶ Alacrima

Congenital absence of tearing occurs in Riley-Day syndrome (familial dysautonomia) and anhidrotic ectodermal dysplasia. Although initially asymptomatic, patients usually develop signs of keratoconjunctivitis sicca. Reduced tear production may occur after damage to the nervus intermedius following surgery in the cerebellopontine angle, such as for vestibular schwannoma (acoustic neuroma), or due to tumors or inflammation of the lacrimal gland.

▶ Lacrimal Hypersecretion

Primary hypersecretion may occur as a result of tumor or inflammation of the lacrimal gland and is a rare cause of tearing. Secondary hypersecretion may be of supranuclear, infranuclear, or reflex etiologies. The most common cause of hypersecretion is reflex lacrimation resulting from ocular surface disease, tear film instability or deficiency. Treatment is therefore directed at stabilizing the underlying disease process. Hypersecretion always needs to be distinguished from tearing due to obstruction of the lacrimal drainage system.

▶ Paradoxic Lacrimation ("Crocodile Tears")

This condition is characterized by tearing while eating. Although it may be congenital, it is usually acquired after Bell's palsy and is the result of aberrant regeneration of the facial nerve. It can be treated by injecting botulinum toxin into the lacrimal gland.

▶ Bloody Tears

Hemolacria is a rare clinical entity attributed to a variety of causes, including conjunctivis, trauma, blood dyscrasias, vascular tumors, and tumors of the lacrimal sac.

▶ Dacryoadenitis

Inflammation of the lacrimal gland can be acute or chronic, and due to infection or systemic disease. **Acute dacryoadenitis** is rare, most often seen in children as a complication of a viral infection including mumps, Epstein-Barr virus, measles, or influenza, but sometimes due to bacterial or fungal infection. In adults, *Neisseria gonorrhea* may be responsible. Symptoms typically evolve over hours or days. There is marked pain, with swelling and redness of the outer portion of the upper eyelid, which often assumes an S-shaped curve. Bacterial infection usually responds to systemic antibiotics, without the need for surgical drainage.

Chronic dacryoadenitis, defined as inflammation for longer than one month, is more common. It can be bilateral and often is painless. It is frequently associated with systemic diseases such as sarcoidosis, Graves' disease, Sjogren syndrome, and lymphoma. When combined with parotid gland swelling, it is called Mikulicz's syndrome. Infectious causes are rare but include syphilis, tuberculosis, leprosy, and trachoma.

▼ LACRIMAL DRAINAGE SYSTEM

The drainage system is composed of the puncta, canaliculi, lacrimal sac, and nasolacrimal duct (see Chapter 1). With each blink, the eyelids close like a zipper—beginning laterally, distributing tears evenly across the cornea, and delivering them to the drainage system on the medial aspect of the lids. Under normal circumstances, tears are produced at about their rate of evaporation, and thus few pass through the drainage system. When tears flood the conjunctival sac, they enter the puncta partially by capillary attraction. With lid closure, the specialized portion of pretarsal orbicularis surrounding the ampulla tightens to prevent their escape. Simultaneously, the lid is drawn toward the posterior lacrimal crest and traction is placed on the fascia surrounding the lacrimal sac, causing the canaliculi to shorten and creating negative pressure within the sac. This dynamic pumping action draws tears into the sac. The tears then pass by gravity and tissue elasticity through the nasolacrimal duct to exit beneath the inferior meatus of the nose. Valve-like folds of the epithelial lining of the duct tend to resist the retrograde flow of tears and air. The most developed of these flaps is the "valve" of Hasner at the distal end. This structure is important because when imperforate it is the commonest cause of congenital nasolacrimal duct obstruction, resulting in epiphora and chronic dacryocystitis.

DISORDERS OF THE DRAINAGE SYSTEM

1. NASOLACRIMAL DUCT OBSTRUCTION AND DACRYOCYSTITIS

Infection of the lacrimal sac is common, most often unilateral, and always secondary to obstruction of the nasolacrimal duct.

In **infantile dacryocystitis** the site of obstruction is usually a persistent membrane covering the valve of Hasner. Failure of canalization of the nasolacrimal duct occurs in up to 87% of newborns, but it usually completes spontaneously being patent at the end of the first month of life in 90% of neonates. Chronic is more common than acute dacryocystitis, but prompt and aggressive treatment of acute dacryocystitis should be instituted because of the risk of orbital cellulitis. Microorganisms involved in chronic and acute infantile dacryocystitis include *Streptococcus pneumoniae*, *Staphylococcus* species, *Haemophilus influenzae*, and Enterobacteriaceae species.

In adults, nasolacrimal duct obstruction typically occurs in postmenopausal women. The cause is often uncertain but generally is attributed to chronic inflammation resulting in fibrosis within the duct. Stasis of tears within the sac leads to secondary infections. Acute and chronic dacryocystitis are usually caused by *S aureus, S epidermidis, Pseudomonas aeruginosa*, or anaerobic organisms such as *Peptostreptococcus* and *Propionibacterium* species. Dacryocystitis is uncommon in other adults unless it follows trauma or is caused by formation of a cast (dacryolith) within the lacrimal sac, in which case spontaneous improvement follows passage of the dacryolith but recurrence is the rule.

▶ Clinical Findings

The chief symptoms of dacryocystitis are tearing and discharge. In the acute form, there is inflammation, pain, swelling, and tenderness beneath the medial canthal tendon in the area of the lacrimal sac (Figure 4–15), and purulent material can be expressed through the lacrimal puncta by pressure directly on the sac. In the chronic form, tearing and matting of lashes are usually the only symptoms, but mucoid material usually can be expressed from the sac.

Dilation of the lacrimal sac (mucocele) indicates obstruction of the nasolacrimal duct. Regurgitation of mucus or pus through the puncta on compression of the enlarged sac establishes patency of the canalicular system. It is important to examine the inside of the nose to determine whether there is adequate drainage space between the septum and the lateral nasal wall.

▶ Treatment

Acute dacryocystitis usually responds to appropriate systemic antibiotics. The infectious agent can be identified by Gram stain and culture of material expressed from the tear sac. Occasionally, incision and drainage of the lacrimal sac may be necessary. Chronic infections can often be kept latent with antibiotic drops. In either case, correction of the obstruction is the definitive cure.

In infants (see Chapter 17), forceful compression of the lacrimal sac will sometimes rupture the membrane and establish patency. If stenosis persists more than 6 months or if there is an episode of acute dacryocystitis, nasolacrimal probing is indicated. One probing is effective in 75% of cases. In the remainder, cure can almost always be achieved by repeated probing, by inward fracture of the inferior turbinate, or by temporary silicone stent intubation or balloon catheter dilation of the lacrimal system. Lacrimal surgery is rarely required. Probing should not be attempted in the presence of acute infection.

In adults, surgical correction of nasolacrimal duct obstruction is usually achieved by **dacryocystorhinostomy**, in which a permanent fistula is formed between the lacrimal sac and the nose. With the traditional approach, exposure is gained by an external incision over the anterior lacrimal crest. Bone is removed from the lateral wall of the nose and incisions are made in the lacrimal sac and adjacent nasal mucosa, sutures then being inserted to fashion the fistula. Various endonasal endoscopic techniques to create the fistula, some using lasers, have been developed, with the advantage of avoiding an external incision but possibly reducing long-term patency rates. Balloon catheter dilation of the distal nasolacrimal duct may also be useful for patients with partial obstruction. Patients with chronic dacryocystitis should undergo lacrimal surgery prior to elective intraocular surgery to reduce the risk of endophthalmitis.

2. CANALICULAR DISORDERS

Congenital anomalies of the canalicular system include imperforate puncta, accessory puncta, canalicular fistulas, and, rarely, agenesis of the canalicular system.

Most cases of canalicular stenosis are acquired and are due to viral, usually varicella zoster, herpes simplex, or adenovirus infection, trauma, conjunctival inflammatory diseases such as Stevens-Johnson syndrome, toxic epidermal necrolysis, erythema multiforme, and cicatricial pemphigoid, or drug therapy, either systemic chemotherapy with fluorouracil or topical idoxuridine.

Canaliculitis is an uncommon chronic unilateral infection caused by *Actinomyces* species (Figure 4–16), *Candida albicans, Aspergillus* species, anaerobic streptococci, or staphylococci. The patient typically complains of a mildly red and irritated eye with a slight discharge. It affects the lower canaliculus more often than the upper, occurs exclusively in adults, and causes a secondary purulent conjunctivitis that frequently escapes etiologic diagnosis. If untreated, it can result in canalicular stenosis.

▶ Clinical Findings

Canalicular probing and irrigation aid in identification of the location and severity of obstruction. Further evidence is provided by compression of the lacrimal sac. No regurgitation of material through the puncta occurring if there is complete obstruction of the common canaliculus or of both the upper and lower canaliculi. Dacryocystography, in which radiographic imaging is performed following injection of contrast media into the lacrimal system, can also assist in localizing the obstruction.

In canaliculitis, the punctum usually pouts and material can be expressed from the canaliculus, with the organism being identifiable by microscopy and culture.

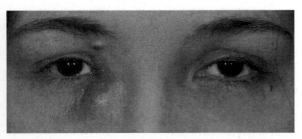

▲ **Figure 4–15.** Acute dacryocystitis.

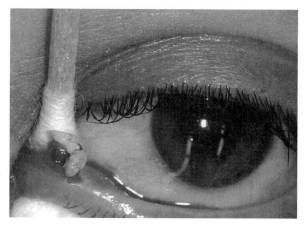

▲ **Figure 4–16.** Actinomyces israelii canaliculitis.

▶ Treatment

Partial common canalicular stenosis may be amenable to intubation with a silicone stent for 3–6 months but severe cases require dacryocystorhinostomy combined with canaliculoplasty and silicone intubation. Total canalicular obstruction necessitates formation of a fistula between the conjunctival sac and the nose (conjunctivodacryocystorhinostomy) with insertion of a Pyrex glass (Lester Jones) tube to maintain its patency, but extrusion of the tube frequently occurs.

For canaliculitis, curettage of material from the involved canaliculus, followed by irrigation, is usually effective in establishing patency, with antibiotic therapy then being determined by microbiological results. Canaliculotomy is sometimes necessary. Recurrence is common.

REFERENCES

Lids

Baroody M, Holds JB, Vick VL: Advances in the diagnosis and treatment of ptosis. Curr Opin Ophthalmol 2005;1:351. [PMID: 16264345] (Review of current concepts of blepharoptosis management.)

Ben Simon GJ et al: External levator advancement vs Müller's muscle-conjunctival resection for correction of upper eyelid involutional ptosis. Am J Ophthalmol 2005;140:426. [PMID: 16083839]

Bleyen I, Dolman PJ: The Wies procedure for management of trichiasis or cicatricial entropion of either upper or lower eyelids. Br J Ophthalmol 2009;93:1612. [PMID: 19574237]

Cates CA, Tyers AG: Results of levator excision followed by fascia lata brow suspension in patients with congenital and jaw-winking ptosis. Orbit 2008;27:83. [PMID: 18415867]

Cetinkaya A, Brannan PA: Ptosis repair options and algorithm. Curr Opin Ophthalmol 2008;19:428. [PMID: 18772677]

Cetinkaya A, Brannan PA: What is new in the era of focal dystonia treatment? Botulinum injections and more. Curr Opin Ophthalmol 2007;18:424. [PMID: 17700237]

Crisponi L et al: The putative forkhead transcription factor FOXL2 is mutated in blepharophimosis/ptosis/epicanthus inversus syndrome. Nat Genet 2001;27:159. [PMID: 11175783]

Demirci H, Frueh BR, Nelson CC: Marcus Gunn jaw-winking synkinesis clinical features and management. Ophthalmology 2010 Feb 24 [Epub ahead of print] [PMID: 20188419]

Engle EC: Genetic basis of congenital strabismus. Arch Ophthalmol 2007;125:189. [PMID: 17296894]

Hallett M et al: Update on blepharospasm: report from the BEBRF International Workshop. Neurology 2008;14;71:1275. [PMID: 18852443]

Jackson WB: Blepharitis: current strategies for diagnosis and management. Can J Ophthalmol 2008;43:170. [PMID: 18347619]

Jones SM et al: Visual outcome and corneal changes in children with chronic blepharokeratoconjunctivitis. Ophthalmology 2007;114:2271. [PMID: 18054641]

Kakizaki H et al: Lower eyelid anatomy: an update. Ann Plast Surg 2009;63:344. [PMID: 19602948]

Kakizaki H, Malhotra R, Selva D: Upper eyelid anatomy: an update. Ann Plast Surg 2009;63:336. [PMID: 19602949]

LeDoux MS: Meige syndrome: what's in a name. Parkinsonism Relat Disord 2009;15:483. [PMID: 19457699]

Lee MJ et al: Frontalis sling operation using silicone rod compared with preserved fascia lata for congenital ptosis a three-year follow-up study. Ophthalmology 2009;116:123. [PMID: 19019443]

Ortisi E et al: Blepharospasm and hemifacial spasm: A protocol for titration of botulinum toxin dose to the individual patient and for the management of refractory cases. Eye 2006;20:916. [PMID: 16531977]

Simpson DM et al: Assessment: Botulinum neurotoxin for the treatment of movement disorders (an evidence-based review): report of the Therapeutics and Technology Assessment Subcommittee of the American Academy of Neurology. Neurology 2008;70:1699. [PMID: 18458230]

Stone DU, Chodosh J: Ocular rosacea: an update on pathogenesis and therapy. Curr Opin Ophthalmol 2004;15:499. [PMID: 15523195]

Eyelid Tumors

Bernardini FP: Management of malignant and benign eyelid lesions. Curr Opin Ophthalmol 2006;17:480. [PMID: 16932064]

Bianciotto C, Demirci H, Shields CL, Eagle RC Jr, Shields JA: Metastatic tumors to the eyelid: report of 20 cases and review of the literature. Arch Ophthalmol 2009;127:999. [PMID: 19667336]

Buitrago W, Joseph AK: Sebaceous carcinoma: the great masquerader: emerging concepts in diagnosis and treatment. Dermatol Ther 2008;21:459. [PMID: 19076624]

Chadha V, Wright M: Small margin excision of periocular basal cell carcinomas. Br J Ophthalmol 2009;93:803. [PMID: 19304655]

Chan FM, O'Donnell BA, Whitehead K, Ryman W, Sullivan TJ: Treatment and outcomes of malignant melanoma of the eyelid: a review of 29 cases in Australia. Ophthalmology 2007;114:187. [PMID: 17140665]

Chi MJ, Baek SH: Clinical analysis of benign eyelid and conjunctival tumors. Ophthalmologica 2006;220:43. [PMID: 16374048]

Coupland SE, Hummel M, Stein H: Ocular adnexal lymphomas: five case presentations and a review of the literature. Surv Ophthalmol 2002;47:470. [PMID: 12431695]

Dasgupta T, Wilson LD, Yu JB: A retrospective review of 1349 cases of sebaceous carcinoma. Cancer 2009;115:158. [PMID: 18988294]

Deokule S, Child V, Tarin S, Sandramouli S: Diagnostic accuracy of benign eyeluid skin lesions in the minor operation theatre. Orbit 2003;22:235. [PMID: 14685896]

Deprez M, Uffer S: Clinicopathologcial features of eyelid skin tumors. A retrospective study of 5504 cases and review of the literature. Am J Dermatopathol 2009;31:256. [PMID: 19384066]

Esmaeli B, Youssef A, Naderi A, Ahmadi MA, Meyer DR, McNab A: Collaborative Eyelid Skin Melanoma Group: margins of excision for cutaneous melanoma of the eyelid skin: the Collaborative Eyelid Skin Melanoma Group Report. Ophthal Plast Reconstr Surg 2003;19:96. [PMID: 12644753]

Frank RC, Cowan BJ, Harrop AR, Astel WF, McPaheln DF: Visual development in infants: visual complicaitons of periocular haemangiomas. J Plast Reconstr Aesthet Surg 2010;632:1. [PMID: 19097831]

Kersten RC, Ewing-Chow D, Kulwin DR, Gallon M: Accuracy of clinical diagnosis of cutaneous eyelid lesions. Ophthalmology 1997;104:479. [PMID: 9082276]

Leibovitch I, Huilgol SC, James CL, Hsuan JD, Davis G, Selva D: Periocular keratoacanthoma: can we always rely upon the clinical diagnosis? Br J Ophthalmol 2005;89:1201. [PMID: 16113382]

Limawararut V, Leibovitch I, Sullivan T, Selva D: Periocular squamous cell carcinoma. Clin Experiment Ophthalmol 2007;35:174. [PMID: 17362462]

Malhotra R, Huilgol SC, Huynh NT, Selva D: The Australia Mohs database, part I: periocular basal cell carcinoma experience over 7 years. Ophthalmology 2004;111:624. [PMID: 15051192]

Narayanan K, Hadid OH, Barnes EA: Mohs micrographic surgery versus surgical excision for periocular basal cell carcinoma. Cochrane Database Syst Rev 2009;2:CD007041. [PMID: 19370670]

Nemet AY, et al: Management of periocular basal and squamous cell carcinoma: a series of 485 cases. Am J Ophthalmol 2006;142:293. [PMID: 16876511]

Pereira PR, et al: Histopathological review of sebaceous carcinoma of the eyelid. J Cutan Pathol 2005;32:496. [PMID: 16008694]

Prabhakaran VC, Gupta A, Huilgol SC, Selva D: Basal cell carcinoma of the eyelids. Compr Ophthalmol Update 2007;8:1. [PMID: 17394754]

Schwartz SR et al: Treatment of capillary hemangiomas causing refractive and occlusional amblyopia. J AAPOS 2007;11:577. [PMID: 17720571]

Shields JA, Demirci H, Marr BP, Eagle RC Jr, Shields CL: Sebaceous carcinoma of the ocular region: a review. Surv Ophthalmol 2005;50:103. [PMID: 15749305]

Shumaker PR et al: Modified Mohs micrographic surgery for periocular melanoma and melanoma in situ: long-term experience at Scripps Clinic. Dermatol Surg 2009;35:1263. [PMID: 19438663]

Sullivan TJ: Squamous cell carcinoma of eyelid, periocular, and perirobital skin. In Ophthalmol Clin 2009;49:17. [PMID: 20348855]

Tildsley J, Diaper C, Herd R: Mohs surgery vs primary excision for eyelid BCCs. Orbit 2010;29:140. [PMID: 20497079]

Weiss AH, Kelly JP: Reappraisal of astigmatism induced by periocular capillary hemangioma and treatment with intralesional corticosteroid injection. Ophthalmology 2008;115:390. [PMID: 17588666]

Lacrimal Apparatus

Casady DR et al: Stepwise treatment paradigm for congenital nasolacrimal duct obstruction. Ophthal Plast Reconstr Surg 2006;22:243. [PMID: 16855492]

Fayers T, Laverde T, Tay E, Oliver JM: Lacrimal surgery success after external dacryocystorhinostomy: functional and anatomical results using strict outcome criteria. Ophthal Plast Reconstr Surg 2009;25:472. [PMID: 19935252]

Leong SC, Macewen CJ, White PS: A systematic review of outcomes after dacrycystorhinostomy in adults. Am J Rhinol Allergy 2010;24:81. [PMID: 20109333]

Onerci M: Dacryocystorhinostomy. Diagnosis and treatment of nasolacrimal canal obstructions. Rhinology 2002;40:49. [PMID: 12091994]

Pediatric Eye Disease Investigator Group: Primary treatment of nasolacrimal duct obstruction with probing in children younger than 4 years. Ophthalmology 2008;115:577. [PMID: 17996306]

Pediatric Eye Disease Investigator Group: Primary treatment of nasolacrimal duct obstruction with nasolacrimal duct intubation in children younger than 4 years of age. J AAPOS 2008;12:445. [PMID: 18595756]

Pediatric Eye Disease Investigator Group: Primary treatment of nasolacrimal duct obstruction with balloon catheter dilation in children younger than 4 years of age. J AAPOS 2008;12:451. [PMID: 18929305]

Poublon RM, Hertoge Kdde R: Endoscopic-assisted reconstructive surgery of the lacrimal duct. Clin Plast Surg 2009;36:399. [PMID: 19505610]

Repka MX et al: Balloon catheter dilation and nasolacrimal duct intubation for treatment of nasolacrimal duct obstruction after failed probing. Arch Ophthalmol 2009;127:633. [PMID: 19433712]

Varma D, Chang B, Musaad S: A case series on chronic canaliculitis. Orbit 2005;24:11. [PMID: 15764110]

Zaldivar RA, Bradley EA: Primary canaliculitis. Ophthal Plast Reconstr Surg 2009;25:481. [PMID: 19935254]

Conjunctiva & Tears

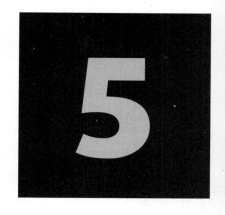

Lisa M. Nijm, MD, JD, Francisco J. Garcia-Ferrer, MD,
Ivan R. Schwab, MD, James J. Augsburger MD, and
Zélia M. Corrêa MD, PhD

5.1. Conjunctiva

Lisa M. Nijm, MD, JD, Francisco J. Garcia-Ferrer, MD, and Ivan R. Schwab, MD

I. CONJUNCTIVITIS

Inflammation of the conjunctiva (conjunctivitis) is the most common eye disease worldwide. It varies in severity from a mild hyperemia with tearing to a severe conjunctivitis with copious purulent discharge. The cause is usually exogenous, but rarely may be endogenous.

CONJUNCTIVITIS DUE TO INFECTIOUS AGENTS

The types of conjunctivitis and their most common causes are summarized in Tables 5–1 and 5–2. Conjunctival inflammation that occurs in the setting of uveitis, or scleral or episcleral inflammation is discussed in Chapter 7.

Because of its location, the conjunctiva is exposed to many microorganisms and other environmental factors. Several mechanisms protect the surface of the eye. In the tear film, the aqueous component dilutes infectious material, mucus traps debris, and a pumping action of the lids constantly flushes the tears to the tear duct. In addition, the tears contain antimicrobial substances, including lysozyme and antibodies (IgG and IgA).

Common pathogens that can cause conjunctivitis include *Streptococcus pneumoniae, Haemophilus influenzae, Staphylococcus aureus, Neisseria meningitidis,* most human adenovirus strains, herpes simplex virus type 1 and type 2, and two picornaviruses. Two sexually transmitted agents that cause conjunctivitis are *Chlamydia trachomatis* and *Neisseria gonorrhoeae.*

▶ Cytology of Conjunctivitis

Damage to the conjunctival epithelium by a noxious agent may be followed by epithelial edema, cellular death and exfoliation, epithelial hypertrophy, or granuloma formation. There may also be edema of the conjunctival stroma (chemosis) and hypertrophy of the lymphoid layer of the stroma (follicle formation). Inflammatory cells, including neutrophils, eosinophils, basophils, lymphocytes, and plasma cells, may be seen and often indicate the nature of the damaging agent. These cells migrate from the conjunctival stroma through the epithelium to the surface. They then combine with fibrin and mucus from the goblet cells to form conjunctival exudate, which is responsible for the "mattering" on the lid margins (especially in the morning).

The inflammatory cells appear in the exudate or in scrapings taken with a sterile platinum spatula from the anesthetized conjunctival surface. The material is stained with Gram's stain (to identify the bacterial organisms) and with Giemsa's stain (to identify the cell types and morphology). A predominance of polymorphonuclear leukocytes is characteristic of bacterial conjunctivitis. Generally, a predominance of mononuclear cells—especially lymphocytes—is characteristic of viral conjunctivitis. If a pseudomembrane or true membrane is present (eg, epidemic keratoconjunctivitis or herpes simplex virus conjunctivitis), neutrophils usually predominate because of coexistent necrosis. In chlamydial conjunctivitis, neutrophils and lymphocytes are generally present in equal numbers.

In allergic conjunctivitis, eosinophils and basophils are frequently present in conjunctival biopsies, but they are less common on conjunctival smears; eosinophils or eosinophilic granules are commonly found in vernal keratoconjunctivitis. High levels of proteins secreted by eosinophils (eg, eosinophil cationic protein) can be found in the tears of patients with vernal, atopic, or allergic conjunctivitis. Eosinophils and

Table 5-1. Causes of Conjunctivitis

Bacterial
  Hyperacute (purulent)
    Neisseria gonorrhoeae
    Neisseria meningitidis
    Neisseria gonorrhoeae subspecies *kochii*
  Acute (mucopurulent)
    Pneumococcus (*Streptococcus pneumoniae*)
     (temperate climates)
    Haemophilus aegyptius (Koch-Weeks bacillus) (tropical climates)
  Subacute
    Haemophilus influenzae (temperate climates)
  Chronic, including blepharoconjunctivitis
    Staphylococcus aureus
    Moraxella lacunata (diplobacillus of Morax-Axenfeld)
  Rare types (acute, subacute, chronic)
    Streptococci
    Moraxella catarrhalis
    Coliforms
    Proteus
    Corynebacterium diphtheriae
    Mycobacterium tuberculosis

Chlamydial
  Trachoma (*C trachomatis* serovars A–C)
  Inclusion conjunctivitis (*C trachomatis* serovars D–K)
  Lymphogranuloma venereum (LGV) (*C trachomatis*
    serovars L1–3)

Viral
  Acute viral follicular conjunctivitis
    Pharyngoconjunctival fever due to adenoviruses types 3 and 7
     and other serotypes
    Epidemic keratoconjunctivitis due to adenovirus types 8 and 19
    Herpes simplex virus
    Acute hemorrhagic conjunctivitis due to enterovirus type 70;
     rarely, coxsackievirus type A24
  Chronic viral follicular conjunctivitis
    Molluscum contagiosum virus
  Viral blepharoconjunctivitis
    Varicella, herpes zoster due to varicella-zoster virus
    Measles virus

Rickettsial (rare)
  Nonpurulent conjunctivitis with hyperemia and minimal infiltration,
    often a feature of rickettsial diseases
    Typhus
    Murine typhus
    Scrub typhus
    Rocky Mountain spotted fever
    Mediterranean fever
    Q fever

Fungal (rare)
  Ulcerative or granulomatous
    Candida
  Granulomatous

  Rhinosporidium seeberi
  Coccidioides immitis (San Joaquin Valley fever)
  Sporothrix schenckii

Parasitic (rare but important)
  Chronic conjunctivitis and blepharoconjunctivitis
    Thelazia californiensis
    Loa loa
    Ascaris lumbricoides
    Trichinella spiralis
    Schistosoma haematobium (bladder fluke)
    Taenia solium (cysticercus)
    Pthirus pubis (*Pediculus pubis*, public louse)
    Fly larvae (*Oestrus ovis*, etc) (ocular myiasis)

Immunologic (allergic)
  Immediate (humoral) hypersensitivity reactions
    Hay fever conjunctivitis (pollens, grasses, animal
     danders, etc)
    Vernal keratoconjunctivitis
    Atopic keratoconjunctivitis
    Giant papillary conjunctivitis
  Delayed (cellular) hypersensitivity reactions
    Phylctenulosis
    Mild conjunctivitis secondary to contact blepharitis
  Autoimmune disease
    Primary and secondary Sjögren's syndrome
    Mucous membrane pemphigoid

Chemical or irritative
  Iatrogenic
    Idoxuridine, brimonidine, apraclonidine, dipivefrin, and other
     topically applied drugs
    Preservatives in eye drops
    Contact lens solutions, particularly their preservatives
  Occupational
    Acids
    Alkalies
    Smoke
    Wind
    Ultraviolet light
  Caterpillar hair

Etiology unknown
  Folliculosis
  Chronic follicular conjunctivitis (Orphan's conjunctivitis,
    Axenfeld's conjunctivitis)
  Ocular rosacea
  Psoriasis
  Stevens–Johnson syndrome, toxic epidermal necrolysis, and
    erythema multiforme
  Dermatitis herpetiformis
  Epidermolysis bullosa
  Superior limbic keratoconjunctivitis
  Ligneous conjunctivitis
  Reiter's syndrome
  Mucocutaneous lymph node syndrome (Kawasaki disease)

(Continued)

Table 5–1. Causes of Conjunctivitis (*continued*)

Associated with systemic disease	Secondary to dacryocystitis or canaliculitis
Thyroid disease (exposure, congestive) Gouty conjunctivitis Carcinoid conjunctivitis Sarcoidosis Tuberculosis Syphilis	Conjunctivitis secondary to dacryocystitis pneumococci or beta-hemolytic streptococci Conjunctivitis secondary to canaliculitis *Actinomyces israelii*, *Candida* species *Aspergillus* species (rarely)

basophils are found in allergic conjunctivitis, and scattered eosinophilic granules and eosinophils are found in vernal keratoconjunctivitis. In all types of conjunctivitis, there are plasma cells in the conjunctival stroma. Unlike other inflammatory cells, they do not migrate through the epithelium, and are therefore not present in smears of exudate or of scrapings from the conjunctival surface unless the epithelium has become necrotic (eg, trachoma). In trachoma, the rupturing of a follicle allows the plasma cells to reach the epithelial surface. As the mature follicles of trachoma rupture easily, the finding of large, pale-staining lymphoblastic (germinal-center) cells in scrapings strongly suggests trachoma.

Symptoms of Conjunctivitis

The important symptoms of conjunctivitis include foreign body sensation, scratching or burning sensation, sensation of fullness around the eyes, itching, and photophobia.

Foreign body sensation and scratching or burning sensation are often associated with the swelling and papillary hypertrophy that normally accompany conjunctival hyperemia. Pain rather than discomfort commonly indicates corneal involvement.

Signs of Conjunctivitis (Table 5–2)

The important signs of conjunctivitis include hyperemia, tearing, exudation, pseudoptosis, papillary hypertrophy, chemosis, follicles, pseudomembranes and membranes, granulomas, and preauricular adenopathy.

Hyperemia is the most conspicuous clinical sign of acute conjunctivitis. The redness is most marked in the fornix and diminishes toward the limbus by virtue of the dilation of the posterior conjunctival vessels. (A perilimbal dilation or ciliary flush suggests inflammation of the cornea or deeper structures.) A brilliant red suggests bacterial conjunctivitis, whereas a milky appearance suggests allergic conjunctivitis. Hyperemia without cellular infiltration suggests irritation from physical causes, such as wind, sun, smoke, etc, but it may occur occasionally with diseases associated with vascular instability (eg, acne rosacea).

Tearing (epiphora) is often prominent in conjunctivitis, the tears resulting from the foreign body sensation, the burning or scratching sensation, or the itching. Mild transudation also arises from the hyperemic vessels and adds to the tearing. An abnormally scant secretion of tears and an increase in mucous filaments suggest dry eye syndrome.

Table 5–2. Differentiation of the Common Types of Conjunctivitis

Clinical Findings and Cytology	Viral	Bacterial	Chlamydial	Allergic
Itching	Minimal	Minimal	Minimal	Severe
Hyperemia	Generalized	Generalized	Generalized	Generalized
Tearing	Profuse	Moderate	Moderate	Moderate
Exudation	Minimal	Profuse	Profuse	Minimal
Preauricular adenopathy	Common	Uncommon	Common only in inclusion conjunctivitis	None
In stained scrapings and exudates	Monocytes	Bacteria, PMNs[1]	PMNs, plasma cells, inclusion bodies	Eosinophils
Associated sore throat and fever	Occasionally	Occasionally	Never	Never

[1]Polymorphonuclear cells.

Exudation is a feature of all types of acute conjunctivitis. The exudate is flaky and amorphous in bacterial conjunctivitis and stringy in allergic conjunctivitis. "Mattering" of the eyelids occurs upon awakening in almost all types of conjunctivitis, and if the exudate is copious and the lids are firmly stuck together, the conjunctivitis is probably bacterial or chlamydial.

Pseudoptosis is a drooping of the upper lid secondary to infiltration and inflammation of Müller's muscle. The condition is seen in several types of severe conjunctivitis, for example trachoma and epidemic keratoconjunctivitis.

Papillary hypertrophy is a nonspecific conjunctival reaction that occurs because the conjunctiva is bound down to the underlying tarsus or limbus by fine fibrils. When the tuft of vessels that forms the substance of the papilla (along with cellular elements and exudates) reaches the basement membrane of the epithelium, it branches over the papilla like the spokes in the frame of an umbrella. An inflammatory exudate accumulates between the fibrils, heaping the conjunctiva into mounds. In necrotizing disease (eg, trachoma), the exudate may be replaced by granulation tissue or connective tissue.

When the papillae are small, the conjunctiva usually has a smooth, velvety appearance. A red papillary conjunctiva suggests bacterial or chlamydial disease (eg, a velvety red palpebral conjunctiva is characteristic of acute trachoma). With marked infiltration of the conjunctiva, giant papillae form. Also called "cobblestone papillae" in vernal keratoconjunctivitis because of their crowded appearance, giant papillae are flat-topped, polygonal, and milky-red in color. On the upper tarsus, they suggest vernal keratoconjunctivitis and giant papillary conjunctivitis with contact lens sensitivities; on the lower tarsus, they suggest atopic keratoconjunctivitis. Giant papillae may also occur at the limbus, especially in the area that is normally exposed when the eyes are open (between 2 and 4 o'clock and between 8 and 10 o'clock). Here they appear as gelatinous mounds that may encroach on the cornea. Limbal papillae are characteristic of vernal keratoconjunctivitis but rarely occur in atopic keratoconjunctivitis.

Chemosis of the conjunctiva strongly suggests acute allergic conjunctivitis but may also occur in acute gonococcal or meningococcal conjunctivitis and especially in adenoviral conjunctivitis. Chemosis of the bulbar conjunctiva is seen in patients with trichinosis. Occasionally, chemosis may appear before there is any gross cellular infiltration or exudation.

Follicles are seen in most cases of viral conjunctivitis, in all cases of chlamydial conjunctivitis except neonatal inclusion conjunctivitis, in some cases of parasitic conjunctivitis, and in some cases of toxic conjunctivitis induced by topical medications such as idoxuridine, brimonidine, apraclonidine, and dipivefrin, or by preservatives in eye drops or contact lens solutions. Follicles in the inferior fornix and at the tarsal margins have limited diagnostic value, but when they are located on the tarsi (especially the upper tarsus), chlamydial, viral, or toxic conjunctivitis (following topical medication) should be suspected.

The follicle consists of a focal lymphoid hyperplasia within the lymphoid layer of the conjunctiva and usually contains a germinal center. Clinically, it can be recognized as a rounded, avascular white or gray structure. On slitlamp examination, small vessels can be seen arising at the border of the follicle and encircling it.

Pseudomembranes and membranes are the result of an exudative process and differ only in degree. A pseudomembrane is a coagulum on the *surface* of the epithelium, and when it is removed, the epithelium remains intact. In contrast, a true membrane is a coagulum involving the *entire* epithelium, and if it is removed, a raw, bleeding surface remains. Both pseudomembranes and membranes may accompany epidemic keratoconjunctivitis, primary herpes simplex virus conjunctivitis, streptococcal conjunctivitis, diphtheria, mucous membrane pemphigoid, Stevens–Johnson syndrome, toxic epidermal necrolysis, and erythema multiforme. They may also be an aftermath of chemical exposure, especially alkali burns.

Ligneous conjunctivitis is a peculiar form of recurring membranous conjunctivitis. It is bilateral, seen mainly in children, and predominantly in females. It may be associated with other systemic findings, including nasopharyngitis and vulvovaginitis.

Granulomas of the conjunctiva always affect the stroma and most commonly are chalazia. Other endogenous causes include sarcoidosis, syphilis, cat-scratch disease, and, rarely, coccidioidomycosis. Parinaud's oculoglandular syndrome includes conjunctival granulomas and a prominent preauricular lymph node, and this group of diseases may require biopsy examination to establish the diagnosis.

Phlyctenules represent a delayed hypersensitivity reaction to microbial antigen, for example staphylococcal or mycobacterial antigens. Phlyctenules of the conjunctiva initially consist of a perivasculitis with lymphocytic cuffing of a vessel. When they progress to ulceration of the conjunctiva, the ulcer bed has many polymorphonuclear leukocytes.

Preauricular lymphadenopathy is an important sign of conjunctivitis. A grossly visible preauricular node is seen in Parinaud's oculoglandular syndrome and, rarely, in epidemic keratoconjunctivitis. A large or small preauricular node, sometimes slightly tender, occurs in primary herpes simplex conjunctivitis, epidemic keratoconjunctivitis, inclusion conjunctivitis, and trachoma. Small but nontender preauricular lymph nodes tend to occur in pharyngoconjunctival fever and acute hemorrhagic conjunctivitis. Occasionally, preauricular lymphadenopathy may be observed in children with infections of the meibomian glands.

BACTERIAL CONJUNCTIVITIS

Two forms of bacterial conjunctivitis are recognized: acute (including hyperacute and subacute) and chronic. Acute bacterial conjunctivitis is usually benign and self-limited, lasting no more than 14 days. Treatment with one of the many available antibacterial agents usually cures the condition within a few days. In contrast, hyper-acute (purulent) conjunctivitis caused by *N gonorrhoeae* or *N meningitidis* may lead to serious ocular complications if not treated promptly. Chronic conjunctivitis is usually secondary to eyelid disease or nasolacrimal duct obstruction.

▶ Clinical Findings

A. Symptoms and Signs

The organisms that account for most cases of bacterial conjunctivitis are listed in Table 5–1. Generally it manifests as bilateral irritation and injection, purulent exudate with sticky lids on waking, and occasionally lid edema. The infection usually starts in one eye and may be spread to the eye by direct contact from the hands. It may be spread from one person to another by fomites.

Hyperacute (purulent) bacterial conjunctivitis (caused by *N gonorrhoeae*, *Neisseria kochii*, and *N meningitidis*) is marked by a profuse purulent exudate (Figure 5–1). Meningococcal conjunctivitis may occasionally be seen in children. Any severe, profusely exudative conjunctivitis demands immediate laboratory investigation and immediate treatment. If there is any delay, there may be severe corneal damage or loss of the eye, or the conjunctiva could become the portal of entry for either *N gonorrhoeae* or *N meningitidis*, leading to septicemia or meningitis.

Acute mucopurulent (catarrhal) conjunctivitis often occurs in epidemic form and is called "pinkeye" by most laymen. It is characterized by an acute onset of conjunctival hyperemia and a moderate amount of mucopurulent discharge. The most common causes are *S pneumoniae* in temperate climates and *Haemophilus aegyptius* in warm climates. Less common causes are staphylococci and other streptococci. The conjunctivitis caused by *S pneumoniae* and *H aegyptius* may be accompanied by subconjunctival hemorrhages. *H aegyptius* conjunctivitis in Brazil has been followed by a fatal purpuric fever produced by a plasmid-associated toxin of the bacteria.

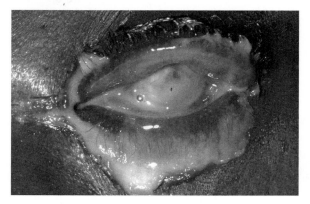

▲ **Figure 5–1.** Gonococcal conjunctivitis. Profuse purulent exudate. (Courtesy of L Schwab.)

Subacute conjunctivitis is caused most often by *H influenzae* and occasionally by *Escherichia coli* and proteus species. *H influenzae* infection is characterized by a thin, watery, or flocculent exudate.

Chronic bacterial conjunctivitis occurs in patients with nasolacrimal duct obstruction and chronic dacryocystitis, which are usually unilateral. It may also be associated with chronic bacterial blepharitis or meibomian gland dysfunction. Patients with floppy lid syndrome or ectropion may develop secondary bacterial conjunctivitis.

Rarely, bacterial conjunctivitis may be caused by *Corynebacterium diphtheriae* and *Streptococcus pyogenes*. Pseudomembranes or membranes caused by these organisms may form on the palpebral conjunctiva. The rare cases of chronic conjunctivitis produced by *Moraxella catarrhalis*, the coliform bacilli, proteus, etc, are as a rule indistinguishable clinically.

B. Laboratory Findings

In most cases of bacterial conjunctivitis, the organisms can be identified by the microscopic examination of conjunctival scrapings stained with Gram's stain or Giemsa's stain; this reveals numerous polymorphonuclear neutrophils. Conjunctival scrapings for microscopic examination and culture are recommended for all cases and are mandatory if the disease is purulent, membranous, or pseudomembranous. Antibiotic sensitivity studies are also desirable, but empirical antibiotic therapy should be started. When the results of antibiotic sensitivity tests become available, specific antibiotic therapy can then be instituted.

▶ Complications & Sequelae

Chronic marginal blepharitis often accompanies staphylococcal conjunctivitis except in very young patients who are not subject to blepharitis. Conjunctival scarring may follow both pseudomembranous and membranous conjunctivitis, and in rare cases corneal ulceration and perforation supervene.

Marginal corneal ulceration may follow infection with *N gonorrhoeae*, *N kochii*, *N meningitidis*, *H aegyptius*, *S aureus*, and *M catarrhalis;* if the toxic products of *N gonorrhoeae* diffuse through the cornea into the anterior chamber, they may cause toxic iritis.

▶ Treatment

Specific therapy of bacterial conjunctivitis depends on identification of the microbiologic agent. While waiting for laboratory reports, the physician can start topical therapy with a broad-spectrum antibacterial agent (eg, polymyxin-trimethoprim). In any purulent conjunctivitis in which the Gram stain shows gram-negative diplococci suggestive of neisseria, both systemic and topical therapy should be started immediately. If there is no corneal involvement, a single intramuscular dose of ceftriaxone, 1 g, is usually adequate systemic therapy. If there is corneal involvement, a 5-day course of parenteral ceftriaxone, 1–2 g daily, is required.

In purulent and mucopurulent conjunctivitis, the conjunctival sac should be irrigated with saline solution as necessary to remove the conjunctival secretions. To prevent spread of the disease, the patient and family should be instructed to give special attention to personal hygiene.

▶ Course & Prognosis

Acute bacterial conjunctivitis is almost always self-limited. Untreated, it may last 10–14 days; if properly treated, 1–3 days. The exceptions are staphylococcal conjunctivitis (which may progress to blepharoconjunctivitis and enter a chronic phase) and gonococcal conjunctivitis (which, when untreated, can lead to corneal perforation and endophthalmitis). Since the conjunctiva may be the portal of entry for the meningococcus to the bloodstream and meninges, septicemia and meningitis may be the end results of meningococcal conjunctivitis.

Chronic bacterial conjunctivitis may not be self-limited and may become a troublesome therapeutic problem.

CHLAMYDIAL CONJUNCTIVITIS

1. TRACHOMA

Although worldwide the number of individuals with profound vision loss from trachoma has dropped from 6 million to 1.3 million, trachoma remains one of the leading causes of preventable blindness. It was first recognized as a cause of trichiasis (misdirected lashes) as early as the 27th century BC. It is usually endemic in regions with poor hygiene, overcrowding, poverty, lack of clean water and poor sanitation. Blinding trachoma occurs in many parts of Africa, in some parts of Asia, among Australian aborigines, and in northern Brazil. Communities with milder nonblinding trachoma occur in the same regions and in some areas of Latin America and the Pacific Islands.

Trachoma usually presents bilaterally and often spreads by direct contact or fomites, most often from other family members, who should also be examined for the disease. Insect vectors, especially flies, may play a role in transmission. The acute forms of the disease are more infectious than the cicatricial forms, and the larger the inoculum, the more severe the disease. Spread is often associated with epidemics of bacterial conjunctivitis and with the dry seasons in tropical and semitropical countries.

▶ Clinical Findings
A. Symptoms and Signs

Trachoma begins as a chronic follicular conjunctivitis of childhood that progresses to conjunctival scarring (Figure 5–2). In severe cases, trichiasis occurs in early adult life as a result of

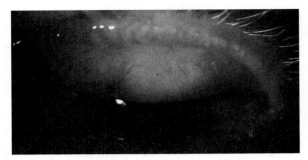

▲ **Figure 5–2.** Conjunctival scarring secondary to trachoma. The superior tarsus is the classic site for subconjunctival scarring in association with trachoma.

severe conjunctival scarring. The constant abrasion of inturned lashes and a defective tear film lead to corneal scarring, usually after the age of 30 years (Figure 5–3).

The incubation period of trachoma averages 7 days but varies from 5–14 days. In an infant or child, the onset is usually insidious, and the disease may resolve with minimal or no complications. In adults, the onset is often subacute or acute, and complications may develop early. At onset, trachoma often resembles other bacterial conjunctivitis. The signs and symptoms usually consist of tearing, photophobia, pain, exudation, edema of the eyelids, chemosis of the bulbar conjunctiva, hyperemia, papillary hypertrophy, tarsal and limbal follicles, superior keratitis, pannus formation, and a small, tender preauricular node.

In established trachoma, there may also be superior epithelial keratitis, subepithelial keratitis, pannus, or superior limbal follicles, and ultimately the pathognomonic cicatricial

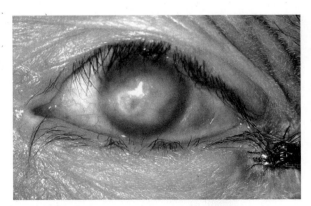

▲ **Figure 5–3.** Advanced trachoma following corneal ulceration and scarring. Note the fly on the temporal aspect of the lower lid. The fly is a principal vector for trachoma.

remains of these follicles, known as **Herbert's pits**—small depressions covered by epithelium at the limbocorneal junction. The associated pannus is a fibrovascular membrane arising from the limbus, with vascular loops extending onto the cornea. All of the signs of trachoma are more severe in the upper than in the lower conjunctiva and cornea.

To establish the presence of endemic trachoma in a family or community, a substantial number of children must have at least two of the following signs:

1. Five or more follicles on the flat palpebral conjunctiva lining the upper eye lid.

2. Typical conjunctival scarring of the upper palpebral conjunctiva.

3. Limbal follicles or their sequelae (Herbert's pits).

4. An even extension of blood vessels on to the cornea, most marked at the upper limbus.

While occasional individuals will meet these criteria, it is the wide distribution of these signs in individual families and in a community that identify the presence of trachoma.

For control purposes, the World Health Organization has developed a simplified method to describe the disease (Table 5–3).

The presence of TF and TI indicates active infectious trachoma and a need for treatment. TS is evidence of damage from the disease. TT is potentially blinding and is an indication for corrective lid surgery. CO is the final blinding lesion of trachoma.

B. Laboratory Findings

Chlamydial inclusion bodies may be found in Giemsa-stained conjunctival scrapings, but they are not always present. Inclusions appear in the Giemsa-stained preparations as particulate, dark purple, or blue cytoplasmic masses that cap the nucleus of the epithelial cell. Fluorescent antibody stains and enzyme immunoassay tests are available commercially and are widely used in clinical laboratories. These and other new tests, including polymerase chain reaction (PCR), have superseded Giemsa staining of conjunctival smears and isolation of chlamydial agent in cell culture.

Table 5–3. WHO Simplified Trachoma Grading System

TF:	Five or more follicles on the upper palpebral conjunctiva.
TI:	Diffuse infiltration and papillary hypertrophy of the upper palpebral conjunctiva obscuring at least 50% of the normal deep vessels.
TS:	Trachomatous conjunctival scarring.
TT:	Trichiasis or entropion (inturned eyelashes).
CO:	Corneal opacity.

The agent of trachoma resembles the agent of inclusion conjunctivitis morphologically, but the two can be differentiated serologically by microimmunofluorescence. Trachoma is usually caused by *C trachomatis* serovars A, B, Ba, or C.

▶ Differential Diagnosis

Epidemiologic and clinical factors to be considered in differentiating trachoma from other forms of follicular conjunctivitis can be summarized as follows:

1. No history of exposure to endemic trachoma speaks against the diagnosis.

2. Viral follicular conjunctivitis (due to infection with adenovirus, herpes simplex virus, picornavirus, and coxsackievirus) usually has an acute onset and is clearly resolving by 2–3 weeks.

3. Infection with genitally transmitted chlamydial strains usually has an acute onset in sexually active individuals.

4. Chronic follicular conjunctivitis with exogenous substances (molluscum nodules of the lids, topical eye medications) resolve slowly when the nodules are removed or the drug is withdrawn.

5. Parinaud's oculoglandular syndrome is manifested by massively enlarged preauricular or cervical lymph nodes, although the conjunctival lesion may be follicular.

6. Young children often have some follicles (like hypertrophied tonsils), a condition known as folliculosis.

7. The atopic conditions vernal conjunctivitis and atopic keratoconjunctivitis are associated with giant papillae that are elevated and often polygonal, with a milky-red appearance. Eosinophils are present in smears.

8. Look for a history of contact lens intolerance in patients with conjunctival scarring and pannus; giant papillae in some contact lens wearers can be confused with trachoma follicles.

▶ Complications & Sequelae

Conjunctival scarring occur as a frequent complication of trachoma and can destroy the accessory lacrimal glands and obliterate the ductules of the lacrimal gland. These effects may drastically reduce the aqueous component of the precorneal tear film, and the film's mucous components may be reduced by loss of goblet cells. The scars may also cause distortion of the upper lid with inward deviation of individual lashes (trichiasis) or of the whole lid margin (entropion), so that the lashes constantly abrade the cornea. This often leads to corneal ulceration, bacterial corneal infections, and corneal scarring.

Ptosis, nasolacrimal duct obstruction, and dacryocystitis are other common complications of trachoma.

Treatment

Striking clinical improvement can usually be achieved with tetracycline, 1–1.5 g/d orally in four divided doses for 3–4 weeks; doxycycline, 100 mg orally twice daily for 3 weeks; or erythromycin, 1 g/d orally in four divided doses for 3–4 weeks. Several courses are sometimes necessary for actual cure. Systemic tetracyclines should not be given to a child under 7 years of age or to a pregnant woman. Tetracycline binds to calcium in the developing teeth and in growing bone and may lead to congenital yellowish discoloration of the permanent teeth and skeletal (eg, clavicular) abnormalities. Recent studies in developing countries have demonstrated that azithromycin is an effective treatment for trachoma given orally as a 1-g dose in children. Because of minimal side effects and ease of administration, this macrolide antibiotic has become the drug of choice for mass treatment campaigns.

Topical ointments or drops, including preparations of sulfonamides, tetracyclines, erythromycin, and rifampin, used four times daily for 6 weeks, are equally effective.

From the time therapy is begun, its maximum effect is usually not achieved for 10–12 weeks. The persistence of follicles on the upper tarsus for some weeks after a course of therapy should therefore not be construed as evidence of therapeutic failure.

Surgical correction of trichiasis is essential to prevent scarring from late trachoma in developing countries. Such surgery is increasingly done by nonspecialist physicians or specially trained auxiliary personnel.

Course & Prognosis

Characteristically, trachoma is a chronic disease of long duration. Under good hygienic conditions (specifically, face-washing of young children), the disease resolves or becomes milder so that severe sequelae are avoided.

2. INCLUSION CONJUNCTIVITIS

Inclusion conjunctivitis is often bilateral and usually occurs in sexually active young people. The chlamydial agent infects the urethra of the male and the cervix of the female. Transmission to the eyes of adults is usually by oral-genital sexual practices or hand to eye transmission. About 1 in 300 persons with genital chlamydial infection develops the eye disease. Indirect transmission has been reported to occur in inadequately chlorinated swimming pools. In newborns, the agent is transmitted during birth by direct contamination of the conjunctiva with cervical secretions. Credé prophylaxis (1% silver nitrate) gives only partial protection against inclusion conjunctivitis.

Clinical Findings
A. Symptoms and Signs

Inclusion conjunctivitis may have an acute or a subacute onset. The patient frequently complains of redness, pseudoptosis, and discharge, especially in the mornings. Newborns

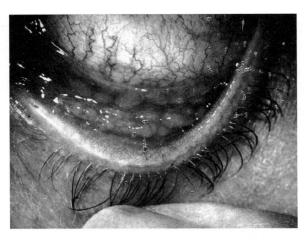

▲ **Figure 5–4.** Acute follicular conjunctivitis caused by inclusion conjunctivitis in a 22-year-old man with urethritis. (Courtesy of K Tabbara.)

have papillary conjunctivitis and a moderate amount of exudate, and in hyper-acute cases, pseudomembranes occasionally form and can lead to scarring. Since the newborn has no adenoid tissue in the stroma of the conjunctiva, there is no follicle formation; but if the conjunctivitis persists for 2–3 months follicles appear, similar to the conjunctival picture in older children and adults. In the newborn, chlamydial infection may cause pharyngitis, otitis media, and interstitial pneumonitis.

In adults, the conjunctiva of both tarsi—especially the lower tarsus—have papillae and follicles (Figure 5–4). Since pseudomembranes do not usually form in the adult, scarring does not usually occur. Superficial keratitis may be noted superiorly and, less often, a small superior micropannus (<1–2 mm). Subepithelial opacities, usually marginal, often develop. Otitis media may occur as a result of infection of the auditory tube.

B. Laboratory Findings

Because of the sexually transmitted nature of adult inclusion conjunctivitis and the need for systemic treatment of the patient and the patient's sexual partners, rapid diagnostic tests such as the direct fluorescent antibody test and enzyme-linked immunosorbent assay (ELISA) and PCR have replaced Giemsa staining in routine clinical practice. In the case of chlamydial ophthalmia neonatorum, rapid diagnosis is also imperative to prevent systemic complications such as chlamydial pneumonitis. Inclusion conjunctivitis is usually caused by *C trachomatis* serovars D–K with occasional isolations of serotype B. Serologic determinations are not useful in the diagnosis of ocular infections, but measurement of IgM antibody levels is extremely valuable in the diagnosis of chlamydial pneumonitis in infants.

▶ Differential Diagnosis

Inclusion conjunctivitis can be clinically differentiated from trachoma on the following grounds:

1. Active, follicular trachoma occurs commonly in young children or others living in or exposed to a community with endemic trachoma; inclusion conjunctivitis occurs in sexually active adolescents or adults.

2. Conjunctival scarring is very rare in adult inclusion conjunctivitis.

3. Herbert's pits serve as a hallmark of previous trachoma infection.

▶ Treatment

A. In Infants

Oral erythromycin suspension, 50 mg/kg/d in four divided doses for at least 14 days may be used to treat infants. Systemic treatment is necessary because chlamydial infection also involves the respiratory and gastrointestinal tracts. Topical antibiotics (tetracyclines, erythromycin, sulfonamides) are not useful in newborns treated with oral erythromycin. Both parents also should be treated with oral tetracycline or erythromycin.

B. In Adults

In adults, cure of chalmydial disease can be achieved with doxycycline, 100 mg orally twice daily for 7 days; erythromycin, 2 g/d for 7 days, or possibly azithromycin 1 g in a single dose. (Systemic tetracyclines should not be given to a pregnant woman or a child under 7 years of age, since they cause epiphysial problems in the fetus or staining of the young child's teeth.) The patient's sexual partners should be examined and treated.

When one of the standard therapeutic regimens is followed, recurrences are rare. If untreated, inclusion conjunctivitis runs a course of 3–9 months or longer with an average duration of 5 months.

3. CONJUNCTIVITIS CAUSED BY OTHER CHLAMYDIAL AGENTS

Lymphogranuloma venereum conjunctivitis is a rare sexually transmitted disease, manifesting as dramatic granulomatous conjunctival reaction with greatly enlarged preauricular nodes (Parinaud's syndrome). It is caused by *C trachomatis* serovars L1, L2, or L3.

Chlamydia psittaci only rarely causes conjunctivitis in humans. Strains from parrots (psittacosis) and cats (feline pneumonitis) have caused follicular conjunctivitis in humans. The prototype strains of *C pneumoniae* were isolated from the conjunctiva but have not been identified as a cause of ocular disease.

VIRAL CONJUNCTIVITIS

Viral conjunctivitis, a common affliction, can be caused by a wide variety of viruses. Severity ranges from severe, disabling disease to mild, rapidly self-limited infection.

1. ACUTE VIRAL FOLLICULAR CONJUNCTIVITIS

▶ Pharyngoconjunctival Fever

Pharyngoconjunctival fever is characterized by fever of 38.3–40°C, sore throat, and a follicular conjunctivitis in one or both eyes. The follicles are often very prominent on both the conjunctiva (Figure 5–5) and the pharyngeal mucosa. The disease can be either bilateral or unilateral. Injection and tearing often occur, and there may be transient superficial epithelial keratitis and occasionally some subepithelial opacities. Preauricular lymphadenopathy (nontender) is characteristic. The syndrome may be incomplete, consisting of only one or two of the cardinal signs (fever, pharyngitis, and conjunctivitis).

Pharyngoconjunctival fever is most frequently caused by adenovirus type 3 and occasionally by types 4 and 7. The virus can be grown on HeLa cells and identified by neutralization tests. As the disease progresses, it can also be diagnosed serologically by a rising titer of neutralizing antibody to the virus. Clinical diagnosis is a simple matter, however, and clearly more practical.

Conjunctival scrapings contain predominantly mononuclear cells, and no bacteria grow in cultures. The condition is more common in children than in adults and can be transmitted in poorly chlorinated swimming pools. The conjunctivitis is self-limited, and as such, only supportive treatment is indicated, with the episode resolving in approximately 10 days.

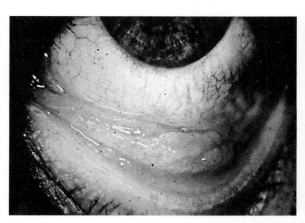

▲ **Figure 5–5.** Acute follicular conjunctivitis due to adenovirus type 3. (Courtesy of P Thygeson.)

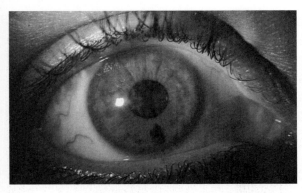

▲ **Figure 5–6.** Corneal findings in EKC. Note the uniform, central round subepithelial opacities present in the cornea. (Courtesy of University of California, Davis, Cornea and External Diseases.)

▶ Epidemic Keratoconjunctivitis

The onset of epidemic keratoconjunctivitis is often unilateral, with both eyes subsequently being affected but the first eye usually being more severely affected. Initial symptoms include conjunctival injection, moderate pain, and tearing. Usually by 5–14 days, photophobia, epithelial keratitis, and round subepithelial opacities have also developed (Figure 5–6). Corneal sensation is normal. A tender preauricular node is characteristic. Edema of the eyelids, chemosis, and conjunctival hyperemia mark the acute phase, with follicles and subconjunctival hemorrhages often appearing within 48 hours. Pseudomembranes (Figure 5–7) (and occasionally true membranes) may occur and may be followed by flat scars or symblepharon formation.

The conjunctivitis usually resolves by 3–4 weeks at most. The subepithelial opacities are concentrated in the central cornea, usually sparing the periphery, and may persist for months but generally heal without scars.

Epidemic keratoconjunctivitis is caused by adenovirus types 8, 19, 29, and 37 (subgroup D of the human adenoviruses). They can be isolated in cell culture and identified by neutralization tests. Scrapings from the conjunctiva show a primarily mononuclear inflammatory reaction (Figure 5–8); when pseudomembranes occur, neutrophils may also be prominent.

Epidemic keratoconjunctivitis in adults is confined to the external eye, but in children there may be systemic symptoms of viral infection as fever, sore throat, otitis media, and diarrhea. Nosocomial transmission during eye examinations takes place all too often by way of the physician's examination, use of improperly sterilized ophthalmic instruments, or use of contaminated solutions. Eye solutions, particularly topical anesthetics, can be contaminated when a dropper tip aspirates infected material from the conjunctiva or cilia. The virus can persist in the solution, which becomes a source of spread.

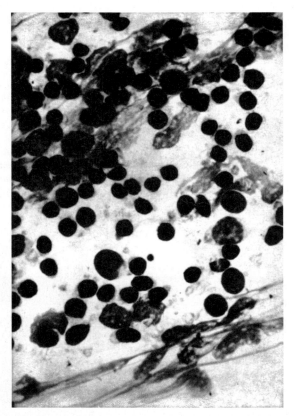

▲ **Figure 5–8.** Mononuclear cell reaction in conjunctival scrapings of a patient with viral conjunctivitis caused by adenovirus type 8. (Courtesy of M Okumoto.)

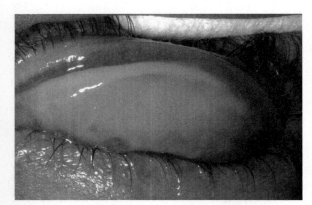

▲ **Figure 5–7.** Thick white pseudomembrane on upper palpebral conjunctiva in epidemic keratoconjunctivitis.

The danger of contaminated solution bottles can be avoided by the use of individual sterile droppers or unit-dose packages of eye drops. Regular hand washing between examinations and careful cleaning and sterilization of instruments that touch the eyes—especially tonometers—are also mandatory. Applanation tonometers should be cleaned by wiping with alcohol or hypochlorite, then rinsing with sterile water and carefully drying.

There is no specific therapy at present, but cold compresses and artificial tears will relieve some symptoms. Corticosteroids utilized during acute conjunctivitis may prolong late corneal involvement and should be avoided whenever possible. Antibacterial agents should be administered if bacterial superinfection occurs.

Herpes Simplex Virus Conjunctivitis

Herpes simplex virus (HSV) conjunctivitis, usually a disease of young children, is an uncommon entity characterized by unilateral injection, irritation, mucoid discharge, pain, and mild photophobia. It occurs during primary infection with HSV or during recurrent episodes of ocular herpes (Figure 5–9). It is often associated with herpes simplex keratitis, in which the cornea shows discrete epithelial lesions that usually coalesce to form single or multiple branching epithelial (dendritic) ulcers (Figure 5–10). The conjunctivitis is follicular or, less often, pseudomembranous. (Patients receiving topical antivirals may develop follicular conjunctivitis that can be differentiated because the herpetic follicular conjunctivitis has an acute onset.) Herpetic vesicles may sometimes appear on the eyelids and lid margins, associated with severe edema of the eyelids. Typically, there is a small tender preauricular node.

No bacteria are found in scrapings or recovered in cultures. If the conjunctivitis is follicular, the predominant inflammatory reaction is mononuclear, but if it is pseudomembranous, the predominant reaction is polymorphonuclear,

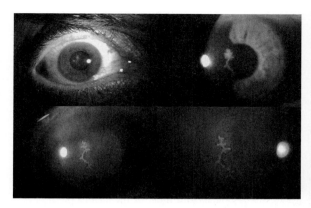

▲ **Figure 5–10.** Dendritic ulcer in HSV keratitis. (Courtesy of University of California, Davis, Cornea and External Diseases.)

owing to the chemotaxis of necrosis. Intranuclear inclusions (because of the margination of the chromatin) can be seen in conjunctival and corneal cells if Bouin fixation and the Papanicolaou stain are used but not in Giemsa-stained smears. The finding of multinucleated giant epithelial cells has diagnostic value.

The virus can be readily isolated by gently rubbing a dry Dacron or calcium alginate swab over the conjunctiva and transferring the infected cells to a susceptible tissue culture.

HSV conjunctivitis may persist for 2–3 weeks, and if it is pseudomembranous, it may leave fine linear or flat scars. Complications consist of corneal involvement (including dendrites) and vesicles on the skin. Although type 1 herpesvirus causes the overwhelming majority of ocular cases, type 2 is the usual cause of herpetic conjunctivitis in newborns and a rare cause in adults. In the newborn, there may be generalized disease with encephalitis, chorioretinitis, hepatitis, etc. Any HSV infection in the newborn must be treated with systemic antiviral therapy (acyclovir) and monitored in a hospital setting.

If the conjunctivitis occurs in a child over 1 year of age or in an adult, it is usually self-limited and may not require therapy. Topical or systemic antivirals should be given, however, to prevent corneal involvement. For corneal ulcers, corneal debridement may be performed by gently wiping the ulcer with a dry cotton swab, applying antiviral drops, and patching the eye for 24 hours. Topical antivirals alone should be applied for 7–10 days (eg, trifluridine every 2 hours while awake). Herpetic keratitis may also be treated with 3% acyclovir ointment (not available in the United States) five times daily for 10 days, or with oral acyclovir, 400 mg five times daily for 7 days. Corticosteroid use is contraindicated since it may aggravate herpetic infections causing a prolonged and usually more severe course.

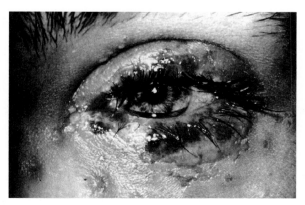

▲ **Figure 5–9.** Primary ocular herpes. (Courtesy of HB Ostler.)

Newcastle Disease Conjunctivitis

Newcastle disease conjunctivitis is a rare disorder characterized by burning, itching, pain, redness, tearing, and (rarely) blurring of vision. It often occurs in small epidemics among poultry workers handling infected birds or among veterinarians or laboratory helpers working with live vaccines or virus.

The conjunctivitis resembles that caused by other viral agents, with chemosis, a small preauricular node, and follicles on the upper and lower tarsus. No treatment is available or necessary for this self-limited disease.

Acute Hemorrhagic Conjunctivitis

All of the continents and most of the islands of the world have had major epidemics of acute hemorrhagic conjunctivitis. It was first recognized in Ghana in 1969. It is caused by enterovirus type 70 and occasionally by coxsackievirus A24.

Characteristically, the disease has a short incubation period (8–48 hours) and course (5–7 days). The usual signs and symptoms are pain, photophobia, foreign-body sensation, copious tearing, redness, lid edema, and subconjunctival hemorrhages (Figure 5–11). Chemosis sometimes also occurs. The subconjunctival hemorrhages are usually diffuse but may be punctate at onset, beginning in the upper bulbar conjunctiva and spreading to the lower. Most patients have preauricular lymphadenopathy, conjunctival follicles, and epithelial keratitis. Anterior uveitis has been reported; fever, malaise, and generalized myalgia have been observed in 25% of cases; and motor paralysis of the lower extremities has occurred in rare cases in India and Japan.

The virus is transmitted by close person-to-person contact and by such fomites as common linens, contaminated optical instruments, and water. Recovery occurs within 5–7 days, and there is no known treatment. In the United States, at times closure of schools has been needed to stop epidemics.

Molluscum Contagiosum Blepharoconjunctivitis

A molluscum nodule on the lid margins or the skin of the lids or brow may produce unilateral chronic follicular conjunctivitis, superior keratitis, and superior pannus that resembles trachoma. The inflammatory reaction is predominantly mononuclear (unlike the reaction in trachoma), and the round, waxy, pearly-white, noninflammatory lesion with an umbilicated center is typical of molluscum contagiosum (Figure 5–12). Biopsy shows eosinophilic cytoplasmic inclusions that fill the entire cytoplasm of the enlarged cell, pushing its nucleus to one side.

Excision or simple incision of the nodule, thus allowing peripheral blood to permeate it, or cryotherapy cures the conjunctivitis. On very rare occasions, molluscum nodules have occurred on the conjunctiva. In these cases, excision of the nodule has also relieved the conjunctivitis. Multiple lid or facial lesions of molluscum contagiosum occur in patients with AIDS.

Varicella-Zoster Blepharoconjunctivitis

Hyperemia and an infiltrative conjunctivitis—associated with the typical vesicular eruption along the dermatomal distribution of the ophthalmic branch of the trigeminal nerve (Figure 5–13) —are characteristic of ophthalmic (herpes) zoster (shingles), due to reactivation of varicella-zoster virus infection. The conjunctivitis is usually papillary, but follicles, pseudomembranes, and transitory vesicles that later ulcerate have all been noted. A tender preauricular lymph node occurs early in the disease. Scarring of the lid, entropion, and the misdirection of individual lashes are sequelae.

The lid lesions of varicella, which are like the skin lesions (pox) elsewhere, may appear on both the lid margins and the

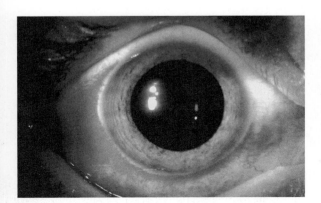

▲ **Figure 5–11.** Acute hemorrhagic conjunctivitis.

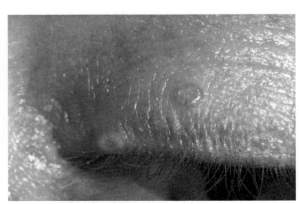

▲ **Figure 5–12.** Molluscum contagiosum of lid margin. Follicular conjunctivitis was present.

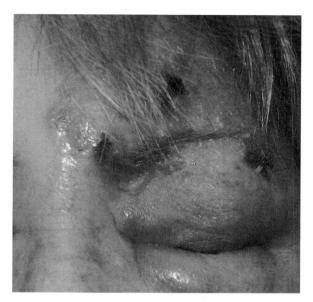

▲ **Figure 5–13.** Characteristic vesicular rash affecting the V1 dermatome in ophthalmic zoster (shingles).

lids and often leave scars. A mild exudative conjunctivitis often occurs, but discrete conjunctival lesions (except at the limbus) are very rare. Limbal lesions resemble phlyctenules and may go through all the stages of vesicle, papule, and ulcer. The adjacent cornea becomes infiltrated and may vascularize.

In both zoster and varicella, scrapings from lid vesicles contain giant cells and a predominance of polymorphonuclear leukocytes; scrapings from the conjunctiva in varicella and from conjunctival vesicles in zoster may contain giant cells and monocytes. The virus can be recovered in tissue cultures of human embryo cells.

In the immunocompetent, oral antiviral therapy (acyclovir 800 mg orally five times daily, famciclovir, 500 mg three times daily, or valacyclovir, 1 g three times daily, all for 7 days), if started within 72 hours after appearance of the rash, reduces the incidence of ocular complications but not necessarily of postherpetic neuralgia. The value of supplementary therapy with oral prednisone, initially 60 mg per day reducing over 3 weeks, is uncertain. In the immunocompromised, oral antiviral therapy should be continued for up to 2 weeks and may need to be given intravenously if there is evidence of progression of disease. Oral prednisone is contraindicated.

▶ Measles Keratoconjunctivitis

The characteristic enanthem of measles frequently precedes the skin eruption. At this early stage, the conjunctiva may have a peculiar glassy appearance, followed within a few days

by swelling of the semilunar fold (Meyer's sign). Several days before the skin eruption, an exudative conjunctivitis with a mucopurulent discharge develops. At the time of the skin eruption, Koplik's spots appear on the conjunctiva and occasionally on the caruncle. At some time (early in children, late in adults), epithelial keratitis supervenes.

In the immunocompetent patient, measles keratoconjunctivitis has few or no sequelae, but in malnourished or otherwise immunocompromised patients, the ocular disease is frequently associated with a secondary HSV or bacterial infection due to *S pneumoniae, H influenzae,* and other organisms. These agents may lead to purulent conjunctivitis with associated corneal ulceration and severe visual loss. Herpes infection can cause severe corneal ulceration with corneal perforation and loss of vision in poorly nourished children in developing countries.

Conjunctival scrapings show a mononuclear cell reaction unless there are pseudomembranes or secondary infection. Giemsa-stained preparations contain giant cells. Since there is no specific therapy, only supportive measures are indicated unless a secondary infection is present.

RICKETTSIAL CONJUNCTIVITIS

All rickettsiae recognized as pathogenic for humans may attack the conjunctiva, and the conjunctiva may be their portal of entry.

Q fever is associated with severe conjunctival hyperemia. Treatment with systemic tetracycline or chloramphenicol is curative.

Marseilles fever (boutonneuse fever) is often associated with ulcerative or granulomatous conjunctivitis and a grossly visible preauricular lymph node.

Endemic (murine) typhus, scrub typhus, Rocky Mountain spotted fever, and **epidemic typhus** have associated, variable, and usually mild conjunctival signs.

FUNGAL CONJUNCTIVITIS

▶ Candidal Conjunctivitis

Conjunctivitis caused by *Candida* species (usually *Candida albicans*) is a rare infection that usually appears as a white plaque. This may occur in diabetics or immunocompromised patients as an ulcerative or granulomatous conjunctivitis.

Scrapings show a polymorphonuclear cell inflammatory reaction. The organism grows readily on blood agar or Sabouraud's medium and can be readily identified as a budding yeast or, rarely, as pseudohyphae.

The infection responds to amphotericin B (3–8 mg/mL) in aqueous (not saline) solution or to applications of nystatin dermatologic cream (100,000 U/g) four to six times daily. The ointment must be applied carefully to ensure that it reaches the conjunctival sac and does not just build up on the lid margins.

Other Fungal Conjunctivitides

Sporothrix schenckii may rarely involve the conjunctiva or the eyelids. It is a granulomatous disease associated with a visible preauricular node. Microscopic examination of a biopsy of the granuloma reveals gram-positive, cigar-shaped conidia (spores).

Rhinosporidium seeberi may rarely affect the conjunctiva, lacrimal sac, lids, canaliculi, and sclera. The typical lesion is a polypoid granuloma that bleeds after minimal trauma. Histologic examination shows a granuloma with enclosed large spherules containing myriad endospores. Treatment is by simple excision and cauterization of the base.

Coccidioides immitis may rarely cause a granulomatous conjunctivitis associated with a grossly visible preauricular node (Parinaud's oculoglandular syndrome). This is not a primary disease but a manifestation of metastatic infection from a primary pulmonary infection (San Joaquin Valley fever). Disseminated disease suggests a poor prognosis.

PARASITIC CONJUNCTIVITIS

Thelazia californiensis Infection

The natural habitat of this roundworm is the eye of the dog, but it can also infect the eyes of cats, sheep, black bears, horses, and deer. Accidental infection of the human conjunctival sac has occurred. The disease can be treated effectively by removing the worms from the conjunctival sac with forceps or a cotton-tipped applicator.

Loa loa Infection

L loa is the eye worm of Africa. It lives in the connective tissue of humans and monkeys, and the monkey may be its reservoir. The parasite is transmitted by the bite of the horse or mango fly. The mature worm may then migrate to the lid, the conjunctiva, or the orbit.

Infection with *L loa* is accompanied by a 60–80% eosinophilia, but diagnosis is made by identifying the worm on removal or by finding microfilariae in blood examined at midday.

Diethylcarbamazine is currently the drug of choice.

Ascaris lumbricoides Infection (Butcher's Conjunctivitis)

Ascaris may cause a rare type of violent conjunctivitis. When butchers or persons performing postmortem examinations cut tissue containing ascaris, the tissue juice of some of the organisms may accidentally splash in the eye. A violent and painful toxic conjunctivitis ensues, marked by extreme chemosis and lid edema. Treatment consists of rapid and thorough irrigation of the conjunctival sac.

Trichinella spiralis Infection

T spiralis does not cause a true conjunctivitis, but in the course of its general dissemination, there may be a doughy edema of the upper and lower eyelids, and over 50% of patients have chemosis—a pale, lemon-yellow swelling most marked over the lateral and medial rectus muscles and fading toward the limbus. The chemosis may last a week or more, and there is often pain on movement of the eyes.

Schistosoma haematobium Infection

Schistosomiasis (bilharziasis) is endemic in Egypt, especially in the region irrigated by the Nile. Granulomatous conjunctival lesions appearing as small, soft, smooth, pinkish-yellow tumors occur, especially in males. The symptoms are minimal. Diagnosis depends on microscopic examination of biopsy material, which shows a granuloma-containing lymphocytes, plasma cells, giant cells, and eosinophils surrounding bilharzial ova in various stages of disintegration.

Treatment consists of excision of the conjunctival granuloma and systemic therapy with antimonials such as niridazole.

Taenia solium Infection

T Solium rarely causes conjunctivitis but more often invades the retina, choroid, or vitreous to produce ocular cysticercosis. As a rule, the affected conjunctiva shows a subconjunctival cyst in the form of a localized hemispherical swelling, usually at the inner angle of the lower fornix, which is adherent to the underlying sclera and painful on pressure. The conjunctiva and lid may be inflamed and edematous.

Diagnosis is based on a positive complement fixation or precipitin test or on demonstration of the organism in the gastrointestinal tract. Eosinophilia is a constant feature.

The best treatment is to excise the lesion. The intestinal condition can be treated by niclosamide.

Pthirus pubis Infection (Pubic Louse Infection)

P. pubis may infest the cilia and margins of the eyelids. Because of its size, the pubic louse seems to require widely spaced hair. For this reason it has a predilection for the widely spaced cilia as well as for pubic hair. The parasites apparently release an irritating substance (probably feces) that produces a toxic follicular conjunctivitis in children and an irritating papillary conjunctivitis in adults. The lid margin is usually red, and the patient may complain of intense itching.

Finding the adult organism or the ova-shaped nits cemented to the eyelashes is diagnostic.

Lindane (Kwell) 1% or RID (pyrethrins), applied to the pubic area and lash margins after removal of the nits, is usually curative. Application of lindane or RID to the lid margins must be undertaken with great care to avoid contact with the eye. Any ointment applied to the lid margin tends to smother the adult organisms. The patient's family and close contacts should be examined and treated. All clothes and fomites should be carefully washed.

Ophthalmomyiasis

Myiasis is infection with larvae of flies. Many different species of flies may produce myiasis. The ocular tissues may be injured by mechanical transmission of disease-producing organisms and by the parasitic activities of the larvae in the ocular tissues. The larvae are able to invade either necrotic or healthy tissue. Many individuals become infected by accidental ingestion of the eggs or larvae or by contamination of external wounds or skin. Infants and young children, alcoholics, and debilitated unattended patients are common targets for infection with myiasis-producing flies.

These larvae may affect the ocular surface, the intraocular tissues, or the deeper orbital tissues.

Ocular surface involvement may be caused by *Musca domestica,* the housefly, *Fannia,* the latrine fly, and *Oestrus ovis,* the sheep botfly. These flies deposit their eggs at the lower lid margin or inner canthus, and the larvae may remain on the surface of the eye, causing irritation, pain, and conjunctival hyperemia.

Treatment of ocular surface myiasis is by mechanical removal of the larvae after topical anesthesia.

▼ IMMUNOLOGIC (ALLERGIC) CONJUNCTIVITIS

IMMEDIATE HUMORAL HYPERSENSITIVITY REACTIONS

1. HAY FEVER CONJUNCTIVITIS

A mild, nonspecific conjunctival inflammation is commonly associated with hay fever (allergic rhinitis). In most cases, there is a history of allergy to pollens, grasses, animal danders, etc. The patient complains of itching, tearing, and redness of the eyes and often states that the eyes seem to be "sinking into the surrounding tissue." There is mild injection of the palpebral and bulbar conjunctiva, and during acute attacks often a severe chemosis, which no doubt accounts for the "sinking" description (Figure 5–14). There may be a small

amount of ropy discharge, especially if the patient has been rubbing the eyes. Eosinophils are difficult to find in conjunctival scrapings. A papillary conjunctivitis may occur if the allergen persists.

Treatment consists of the instillation of topical antihistamine-vasoconstrictor preparations. Cold compresses are helpful to relieve itching, and antihistamines by mouth are of some value. The immediate response to treatment is satisfactory, but recurrences are common unless the antigen is eliminated. Fortunately, the frequency of the attacks and the severity of the symptoms tend to moderate as the patient ages.

2. VERNAL KERATOCONJUNCTIVITIS

Vernal keratoconjunctivitis, also known as "spring catarrh," "seasonal conjunctivitis" or "warm weather conjunctivitis," is an uncommon bilateral allergic disease that usually begins in the prepubertal years and lasts for 5–10 years. It occurs much more often in boys than in girls. The specific allergen or allergens are difficult to identify, but patients with vernal keratoconjunctivitis usually show other manifestations of allergy known to be related to grass pollen sensitivity. The disease is less common in temperate than in warm climates and is almost nonexistent in cold climates. It is almost always more severe during the spring, summer, and fall than in the winter. It is most commonly seen in sub-Saharan Africa and the Middle East.

The patient usually complains of extreme itching and a ropy discharge. There is often a family history of allergy (hay fever, eczema, etc), and sometimes there is a history of allergy in the young patient as well. The conjunctiva has a milky appearance with many fine papillae in the lower palpebral conjunctiva. The upper palpebral conjunctiva often has giant papillae that give a cobblestone appearance (Figure 5–15). Each giant papilla is polygonal, has a flat top, and contains tufts of capillaries.

A stringy conjunctival discharge and a fine, fibrinous pseudomembrane (Maxwell-Lyons sign) may be noted, especially on the upper tarsus on exposure to heat. In some cases, especially in persons of black African ancestry, the most prominent lesions are located at the limbus, where gelatinous

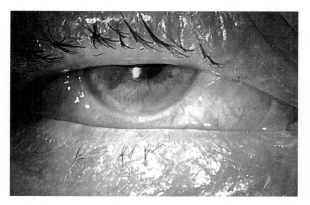

▲ **Figure 5–14.** Hay fever conjunctivitis with moderate to marked chemosis, mild injection of the conjunctiva, and the appearance of the eye "sinking" into the surrounding tissue.

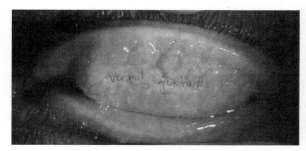

▲ **Figure 5–15.** "Cobblestone" papillae on the superior palpebral conjunctiva in vernal keratoconjunctivitis.

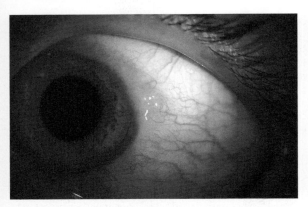

▲ **Figure 5–16.** Limbal papillae associated with vernal keratoconjunctivitis in a young male. (Courtesy of University of California, Davis, Cornea and External Diseases.)

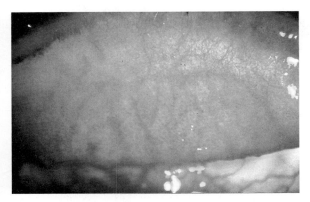

▲ **Figure 5–17.** Moderate to marked papillary response of upper palpebral conjunctiva in atopic keratoconjunctivitis.

swellings (papillae) are noted (Figure 5–16). A pseudogerontoxon (arcus-like haze) is often noted in the cornea adjacent to the limbal papillae. Trantas' dots are whitish dots seen at the limbus in some patients with vernal keratoconjunctivitis during the active phase of the disease. Many eosinophils and free eosinophilic granules are found in Giemsa-stained smears of the conjunctival exudate and in Trantas' dots.

Micropannus is often seen in both palpebral and limbal vernal keratoconjunctivitis, but gross pannus is unusual. Conjunctival scarring usually does not occur unless the patient has been treated with cryotherapy, surgical removal of the papillae, irradiation, or other damaging procedure. Superficial corneal ("shield") ulcers (oval and located superiorly) may form and may be followed by mild corneal scarring. A characteristic diffuse epithelial keratitis frequently occurs. None of the corneal lesions respond well to standard treatment.

The disease may also be associated with keratoconus.

▶ Treatment

Since vernal keratoconjunctivitis is a self-limited disease, it must be recognized that the medication used to treat the symptoms may provide short-term benefit but long-term harm. Topical and systemic steroids, which relieve the itching, affect the corneal disease only minimally, and their side effects (glaucoma, cataract, and other complications) can be severely damaging. Newer mast cell stabilizer-antihistamine combinations are useful prophylactic and therapeutic agents in moderate to severe cases. Vasoconstrictors, cold compresses, and ice packs are helpful, and sleeping (and, if possible, working) in cool, air-conditioned rooms can keep the patient reasonably comfortable. Probably the best remedy of all is to relocate to a cool, moist climate. Patients able to do so benefit from a marked reduction in symptoms, if not a complete cure.

The acute symptoms of an extremely photophobic patient who is unable to function can often be relieved by a short course of topical or systemic steroids followed by vasoconstrictors, cold packs, and regular use of histamine-blocking eye drops. Topical nonsteroidal anti-inflammatory agents, such as ketorolac, mast cell stabilizers, such as lodoxamide, and topical antihistamines (see Chapter 22) may provide significant symptomatic relief but may slow the reepithelialization of a shield ulcer. As has already been indicated, the prolonged use of steroids should be avoided. Recent clinical studies have shown that topical 2% cyclosporine eye drops are effective in severe unresponsive cases. Supratarsal injection of depot corticosteroids with or without surgical excision of giant papillae has been demonstrated to be effective for vernal shield ulcers.

Desensitization to grass pollens and other antigens has not been rewarding. Staphylococcal blepharitis and conjunctivitis are frequent complications and should be treated. Recurrences are the rule, particularly in the spring and summer; but after a number of recurrences, the papillae disappear completely, leaving no scars.

3. ATOPIC KERATOCONJUNCTIVITIS

Patients with atopic dermatitis (eczema) often also have atopic keratoconjunctivitis. The symptoms and signs are a burning sensation, mucoid discharge, redness, and photophobia. The lid margins are erythematous, and the conjunctiva has a milky appearance. There are fine papillae (Figure 5–17), but giant papillae are less developed than in vernal keratoconjunctivitis and occur more frequently on the lower rather than upper palpebral conjunctiva. Severe corneal signs appear late in the disease after repeated exacerbations of the conjunctivitis. Superficial peripheral keratitis develops and is followed by vascularization. In severe cases, the entire cornea becomes hazy and vascularized, and visual acuity is reduced.

There is usually a history of allergy (hay fever, asthma, or eczema) affecting the patient or the patient's family. Most patients have had atopic dermatitis since infancy. Scarring of the flexure creases of the antecubital folds and of the wrists and knees is common. Like the dermatitis with which it is associated, atopic keratoconjunctivitis has a protracted course and is subject to exacerbations and remissions. As in vernal keratoconjunctivitis, it tends to become less active when the patient reaches the fifth decade.

Scrapings of the conjunctiva show eosinophils, though not nearly as many as are seen in vernal keratoconjunctivitis. Scarring of both the conjunctiva and cornea is often seen, and an atopic cataract, a posterior subcapsular plaque, or an anterior shield-like cataract may develop. Keratoconus, retinal detachment, and herpes simplex keratitis are all more likely than usual in patients with atopic keratoconjunctivitis, and there are many cases of secondary bacterial blepharitis and conjunctivitis, usually staphylococcal.

The management of atopic keratoconjunctivitis is often discouraging. Any secondary infection must be treated. Environmental control should be considered. Chronic topical therapy with mast cell stabilizers, antihistamines, and nonsteroidal anti-inflammatory agents (see Chapter 22) is the mainstay in treatment. Oral antihistamines are also beneficial. A short course of topical steroids may also relieve symptoms. In severe cases, plasmapheresis or systemic immunosuppression may be an adjunct to therapy. In advanced cases with severe corneal complications, corneal transplantation may be needed to improve the visual acuity.

4. GIANT PAPILLARY CONJUNCTIVITIS

Giant papillary conjunctivitis with signs and symptoms resembling those of vernal conjunctivitis may develop in patients wearing plastic artificial eyes or contact lenses (Figure 5–18). It is probably a basophil-rich delayed hypersensitivity disorder (Jones-Mote hypersensitivity), perhaps with an IgE humoral component. Use of glass instead of plastic for prostheses and spectacle lenses instead of contact lenses is curative. If the goal is to maintain contact lens wear, additional therapy will be required. Careful contact lens care, including preservative-free agents, is essential. Hydrogen peroxide disinfection and enzymatic cleaning of contact lenses may also help. Alternatively, changing to a weekly disposable or daily disposable contact lens system may be beneficial. If these treatments are unsuccessful, use of contact lenses should be discontinued.

DELAYED HYPERSENSITIVITY REACTIONS

1. PHLYCTENULOSIS

Phlyctenular keratoconjunctivitis is a Type IV delayed hypersensitivity response to microbial proteins, including the proteins of the tubercle bacillus, *Staphylococcus* species, *C albicans, Coccidioides immitis, H aegyptius,* and *C trachomatis* serovars L1, L2, and L3. Until recently, by far the most frequent cause of phlyctenulosis in the United States was delayed hypersensitivity to the protein of the human tubercle bacillus. This is still the most common cause in regions where tuberculosis is still prevalent. In the United States, however, most cases are now associated with delayed hypersensitivity to *S. aureus.*

The conjunctival phlyctenule begins as a small lesion (usually 1–3 mm in diameter) that is hard, red, elevated, and surrounded by a zone of hyperemia. At the limbus it is often triangular in shape, with its apex toward the cornea (Figure 5–19). In this location it develops a grayish-white center that soon ulcerates and then subsides within 10–12 days. The patient's first phlyctenule and most of the recurrences develop at the limbus, but there may also be corneal, bulbar, and, very rarely, even tarsal phlyctenules.

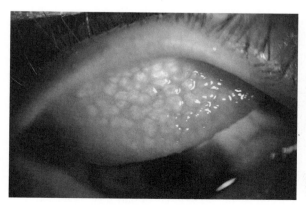

▲ **Figure 5–18.** Giant papillary conjunctivitis associated with soft contact lens wear.

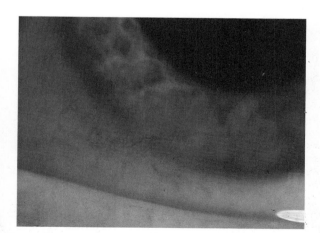

▲ **Figure 5–19.** Mild Phlyctenule probably secondary to staph marginal disease in a 30-year-old female that improved with corticosteroid treatment.

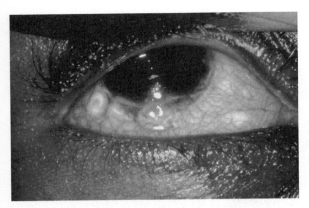

▲ **Figure 5–20.** Phlyctenulosis with three phlyctenules along the inferior limbus, each with an umbilicated center.

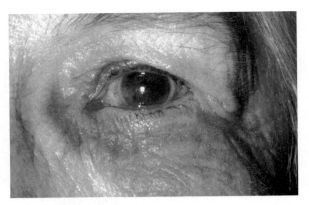

▲ **Figure 5–21.** Contact dermatitis secondary to neomycin, with particular involvement of the lower eyelid.

Unlike the conjunctival phlyctenule, which leaves no scar, the corneal phlyctenule develops as an amorphous gray infiltrate and always leaves a scar. Consistent with this difference is the fact that scars form on the corneal side of the limbal lesion and not on the conjunctival side. The result is a triangular scar with its base at the limbus—a valuable sign of old phlyctenulosis when the limbus has been involved.

Conjunctival phlyctenules usually produce only irritation and tearing, but corneal and limbal phlyctenules are usually accompanied by intense photophobia. Phlyctenulosis is often triggered by active blepharitis, acute bacterial conjunctivitis, and dietary deficiencies (Figure 5–20). Phlyctenular scarring, which may be minimal or extensive, is often followed by Salzmann's nodular degeneration.

Histologically, the phlyctenule is a focal subepithelial and perivascular infiltration of small round cells, followed by a preponderance of polymorphonuclear cells when the overlying epithelium necrotizes and sloughs—a sequence of events characteristic of the delayed tuberculin-type hypersensitivity reaction.

Phlyctenulosis induced by tuberculoprotein and the proteins of other systemic infections responds dramatically to topical corticosteroids. A major reduction of symptoms occurs within 24 hours and disappearance of the lesion in another 24 hours. Phlyctenulosis produced by staphylococcal proteins responds somewhat more slowly. Topical antibiotics should be added for active staphylococcal blepharoconjunctivitis. Treatment should be aimed at the underlying disease, and steroids, when effective, should be used only to control acute symptoms and persistent corneal scarring. Severe corneal scarring may require corneal transplantation.

2. MILD CONJUNCTIVITIS SECONDARY TO CONTACT BLEPHARITIS

Contact blepharitis caused by atropine, neomycin, broad-spectrum antibiotics, and other topically applied medications, or the preservatives in them, is often followed by a mild infiltrative conjunctivitis that produces hyperemia, mild papillary hypertrophy, a mild mucoid discharge, and some irritation (Figure 5–21). Examination of Giemsa-stained scrapings often discloses only a few degenerated epithelial cells, a few polymorphonuclear and mononuclear cells, and no eosinophils.

Treatment should be directed toward finding the offending agent and eliminating it. The contact blepharitis may clear rapidly with topical corticosteroids, but their use should be limited. Long-term use of steroids on the lids may lead to steroid glaucoma and to skin atrophy with disfiguring telangiectasis.

CONJUNCTIVITIS DUE TO AUTOIMMUNE DISEASE

SJÖGREN'S SYNDROME

Sjögren's syndrome is an autoimmune disease characterized by dry eye syndrome (keratoconjunctivitis sicca) and dry mouth (xerostomia). When associated with a generalized autoimmune disease, usually rheumatoid arthritis, it is known as secondary rather than primary Sjögren's syndrome. The syndrome is overwhelmingly more common in women at or beyond the menopause than in other groups, although men and younger women may also be affected. The lacrimal gland is infiltrated with lymphocytes and occasionally with plasma cells, leading to atrophy and destruction of the glandular structures.

Dry eye syndrome is characterized by bulbar conjunctival hyperemia (especially in the palpebral aperture) and symptoms of irritation that are out of proportion to the mild inflammatory sign, pain increasing by the afternoon and evening but being absent or only slight in the morning. It often begins as a mild conjunctivitis with a mucoid discharge. Blotchy epithelial lesions appear on the cornea, more

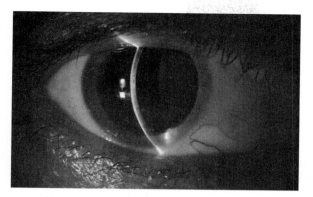

▲ **Figure 5–22.** Demonstration with fluorescein staining of punctuate epithelial erosions found in dry eye syndrome due to Sjogren's syndrome, with greater distribution of epithelial lesions inferiorly. See color insert. (Courtesy of University of California, Davis, Cornea and External Diseases.)

prominently in its lower half (Figure 5–22), and filaments may be seen. Rose bengal or lissamine green staining of the cornea and conjunctiva in the palpebral aperture is a helpful diagnostic test. The tear film is diminished and often contains shreds of mucus. Results of the Schirmer test are abnormal.

The diagnosis is confirmed by demonstrating lymphocytic and plasma cell infiltration of the accessory salivary glands in a labial biopsy obtained by means of a simple surgical procedure (Figure 5–23).

Treatment should be directed toward preserving and improving the quality of the tear film with artificial tears, with obliteration of the puncta, and with side shields, moisture chambers, and Buller shields. Recent clinical studies have demonstrated the efficacy of preservative-free, low-dose corticosteroid preparations and topical cyclosporine in the treatment of Sjögren's syndrome. As a rule, the simpler measures should be tried first.

(Dry eye syndrome [keratoconjunctivitis sicca] is also discussed in the subsequent section on Tears.)

MUCOUS MEMBRANE (OCULAR CICATRICIAL) PEMPHIGOID

Mucous membrane pemphigoid usually begins as a nonspecific chronic conjunctivitis that is resistant to therapy. The conjunctiva may be affected alone or, as indicated by its name, in combination with the mouth, nose, esophagus, vulva, and skin. The conjunctivitis leads to progressive scarring, obliteration of the fornices (especially the lower fornix), symblepharon formation (Figure 5–24), and entropion with trichiasis. The patient complains of pain, irritation, and blurring of vision. The cornea is affected only secondarily as a result of trichiasis and lack of the precorneal tear film. The disease is often more severe in women than in men and typically occurs in middle life, very rarely before age 45. In women, it may progress to blindness in a year or less; in men, progress is slower, and spontaneous remission sometimes occurs.

Conjunctival biopsies may contain eosinophils, and the basement membrane will stain positively with certain immunofluorescent stains (IgG, IgM, IgA complement). Active inflammatory disease may respond to dapsone or conventional immunosuppressant therapy but newer agents, such as tumor necrosis factor (TNF) antagonist, increasingly are being used. The secondary consequences, such as tear deficiency,

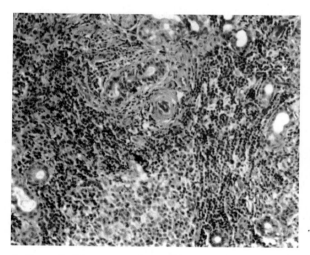

▲ **Figure 5–23.** Mononuclear infiltration of the accessory salivary glands of a patient with Sjögren's syndrome. (Courtesy of K Tabbara.)

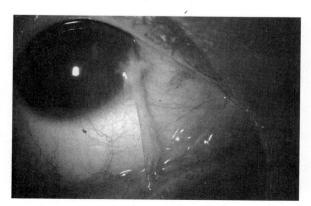

▲ **Figure 5–24.** Symblepharon formation in mucous membrane pemphigoid.

trichiais, and ocular toxicity need to be recognized and treated appropriately. Generally, the course is long and the prognosis poor, with blindness due to complete symblepharon and corneal desiccation.

▼ CHEMICAL OR IRRITATIVE CONJUNCTIVITIS

IATROGENIC CONJUNCTIVITIS FROM TOPICALLY APPLIED DRUGS

A toxic follicular conjunctivitis or an infiltrative, nonspecific conjunctivitis, followed by scarring, is often produced by the prolonged administration of topical medications such as idoxuridine, brimonidine, apraclonidine, and dipivefrin, or by preservatives in eye drops. Silver nitrate instilled into the conjunctival sac at birth (Credë prophylaxis) is a frequent cause of mild chemical conjunctivitis. If tear production is reduced by continual irritation, the conjunctiva can be further damaged by the lack of dilution of the noxious agent as it is instilled into the conjunctival sac.

Conjunctival scrapings often contain keratinized epithelial cells, a few polymorphonuclear neutrophils, and an occasional oddly shaped cell. Treatment consists of stopping the offending agent and using bland drops or none at all. Often the conjunctival reaction persists for weeks or months after its cause has been eliminated.

OCCUPATIONAL CONJUNCTIVITIS FROM CHEMICALS & IRRITANTS

Acids, alkalies, smoke, wind, and almost any irritating substance that enters the conjunctival sac may cause conjunctivitis. Some common irritants are fertilizers, soaps, deodorants, hair sprays, tobacco, makeup preparations (mascara, etc), and various acids and alkalies. In certain areas, smog has become the most common cause of mild chemical conjunctivitis. The specific irritant in smog has not been positively identified, and treatment is nonspecific. There are no permanent ocular effects, but affected eyes are frequently chronically red and irritated.

In acid burns, the acids denature the tissue proteins and the effect is immediate. Alkalies do not denature the proteins, but tend to penetrate the tissues deeply and rapidly and to linger in the conjunctival tissue. Once in contact with the ocular surface, alkalies saponify fatty acids and continue to inflict damage for hours or days, depending on the molar concentration of the alkali and the amount introduced. Adhesions between the bulbar and palpebral conjunctiva (symblepharon) and corneal scarring are more likely to occur if the offending agent is an alkali. In either event, pain, injection, photophobia, and blepharospasm are the principal symptoms of caustic burns. A careful history will usually the identify the precipitating event.

Immediate and profuse irrigation of the conjunctival sac with water or saline solution is of great importance, and any solid material should be removed mechanically. Do not use chemical antidotes. Further treatment may involve intensive topical steroids, ascorbate and citrate eyedrops, cycloplegics, antiglaucoma treatment as necessary, cold compresses, and systemic analgesics (see Chapter 19). Bacterial conjunctivitis may be treated with appropriate antibacterial agents. Corneal scarring may require corneal transplantation, and symblepharon may require reconstruction of the conjunctiva. Severe conjunctival and corneal burns have a poor prognosis even with surgery, but if proper treatment is started immediately, scarring may be minimized and the prognosis improved.

CATERPILLAR HAIR CONJUNCTIVITIS (OPHTHALMIA NODOSUM)

On rare occasions, caterpillar hairs are introduced into the conjunctival sac, where they produce one or many granulomas (ophthalmia nodosum). Under magnification, each granuloma is seen to contain a small foreign body.

Treatment by removal of each hair individually is effective. If a hair is retained, invasion of the sclera and uveal tract may occur.

▼ CONJUNCTIVITIS OF UNKNOWN CAUSE

FOLLICULOSIS

Folliculosis is a widespread benign, bilateral noninflammatory conjunctival condition characterized by follicular hypertrophy. It is more common in children than in adults, and the symptoms are minimal. The follicles are more numerous in the lower than in the upper cul-de-sac and palpebral conjunctiva. There is no associated inflammation or papillary hypertrophy, and complications do not occur.

There is no treatment for folliculosis, which disappears spontaneously after a course of 2–3 years. The cause is unknown, but folliculosis may be only a manifestation of a generalized adenoidal hypertrophy.

CHRONIC FOLLICULAR CONJUNCTIVITIS (AXENFELD'S CONJUNCTIVITIS)

Chronic follicular conjunctivitis is a bilateral transmissible disease of children characterized by numerous follicles in the upper and lower palpebral conjunctiva. There are minimal conjunctival exudates and minimal inflammation but no complications. Treatment is ineffective, but the disease is self-limited within 2 years.

OCULAR ROSACEA

Ocular rosacea is a common complication of acne rosacea and probably occurs more often in light-skinned people, especially those of northern European ancestry. It is usually a blepharoconjunctivitis, but in severe cases, corneal ulceration and scarring may also occur. The patient generally complains of mild injection and irritation but discomfort increases if there is acute corneal involvement.

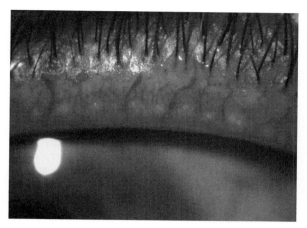

▲ **Figure 5–25.** Dilation of the blood vessels of the eyelid margin in the blepharitis of ocular rosacea.

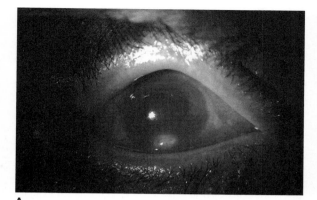

A

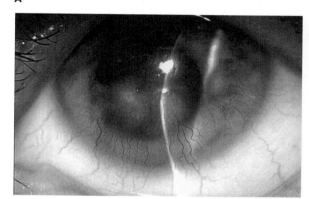

B

▲ **Figure 5–26.** Keratitis in ocular rosacea. **A:** inferior acute corneal ulceration with narrow base at the limbus and wider infiltrate centrally. **B:** chronic inferior keratopathy with segmental pannus and scarring.

There is dilation of the blood vessels of the eyelid margin (Figure 5–25) and frequently an accompanying staphylococcal blepharitis. The conjunctiva is hyperemic, especially in the exposed interpalpebral region. Less often, there may be a nodular conjunctivitis with small gray nodules on the bulbar conjunctiva, especially near the limbus, which may ulcerate superficially. The lesions can be differentiated from phlyctenules by the fact that even after they subside, large dilated vessels persist. Microscopic examination of the nodules shows lymphocytes and epithelial cells.

The peripheral cornea may ulcerate, characteristically with a narrow base at the limbus and a wider infiltrate centrally; vascularize, the resulting pannus often being wedge or spade-shaped and situated predominantly inferiorly; and scar (Figure 5–26).

Treatment of ocular rosacea consists of the elimination of hot, spicy foods and of alcoholic beverages, which are responsible for dilation of the facial vessels (Figure 5–27). Any secondary staphylococcal infection, which may also result in conjunctival concretions (Figure 5–28), should be treated. A course of oral tetracycline, standard doxycycline, or sustained release doxycycline may be used, with a maintenance dose often being needed to control more severe disease.

Ocular rosacea is a chronic, recurrent disease and may respond poorly to treatment. If the cornea is not affected, the visual prognosis is good; but corneal lesions tend to recur and progress, and the vision grows steadily worse over a period of years.

PSORIASIS

Psoriasis vulgaris usually affects the areas of the skin not exposed to the sun, but in about 10% of cases, lesions appear on the skin of the eyelids, and the plaques may extend to the conjunctiva, where they cause irritation, a foreign body sensation, and tearing. Psoriasis also causes nonspecific chronic conjunctivitis with

considerable mucoid discharge. Rarely, the cornea may show marginal ulceration or a deep, vascularized opacity.

The conjunctival and corneal lesions wax and wane with the skin lesions and are not affected by specific treatment. In rare cases, conjunctival scarring (symblepharon, trichiasis), corneal scarring, and occlusion of the nasolacrimal duct have occurred.

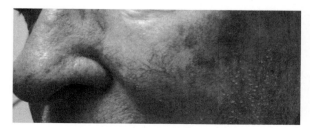

▲ **Figure 5–27.** Skin lesions in acne rosacea.

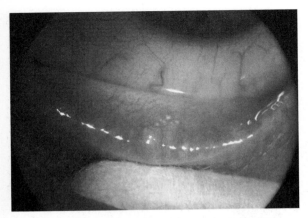

▲ **Figure 5–28.** Multiple concretions on the inferior tarsus. These are often associated with chronic lid disease caused by staphylococcal species.

STEVENS–JOHNSON SYNDROME, TOXIC EPIDERMAL NECROLYSIS, AND ERYTHEMA MULTIFORME

Stevens–Johnson syndrome and **toxic epidermal necrolysis,** the more extensive variant of the same disease, as well as **erythema multiforme,** cause skin and mucous membrane lesions, the latter possibly leading to cicatrizing conjunctivitis with the potential for severe corneal dryness and scarring (see Chapter 16). The skin lesion is an erythematous, urticarial bullous eruption that appears suddenly and is often distributed symmetrically. Bilateral conjunctivitis, often membranous, is a common manifestation. The patient complains of pain, irritation, discharge, and photophobia. The cornea becomes affected secondarily, and vascularization and scarring may seriously reduce vision.

Cultures are negative for bacteria and conjunctival scrapings show a preponderance of polymorphonuclear cells. Systemic steroids are thought to shorten the course of the systemic disease but have little or no effect on the eye lesions. Careful cleansing of the conjunctiva to remove the accumulated secretion is helpful, however, and tear replacement may be indicated. If trichiasis and entropion supervene, they should be corrected. Topical steroids probably have no beneficial effect, and their protracted use can cause corneal melting and perforation.

The acute episode usually lasts about 6 weeks, but the conjunctival scarring, loss of tears, and complications from entropion and trichiasis may result in prolonged morbidity and progressive corneal cicatrization.

DERMATITIS HERPETIFORMIS

Dermatitis herpetiformis is a rare skin disorder characterized by symmetrically grouped erythematous papulovesicular, vesicular, or bullous lesions. The disease has a predilection

for the posterior axillary fold, the sacral region, the buttocks, and the forearms. Itching is often severe. Rarely, a pseudomembranous conjunctivitis occurs and may result in cicatrization resembling that seen in mucous membrane pemphigoid. The skin eruption and conjunctivitis usually respond readily to systemic sulfones or sulfapyridine.

EPIDERMOLYSIS BULLOSA

This is a rare hereditary disease characterized by vesicles, bullae, and epidermal cysts. The lesions occur chiefly on the extensor surfaces of the joints and other areas exposed to trauma. The severe dystrophic type that leads to scarring may also produce conjunctival scars similar to those seen in dermatitis herpetiformis and mucous membrane pemphigoid. No known treatment is satisfactory.

SUPERIOR LIMBIC KERATOCONJUNCTIVITIS

Superior limbic keratoconjunctivitis is usually bilateral and limited to the upper tarsus and upper limbus. The principal complaints are irritation and hyperemia. The signs are papillary hypertrophy of the upper tarsus, redness of the superior bulbar conjunctiva, thickening and keratinization of the superior limbus, epithelial keratitis, recurrent superior filaments, and superior micropannus. Rose bengal staining is a helpful diagnostic test (Figure 5–29). The keratinized epithelial cells and mucous debris pick up the stain. Scrapings from the upper limbus show keratinizing epithelial cells.

In about 50% of cases, the condition has been associated with abnormal function of the thyroid gland. Applying 0.5% or 1% silver nitrate to the upper palpebral conjunctiva and allowing the tarsus to drop back onto the upper limbus usually result in shedding of the keratinizing cells and relief of symptoms for 4–6 weeks. This treatment can be repeated. There are no complications, and the disease usually runs a course of 2–4 years.

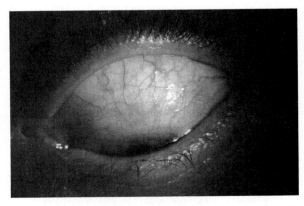

▲ **Figure 5–29.** Superior limbic keratoconjunctivitis with staining with rose bengal. See color insert.

In severe cases, one may consider 5-mm resection of the perilimbal superior conjunctiva.

LIGNEOUS CONJUNCTIVITIS

This is a rare bilateral, chronic or recurrent, pseudomembranous or membranous conjunctivitis that arises early in life, predominantly in young girls, and often persists for many years. Granulomas are often associated with it, and the lids may feel very hard. Recent studies have shown an underlying type 1 plasminogen deficiency in patients suffering from ligneous conjunctivitis. Cyclosporine has been an effective treatment. Future therapies will focus on topical delivery of plasminogen.

REITER'S SYNDROME

A triad of disease manifestations—nonspecific urethritis, arthritis, and conjunctivitis—constitutes Reiter's syndrome. Iritis can also occur, but tends to be a late complication. The syndrome occurs much more often in men than in women and has been found in association with HLA-B27 antigen. The conjunctivitis is papillary in type and usually bilateral. Conjunctival scrapings contain polymorphonuclear cells. No bacteria grow in cultures. The arthritis usually affects the large weight-bearing joints. There is no satisfactory treatment, although nonsteroidal anti-inflammatory agents may be effective. Corticosteroids usually help in resolution of iridocyclitis if present.

MUCOCUTANEOUS LYMPH NODE SYNDROME (KAWASAKI DISEASE)

This disease of unknown cause was first described in Japan in 1967. Conjunctivitis is one of its six diagnostic features, of which the others are (1) fever that fails to respond to antibiotics; (2) changes in the lips and oral cavity; (3) such changes in the extremities as erythema of the palms and soles, indurative edema, and membranous desquamation of the fingertips; (4) polymorphous exanthem of the trunk; and (5) acute nonpurulent swelling of the cervical lymph nodes.

The disease occurs almost exclusively in prepubertal children and carries a 1–2% mortality rate from cardiac failure. The conjunctivitis has not been severe, and no corneal lesions have been reported.

Recent findings suggest a possible infectious cause of Kawasaki disease.

Treatment is supportive only.

▼ CONJUNCTIVITIS ASSOCIATED WITH SYSTEMIC DISEASE

CONJUNCTIVITIS IN THYROID DISEASE

In orbital Graves' disease, the conjunctiva may be red and chemotic and the patient may complain of copious tearing. As the disease progresses, the chemosis increases, and in advanced cases the chemotic conjunctiva may extrude between the lids (Figure 5–30).

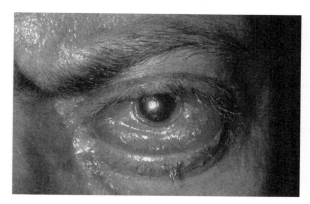

▲ **Figure 5–30.** Graves' disease. Note conjunctival prolapse, keratinization, and marked chemosis and injection.

Treatment is directed toward control of the thyroid disease, and every effort must be made to protect the conjunctiva and cornea by bland ointment, surgical lid adhesions (tarsorrhaphy) if necessary, or even orbital decompression if the lids do not close enough to cover the cornea and conjunctiva.

GOUTY CONJUNCTIVITIS

Patients with gout often complain of a "hot eye" during attacks. On examination, a mild conjunctivitis is found that is less severe than suggested by the symptoms. Gout may also be associated with episcleritis or scleritis, iridocyclitis, keratitis, vitreous opacities, and retinopathy. Treatment is aimed at controlling the gouty attack with colchicine and allopurinol.

CARCINOID CONJUNCTIVITIS

In carcinoid, the conjunctiva is sometimes congested and cyanotic as a result of the secretion of serotonin by the chromaffin cells of the gastrointestinal tract. The patient may complain of a "hot eye" during such attacks.

▼ CONJUNCTIVITIS SECONDARY TO DACRYOCYSTITIS OR CANALICULITIS

CONJUNCTIVITIS SECONDARY TO DACRYOCYSTITIS

Both pneumococcal conjunctivitis (often unilateral and unresponsive to treatment) and beta-hemolytic streptococcal conjunctivitis (often hyperacute and purulent) may be secondary to chronic dacryocystitis (see Chapter 4). The nature and source of the conjunctivitis in both instances are often missed until the lacrimal system is investigated.

CONJUNCTIVITIS SECONDARY TO CANALICULITIS

Canaliculitis due to canalicular infection with *A israelii* or *Candida* species (or, very rarely, *Aspergillus* species) may cause unilateral mucopurulent conjunctivitis, often chronic (see Chapter 4). The source of the condition is often missed unless the characteristic hyperemic, pouting punctum is noted. Expression of the canaliculus (upper or lower, whichever is involved) is curative provided the entire concretion is removed.

Conjunctival scrapings show a predominance of polymorphonuclear cells. Cultures (unless anaerobic) are usually negative. Candida grows readily on ordinary culture media, but almost all of the infections are caused by *A israelii*, which requires an anaerobic medium.

II. DEGENERATIVE DISEASES OF THE CONJUNCTIVA

PINGUECULA

Pingueculae are extremely common in adults. They appear as yellow nodules on both sides of the cornea (more commonly on the nasal side) in the area of the palpebral aperture. The nodules, consisting of hyaline and yellow elastic tissue, rarely increase in size, but inflammation is common. In general, no treatment is required, but in certain cases of pingueculitis, weak topical steroids (eg, prednisolone 0.12%) or topical nonsteroidal anti-inflammatory agents may be given (Figure 5–31).

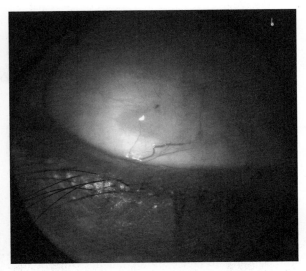

▲ **Figure 5–31.** Pinguecula. Note elevated nodule present nasally without involvement of the cornea.

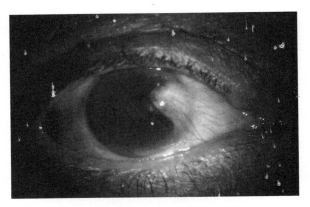

▲ **Figure 5–32.** Pterygium encroaching on the cornea and invading the visual axis.

PTERYGIUM

A pterygium is a fleshy, triangular encroachment of a pinguecula onto the cornea, usually on the nasal side bilaterally (Figure 5–32). It is thought to be an irritative phenomenon due to ultraviolet light, drying, and windy environments, since it is common in persons who spend much of their lives out of doors in sunny, dusty, or sandy, windblown surroundings. The pathologic findings in the conjunctiva are the same as those of pinguecula. In the cornea, there is replacement of Bowman's layer by hyaline and elastic tissue.

If the pterygium is enlarging and encroaches on the pupillary area, it should be removed surgically along with a small portion of superficial clear cornea beyond the area of encroachment. Conjunctival autografts combined with surgical excision have been shown to reduce the risk of recurrent disease.

CLIMATIC DROPLET KERATOPATHY (BIETTI'S BAND-SHAPED NODULAR DYSTROPHY, LABRADOR KERATOPATHY, SPHEROIDAL DEGENERATION)

Climatic droplet keratopathy is an uncommon degenerative disorder of the cornea characterized by aggregates of yellowish-golden spherules that accumulate in the subepithelial layers. The cause is unknown, but certain factors such as exposure to ultraviolet light, aridity, and microtrauma are recognized predisposing factors. The deposits may result in elevation of the epithelium in a band-shaped configuration. The condition is more common in geographic regions with high levels of direct and reflected sunlight.

III. MISCELLANEOUS DISORDERS OF THE CONJUNCTIVA

LYMPHANGIECTASIS

Lymphangiectasis is characterized by localized small, clear, tortuous dilations in the conjunctiva. They are merely dilated

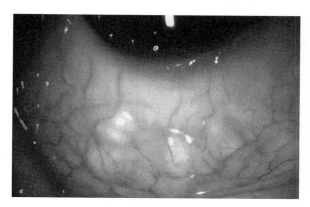

▲ **Figure 5–33.** Conjunctival lymphangiectasis. Note the clear tortuous dilations in the conjunctiva.

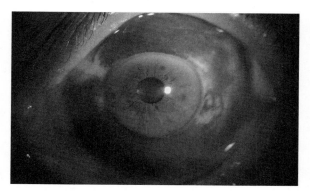

▲ **Figure 5–34.** Spontaneous subconjunctival hemorrhage while on warfarin. See color insert. (Courtesy of University of California, Davis, Cornea and External Diseases.)

lymph vessels, and no treatment is indicated unless they are irritating or cosmetically objectionable. They can then be cauterized or excised (Figure 5–33).

CONGENITAL CONJUNCTIVAL LYMPHEDEMA

This is a rare entity, unilateral or bilateral, and characterized by pinkish, fleshy edema of the bulbar conjunctiva. Usually observed as an isolated entity at birth, the condition is thought to be due to a congenital defect in the lymphatic drainage of the conjunctiva. It has been observed in chronic hereditary lymphedema of the lower extremities (Milroy's disease) and is thought to be an ocular manifestation of this disease rather than an associated anomaly.

CYSTINOSIS

Cystinosis is a rare congenital disorder of amino acid metabolism characterized by widespread intracellular deposition of cystine crystals in various body tissues, including the conjunctiva and cornea. Three types are recognized: childhood, adolescent, and adult. Life expectancy is reduced in the first two types.

SUBCONJUNCTIVAL HEMORRHAGE

This common disorder may occur spontaneously, usually in only one eye, in any age group. Its sudden onset and bright-red appearance usually alarm the patient. The hemorrhage is caused by rupture of a small conjunctival vessel, sometimes preceded by a bout of severe coughing or sneezing (Figure 5–34).

The best treatment is reassurance. The hemorrhage usually absorbs in 2–3 weeks.

In rare instances, if the hemorrhages are bilateral or recurrent; the possibility of blood dyscrasias should then be ruled out.

OPHTHALMIA NEONATORUM

Ophthalmia neonatorum in its broad sense refers to any infection of the newborn conjunctiva. In its narrow and commonly used sense, however, it refers to a conjunctival infection, chiefly gonococcal, that follows contamination of the baby's eyes during its passage through the mother's cervix and vagina or during the postpartum period. Because gonococcal conjunctivitis can rapidly cause blindness, the cause of all cases of ophthalmia neonatorum should be verified by examination of smears of exudate, epithelial scrapings, cultures, and rapid tests for gonococci.

Gonococcal neonatal conjunctivitis causes corneal ulceration and blindness if not treated immediately. Chlamydial neonatal conjunctivitis (inclusion blennorrhea) is less destructive but can last months if untreated and may be followed by pneumonia. Other causes include infections with staphylococci, pneumococci, haemophilus, and herpes simplex virus and silver nitrate prophylaxis.

The time of onset is important but not entirely reliable in clinical diagnosis since the two principal types, gonorrheal ophthalmia and inclusion blennorrhea, have widely differing incubation periods: gonococcal disease 2–3 days and chlamydial disease 5–12 days. The third important birth-canal infection (HSV-2 keratoconjunctivitis) has a 2- to 3-day incubation period and is potentially quite serious because of the possibility of systemic dissemination.

Treatment for neonatal gonococcal conjunctivitis is with ceftriaxone, 125 mg as a single intramuscular dose; a second choice is kanamycin, 75 mg intramuscularly. To treat chlamydial conjunctivitis in newborns, erythromycin oral suspension is effective at a dosage of 50 mg/kg/d in four divided doses for 2 weeks. In both gonococcal and chlamydial conjunctivitis, the parents need to be treated. Herpes simplex keratoconjunctivitis is treated with acyclovir, 30 mg/kg/d in three divided doses for 14 days. Neonatal disease from HSV requires hospitalization because of the potential neurologic or systemic manifestations. Other types of neonatal conjunctivitis are treated with erythromycin, gentamicin, or tobramycin ophthalmic ointment four times daily.

Credé 1% silver nitrate prophylaxis is effective for the prevention of gonorrheal ophthalmia but not inclusion blennorrhea or herpetic infection. The slight chemical conjunctivitis induced by silver nitrate is minor and of short duration. Accidents with concentrated solutions can be avoided by using wax ampules specially prepared for Credé prophylaxis. Tetracycline and erythromycin ointment are effective substitutes.

OCULOGLANDULAR DISEASE (PARINAUD'S OCULOGLANDULAR SYNDROME)

This is a group of conjunctival diseases, usually unilateral, characterized by low-grade fever, grossly visible preauricular adenopathy, and one or more conjunctival granulomas (Figure 5–35). The most common cause is cat-scratch disease, but there are many other causes, including *M tuberculosis*, *Treponema pallidum, Francisella tularensis, Pasteurella (Yersinia) pseudo-tuberculosis, C trachomatis* serovars L1, L2, and L3, and *Coccidioides immitis*.

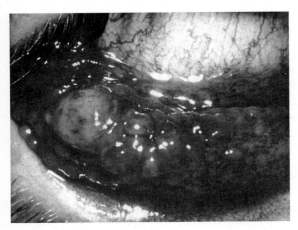

▲ **Figure 5–35.** Conjunctival granuloma. (Courtesy of P Thygeson.)

▶ Conjunctival Cat-Scratch Disease

This protracted but benign granulomatous conjunctivitis is found most commonly in children who have been in intimate contact with cats. The child often runs a low-grade fever and develops a reasonably enlarged preauricular node and one or more conjunctival granulomas. These may show focal necrosis and may sometimes ulcerate. The regional adenopathy does not suppurate. The clinical diagnosis is supported by serology.

The disease appears to be caused by a slender pleomorphic gram-negative bacillus (*Bartonella* [formerly *Rochalimaea*] *henselae*), which grows in the walls of blood vessels. With special stains, this organism can be seen in biopsies of conjunctival tissue. The organism closely resembles *Leptotrichia buccalis*, and the disease was previously known as leptotrichosis conjunctivae (Parinaud's conjunctivitis). The organism is commonly found in the mouth in humans and always in the mouth in cats. The eye may be contaminated by saliva on the child's fingers or by cat saliva on the child's pillow. *Afipia felis* has been incriminated also and may still play a role.

The disease is self-limited (without corneal or other complications) and resolves in 2–3 months. The conjunctival nodule can be excised; in the case of a solitary granuloma, this may be curative. Systemic tetracyclines may shorten the course but should not be given to children under 7 years of age.

▶ Conjunctivitis Secondary to Neoplasms (Masquerade Syndrome)

When examined superficially, a neoplasm of the conjunctiva or lid margin is often misdiagnosed as a chronic infectious conjunctivitis or keratoconjunctivitis. Since the underlying lesion is often not recognized, the condition has been referred to as masquerade syndrome. The masquerading neoplasms on record are conjunctival capillary carcinoma, conjunctival carcinoma in situ, infectious papilloma of the conjunctiva, sebaceous gland carcinoma, and verrucae. Verrucae and molluscum tumors of the lid margin may desquamate toxic tumor material that produces a chronic conjunctivitis, keratoconjunctivitis, or (rarely) keratitis alone.

5.2. Conjunctival Tumors
James J. Augsburger, MD, and Zélia M. Corrêa, MD, PhD

This section presents an overview of the most common and most important neoplasms, hamartomas, and choristomas of the conjunctiva. Readers are referred to other sections of this chapter for information about inflammatory and degenerative lesions of the conjunctiva (eg, pingueculum and pterygium) that can simulate conjunctival neoplasms.

BENIGN TUMORS OF CONJUNCTIVA

Benign neoplasms are acquired tumors of cells that are atypical but not sufficient to be classified as malignant. They may enlarge slowly, but have little or no invasive potential and no metastatic capability. **Hamartomas** are congenital tumors composed of normal or near-normal cells and tissues for the anatomic site but in excessive amounts. **Choristomas** are congenital tumors consisting of normal cells and tissue elements but not occurring normally at the anatomic site.

Melanocytic Nevus of Conjunctiva

Melanocytic nevus of the conjunctiva (conjunctival nevus) is a benign acquired, rarely congenital, neoplasm arising from melanocytes that are present normally in limited numbers within the basal layers of the conjunctival stratified squamous epithelium. It is probably the most commonly encountered conjunctival neoplasm, but its exact incidence has never been calculated. It affects men and women equally. It is almost always a unilateral unifocal lesion. It is usually first noted by the child's parents during the first decade of life, but occasionally it does not become apparent until the teenage years or even later. It manifests as a dark brown to tan lesion, most characteristically located adjacent the limbus in the inter-palpebral fissure (Figure 5–36). Less frequently, it involves the semilunar fold or caruncle. Slitlamp biomicroscopy frequently reveals intralesional cysts and fine blood vessels. The lesion can grow to over 5 mm in diameter and over 1 mm in thickness, especially if it contains multiple microcysts. Treatment consists of surgical excision of the entire lesion.

Conjunctival Choristomas

Limbal dermoid is the commonest conjunctival choristoma, characteristically located inferotemporally in one or both eyes. It consists of a variety of cells and tissues of mesenchymal (mesodermal) origin, including fat cells, fibroblasts, and hair follicles, and manifests as a slightly elevated dome-shaped white mass straddling the limbus, thus involving the cornea as well as the conjunctiva (Figure 5–37). On slitlamp

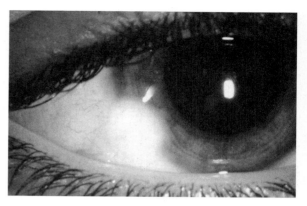

▲ **Figure 5–37.** Limbal dermoid exhibiting typical off-white color and inferotemporal location.

biomicroscopy, fine hair shafts are frequently evident on the surface. Unilateral unifocal lesions frequently occur as isolated abnormalities. Bilateral limbal dermoids are usually a sign of Goldenhaar syndrome. Small lesions can usually be left alone. Larger ones that extend to or near the visual axis, or cause pronounced irregular astigmatism, are usually treated by penetrating or lamellar keratoplasty.

Conjunctival dermolipoma is composed principally of fat cells and other dermal elements, the most common of which are hair follicles. It typically occurs in the forniceal conjunctiva superotemporally, manifesting as a pale pink to golden subepithelial mass that is soft and non-tender. It is frequently not recognized until teenage to adult years and in most cases can be left alone. Surgical excision may be performed to remove or reduce the size of the lesion.

Benign Lymphoid Hyperplasia of Conjunctiva

Benign lymphoid hyperplasia of the conjunctiva is composed of mildly atypical lymphocytic cells within the conjunctival substantia propria. Usually it does not develop until middle age. It affects both men and women, and it can be unifocal, multifocal, or diffuse in one or both eyes. The individual lesion appears as an ill-defined pink mass within the bulbar or forniceal conjunctiva, which cannot be distinguished clinically from a malignant lymphoid tumor (see later in the chapter). Incisional or excisional biopsy thus may be indicated to exclude lymphoma.

Conjunctival Hemangioma

Conjunctival hemangioma is a hamartoma of the conjunctival blood vessels. It is present at birth but may not become apparent until it enlarges. It is virtually always unilateral and manifests as a prominent collection of large caliber blood vessels thickening the conjunctiva (Figure 5–38). On slitlamp biomicroscopy, some of the deeper blood vessels may be seen

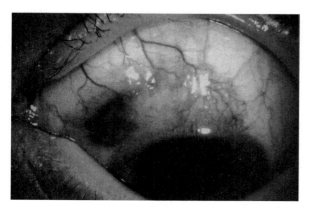

▲ **Figure 5–36.** Conjunctival nevus of superior limbal and bulbar conjunctiva with variable intensity of melanotic pigmentation and microcysts visible in the less pigmented areas.

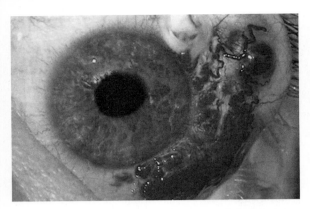

▲ **Figure 5–38.** Cavernous hemangioma of conjunctiva, composed of large caliber blood vessels, some of which appear to extend into the underlying sclera.

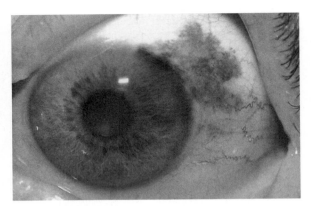

▲ **Figure 5–39.** Conjunctival primary acquired melanosis (PAM).

to extend into the sclera. Unlike capillary hemangiomas of the eyelids and orbit, conjunctival hemangiomas rarely regress spontaneously. The principal indication for treatment is unsightly appearance, but no treatment has been shown to be both safe and effective. Surgical excision can be complicated by difficult to control bleeding and incomplete removal that fails to improve or worsens the appearance. Double freeze-thaw cryotherapy is sometimes effective in inducing at least partial regression.

▶ Conjunctival Lymphangioma

Conjunctival lymphangioma is a hamartoma composed of conjunctival lymphatic channels lined by endothelial cells. Although congenital, it frequently does not manifest until older childhood. It often enlarges abruptly during episodes of upper respiratory infection and may even fill with blood. Like conjunctival hemangioma, it is notoriously difficult if not impossible to eradicate by surgical excision.

CONJUNCTIVAL TUMORS INTERMEDIATE BETWEEN BENIGN AND MALIGNANT

The tumors described are categorized as neoplasms of borderline malignancy because clinically they cannot be categorized reliably as either benign or malignant. If a biopsy is performed, pathologic studies may reveal benign cells, malignant cells, or cells deemed to be borderline even by cytologic criteria. Tumors that cannot be classified unequivocally as either completely benign or definitely malignant are frequently referred to as pre-malignant or precancerous lesions.

▶ Conjunctival Primary Acquired Melanosis

Primary acquired melanosis (PAM) of the conjunctiva represents hyperplasia of conjunctival melanocytes. It is almost exclusively a unilateral unifocal lesion. It affects men and women with equal frequency. It rarely develops before middle age and most commonly manifests in older individuals. It can arise from the limbal, bulbar, forniceal or even palpebral conjunctiva. Clinically, it appears as a flat to minimally elevated dark brown patch of conjunctiva in an area that was normal in appearance previously (Figure 5–39). If it involves the limbal conjunctiva, it may extend into the corneal epithelium. The lesion usually enlarges slowly over several years. Prominent patches of PAM occasionally give rise to conjunctival melanomas (see later in the chapter), so they should be regarded as pre-malignant lesions. Suspicious lesions should be excised or biopsied for histopathologic study. The crucial pathologic features are the degree of atypia of the melanocytic cells and the extent of their replacement of the conjunctival epithelial cells. High-risk PAM that cannot be excised completely may benefit from topical drug therapy using mitomycin C, 5-fluorouracil, or interferon alpha 2b.

▶ Dysplasia of Conjunctival Stratified Squamous Epithelium

Dysplasia of the conjunctival stratified squamous epithelium is a disordered growth and maturation of the epithelium that can be a precursor to squamous cell carcinoma (see later in the chapter). The disease is almost always unilateral, unifocal, and involving the limbus in the interpalpebral fissure, ie sun exposed area, and virtually always occurs in older middle aged or elderly individuals. Typically it appears as an irregular off-white thickening of the limbal conjunctiva. Accumulation of keratin sometimes results in focal leukoplakia (white patch of hyperkeratotic epithelium). Because it is not possible to distinguish the lesion clinically from squamous cell carcinoma, surgical excision is usually recommended.

▶ Conjunctival and/or Corneal Intraepithelial Neoplasia

Conjunctival and/or corneal intraepithelial neoplasia (CIN) is a pre-malignant to in situ malignant disorder affecting the

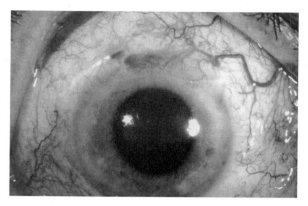

▲ **Figure 5–40.** Corneal and conjunctival intraepithelial neoplasia (CIN) predominantly manifesting as mild translucency of the upper two thirds of the corneal epithelium.

conjunctival and/or corneal stratified squamous epithelium. It occurs in middle-aged to older adults and is most evident in the corneal epithelium. On slitlamp biomicroscopy, CIN appears as a translucent area of mild corneal epithelial thickening without vascularization or hyperkeratosis (Figure 5–40). It may be limited to the peripheral cornea or extend across the visual axis. It is frequently associated with one or more foci of conjunctival squamous cell carcinoma (see later in the chapter). It can be managed by surgical removal of the visibly abnormal epithelial cells and/or topical therapy with mitomycin-C, 5-fluorouracil, or interferon-alpha 2b.

▶ Atypical Lymphoid Hyperplasia of Conjunctiva

Atypical lymphoid hyperplasia of the conjunctiva is composed of moderately atypical lymphocytic cells within the conjunctival substantia propria. It is generally regarded as part of the spectrum of conjunctival lymphocytic infiltrates, intermediate between benign lymphoid hyperplasia (see earlier in the chapter) and malignant lymphoma (see later in the chapter). It usually does not develop until middle age. It affects both men and women, and can be unifocal, multifocal, or diffuse in one or both eyes, manifesting as a pink mass within the bulbar or forniceal conjunctiva. It cannot be distinguished clinically from benign lymphoid hyperplasia or malignant lymphoma of the conjunctiva. If the lesion is prominent, incisional or excisional biopsy is indicated to exclude lymphoma. Some patients with lesions classified pathologically as atypical lymphoid hyperplasia eventually develop extra-ophthalmic foci of systemic lymphoma, so patients with this type of conjunctival lesion are usually treated with relatively low dose external beam radiation therapy to the affected eye(s) and monitored periodically over the ensuing years for signs of systemic lymphoma.

MALIGNANT CONJUNCTIVAL TUMORS

Malignant conjunctival tumors consist of morphologically abnormal cells and tissues. Invasive features are generally evident clinically and pathologically, and regional and distant metastases are potential sequelae.

▶ Conjunctival Squamous Cell Carcinoma and Its Variants

Squamous cell carcinoma of the conjunctiva is composed of very atypical neoplastic cells arising from the stratified squamous epithelium. It tends to occur in middle-aged to elderly persons, except in xeroderma pigmentosum when it tends to develop early in life. It is almost exclusively unilateral and unifocal, occurring more commonly in men than women. It usually develops at the limbus in the interpalpebral fissure.

Clinically, squamous cell carcinoma of the conjunctival manifests in most cases as (1) a focal leukoplakic lesion (Figure 5–41), (2) a gelatinous conjunctival mass (Figure 5–42), or (3) a papillary tumor (Figure 5–43). If neglected or particularly aggressive, conjunctival squamous cell carcinoma can invade the sclera and extend intraocularly, or invade the orbit. Excision of the lesion is generally regarded to be the treatment of choice. Double freeze-thaw cryotherapy to the conjunctiva and sclera immediately surrounding the excised tissue, and even supplemental excision of lamellar sclera and peripheral cornea underlying the site of the tumor, are frequently employed to reduce the chance of local recurrence. If clinical examination, or pathologic study of the excised specimen, suggests residual conjunctival or corneal intraepithelial neoplasia, topical therapy with mitomycin-C, 5-fluorouracil, or interferon-alpha 2b is probably indicated. If intraocular extension is evident, plaque radiotherapy to the intraocular tumor or attempted en bloc resection of the

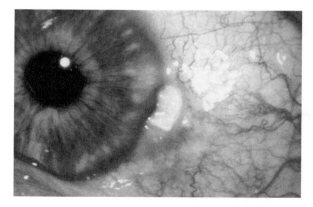

▲ **Figure 5–41.** Leukoplakic type of squamous cell carcinoma of the limbal conjunctiva, the surface white plaque (leukoplakia) being due to focal hyperkeratosis.

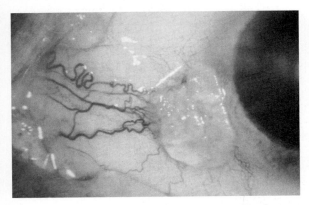

▲ **Figure 5-42.** Gelatinous type of squamous cell carcinoma of the limbal conjunctiva, with prominent conjunctival blood vessels extending to the tumor.

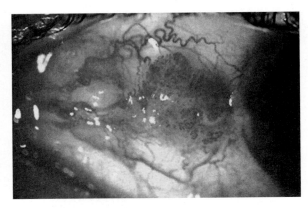

▲ **Figure 5-44.** Mucoepidermoid carcinoma of conjunctiva, manifesting as papillary type anteriorly and subepithelial nodule posteriorly.

tumor and adjacent conjunctiva, cornea, and sclera, with insertion of donor cornea and/or sclera may be attempted to salvage the eye. If the intraocular involvement is too extensive or cannot be eradicated by these methods, the eye is usually enucleated. If the orbit is involved, exenteration is usually recommended.

Mucoepidermoid carcinoma of the conjunctiva is a particularly aggressive variant of conjunctival squamous cell carcinoma. The tumor tends to be ill-defined and lumpy and frequently exhibits a yellowish color (Figure 5–44). It tends to be highly invasive and frequently extends into the orbit by the time it is diagnosed. In most cases, exenteration is required.

▶ Conjunctival Melanoma

Conjunctival melanoma arises from the intraepithelial melanocytes of the conjunctiva. It is almost exclusively unilateral, but may be multifocal if it arises from pre-existing primary acquired melanosis (see earlier in the chapter). It usually affects middle-aged or older individuals. It affects both men and women with equal frequency. It is much more common in Caucasians.

Conjunctival melanoms can arise from any region of the conjunctiva (limbal, bulbar, forniceal, palpebral, or caruncular), but is most common near the limbus in the interpalpebral area. It typically manifests as a dark brown nodular mass, which tends to be densely vascularized by conjunctival blood vessels (Figure 5–45). It frequently

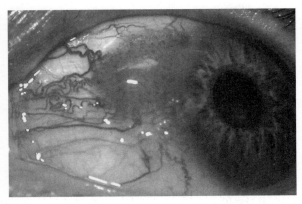

▲ **Figure 5-43.** Papillary type of squamous cell carcinoma of the limbal conjunctiva with prominent conjunctival blood vessels extending to the tumor.

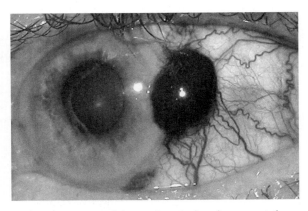

▲ **Figure 5-45.** Nodular conjunctival melanoma at the limbus, with prominent conjunctival blood vessels extending to the tumor, and a small patch of primary acquired melanosis inferiorly.

attains a thickness of 1 to 3 mm before it is recognized. It has the capability of invading the conjunctival stromal, extending into the conjunctival lymphatics, and metastasizing to regional lymph nodes in the head and neck and then to distant organs. Unfavorable prognostic factors for metastasis and metastatic death include larger tumor size, involvement of the fornix or caruncle, and local recurrence following surgical excision. Treatment usually consists of wide surgical excision followed by conjunctival closure using sliding or transpostion flaps or a mucous membrane graft. Supplemental cryotherapy to the adjacent conjunctiva or topical therapy with mitomycin-C, 5-fluorouracil, or interferon-alpha 2b is frequently performed to reduce the likelihood of local recurrence. Ruthenium plaque radiation therapy has also been employed in a few centers, with success rates similar to those after excision plus supplemental treatments. Regional lymph node dissection at the time of initial treatment is being performed in some centers, but the benefits of this treatment have not yet been identified. There is no evidence that exenteration of the orbit improves the survival prognosis of patients with orbital invasion by conjunctival melanoma. Thus exenteration is usually limited to patients with massive orbital involvement without evidence of distant metastasis. A substantial proportion of patients with larger conjunctival melanomas involving the fornix or caruncle at the time of initial treatment will eventually die from metastatic disease despite aggressive local therapy.

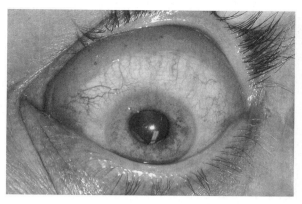

▲ **Figure 5–46.** Conjunctival lymphoma involving 180° of the superior forniceal conjunctiva, found to be malignant by histopathologic and immunohistochemical analysis.

▶ Conjunctival Lymphoma

Malignant lymphoma of the conjunctiva is composed of an abnormal proliferation of atypical lymphocytic cells within the conjunctival stroma. It usually occurs in middle aged and older persons. It affects both men and women, and it can be unifocal, multifocal or diffuse in one or both eyes. The individual lesion manifests as a pink mass within the bulbar or forniceal conjunctiva (Figure 5–46), which cannot be distinguished clinically from benign or atypical lymphoid hyperplasia of the conjunctiva (see earlier in the chapter). If the lesion is prominent clinically, incisional or excisional biopsy is indicated to establish the diagnosis. Approximately 20% of patients with lesions classified pathologically as malignant lymphoma eventually develop extra-ophthalmic foci of systemic lymphoma, so patients are usually treated with fractionated external beam radiation therapy to the affected eye(s) and monitored periodically over the ensuing years for signs of systemic lymphoma.

▶ Conjunctival Kaposi Sarcoma

Kaposi sarcoma of the conjunctiva is composed of pleomorphic, malignant cells that become densely vascularized. Most commonly it develops in individuals with AIDS, and in middle-aged or older men. It is usually unilateral and unifocal but can be bilateral and multifocal. Typical Kaposi sarcoma of the conjunctiva manifests as a nodular red mass that is frequently hemorrhagic. Focal treatment can be performed by excision, cryotherapy, or even radiation therapy, but whole body therapy is generally indicated because lesions eventually develop in many sites in individuals with AIDS.

5.3. Tears

Lisa M. Nijm, MD, JD, Francisco J. Garcia-Ferrer, MD, and Ivan R. Schwab, MD

Tears form a thin layer approximately 7–10 μm thick that covers the corneal and conjunctival epithelium. The functions of this ultrathin layer are (1) to make the cornea a smooth optical surface by abolishing minute surface epithelial irregularities; (2) to wet and protect the delicate surface of the corneal and conjunctival epithelium; (3) to inhibit the growth of microorganisms by mechanical flushing and antimicrobial action; and (4) to provide the cornea with necessary nutrient substances.

LAYERS OF THE TEAR FILM

The tear film is composed of three primary layers (Figure 5–47).

1. The superficial lipid layer is a monomolecular film derived from meibomian glands. It is thought to retard evaporation and form a watertight seal when the lids are closed.

2. The middle aqueous layer is elaborated by the major and minor lacrimal glands and contains water-soluble substances (salts and proteins).

3. The deep mucinous layer is composed of glycoprotein and overlies the corneal and conjunctival epithelial cells. The epithelial cell membranes are composed mainly of lipoproteins and are therefore relatively hydrophobic. Mucin is partly adsorbed onto the corneal epithelial cell membranes and is anchored by the microvilli of the surface epithelial cells. This provides a new hydrophilic surface for the aqueous tears to spread over, which is wetted by a lowering of surface tension.

COMPOSITION OF TEARS

The normal tear volume is estimated to be 7 ± 2 μL in each eye. Albumin accounts for 60% of the total protein in tear fluid. Immunoglobulins IgA, IgG, and IgE as well as lysozymes make up the remaining 40% of total protein. IgA predominates and differs from serum IgA in that it is not

only transudated from serum but is produced by plasma cells located in the lacrimal gland. In certain allergic conditions such as vernal conjunctivitis, the IgE concentration of tear fluid increases. Tear lysozymes form 21–25% of the total protein and—acting synergistically with gamma globulins and other nonlysozyme antibacterial factors—represent an important defense mechanism against infection. Other tear enzymes may also play a role in diagnosis of certain clinical entities, for example hexoseaminidase assay for diagnosis of Tay–Sachs disease.

K^+, Na^+, and Cl^- also occur in higher concentrations in tears than in plasma. Tears contain a small amount of glucose (5 mg/dL) and urea (0.04 mg/dL), and changes in blood concentration parallel changes in tear glucose and urea levels. The average pH of tears is 7.35, although a wide normal variation exists (5.20–8.35). Under normal conditions, tear fluid is isotonic. Tear film osmolarity ranges from 295 to 309 mosm/L.

DRY EYE SYNDROME (KERATOCONJUNCTIVITIS SICCA)

Dryness of the eye may result from any disease associated with deficiency of the tear film components (aqueous, mucin, or lipid), lid surface abnormalities, or epithelial abnormalities. Hence there are many causes of dry eye syndrome (keratoconjunctivitis sicca) (Table 5–4). Primary Sjögren's syndrome, an immune-mediated disorder of the lacrimal and salivary glands, characteristically manifesting as dry mouth as well as dry eyes, is an important specific disease entity that predominantly presents in women in the 5th to 7th decades of life. When associated with rheumatoid arthritis or other autoimmune diseases, it is known as secondary Sjögren's syndrome.

▶ Etiology

Many of the causes of dry eye syndrome affect more than one component of the tear film or lead to ocular surface alterations that secondarily cause tear film instability. Histopathologic features include the appearance of dry spots on the corneal and conjunctival epithelium, formation of filaments, loss of conjunctival goblet cells, abnormal enlargement of nongoblet epithelial cells, increased cellular stratification, and increased keratinization.

▶ Clinical Findings

Patients with dry eyes complain most frequently of a scratchy or sandy (foreign body) sensation. Other common symptoms are itching, excessive mucus secretion, inability to produce tears, a burning sensation, photosensitivity, redness, pain, and difficulty in moving the lids. On gross examination the eyes may appear normal, but on careful slit lamp examination, subtle indications of the presence of chronic dryness and irritation are found. The most characteristic

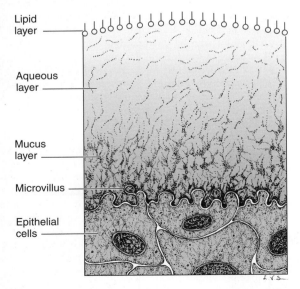

Lipid layer

Aqueous layer

Mucus layer

Microvillus

Epithelial cells

▲ **Figure 5–47.** The three primary layers of the tear film covering the superficial epithelial layer of the cornea.

Table 5–4. Etiology and Diagnosis of Dry Eye Syndrome

I. Etiology
  A. Conditions characterized by hypofunction of the lacrimal gland:
    1. Congenital
      a. Familial dysautonomia (Riley-Day syndrome)
      b. Aplasia of the lacrimal gland (congenital alacrima)
      c. Ectodermal dysplasia
    2. Acquired
      a. Systemic diseases
        (1) Primary and secondary Sjögren's syndrome
        (2) Progressive systemic sclerosis
        (3) Sarcoidosis
        (4) Leukemia, lymphoma
        (5) Amyloidosis
        (6) Hemochromatosis
      b. Infection
        (1) Mumps
      c. Injury
        (1) Surgical removal of, or damage to, lacrimal gland
        (2) Irradiation
        (3) Chemical burn
      d. Medications
        (1) Antihistamines
        (2) Antimuscarinics: atropine, scopolamine
        (3) Beta-adrenergic blockers: timolol
      e. Neurogenic (eg, facial nerve palsy)
  B. Conditions characterized by mucin deficiency:
    1. Avitaminosis A
    2. Stevens-Johnson syndrome, toxic epidermal necrolysis and erythema multiforme
    3. Mucous membrane pemphigoid
    4. Chronic conjunctivitis, eg, trachoma
    5. Chemical burns
    6. Medications—Antihistamines, antimuscarinic agents, beta-adrenergic blocking agents, eyedrop preservatives
    7. Folk remedies, eg, kermes
	C. Conditions Characterized by Lipid Deficiency:
	    1. Lid margin scarring
	    2. Blepharitis
	  D. Defective spreading of the tear film:
	    1. Eyelid abnormalities
	      a. Defects, coloboma
	      b. Ectropion or entropion
	      c. Keratinization of lid margin
	      d. Decreased or absent blinking
	        (1) Neurologic disorders (eg, facial nerve palsy)
	        (2) Hyperthyroidism
	        (3) Contact lens
	        (4) Drugs
	        (5) Herpes simplex keratitis
	        (6) Leprosy
	      e. Lagophthalmos
	        (1) Nocturnal lagophthalmos
	        (2) Hyperthyroidism
	        (3) Leprosy
	    2. Conjunctival abnormalities
	      a. Pterygium
	      b. Symblepharon
	    3. Proptosis
	II. Diagnostic Tests:
	  A. Schirmer test without anesthesia
	  B. Tear break-up time
	  C. Ocular ferning test
	  D. Impression cytology
	  E. Fluorescein staining
	  F. Rose bengal and lissamine green staining
	  G. Tear lysozyme
	  H. Tear film osmolality
	  I. Tear lactoferrin

feature is interruption or absence of the tear meniscus at the lower lid margin. Tenacious yellowish mucus strands are sometimes seen in the lower conjunctival fornix. The bulbar conjunctiva loses its normal luster and may be thickened, edematous, and hyperemic.

The corneal epithelium shows varying degrees of fine punctate stippling in the interpalpebral fissure. The damaged corneal and conjunctival epithelial cells stain with 1% rose bengal, and defects in the corneal epithelium stain with fluorescein (Figures 5–22 and 5–48). In the late stages of keratoconjunctivitis sicca, filaments may be seen—one end of each filament attached to the corneal epithelium and the other end moving freely (Figure 5–49).

In Sjögren's syndrome conjunctival scrapings may show increased numbers of goblet cells. Lacrimal gland enlargement occurs uncommonly in patients with Sjögren's syndrome. The principal diagnostic investigations in Sjögren's syndrome are detection of antibodies against Ro (SSA) and La (SSB) or histopathologic features in salivary gland biopsy.

Accurate diagnosis and grading of dry eye syndrome can be achieved using various diagnostic tests (Table 5–4).

A. Schirmer Test

Schirmer strips (Whatman filter paper No. 41) are inserted into the lower conjunctival cul-de-sac at the junction of the

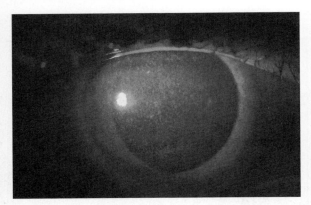

▲ **Figure 5–48.** Staining of the corneal epithelium with fluorescein in a patient with dry eye syndrome secondary to contact lens overuse.

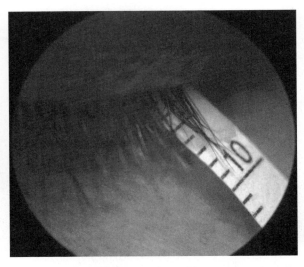

▲ **Figure 5-50.** Schirmer testing with 7 mm wetting of the filter paper strip.

mid and temporal thirds of the lower lid (Figure 5-50). The moistened exposed portion is measured 5 minutes after insertion. When performed without anesthesia, the test measures the function of the main lacrimal gland, whose secretory activity is stimulated by the irritating nature of the filter paper. Less than 10 mm of wetting without anesthesia is considered abnormal.

Schirmer tests can be performed after topical anesthesia (0.5% tetracaine) to measure the function of the accessory lacrimal glands, but the test is considered unreliable. Less than 5 mm in 5 minutes is abnormal.

The Schirmer test is a screening test for assessment of tear production. False-positive and false-negative results occur. Low readings are sporadically found in normal eyes, and normal tests may occur in dry eyes—especially those secondary to mucin deficiency.

B. Tear Film Break-Up Time

Measurement of the tear film break-up time may sometimes be useful to estimate the mucin content of tear fluid. Deficiency in mucin may not affect the Schirmer test, which quantifies tear production, but may lead to instability of the tear film, resulting in its rapid break-up. "Dry spots" (Figure 5–51) are formed in the tear film, followed by exposure of the corneal or conjunctival epithelium. This process ultimately damages the epithelial cells, which can then be stained with rose bengal. Damaged epithelial cells may be shed from the cornea, leaving areas susceptible to punctate staining when the corneal surface is flooded with fluorescein.

The tear film break-up time is measured by applying a slightly moistened fluorescein strip to the bulbar conjunctiva and asking the patient to blink. The tear film is then scanned with the aid of the cobalt filter on the slit-lamp while the patient refrains from blinking. The time that elapses before the first dry spot appears in the corneal fluorescein layer is the tear film break-up time. Normally it is over 15 seconds, but it will be reduced appreciably by the use of local anesthetics, by manipulating the eye, or by holding the lids open. Tear film

Filaments

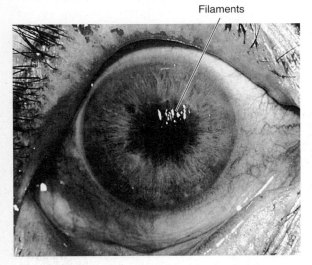

▲ **Figure 5–49.** Corneal filaments in a 56-year-old patient with dry eye syndrome.

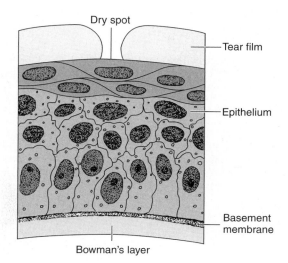

▲ Figure 5–51. Baring of the corneal epithelium following formation of a dry spot in the tear film.

break-up time is reduced in eyes with aqueous tear deficiency and is always shorter than normal in eyes with mucin deficiency.

C. Ocular Ferning Test

A simple and inexpensive qualitative test for the study of conjunctival mucus is performed by drying conjunctival scrapings on a clean glass slide. Microscopic arborization (ferning) is observed in normal eyes. In patients with cicatrizing conjunctivitis (mucous membrane pemphigoid, Stevens–Johnson syndrome, toxic epidermal necrolysis, erythema multiforme, diffuse conjunctival cicatrization), ferning of the mucus is reduced or absent.

D. Impression Cytology

Impression cytology is a method by which goblet cell densities on the conjunctival surface can be counted. In normal persons, the goblet cell population is highest in the infranasal quadrant. Loss of goblet cells has been documented in trachoma, mucous membrane pemphigoid, Stevens–Johnson syndrome, and avitaminosis A.

E. Fluorescein Staining

Touching the conjunctiva with a dry strip of fluorescein is a good indicator of wetness, and the tear meniscus can be seen easily. Fluorescein will stain the eroded and denuded areas as well as microscopic defects of the corneal epithelium (Figures 5–22 and 5–48).

F. Rose Bengal and Lissamine Green Staining

Rose bengal (Figure 5–29) and lissamine green are equally sensitive for staining the conjunctiva. Both dyes will stain all desiccated nonvital epithelial cells of the conjunctiva and to a lesser extent the cornea. Unlike rose bengal, lissamine green does not cause significant irritation.

G. Tear Lysozyme Assay

Reduction in tear lysozyme concentration usually occurs early in the course of Sjögren's syndrome and is helpful in diagnosis. Tears can be collected on Schirmer strips and assayed, usually by spectrophotometric methods.

H. Tear Osmolality

Hyperosmolality of tears has been documented in dry eye syndrome and in contact lens wearers, and is thought to be a consequence of decreased corneal sensitivity. Reports claim that hyperosmolality is the most specific test for dry eye syndrome. Hyperosmolality may be found even when Schirmer test and staining with rose bengal and lissamine green are normal.

I. Lactoferrin

Tear lactoferrin is low in patients with hyposecretion of the lacrimal gland. Testing kits are commercially available.

▶ Complications

Early in the course of dry eye syndrome, vision is slightly impaired. As the condition worsens, discomfort can become disabling. In advanced cases, corneal ulceration, corneal thinning, and perforation may develop. Secondary bacterial infection occasionally occurs, and corneal scarring and vascularization may result in marked reduction in vision. Early treatment may prevent these complications.

▶ Treatment

The patient should understand that dry eye syndrome is a chronic condition and complete relief is unlikely except in mild cases when the corneal and conjunctival epithelial changes are reversible. Artificial tears, particularly preservative-free tears in more advanced cases, are the mainstay of treatment. Ointment is useful for prolonged lubrication, especially when sleeping. Additional relief can be achieved by using humidifiers, moisture-chamber spectacles, or swim goggles.

The primary function of these measures is fluid replacement. Restoration of mucin is a more formidable task. In recent years, high-molecular-weight water-soluble polymers have been added to artificial tears in an attempt to improve and prolong surface wetting. Other mucomimetic agents include sodium hyaluronate and autologous serum. If the mucus is tenacious, as in Sjögren's syndrome, mucolytic agents (eg, acetylcysteine 10%) are helpful.

Patients with excessive tear lipids may require specific instructions for removal of lipid strands from the eyelid margin. Antibiotics topically or systemically may be necessary. Dietary supplementation with omega-3 fatty acids or flax seed oil has been advocated to modulate favorably meibomian gland secretion. Topical vitamin A may be useful in reversing ocular surface metaplasia.

Recent clinical studies have demonstrated the efficacy of preservative-free, low-dose corticosteroid preparations in the treatment of Sjögren's syndrome. Presumably due to its effects on ocular surface and lacrimal gland inflammation, cyclosporine 0.05% ophthalmic emulsion (Restasis) twice a day has been shown to be beneficial in moderate and severe dry eye syndrome with few adverse effects even in individuals treated for up to 4 years. Oral hydroxychloroquine is reported to improve tear production in Sjögren's syndrome.

All chemical preservatives in artificial tears induce a certain amount of corneal toxicity. Benzalkonium chloride is the most damaging of the commonly used preparations. Patients who require frequent drops fare better with non-preserved solutions. Preservatives can also cause idiosyncratic reactions. This is most common with thimerosal.

Patients with dry eyes from any cause are more likely to have concurrent infections. Chronic blepharitis is common and should be treated with appropriate lid hygiene and topical antibiotics as needed. If there is acne rosacea treatment with systemic doxycycline may be helpful.

Surgical treatment for dry eyes includes insertion of temporary (collagen) or extended (silicone) punctal plugs to retain lacrimal secretions. Permanent closure of the puncta and canaliculi can be achieved by thermal, electrocautery, or laser treatment. Injection of botulinum toxin into the medial lower eyelid is reported to improve discomfort by reducing tear drainage.

REFERENCES

Conjunctiva

Adebayo A, Parikh JG, McCormick SA, et al: Shifting trends in in vitro antibiotic susceptibilities for common bacterial conjunctival isolates in the last decade at the New York Eye and Ear Infirmary. Graefes Arch Clin Exp Ophthalmol 2010 Jun 8. [Epub ahead of print] [PMID: 20532549]

Biebesheimer JB, House J, Hong KC, et al: Complete local elimination of infectious trachoma from severely affected communities after six biannual mass azithromycin distributions. Ophthalmology 2009;116:2047. [PMID: 19744717]

Bradley JC, Yang W, Bradley RH, Reid TW, Schwab IR: The science of pterygia. Br J Ophthalmol 2010;94:815. [PMID: 19515643]

Burton MJ, Mabey DC: The global burden of trachoma: a review. PLoS Negl Trop Dis 2009;3:e460. [PMID: 19859534]

Chen YM, Hu FR, Hou YC: Effect of oral azithromycin in the treatment of chlamydial conjunctivitis. Eye 2010;24:985. [PMID: 19893589]

De Rojas MV, Dart JK, Saw VP: The natural history of Stevens–Johnson syndrome: patterns of chronic ocular disease and the role of systemic immunosuppressive therapy. Br J Ophthalmol 2007;91:1048. [PMID: 17314145]

Donnenfeld E, Pflugfelder SC: Topical ophthalmic cyclosporine: pharmacology and clinical uses. Surv Ophthalmol 2009;54:321. [PMID: 19422961]

Dosso AA, Rungger-Brändle E: Clinical course of epidemic keratoconjunctivitis: evaluation by in vivo confocal microscopy. Cornea 2008;27:263. [PMID: 18362649]

Gayton JL. Etiology, prevalence, and treatment of dry eye disease. Clin Ophthalmol 2009;3:405. [PMID: 19688028]

Gichuhi S, Bosire R, Mbori-Ngacha D, et al: Risk factors for neonatal conjunctivitis in babies of HIV-1 infected mothers. Ophthalmic Epidemiol 2009;16:337. [PMID: 19995198]

Granet D: Allergic rhinoconjunctivitis and differential diagnosis of the red eye. Allergy Asthma Proc 2008;29:565. [PMID: 19173783]

Huguet P, Bella L, Einterz EM, Goldschmidt P, Bensaid P: Mass treatment of trachoma with azithromycin 1.5% eye drops in the Republic of Cameroon: feasibility, tolerance and effectiveness. Br J Ophthalmol 2010;94:157. [PMID: 19692356]

Latkany R. Dry eyes: etiology and management. Curr Opin Ophthalmol 2008;19:287. [PMID: 18545008]

Mantelli F, Lambiase A, Bonini S: A simple and rapid diagnostic algorithm for the detection of ocular allergic diseases. Curr Opin Allergy Clin Immunol 2009;9:471. [PMID: 19638928]

Mariotti SP, Pascolini D, Rose-Nussbaumer J: Trachoma: global magnitude of a preventable cause of blindness. Br J Ophthalmol 2009;93:563. [PMID: 19098034]

Ngondi J, Gebre T, Shargie EB, et al: Estimation of effects of community intervention with antibiotics, facial cleanliness, and environmental improvement (A,F,E) in five districts of Ethiopia hyperendemic for trachoma. Br J Ophthalmol 2010;94:278. [PMID: 19897474]

Nithyanandam S, Stephen J, Joseph M, Dabir S: Factors affecting visual outcome in herpes zoster ophthalmicus: a prospective study. Clin Experiment Ophthalmol 2010 Jun 21. [Epub ahead of print] [PMID: 20572824]

O'Brien TP, Jeng BH, McDonald M, Raizman MB: Acute conjunctivitis: truth and misconceptions. Curr Med Res Opin 2009;25:1953. [PMID: 19552618]

Oliver GF, Wilson GA, Everts RJ: Acute infective conjunctivitis: evidence review and management advice for New Zealand practitioners. N Z Med J 2009;122:69. [PMID: 19680306]

Opstelten W, Eekhof J, Neven AK, Verheij T: Treatment of herpes zoster. Can Fam Physician 2008;54:373. [PMID: 18337531]

Origlieri C, Bielory L: Emerging drugs for conjunctivitis. Expert Opin Emerg Drugs 2009;14:523. [PMID: 19708819]

Porco TC, Gebre T, Ayele B, et al: Effect of mass distribution of azithromycin for trachoma control on overall mortality in Ethiopian children: a randomized trial. JAMA 2009;302:962. [PMID: 19724043]

Rose P: Management strategies for acute infective conjunctivitis in primary care: a systematic review. Expert Opin Pharmacother 2007;8:1903. [PMID: 17696792]

Rours IG, Hammerschlag MR, Ott A, et al: Chlamydia trachomatis as a cause of neonatal conjunctivitis in Dutch infants. Pediatrics 2008;121:e321. [PMID: 18245405]

Saw VP, Dart JK: Ocular mucous membrane pemphigoid: diagnosis and management strategies. Ocul Surf 2008;6:128. [PMID: 18781259]

Silva LR, Gurgel RQ, Lima DR, Cuevas LE: Current usefulness of Credé's method of preventing neonatal ophthalmia. Ann Trop Paediatr 2008;28:45. [PMID: 18318948]

Smith AF, Waycaster C. Estimate of the direct and indirect annual cost of bacterial conjunctivitis in the United States. BMC Ophthalmol 2009;9:13. [PMID: 19939250]

Tarabishy AB, Jeng BH: Bacterial conjunctivitis: a review for internists. Cleve Clin J Med 2008;75:507. [PMID: 18646586]

Taylor HR, Fox SS, Xie J, et al: The prevalence of trachoma in Australia: the National Indigenous Eye Health Survey. Med J Aust 2010;192:248. [PMID: 20201757]

Visscher KL, Hutnik CM, Thomas M: Evidence-based treatment of acute infective conjunctivitis: breaking the cycle of antibiotic prescribing. Can Fam Physician 2009;55:1071. [PMID: 19910590]

Woreta TA, Munoz BE, Gower EW, Alemayehu W, West SK: Effect of trichiasis surgery on visual acuity outcomes in Ethiopia. Arch Ophthalmol 2009;127:1505. [PMID: 19901217]

Conjunctival Tumors

Ballalai PL, Erwenne CM, Martins MC, et al: Long-term results of topical mitomycin C 0.02% for primary and recurrent conjunctival-corneal intraepithelial neoplasia. Ophthal Plast Reconstr Surg 2009;25:296. [PMID: 19617789]

Chalasani R, Giblin M, Conway RM: Role of topical chemotherapy for primary acquired melanosis and malignant melanoma of the conjunctiva and cornea: review of the evidence and recommendations for treatment. Clin Experiment Ophthalmol 2006;34:708. [PMID: 16970772]

Damato B, Coupland SE: Conjunctival melanoma and melanosis: a reappraisal of terminology, classification and staging. Clin Experiment Ophthalmol 2008;36:7865. [PMID: 19128387]

Damato B, Coupland SE: Management of conjunctival melanoma. Expert Rev Anticancer Ther 2009;9:1227. [PMID: 19761427]

Doganay S, Er H, Tasar A, Gürses I: Surgical excision, cryotherapy, autolimbal transplantation and mitomycin-C in treatment of conjunctival-corneal intraepithelial neoplasia. Int Ophthalmol 2005;26:53. [PMID: 16779567]

Guech-Ongey M, Engels EA, Goedert JJ, Biggar RJ, Mbulaiteye SM: Elevated risk for squamous cell carcinoma of the conjunctiva among adults with AIDS in the United States. Int J Cancer 2008;122:2590. [PMID: 18224690]

Hamam R, Bhat P, Foster CS: Conjunctival/corneal intraepithelial neoplasia. Int Ophthalmol Clin 2009;49:63. [PMID: 19125065]

Kim JW, Abramson DH: Topical treatment options for conjunctival neoplasms. Clin Ophthalmol 2008;2:503. [PMID: 19668748]

Levecq L, De Potter P, Jamart J: Conjunctival nevi clinical features and therapeutic outcomes. Ophthalmology 2010;117:35. [PMID: 19896191]

Qureshi YA, Karp CL, Dubovy SR: Intralesional interferon alpha-2b therapy for adnexal Kaposi sarcoma. Cornea 2009;28:941. [PMID: 19654515]

Robinson JW, Brownstein S, Jordan DR, Hodge WG: Conjunctival mucoepidermoid carcinoma in a patient with ocular cicatricial pemphigoid and a review of the literature. Surv Ophthalmol 2006;51:513. [PMID: 16950250]

Shields CL, Demirci H, Karatza E, Shields JA: Clinical survey of 1643 melanocytic and nonmelanocytic conjunctival tumors. Ophthalmology 2004;111:1747. [PMID: 15350332]

Shields CL, Shields JA: Conjunctival tumors in children. Curr Opin Ophthalmol 2007;18:351. [PMID: 17700226]

Shields CL, Shields JA: Ocular melanoma: relatively rare but requiring respect. Clin Dermatol 2009;27:122. [PMID: 19095158]

Shields CL, Shields JA, Carvalho C, et al: Conjunctival lymphoid tumors: clinical analysis of 117 cases and relationship to systemic lymphoma. Ophthalmology 2001;108:979. [PMID: 11320031]

Shields JA, Shields CL, Mashayekhi A, et al: Primary acquired melanosis of the conjunctiva: experience with 311 eyes. Trans Am Ophthalmol Soc 2007;105:61. [PMID: 18427595]

Tsai PS, Colby KA: Treatment of conjunctival lymphomas. Semin Ophthalmol 2005;20:239. [PMID: 16352495]

Verma V, Shen D, Sieving PC, Chan CC: The role of infectious agents in the etiology of ocular adnexal neoplasia. Surv Ophthalmol 2008;53:312. [PMID: 18572051]

Tears

Akpek EK, Klimava A, Thorne JE, et al: Evaluation of patients with dry eye for presence of underlying Sjögren syndrome. Cornea 2009;28:493. [PMID: 19421051]

Baroody M, Holds JB, Vick VL: Advances in the diagnosis and treatment of ptosis. Curr Opin Ophthalmol 2005;1:351. [PMID: 16264345]

Caffery B, Simpson T, Wang S, et al: Rose bengal staining of the temporal conjunctiva differentiates Sjögren's syndrome from keratoconjunctivitis sicca. Invest Ophthalmol Vis Sci 2010;51:2381. [PMID: 20107179]

Donnenfeld E, Pflugfelder SC: Topical ophthalmic cyclosporine: pharmacology and clinical uses. Surv Ophthalmol 2009;54:321. [PMID: 19422961]

Foulks GN: The Correlation between the tear film lipid layer and dry eye disease. Surv Ophthalmol 2007;52:369. [PMID: 17574063]

Gayton JL: Etiology, prevalence, and treatment of dry eye disease. Clin Ophthalmol 2009;3:405. [PMID: 19688028]

Geerling G, Tost FH: Surgical occlusion of the lacrimal drainage system. Dev Ophthalmol 2008;41:213. [PMID: 18453771]

Latkany R: Dry eyes: etiology and management. Curr Opin Ophthalmol 2008;19:287. [PMID: 18545008]

Lee GA, Chen SX: Autologous serum in the management of recalcitrant dry eye syndrome. Clin Experiment Ophthalmol 2008;36:119. [PMID: 18352867]

Perry HD, Solomon R, Donnenefeld ED, et al: Evaluation of topical cyclosporine for the treatment of dry eye disease. Arch Ophthalmol 2008;126:1046. [PMID: 18695097]

Rihl M, Ulbricht K, Schmidt RE, Witte T: Treatment of sicca symptoms with hydroxychloroquine in patients with Sjögren's syndrome. Rheumatology 2009;48:796. [PMID: 19433433]

Sahlin, Linderoth R: Eyelid botulinum toxin injections for the dry eye. Dev Ophthalmol 2008;41:187– 192. [PMID: 18453769]

Tost FH, Geerling G: Plugs for occlusion of the lacrimal drainage system. Dev Ophthalmol 2008;41:193. [PMID: 18453770]

Whitcher JP. The treatment of dry eyes. Br J Ophthalmol 2004;88:603. [PMID: 15090407]

Whitcher JP, Shiboski CH, Shiboski SC, et al: A simplified quantitative method for assessing keratoconjunctivitis sicca from the Sjögren's Syndrome International Registry. Am J Ophthalmol 2010;149:405. [PMID: 20035924]

Witte T: Diagnostic markers of Sjögren's syndrome. Dev Ophthalmol 2010;45:123. [.PMID: 20502032]

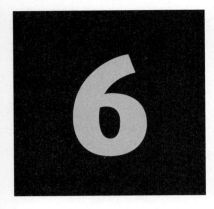

Cornea

6

Roderick Biswell, MD

PHYSIOLOGY

The cornea functions both as a protective barrier and as a "window" through which light rays pass to the retina. Its transparency is due to its uniform structure, avascularity, and deturgescence (see Chapter 1). Deturgescence, or the state of relative dehydration of the corneal tissue, is maintained by the bicarbonate "pump" provided by the endothelium and the barrier function of the epithelium and endothelium. The endothelium is more important than the epithelium in the mechanism of dehydration, and damage to the endothelium is far more serious than damage to the epithelium. Destruction of the endothelial cells causes edema of the cornea and loss of transparency, which is more likely to persist because of the limited potential for recovery of endothelial function. Damage to the epithelium usually causes only transient, localized edema of the corneal stroma that clears with the rapid regeneration of epithelial cells. Evaporation of water from the precorneal tear film produces hypertonicity of the film. Together with direct evaporation, this draws water from the superficial corneal stroma in order to maintain the state of dehydration.

Penetration of the intact cornea by drugs is biphasic. Fat-soluble substances can pass through intact epithelium, and water-soluble substances can pass through intact stroma. Therefore, to pass through the cornea, drugs must be soluble in both lipids and water.

CORNEAL RESISTANCE TO INFECTION

The epithelium is an efficient barrier to the entrance of microorganisms into the cornea. If the epithelium is defective, the avascular stroma and Bowman's layer become susceptible to infection with a variety of organisms, including bacteria, *Acanthamoeba*, and fungi. *Streptococcus pneumoniae* (the pneumococcus) is a true bacterial corneal pathogen; other pathogens require a heavy inoculum, compromised barrier function, or a relative immune deficiency to produce infection.

Moraxella liquefaciens, which occurs mainly in alcoholics (as a result of pyridoxine depletion), is a classic example of the bacterial opportunist, and in recent years a number of new corneal opportunists have been identified. Among them are *Serratia marcescens*, *Mycobacterium fortuitum-chelonei* complex, viridans streptococci, *Staphylococcus epidermidis*, and various coliform and proteus organisms, along with viruses, *Acanthamoeba*, and fungi.

Local or systemic corticosteroids modify the host immune reaction in several ways and may allow opportunistic organisms to invade and flourish.

PHYSIOLOGY OF SYMPTOMS

Since the cornea has many pain fibers, most superficial or deep corneal lesions cause pain and photophobia. The pain of epithelial disease is worsened by movement of the lids (particularly the upper lid) over the cornea and usually persists until healing occurs. Since the cornea serves as the "window" of the eye and refracts light rays, corneal lesions usually blur vision, especially if centrally located.

Photophobia in corneal disease is the result of painful contraction of an inflamed iris. Dilation of iris vessels is a reflex phenomenon caused by irritation of the corneal nerve endings. Photophobia, severe in most corneal disease, is minimal in herpetic keratitis because of the hypesthesia associated with the disease, which can be a valuable diagnostic sign.

Although tearing and photophobia commonly accompany corneal disease, there is usually no discharge except in purulent bacterial ulcers.

INVESTIGATION OF CORNEAL DISEASE

▶ Symptoms & Signs

Obtaining a thorough history is important. A history of trauma can often be elicited, foreign bodies and abrasions being the two most common corneal lesions, and eliciting any history of corneal disease in the patient or the family can be critical. The keratitis of herpes simplex infection is often recurrent, but since recurrent erosion is extremely painful and herpetic keratitis is not, these disorders can be differentiated by their symptoms. The patient's use of topical medications should be investigated, since corticosteroids may have been used and may have predisposed to bacterial, fungal, or viral disease, especially herpes simplex keratitis. Immunosuppression also occurs with systemic diseases, such as diabetes, AIDS, and malignant disease, as well as with specific immunosuppressive therapy. All medications and preservatives can cause contact dermatitis or corneal toxicity; the importance of toxicity as a cause of corneal and conjunctival disease should not be underestimated.

The keys to examination of the cornea are adequate illumination and magnification. The slitlamp is essential in proper examination of the cornea; in its absence, a loupe and bright illumination can be used for gross inspection. Examining the light reflection, while moving the light carefully over the entire cornea, will identify rough areas indicative of epithelial defects. Fluorescein staining can highlight superficial epithelial lesions that might otherwise not be apparent. Examination, particularly after trauma, is often facilitated by instillation of a local anesthetic, but sterile drops must be used. Confocal microscopy assists diagnosis, particularly in suspected *Acanthamoeba* or fungal infection.

▶ Laboratory Studies

To select the proper therapy for corneal infections, especially due to bacteria, fungi, or *Acanthamoeba* laboratory aid is essential. Since a delay in identifying the correct organism may severely compromise the ultimate visual result, it should be achieved as soon as possible. Examination of corneal scrapings, stained with Gram's and Giemsa's stains, may allow identification of the organism, particularly bacteria, while the patient waits. Polymerase chain reaction (PCR) may provide rapid identification of herpes viruses, *Acanthamoeba,* and fungi. Cultures for bacteria are usually obtained in all cases at first presentation. Cultures for fungi, *Acanthamoeba,* or viruses may be undertaken if the clinical features are typical or there is lack of response to treatment for bacterial infection. Appropriate therapy is instituted as soon as the necessary specimens have been obtained. It is important that therapy is not withheld if an organism cannot be identified on microscopic examination of corneal scrapings, although it may have to be empirical based upon the clinical features.

▶ Morphologic Diagnosis of Corneal Lesions
A. Epithelial Keratitis

The corneal epithelium is involved in most types of conjunctivitis and keratitis and in rare cases may be the only tissue involved (eg, in superficial punctate keratitis). The epithelial changes vary widely from simple edema and vacuolation to minute erosions, filament formation, partial keratinization, etc. The lesions vary also in their location on the cornea. All of these features have important diagnostic significance (Figure 6–1), and slitlamp examination with and without fluorescein staining should be a part of every external eye examination.

Minute fluorescein-staining erosions; lower third of the cornea affected predominantly.	Typically dendritic (occasionally round or oval) with edema and degeneration.	More diffuse than lesions of HSK; occasionally linear (pseudodendrites).
		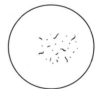
1. Staphylococcal keratitis	2. Herpetic keratitis (HSK)	3. Varicella-zoster keratitis
Minute fluorescein-staining erosions; diffuse but most conspicuous in pupillary area.	Minute pleomorphic, fluorescein-staining, damaged epithelium and erosions; epithelial and mucous filaments are typical; lower half of cornea affected predominantly.	Minute fluorescein-staining irregular erosions; lower half of cornea affected predominantly.
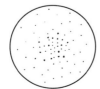	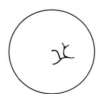	
4. Adenovirus keratitis	5. Keratitis of Sjögren's syndrome	6. Exposure keratitis—due to lagophthalmous or exophthalmous

▲ **Figure 6–1.** Principal types of epithelial keratitis (in order of frequency of occurrence).

Blotchy gray, opaque, synctium-like lesions, most conspicuous in upper pupillary area. Sometimes a plaque of opaque epithelium forms.

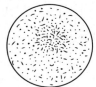

7. Vernal keratoconjunctivitis

Blotchy epithelial edema; diffuse but predominant in palpebral fissure, 9–3 o'clock.

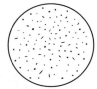

8. Neurotrophic keratitis—sequela of herpes simplex, herpes zoster, and gasserian ganglion destruction

Minute fluorescein-staining erosions with spotty cellular edema; epithelial whorls.

9. Drug-induced keratitis—especially by many antibiotics and preservatives

Foci of edematous epithelial cells, round or oval; elevated when disease is active.

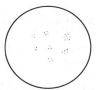

10. Superficial punctate keratitis (SPK)

Minute fluorescein-staining erosions of upper third of cornea; filaments during exacerbations; bulbar hyperemia, thickened keratinized limbus, micropannus.

11. Superior limbic keratoconjunctivitis

Virus-type lesions like those of SPK; in pupillary area.

12. Rubeola, rubella, and mumps keratitis

Minute fluorescein-staining epithelial erosions affecting upper third of cornea.

13. Trachoma

Spotty gray opacification of individual epithelial cells due to partial keratinization; associated with Bitot's spots.

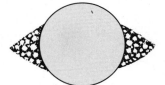

14. Vitamin A deficiency keratitis

▲ **Figure 6–1.** (*Continued*)

B. Subepithelial Keratitis

There are a number of important types of discrete subepithelial lesions, often secondary to epithelial keratitis (eg, the subepithelial infiltrates of epidemic keratoconjunctivitis, caused by adenoviruses 8 and 19).

C. Stromal Keratitis

The responses of the corneal stroma to disease include infiltration, representing accumulation of inflammatory cells; edema manifested as corneal thickening, opacification, or scarring; "melting" or necrosis, which may lead to thinning or perforation; and vascularization. The patterns of these responses are less specific for disease entities than those seen in epithelial keratitis, and the clinician often must rely on other clinical information and laboratory studies for clear identification of causes.

D. Endothelial Keratitis

Dysfunction of the corneal endothelium results in corneal edema, initially involving the stroma and later the epithelium. Stromal edema often produces "folds" or "wrinkles" in Descemet's membrane. This contrasts with corneal edema due to raised intraocular pressure, in which the epithelium is affected before the stroma. As long as the cornea is not too edematous, it is often possible to visualize morphologic abnormalities of the corneal endothelium with the slitlamp.

Inflammatory cells on the endothelium (keratic precipitates or "KPs") are less commonly an indication of endothelial disease, when they are usually localized, than due to anterior uveitis, which may or may not accompany stromal keratitis, when they tend to be more generally distributed.

▼ CORNEAL ULCERATION

Cicatrization due to corneal ulceration is a major cause of blindness and impaired vision throughout the world (see Chapter 20). Most of this visual loss is avoidable by early diagnosis and prompt appropriate treatment, but also by minimizing predisposing factors.

INFECTIOUS CORNEAL ULCERS

Central ulcers usually are infectious ulcers secondary to corneal epithelial damage. The lesion is situated centrally, away from the vascularized limbus. It is often accompanied by hypopyon, a collection of inflammatory cells seen as a pale layer in the inferior anterior chamber that also occurs in severe anterior uveitis (see Chapter 7). Although hypopyon is sterile in bacterial corneal ulcers unless there has been a rupture of Descemet's membrane, in fungal ulcers it may contain fungal elements.

Central suppurative ulceration was once caused almost exclusively by *S pneumoniae* infection complicating corneal trauma, particularly occurring in patients with obstructed nasolacrimal ducts. The commonest predisposing factor in developed countries has become contact lens wear, being particularly associated with *Pseudomonas* and *Acanthamoeba* keratitis. More widespread use of compromising systemic and local medications has increased the incidence of corneal ulcers due to opportunistic bacteria, fungi, and viruses.

1. BACTERIAL KERATITIS

Many types of bacterial corneal ulcers look alike and vary only in severity. This is especially true of ulcers caused by opportunistic bacteria (eg, alpha-hemolytic streptococci, *Staphylococcus aureus*, *S epidermidis*, *Nocardia*, and *M fortuitum-chelonei*), which often cause indolent corneal ulcers that tend to spread slowly and superficially.

▶ *Streptococcus pneumoniae* (pneumococcal) Corneal Ulcer (Figure 6–2)

Pneumococcal corneal ulcer usually manifests 24–48 hours after inoculation of an abraded cornea. It typically produces a gray, fairly well-circumscribed ulcer that tends to spread erratically from the original site of infection toward the center of the cornea. The advancing border shows active ulceration and infiltration as the trailing border begins to heal. (This creeping effect gave rise to the term "acute serpiginous ulcer.") The superficial corneal layers become involved first,

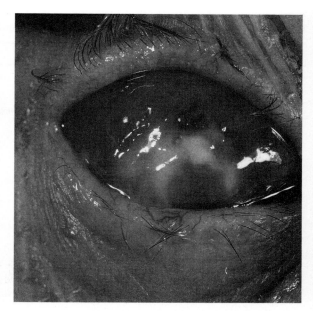

▲ **Figure 6–2.** Pneumococcal corneal ulcer with iris prolapsing through superior peripheral corneal perforation.

and then the deep parenchyma. The cornea surrounding the ulcer is often clear. Hypopyon is common. Scrapings from the leading edge of a pneumococcal corneal ulcer usually contain gram-positive lancet-shaped diplococci. Drugs recommended for use in treatment are listed in Tables 6–1 and 6–2. Concurrent dacryocystitis and nasolacrimal duct obstruction should also be treated.

▶ *Pseudomonas aeruginosa* Corneal Ulcer

Pseudomonas corneal ulcer begins as a gray or yellow infiltrate at the site of a break in the corneal epithelium (Figure 6–3). Severe pain is common. The lesion tends to spread rapidly in all directions because of the proteolytic enzymes produced by the organisms. Although superficial at first, the ulcer may quickly affect the entire cornea with devastating consequences, including corneal perforation and severe intraocular infection. There is often a large hypopyon that tends to increase in size as the ulcer progresses. The infiltrate and exudate may have a bluish-green color. This is due to a pigment produced by the organism and is pathognomonic of *P aeruginosa* infection.

Today, especially in developed countries, *Pseudomonas* corneal infection often is associated with soft contact lenses—especially extended-wear lenses. The organism has been shown to adhere to the surface of soft contact lenses. Some cases have been reported following the use of contaminated fluorescein solution or eye drops. It is mandatory that the clinician use sterile medications and sterile technique when caring for patients with corneal injuries.

Table 6–1. Treatment of Bacterial, Fungal, or Amebic Keratitis[1]

Organisms	Initial Therapies[2]	Alternative Therapies[2]
No organisms identified; ulcer suggestive of bacterial infection	Moxifloxacin, gatifloxacin, or tobramycin with cefazolin	Ciprofloxacin, levofloxacin, gentamicin, ceftazidime, or vancomycin
Gram-positive cocci: lancet-shaped with capsule = *S pneumoniae*	Moxifloxacin, gatifloxacine, or cefazolin	Levofloxacin, penicillin G, vancomycin, or ceftaxidime
Gram-positive cocci: methacillin-resistant *S aureus* (MRSA)	Vancomycin	
Gram-positive rods: slender and varying in length—*Mycobacterium fortuitum, Nocardia* species, *Actinomyces* species	Amikacine, moxifloxacin, or gatifloxacin	Other fluoroquinolones
Other gram-positive organisms: cocci or rods	Cefazolin, moxifloxacin, or gatifloxacin	Other fluoroquinolones, penicillin G, vancomycin, or ceftazidime
Gram-negative cocci[3]	Ceftriaxone[3]	Penicillin G, cefazolin, or vancomycin
Gram-negative rods: thin = *Pseudomonas*	Moxifloxacin, gatifloxacin, ciprofloxaxin, tobramycin, or gentamicin	Other fluoroquinolones, polymyxin B, or carbenicillin
Gram-negative rods: large, a square-ended diplobacilli = *Moraxella*	Moxifloxacin, gatifloxacin, or ciprofloxacin	Tobramyin or getamicin with cefazolin, or penicillin G
Other gram-negative rods	Moxifloxacin, gatifloxacin, or tobramycin	Ceftazidime, getamicin, or carbenicillin
No organism identified; ulcer suggestive of fungal infection	Natamycin, voriconazole, or posaconazole	Amphotericin B, nystatin, miconazole, or flucytosine
Yeast-like organism = *Candida* species[4]	Amphotericin B, voriconazole, or posaconazole	Amphotericin B, nystatin, miconazole, or flucytosine
Hyphae-like organisms = fungal ulcer	Natamycin, voriconazole, or posaconazole	Amphotericin B or nystatin
Cyst, trophozoites = *Acanthamoeba*	Propamidine and/or polyhexamethylene biguanide	Chlorhexidine or neomycin

[1]Intensive topical treatment, every hour during the day and every 2 hours during the night for at least the first 48 hours and then gradually reducing, is essential in all but the mildest cases. Subconjunctival injections may be necessary if there are concerns about compliance with topical therapy or in the treatment of severe disease. Systemic therapy is not generally required. It may be used if the corneal ulcer encroaches on the limbus or if there is associated scleritis or endophthalmitis.
[2]Change in treatment is only necessary if there is a lack of response and can be guided by antibiotic sensitivity of any organism isolated.
[3]Suspected gonococcal keratitis must be treated with systemic therapy (parenteral ceftriaxone, 1–2 g daily for 5 days).
[4]Rarely, *Pityrosporum ovale* or *Pityrosporum orbiculare* may be confused with *Candida* species.

Scrapings from the ulcer may contain long, thin Gram-negative rods that are often few in number. Drugs recommended for use in treatment are listed in Tables 6–1 and 6–2.

▶ *Moraxella liquefaciens* Corneal Ulcer

M liquefaciens (diplobacillus of Petit) causes an indolent oval ulcer that usually affects the inferior cornea and progresses into the deep stroma over a period of days. There is usually no hypopyon or only a small one, and the surrounding cornea is usually clear. *M liquefaciens* ulcer often occurs in a patient with alcoholism, diabetes mellitus, or other causes of immunosuppression. Scrapings may contain large, square-ended Gram-negative diplobacilli. Drugs recommended for use in treatment are listed in Tables 6–1 and 6–2. Treatment can be difficult and prolonged.

▶ Group A *Streptococcus* Corneal Ulcer

Central corneal ulcers caused by beta-hemolytic streptococci have no identifying features. The surrounding corneal stroma is often infiltrated and edematous, and there is usually a

Table 6–2.   Drug Concentrations and Dosages for Treatment of Bacterial or Fungal Keratitis

Drug	Topical[1]	Subconjunctival	Systemic
Amikacin	50–100 mg/mL	25 mg/0.5 mL/dose	10–15 mg/kg/d IV or IM in two doses
Amphotericin B	1.5–3 mg/mL	0.5–1 mg	...
Carbenicillin	4 mg/mL	125 mg/0.5 mL/dose	100–200 mg/kg/d IV in four doses
Cefazolin	50 mg/mL	100 mg/0.5 mL/dose	15 mg/kg/d IV in four doses
Ceftazidime	50 mg/mL	250 mg (0.5 mL)	1 g IV or IM every 8–12 hours (adult dose)
Ceftriaxone	...	...	1–2 g/d IV or IM
Ciprofloxacin	3 mg/mL	...	500–750 mg orally every 12 hours
Flucytosine	1% solution	...	50–150 mg/kg/d orally in four doses
Gatifloxacin	3 mg/mL solution	...	...
Gentamicin	10–20 mg/mL (fortified)	20 mg/0.5–1 mL/dose	...
Miconazole	1% solution or 2% ointment	5–10 mg; 0.5–1 mL/dose	...
Moxifloxacin	5 mg/mL solution	...	...
Natamycin	5% suspension	...	...
Neomycin	20 mg/mL	...	...
Nystatin	50,000 units/mL or cream (100,000 units/g)	...	...
Paromomyocin	10 mg/mL	...	...
Penicillin G	100,000 units/mL	1 million units/dose (painful)	40,000–50,000 units/kg IV in four doses; or continuously, 2–6 million units IV every 4–6 hours
Polyhexamethylene biguanide	0.01%–0.02% solution	...	...
Polymyxin B	1–2 mg/mL	10 mg/0.5 mL dose	...
Posaconazole	1% solution		400 mg orally every 12 hours
Propamidine	0.1 mg/mL solution; 0.15% ointment	...	...
Tobramycin	10–20 mg/mL (fortified)	20 mg/0.5 mL/dose	...
Vancomycin	50 mg/mL	25 mg/0.5mL/dose	...
Voriconazole	1% solution		200–300 mg orally every 12 hours; or 200 mg every 12 hours IV

[1]Topical: Every hour during the day and every 2 hours during the night for at least 48 hours and then gradually reducing. Many of the preparations listed must be prepared by pharmacists with special training.

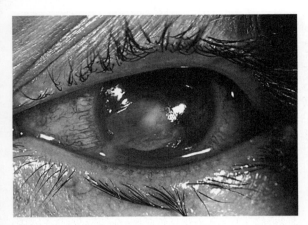

▲ **Figure 6–3.** *Pseudomonas* ulcer related to 24-hour contact lens wear.

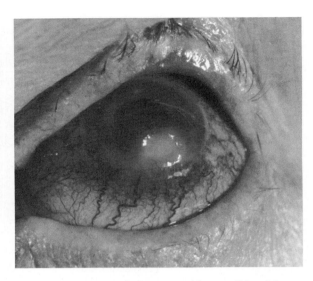

▲ **Figure 6–4.** Corneal ulcer caused by *Candida albicans.*

moderately large hypopyon. Scrapings often contain gram-positive cocci in chains. Drugs recommended for use in treatment are listed in Tables 6–1 and 6–2.

▶ *Staphylococcus aureus, Staphylococcus epidermidis,* & Alpha-Hemolytic *Streptococcus* Corneal Ulcers

Central corneal ulcers caused by these organisms are now being seen more often, many of them in corneas compromised by topical corticosteroid use. The ulcers are often indolent, but may be associated with hypopyon and some surrounding corneal infiltration. They are often superficial, and the ulcer bed feels firm when scraped. Scrapings may contain Gram-positive cocci—singly, in pairs, or in chains. Infectious crystalline keratopathy (in which the cornea has a crystalline appearance) has been described in patients receiving long-term therapy with topical corticosteroids; the disease is often caused by alpha-hemolytic streptococci as well as nutritionally deficient streptococci. Tables 6–1 and 6–2 show recommended drug regimens.

▶ *Mycobacterium fortuitum-chelonei* & *Nocardia* Corneal Ulcers

Ulcers due to *M fortuitum-chelonei* and *Nocardia* are rare. They often follow trauma and are often associated with contact with soil. The ulcers are indolent, and the bed of the ulcer often has radiating lines that make it look like a cracked windshield. Hypopyon may or may not be present. Scrapings may contain acid-fast slender rods (*M fortuitum-chelonei*) or gram-positive filamentous, often branching organisms (*Nocardia*). See Tables 6–1 and 6–2 for recommended drug regimens.

2. FUNGAL KERATITIS

Fungal corneal ulcers once were seen only in agricultural settings, but with the advent of contact lenses, immunosuppressive

disease and corticosteroid use, these infections are seen in a variety of populations. The use of corticosteroids is not indicated in fungal disease; by altering the natural immune response and enhancing collagenase activity, these drugs are counterproductive.

Fungal ulcers are indolent and have a gray infiltrate with irregular edges, often a hypopyon, marked inflammation of the globe, superficial ulceration, and satellite lesions (usually infiltrates at sites distant from the main area of ulceration) (Figure 6–4). Underlying the principal lesion—and the satellite lesions as well—there is often an endothelial plaque associated with a severe anterior chamber reaction. Corneal abscesses frequently occur.

Most fungal ulcers are caused by opportunists such as *Candida, Fusarium, Aspergillus, Penicillium, Cephalosporium,* and others. There are no identifying features that help to differentiate one type of fungal ulcer from another.

Scrapings from fungal corneal ulcers, except those caused by *Candida,* contain hyphal elements; scrapings from *Candida* ulcers usually contain pseudohyphae or yeast forms that show characteristic budding. Tables 6–1 and 6–2 list the drugs recommended for the treatment of fungal ulcers.

3. VIRAL KERATITIS

▶ Herpes Simplex Keratitis

Herpes simplex keratitis occurs in two forms: primary and recurrent. It is the most common cause of both corneal ulceration and corneal blindness in the United States. The epithelial form is the ocular counterpart of labial herpes, with which it shares immunologic and pathologic features as well as having a similar time course. The only difference is that the clinical course of the keratitis may be prolonged because of the avascularity of the corneal stroma, which retards the migration of lymphocytes and macrophages to the lesion. Herpes simplex virus (HSV) ocular infection in the immunocompetent host is often self-limited, but in the immunologically compromised host, including patients treated with topical corticosteroids, its course can be chronic and damaging. Stromal and endothelial disease has previously been thought to be a purely immunologic response to virus particles or virally induced cellular changes. However, there is increasing evidence that active viral infection can occur within stromal and possibly endothelial cells as well as in other tissues within the anterior segment, such as the iris and trabecular endothelium. This highlights the need to assess the relative role of viral replication and host immune responses prior to and during therapy for herpetic disease. Topical corticosteroids may control damaging inflammatory responses but at the expense of facilitation of viral replication. Thus, whenever topical corticosteroids are to be used, antivirals are likely to be necessary. Any patient undergoing topical corticosteroid therapy for herpetic eye disease must be under the supervision of an ophthalmologist.

Serologic studies suggest that most adults have been exposed to the virus, although many do not recollect any episodes of clinical disease. Following primary infection, the virus establishes latency in the trigeminal ganglion. The factors influencing the development of recurrent disease, including its site, have yet to be unraveled. There is increasing evidence that the severity of disease is at least partly determined by the strain of virus involved. Most HSV infections of the cornea are still caused by HSV type 1 (the cause of labial herpes), but in both infants and adults, a few cases caused by HSV type 2 (the cause of genital herpes) have been reported. The corneal lesions caused by the two types are indistinguishable.

Scrapings of the epithelial lesions of HSV keratitis and fluid from skin lesions contain multinucleated giant cells. The virus can be cultivated on the chorioallantoic membrane of embryonated hens' eggs and in many tissue cell lines—for example, HeLa cells, on which it produces characteristic plaques. In most cases, however, diagnosis can be made clinically on the basis of characteristic dendritic or geographic ulcers and greatly reduced or absent corneal sensation. PCR methods are used for accurate identification of HSV from tissue and fluid as well as from corneal epithelial cells.

A. Clinical Findings

Primary ocular herpes simplex is infrequently seen, but manifests as a vesicular blepharoconjunctivitis, occasionally with corneal involvement, and usually occurs in young children. It is generally self-limited, without causing significant ocular damage. Topical antiviral therapy may be used as prophylaxis against corneal involvement and as therapy for corneal disease.

Attacks of the common recurrent type of herpetic keratitis (Figure 6–5) are triggered by fever, overexposure to ultraviolet

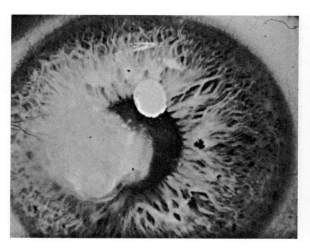

▲ **Figure 6–5.** Corneal scar caused by recurrent herpes simplex keratitis. (Courtesy of A Rosenberg.)

light, trauma, the onset of menstruation, or some other local or systemic source of immunosuppression. Unilaterality is the rule, but bilateral lesions develop in 4%–6% of cases and are seen most often in atopic patients.

1. **Symptoms**—The first symptoms of an HSV infection are usually irritation, photophobia, and tearing. When the central cornea is affected, there is also some reduction in vision. Since corneal anesthesia usually occurs early in the course of the infection, the symptoms may be minimal and the patient may not seek medical advice. There is often a history of fever blisters or other herpetic infection, but corneal ulceration can occasionally be the only sign of a recurrent herpetic infection.

2. **Lesions**—The most characteristic lesion is the **dendritic ulcer,** which occurs in the corneal epithelium, has a typical branching, linear pattern with feathery edges, and has terminal bulbs at its ends (Figure 6–6). Fluorescein staining makes the dendrite easy to identify, but unfortunately herpetic keratitis can also simulate many corneal infections and must be considered in the differential diagnosis of many corneal lesions.

Geographic ulceration is a form of chronic dendritic disease in which the delicate dendritic lesion takes a broader form. The edges of the ulcer lose their feathery quality. Corneal sensation, as with dendritic disease, is diminished. The clinician should always test for this sign.

Other corneal epithelial lesions that may be caused by HSV are a blotchy epithelial keratitis, stellate epithelial keratitis, and filamentary keratitis. All of these are usually transitory, however, and often become typical dendrites within a day or two.

Subepithelial opacities can be caused by HSV infection. A ghost-like image, corresponding in shape to the original

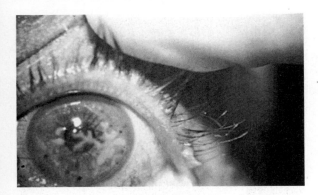

▲ **Figure 6–6.** Dendritic figures seen in herpes simplex keratitis.

epithelial defect but slightly larger, can be seen in the area immediately underlying the epithelial lesion. The "ghost" remains superficial but is often enhanced by the use of antiviral drugs, especially idoxuridine. As a rule, these subepithelial lesions do not persist for more than a year.

Disciform keratitis is the most common form of stromal disease in HSV infection. The stroma is edematous in a central, disk-shaped area, without significant infiltration and usually without vascularization. The edema may be sufficient to produce folds in Descemet's membrane. Keratic precipitates may lie directly under the disciform lesion but may also involve the entire endothelium because of the frequently associated anterior uveitis. The pathogenesis of disciform keratitis is generally regarded as an immunologic reaction to viral antigens in the stroma or endothelium, but active viral disease cannot be ruled out. Like most herpetic lesions in immunocompetent individuals, disciform keratitis is normally self-limited, lasting weeks to months. Edema is the most prominent sign, and healing can occur with minimal scarring and vascularization. A similar clinical appearance is seen with **primary endothelial keratitis (endothelitis)**, which can be associated with anterior uveitis together with raised intraocular pressure and a focal inflammation of the iris. This is thought to be due to viral replication within the various anterior chamber structures.

Stromal HSV keratitis in the form of focal areas of infiltration and edema, often accompanied by vascularization, is likely to be predominantly due to viral replication. Corneal thinning, necrosis, and perforation may develop rapidly, particularly if topical corticosteroids are being used. If there is stromal disease in the presence of epithelial ulceration, it may be difficult to differentiate bacterial or fungal superinfection from herpetic disease. The features of the epithelial disease need to be carefully scrutinized for herpetic characteristics, but a bacterial or fungal component may be present and the patient must be managed accordingly. Stromal necrosis also may be caused by an acute immune reaction,

again complicating the diagnosis with regard to active viral disease. Hypopyon may be seen with necrosis as well as secondary bacterial or fungal infection.

Peripheral lesions of the cornea can also be caused by HSV. They are usually linear and show a loss of epithelium before the underlying corneal stroma becomes infiltrated. (This is in contrast to the marginal ulcer associated with bacterial hypersensitivity, for example, to *S aureus* in staphylococcal blepharitis, in which the infiltration precedes the loss of the overlying epithelium.) Separation of the two disorders is important since the treatment of marginal immune ulcers can include use of corticosteroids, a medication not indicated the treatment of active viral infection. Testing for corneal sensation is unreliable in peripheral herpetic disease. The patient is apt to be far less photophobic than a patient with nonherpetic corneal disease.

B. Treatment

The treatment of HSV keratitis should be directed at eliminating viral replication within the cornea while minimizing the damaging effects of the inflammatory response.

1. **Debridement**—An effective way to treat dendritic keratitis is epithelial debridement, since the virus is located in the epithelium and debridement will also reduce the viral antigenic load to the corneal stroma. Healthy epithelium adheres tightly to the cornea, but infected epithelium is easy to remove. Debridement is accomplished with a tightly wound cotton-tipped applicator. A cycloplegic/mydriatic agent such as homatropine 5% is then instilled into the conjunctival sac, and a pressure dressing is applied. The patient should be examined daily and the dressing changed until the corneal defect has healed, usually within 72 hours. Adjunctive therapy with a topical antiviral accelerates epithelial healing. Topical drug therapy without epithelial debridement for epithelial keratitis offers the advantage of not requiring patching but involves a hazard of drug toxicity.

2. **Drug therapy**—The topical antiviral agents used in herpetic keratitis are idoxuridine, trifluridine, vidarabine, ganciclovir, and acyclovir. (Topical acyclovir for ophthalmic use is not approved in the United States.) Ganciclovir and acyclovir are much more effective in stromal disease than the others. Idoxuridine and trifluridine are frequently associated with toxic epitheliopathy. Oral antivirals like acyclovir are of critical importance in the treatment of herpetic eye disease, particularly in atopic individuals who are susceptible to aggressive ocular and dermal (eczema herpeticum) herpetic disease. Dosage for active disease is 400 mg five times daily in nonimmunocompromised patients and 800 mg five times daily in compromised and atopic patients. Prophylactic dosage in recurrent disease is 400 mg twice daily. Famciclovir or valacyclovir may also be used.

Viral replication in the immunocompetent patient, particularly when confined to the corneal epithelium, usually is self-limited and scarring is minimal. It is thus unnecessary and potentially highly damaging to use topical corticosteroids. Regrettably, particularly when there is stromal disease, concerns about permanent scarring due to the corneal inflammation often result in the use of topical corticosteroids, but this is based on the misconception that reducing inflammation reduces disease severity. Even when the inflammatory response is thought to be purely immunologically driven, such as in disciform keratitis, topical corticosteroids are often best avoided if the episode is likely to be self-limited. Once topical corticosteroids have been used, this usually commits the patient to requiring the drug to control further episodes of keratitis, with the potential for uncontrolled viral replication and other steroid-related side effects, such as bacterial and fungal superinfection, glaucoma, and cataract. Topical corticosteroids may also accelerate corneal thinning, thus increasing the risk of corneal perforation. If it becomes necessary to use topical corticosteroids because of the severity of the inflammatory response, it is absolutely essential that appropriate antiviral therapy be used to control viral replication. Problems in the management of HSV keratitis are often due to inappropriate use of multiple topical treatments, including antivirals, antibiotics, and corticosteroids, resulting in adverse effects including epithelial toxicity. Frequently, using oral antivirals and tapering the corticosteroids will result in marked improvement.

3. **Surgical treatment**—Penetrating keratoplasty may be indicated for visual rehabilitation in patients with severe corneal scarring, but it should not be undertaken until the herpetic disease has been inactive for many months. Postoperatively, recurrent herpetic infection may occur as a result of the surgical trauma and the topical corticosteroids necessary to prevent corneal graft rejection. It may also be difficult to distinguish corneal graft rejection from recurrent stromal disease. Systemic antiviral agents should be used for several months after keratoplasty to cover the use of topical corticosteroids.

Corneal perforation due to progressive herpetic stromal disease or superinfection with bacteria or fungi may necessitate emergency penetrating keratoplasty. Cyanoacrylate glue can be used to seal a small perforation (Figure 6–7), and lamellar "patch" grafts have been successful in selected cases. Lamellar keratoplasty has the advantage over penetrating keratoplasty of reduced potential for corneal graft rejection. A therapeutic soft contact lens, tarsorrhaphy, or amniotic membrane may be required to heal persistent epithelial defects in HSV keratitis.

4. **Control of trigger mechanisms that reactivate HSV infection**—Recurrent HSV infections of the eye are common, occurring in about one-third of cases within 2 years after the first attack. A trigger mechanism can often be discovered by careful questioning of the patient. Once identified, the trigger can often be avoided. Aspirin can be

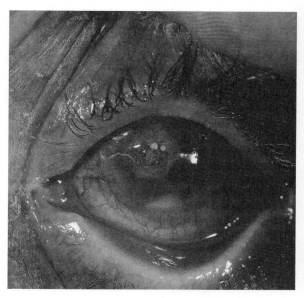

▲ **Figure 6–7.** Medical grade cyanoacrylate glue sealing small paracentral corneal perforation. See color insert.

used to avoid fever, excessive exposure to the sun or ultraviolet light can be avoided, and aspirin can be taken just prior to the onset of menstruation.

▶ Varicella-Zoster Viral Keratitis

Varicella-zoster virus (VZV) infection occurs in two forms: primary (varicella) and recurrent (herpes zoster). Ocular manifestations are uncommon in varicella but common in ophthalmic zoster. In varicella (chicken-pox), the usual eye lesions are pocks on the lids and lid margins. Rarely, keratitis occurs (typically a peripheral stromal lesion with vascularization), and still more rarely, epithelial keratitis occurs with or without pseudodendrites. Disciform keratitis, with uveitis of varying duration, has been reported.

In contrast to the rare and benign corneal lesions of varicella, the relatively frequent ophthalmic herpes zoster is often accompanied by keratouveitis that varies in severity according to the immune status of the patient. Thus, although children with zoster keratouveitis usually have benign disease, the aged have severe and sometimes blinding disease. Corneal complications in ophthalmic zoster often occur if there is a skin eruption in areas supplied by the branches of the nasociliary nerve.

Unlike recurrent HSV keratitis that usually affects only the epithelium, VZV keratitis affects the stroma and anterior uvea at onset. The epithelial lesions are blotchy and amorphous except for an occasional linear pseudodendrite that only vaguely resembles the true dendrites of HSV keratitis. Stromal opacities consist of edema and mild cellular infiltration and initially are subepithelial. Deep stromal disease can follow with

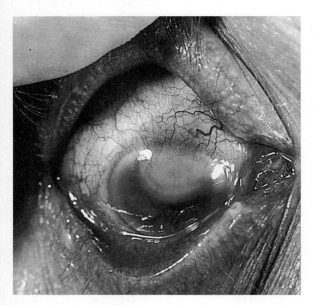

▲ **Figure 6–8.** Herpes zoster keratitis.

necrosis and vascularization (Figure 6–8). A disciform keratitis sometimes develops and resembles HSV disciform keratitis. Loss of corneal sensation, with the risk of neurotrophic keratitis (see later), is always a prominent feature and often persists for months after the corneal lesion appears to have healed. The associated uveitis tends to persist for weeks or months, but with time it eventually heals. Scleritis (sclerokeratitis) can be a serious feature of VZV ocular disease.

Intravenous and oral antivirals have been used successfully for the treatment of herpes zoster ophthalmicus, particularly in immunocompromised patients. The oral dosage for acyclovir is 800 mg five times daily for 10–14 days; for valacyclovir, 1 g three times daily for 7–10 days; for famciclovir, 500 mg every 8 hours for 7–10 days. Therapy needs to be started within 72 hours after appearance of the rash. The role of topical antivirals is less certain. Topical corticosteroids may be necessary to treat severe keratitis, uveitis, and secondary glaucoma. The use of systemic corticosteroids is controversial. They may be indicated in reducing the incidence and severity of postherpetic neuralgia, but the risk of steroid complications is significant. Unfortunately, systemic acyclovir has little influence on the development of postherpetic neuralgia. However, the condition is self-limited, and reassurance can be helpful as a supplement to analgesics. Patients with facial and scalp lesions should be seen for several months after the skin lesions arise because the onset of keratitis can be delayed.

4. ACANTHAMOEBA KERATITIS

Acanthamoeba is a free-living protozoan that thrives in polluted water containing bacteria and organic material. Corneal infection with *Acanthamoeba* is usually associated with soft contact lens wear, including silicone hydrogel lenses, or overnight wear of rigid (gas-permeable) contact lenses to correct refractive errors (orthokeratology). There have been cases associated with a particular contact lens solution, probably related to insufficient anti-*Acanthamoeba* efficacy. It may also occur in non–contact lens wearers after exposure to contaminated water or soil.

The initial symptoms are pain out of proportion to the clinical findings, redness, and photophobia. The characteristic clinical signs are indolent corneal ulceration, a stromal ring, and perineural infiltrates, but patients often present with changes confined to the corneal epithelium.

The diagnosis is established by culturing on specially prepared media (non-nutrient agar with an overlay of *E scherichia coli*). Better results are obtained by corneal biopsy than corneal scraping, since histopathologic examination for amebic forms (trophozoites or cysts) can also be undertaken. Impression cytology and confocal microscopy are newer diagnostic techniques. Contact lens cases and solutions should be cultured. Often the amebic forms can be identified in the contact lens case fluid.

The differential diagnosis includes herpetic keratitis, with which it is frequently confused, fungal keratitis, mycobacterial keratitis, and *Nocardia* infection of the cornea.

In the early stages of the disease, epithelial debridement may be beneficial. Medical treatment is usually started with intensive topical propamidine isethionate (1% solution) and either polyhexamethylene biguanide (0.01%–0.02% solution) or fortified neomycin eyedrops (Tables 6–1 and 6–2). *Acanthamoeba* species may have variable drug sensitivities and may acquire drug resistance. Treatment is also hampered by the organisms' ability to encyst within the corneal stroma, necessitating prolonged treatment. Corticosteroids are not indicated in the treatment of *Acanthamoeba* corneal disease unless required to control severe inflammation.

Keratoplasty may be necessary in advanced disease to arrest progression of the infection or after resolution and scarring to restore vision. Amniotic membrane transplants may be helpful for persistent epithelial defects. If the organism reaches the sclera, medical and surgical treatments are usually fruitless.

NONINFECTIOUS CORNEAL ULCERS

1. MARGINAL INFILTRATES & ULCERS

The majority of marginal corneal ulcers are benign but extremely painful. They are secondary to acute or chronic bacterial conjunctivitis, particularly staphylococcal blepharoconjunctivitis and less often Koch-Weeks (*Haemophilus aegyptius*) conjunctivitis. They are not an infectious process, however, and scrapings do not contain the causal bacteria. They are the result of sensitization to bacterial products,

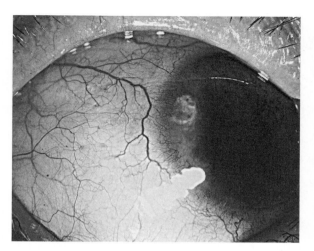

▲ **Figure 6–9.** Marginal ulcer of temporal cornea, right eye. (Courtesy of P Thygeson.)

antibody from the limbal vessels reacting with antigen that has diffused through the corneal epithelium.

Marginal infiltrates and ulcers (Figure 6–9) start as oval or linear infiltrates, separated from the limbus by a lucid interval, and only later may ulcerate and vascularize. They are self-limited, usually lasting from 7 to 10 days, but those associated with staphylococcal blepharoconjunctivitis usually recur. Treatment for blepharitis (shampoo scrubs, antimicrobials) usually will clear the problem; topical corticosteroids may be needed for severe cases. Topical corticosteroid preparations shorten their course and relieve symptoms, which are often severe, but treatment of the underlying blepharoconjunctivitis is essential if recurrences are to be prevented. Before starting corticosteroid therapy, great care must be taken to distinguish this entity from marginal herpetic keratitis. Marginal herpetic keratitis is usually almost symptomless because of corneal anesthesia, whereas hypersensitivity-type marginal ulcer is painful.

2. MOOREN'S ULCER (FIGURE 6–10)

The cause of Mooren's ulcer is still unknown, but an autoimmune origin is suspected. It is a marginal ulcer, unilateral in 60%–80% of cases and characterized by painful, progressive excavation of the limbus and peripheral cornea that often leads to loss of the eye. It occurs most commonly in old age but does not seem to be related to any of the systemic diseases that most often afflict the aged. It is unresponsive to both antibiotics and topical corticosteroids. Surgical excision of the limbal conjunctiva in an effort to remove sensitizing substances has recently been advocated. Lamellar tectonic keratoplasty has been used with success in selected cases. Systemic immunosuppressive therapy often is necessary to control moderate or advanced disease.

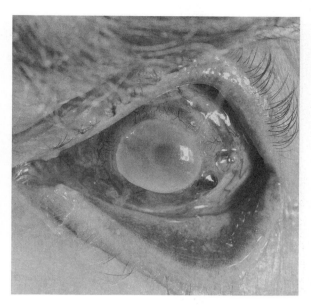

▲ **Figure 6–10.** Advanced Mooren's ulcer.

3. PHLYCTENULAR KERATOCONJUNCTIVITIS

Phlyctenules are localized accumulations of lymphocytes, monocytes, macrophages, and also neutrophils. They appear first at the limbus, but in recurrent attacks they may involve the bulbar conjunctiva and cornea. Corneal phlyctenules, often bilateral, cicatrize and vascularize, but conjunctival phlyctenules leave no trace.

Phlyctenular keratoconjunctivitis is a delayed hypersensitivity response, in most cases in developed countries to *S aureus* or other bacteria that proliferate on the lid margin in association with blepharitis. It may also occur in response to *Mycobacterium tuberculosis,* which was formerly a major cause of visual loss in the United States, particularly among Native Americans. The attack may be triggered by an acute bacterial conjunctivitis but is associated typically with a transient increase in the activity of childhood tuberculosis. Phlyctenules, rarely causing visual disability, also occur in San Joaquin Valley fever, a result of hypersensitivity to a primary infection with *Coccidioides immitis.*

Untreated phlyctenules spontaneously regress after 10–14 days. Topical corticosteroid therapy shortens their duration and decreases scarring and vascularization. In the staphylococcal type, the acute staphylococcal infection and chronic blepharitis need to be treated.

4. MARGINAL KERATITIS IN AUTOIMMUNE DISEASE (FIGURE 6–11)

The peripheral cornea receives its nourishment from the aqueous humor, the limbal capillaries, and the tear film. It is

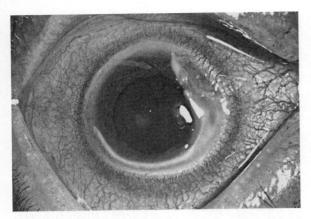

▲ **Figure 6–11.** Marginal keratitis. (Courtesy of M Hogan.)

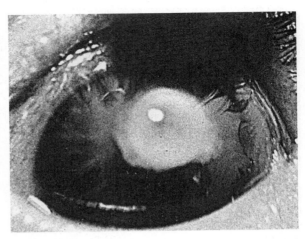

▲ **Figure 6–12.** Keratomalacia with ulceration associated with xerophthalmia (dietary) in an infant. (Photo by Diane Beeston.)

contiguous with the subconjunctival lymphoid tissue and the lymphatic arcades at the limbus. The perilimbal conjunctiva appears to play an important role in the pathogenesis of corneal lesions that arise both from local ocular disease and from systemic disorders, particularly those of autoimmune origin. There is a striking similarity between the limbal capillary network and the renal glomerular capillary network. On the endothelial basement membranes of the capillaries of both networks, immune complexes are deposited and immunologic disease results. Thus, the peripheral cornea often participates in such autoimmune diseases as rheumatoid arthritis, polyarteritis nodosa, systemic lupus erythematosus, scleroderma, midline lethal and Wegener's granulomatosis, ulcerative colitis, Crohn's disease, and relapsing polychondritis. The corneal changes are secondary to scleral inflammation, with or without scleral vascular closure (see Chapter 7). The clinical signs include vascularization, infiltration and opacification, and peripheral guttering that may progress to perforation. Mooren's ulcer may be an example of advanced marginal keratitis. Treatment is directed toward control of the associated systemic disease; topical therapy usually is ineffective, and systemic use of potent immunosuppressive drugs often is required. Corneal perforation may require cyanoacrylate glue (Figure 6–7), lamellar patch grafting, or a full-thickness keratoplasty.

5. CORNEAL ULCER DUE TO VITAMIN A DEFICIENCY

The typical corneal ulcer associated with avitaminosis A is centrally located and bilateral, gray and indolent, with a definite lack of corneal luster in the surrounding area (Figure 6–12). The cornea becomes soft and necrotic (hence the term "keratomalacia"), and perforation is common. The epithelium of the conjunctiva is keratinized, as evidenced by the presence of a Bitot's spot. This is a foamy, wedge-shaped area

in the conjunctiva, usually on the temporal side, with the base of the wedge at the limbus and the apex extending toward the lateral canthus. Within the triangle the conjunctiva is furrowed concentrically with the limbus, and dry flaky material can be seen falling from the area into the inferior cul-de-sac. A stained conjunctival scraping from a Bitot's spot will show many saprophytic xerosis bacilli (*Corynebacterium xerosis;* small curved rods) and keratinized epithelial cells.

Avitaminosis A corneal ulceration results from dietary lack of vitamin A or impaired absorption from the gastrointestinal tract and impaired utilization by the body. It may develop in an infant who has a feeding problem; in an adult who is on a restricted or generally inadequate diet; or in any person with a biliary obstruction, since bile in the gastrointestinal tract is necessary for the absorption of vitamin A, or other causes of mal-absorption. Lack of vitamin A causes a generalized keratinization of the epithelium throughout the body. The conjunctival and corneal changes together are known as **xerophthalmia.** Since the epithelium of the air passages is affected, many patients, if not treated, will die of pneumonia. Avitaminosis A also causes a generalized retardation of osseous growth. This is extremely important in infants; for example, if the skull bones do not grow and the brain continues to grow, increased intracranial pressure and papilledema can result.

Mild vitamin A deficiency should be treated in adults with a dose of 30,000 U/d for 1 week. Advanced cases will require much higher doses initially (20,000 U/kg/d). Sulfonamide or antibiotic ointment can be used locally in the eye to prevent secondary bacterial infection. The average daily requirement of vitamin A is 1500–5000 IU for children, according to age, and 5000 IU for adults. Highly pigmented vegetables are the best source of dietary vitamin A.

6. NEUROTROPHIC KERATITIS

Trigeminal nerve dysfunction, due to trauma, surgery, tumor, inflammation, or any other cause, may result in corneal anesthesia with loss of the blink reflex, one of the cornea's defense mechanisms, as well as lack of trophic factors important for epithelial function. In the early stages of neurotrophic keratitis, there is diffuse blotchy epithelial edema. Subsequently there is loss of the epithelium (neurotrophic ulcer), which may extend over a large area of the cornea.

In the absence of corneal sensation, even a severe keratitis may produce little discomfort. Patients must be warned to look out for redness of the eye, reduced vision, or increased conjunctival discharge and to seek ophthalmic care as soon as any of these develop. Keeping the cornea moist with artificial tears and lubricant ointments may help to protect it. Swim goggles may be useful at night (Figure 6–13).

Once neurotrophic keratitis develops, it must be treated promptly. The most effective management is to keep the eye closed by careful horizontal taping of the eyelids, by tarsorrhaphy, or by means of ptosis induced with botulinum toxin. Secondary corneal infection must be treated promptly.

7. EXPOSURE KERATITIS

Exposure keratitis may develop in any situation in which the cornea is not properly moistened and covered by the eyelids. Examples include exophthalmos from any cause, ectropion, floppy lid syndrome, the absence of part of an eyelid as a result of trauma, and inability to close the lids properly, as in Bell's palsy. The two factors at work are the drying of the

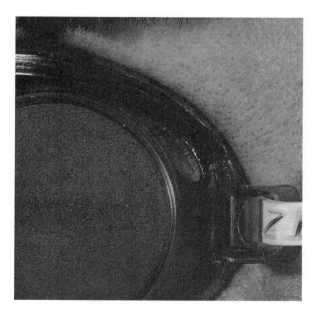

▲ **Figure 6–13.** Swim goggles are used at night to reduce corneal evaporation.

cornea and its exposure to minor trauma. The uncovered cornea is particularly subject to drying during sleeping hours and swim goggles may be useful at night (Figure 6–13). If an ulcer develops, it usually follows minor trauma and occurs in the inferior third of the cornea. Exposure keratitis is sterile but can become secondarily infected.

The therapeutic objective is to provide protection and moisture for the entire corneal surface. The treatment method depends on the underlying condition: eyelid surgery, correction of exophthalmos, an eye shield, or the options mentioned above in the discussion of neurotrophic keratitis. The combination of corneal anesthesia and exposure is particularly likely to result in severe keratitis.

▼ EPITHELIAL KERATITIS

CHLAMYDIAL KERATITIS

All five principal types of chlamydial conjunctivitis (trachoma, inclusion conjunctivitis, primary ocular lymphogranuloma venereum, parakeet or psittacosis conjunctivitis, and feline pneumonitis conjunctivitis) may be accompanied by corneal lesions. Only in trachoma and lymphogranuloma venereum, however, are they blinding or visually damaging. The corneal lesions of trachoma have been extensively studied and are of great diagnostic importance. In order of appearance, they consist of (1) epithelial microerosions affecting the upper third of the cornea; (2) micropannus; (3) subepithelial round opacities, commonly called trachoma pustules; (4) limbal follicles and their cicatricial remains, known as Herbert's peripheral pits; (5) gross pannus; and (6) extensive, diffuse, subepithelial cicatrization. Mild cases of trachoma may have only epithelial keratitis and micropannus and may heal without impairing vision.

The rare cases of lymphogranuloma venereum have far fewer characteristic changes but are known to have developed blindness secondary to diffuse corneal scarring and total pannus. The remaining types of chlamydial infection cause only micropannus, epithelial keratitis, and, rarely, subepithelial opacities that are not visually significant. Several methods of identifying chlamydia are available through any competent laboratory.

Chlamydial keratoconjunctivitis responds to systemic tetracyclines, for example, doxycycline, erythromycin, and azithromycin (see Chapter 5). Topical sulfonamides, tetracyclines, erythromycin, and rifampin are also effective.

DRUG-INDUCED EPITHELIAL KERATITIS

Epithelial keratitis is not uncommonly seen in patients using antiviral medications (idoxuridine and trifluridine) and several of the broad-spectrum and medium-spectrum antibiotics, such as neomycin, gentamicin, and tobramycin. It is usually a coarse superficial keratitis affecting predominantly the lower half of the cornea and interpalpebral fissure and may cause permanent scarring. The preservatives in eyedrops, particularly benzalkonium chloride (BAK) and thimerosal, are common causes of toxic keratitis.

KERATOCONJUNCTIVITIS SICCA (INCLUDING SJÖGREN'S SYNDROME)

Epithelial filaments in the lower half of the cornea are the cardinal signs of this autoimmune disease, in which secretion of the lacrimal and accessory lacrimal glands is diminished or eliminated. There is also a blotchy epithelial keratitis that affects mainly the lower half. Severe cases develop mucous pseudofilaments that stick to the corneal epithelium.

This pattern of keratitis also occurs in cicatrizing conjunctival diseases such as ocular pemphigoid, in which destruction of goblet cells of the conjunctiva results in mucus deficiency, such that any tears fail to wet the corneal epithelium effectively.

Treatment of keratoconjunctivitis sicca calls for the frequent use of tear substitutes and lubricating ointments, of which there are many commercial preparations. Fish or flaxseed oil has been found to be helpful (1000 mg bid). Mucus deficiency requires treatment with mucus substitutes in addition to artificial tears. Topical vitamin A may help to reverse epithelial keratinization. Moisture chambers or swim goggles may be required (Figure 6–13). Lacrimal punctal plugs and punctal occlusion are important in the management of advanced cases, as are room humidifiers. Cyclosporine (a T-cell inhibitor), 0.05% applied topically, occasionally can reestablish goblet cell (mucin) density. Preservative-free artificial tears are often indicated.

ADENOVIRUS KERATITIS

Keratitis usually accompanies all types of adenoviral conjunctivitis, reaching its peak 5–7 days after onset of the conjunctivitis. It is a fine epithelial keratitis best seen with the slitlamp after instillation of fluorescein. The minute lesions may group together to make up larger ones.

The epithelial keratitis is often followed by subepithelial opacities. In epidemic keratoconjunctivitis (EKC), which is due to adenovirus types 8 and 19, the subepithelial lesions are round and grossly visible (see Figure 5–6). They appear 8–15 days after onset of the conjunctivitis and may persist for months or even (rarely) for several years. Similar lesions occur very exceptionally in other adenoviral infections, eg, those caused by types 3, 4, and 7, but tend to be transitory and mild, lasting a few weeks at most.

Although the corneal opacities of adenoviral keratoconjunctivitis tend to fade temporarily with the use of topical corticosteroids so that the patient is temporarily more comfortable, corticosteroid therapy can prolong the corneal disease and is therefore not recommended.

OTHER VIRAL KERATITIDES

A fine epithelial keratitis may be seen in other viral infections, such as measles (in which the central cornea is affected predominantly), rubella, mumps, infectious mononucleosis, acute hemorrhagic conjunctivitis, Newcastle disease conjunctivitis, and verruca of the lid margin. A superior epithelial keratitis and pannus often accompany molluscum contagiosum nodules on the lid margin, which is a feature of HIV infection.

▼ DEGENERATIVE CORNEAL CONDITIONS

KERATOCONUS

Keratoconus is an uncommon degenerative bilateral disease that may be inherited as an autosomal recessive or autosomal dominant trait. Unilateral cases of unknown cause occur rarely. Symptoms appear in the second decade of life. The disease affects all races. Keratoconus has been associated with a number of diseases, including Down's syndrome, atopic dermatitis, retinitis pigmentosa, aniridia, vernal catarrh, Marfan's syndrome, Alport's syndrome, and Ehlers–Danlos syndrome. Pathologically, there are disruptive changes in Bowman's layer with keratocyte degeneration and ruptures in Descemet's membrane.

Blurred vision is the only symptom. Many patients present with rapidly increasing myopic astigmatism. Signs include cone-shaped cornea (Figure 6–14A); linear narrow folds centrally in Descemet's membrane (Vogt's lines), which are pathognomonic; an iron ring around the base of the cone (Fleischer's ring); and, in extreme cases, indentation of the lower lid by the cornea when the patient looks down (Munson's sign). There is an irregular or scissor reflex on retinoscopy and a distorted corneal reflection with Placido's disk or the keratoscope even early in the disease. Color-coded topography provides earlier and more accurate information on the degree of corneal distortion (Figure 2–24). Early topographic signs of keratoconus (forme fruste) suggests an unstable cornea and possibly an unsuitable candidate for laser refractive surgery. Often, the fundi cannot be clearly seen because of corneal astigmatism.

Acute hydrops of the cornea may occur, manifested by sudden diminution of vision associated with central corneal edema (Figure 6–14B). This arises as a consequence of rupture of Descemet's membrane. Usually it clears gradually without treatment but often leaves apical and Descemet membrane scarring.

Rigid contact lenses will markedly improve vision in the early stages by correcting irregular astigmatism. Keratoconus is one of the most common indications for corneal transplantation, traditionally penetrating keratoplasty but possibly deep lamellar keratoplasty (DLK), which avoids the risk of endothelial rejection. Surgery is indicated when a contact lens can no longer be effectively worn or when peripheral thinning will affect the surgery.

Keratoconus is often slowly progressive between the ages of 20 and 60, although an arrest in progression of the keratoconus may occur at any time. If a corneal transplant is done

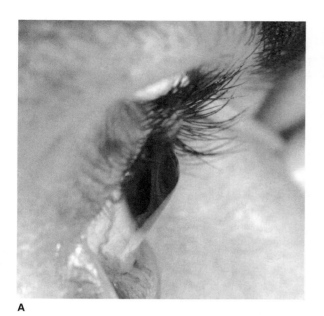

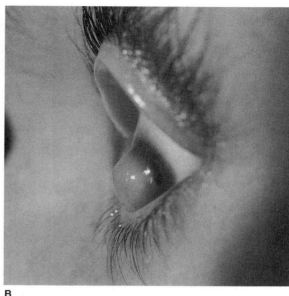

A

B

▲ **Figure 6–14.** **(A)** Keratoconus. **(B)** Acute corneal hydrops due to keratoconus.

before extreme corneal thinning occurs, the prognosis is excellent; good best-corrected vision is achieved in over 85% of eyes after 4 years and in over 70% of eyes after 14 years. Best vision after deep lamellar or penetrating keratoplasty often will require use of a rigid contact lens. Insertion of intracorneal (stromal) ring segments (Intacs) may delay the need for corneal transplantation, being suitable for patients with moderate keratoconus intolerant of contact lenses.

CORNEAL DEGENERATION

The corneal degenerations are a rare group of slowly progressive, bilateral, degenerative disorders that usually appear in the second or third decades of life. Some are hereditary. Other cases follow ocular inflammatory disease, and some are of unknown cause.

▶ Terrien's Disease

Terrien's disease is a rare bilateral symmetric degeneration characterized by marginal thinning of the upper nasal quadrants of the cornea. Men are more commonly affected than women, and the condition occurs more frequently in the third and fourth decades. There are no symptoms except for mild irritation during occasional inflammatory episodes, and the condition is slowly progressive. The clinical picture consists of marginal thinning and peripheral vascularization with lipid deposition. Perforation is a complication, especially from trauma. Tectonic (structural) keratoplasty may be required. Histopathologic studies of affected corneas have revealed vascularized connective tissue with fibrillary degeneration and

fatty infiltration of collagen fibers. Because the course of progression is slow and the central cornea is spared, the prognosis is reasonably good.

▶ Band (Calcific) Keratopathy (Figure 6–15)

Band keratopathy is characterized by the deposition of calcium salts in a band-like pattern in the anterior layers of the cornea. The keratopathy is usually limited to the interpalpebral area. The calcium deposits are noted in the basement membrane, Bowman's layer, and anterior stromal lamellas. A clear margin separates the calcific band from the limbus, and clear holes may be seen in the band, giving a Swiss-cheese appearance. Symptoms include irritation, injection, and blurring of vision.

Calcific band keratopathy has been described in a number of inflammatory, metabolic, and degenerative conditions. It is characteristically associated with juvenile idiopathic arthritis. It has been described in long-standing inflammatory conditions of the eye, glaucoma, and chronic cyclitis. Band keratopathy may also be associated with hyperparathyroidism, vitamin D intoxication, sarcoidosis, and leprosy. The standard method of removing band keratopathy consists of removal of the corneal epithelium by curettage under topical anesthesia followed by irrigation of the cornea with a sterile 0.01-molar solution of ethylenediaminetetraacetic acid (EDTA) (edetate calcium) or application of EDTA with a cotton-tip applicator. The rigid sheets of calcium deposits can be lifted and dissected away with a sharp blade. Final smoothing of the area is accomplished best with the excimer laser (photo-therapeutic keratectomy—PTK).

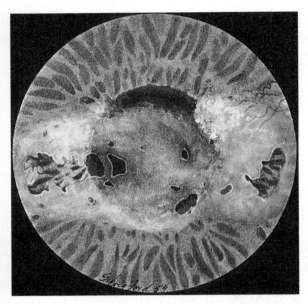

▲ **Figure 6-15.** Calcific band keratopathy. (Courtesy of M Hogan.)

▶ Climatic Droplet Keratopathy (Labrador Keratopathy, Spheroid Degeneration of the Cornea) (Figure 6–16)

Climatic droplet keratopathy affects mainly people who work out of doors. The corneal degeneration is thought to be caused by exposure to ultraviolet light and is characterized in the early stages by fine subepithelial yellow droplets in the peripheral cornea. As the disease advances, the droplets become central, with subsequent corneal clouding causing blurred vision. Treatment in advanced cases is corneal transplantation.

▶ Salzmann's Nodular Degeneration

This disorder is usually preceded by corneal inflammation, particularly phlyctenular keratoconjunctivitis or trachoma. Symptoms include redness, irritation, and blurring of vision. There is degeneration of the superficial cornea that involves the stroma, Bowman's layer, and epithelium, with superficial whitish-gray elevated nodules sometimes occurring in chains.

Rigid contact lenses will significantly improve visual acuity in most cases. Corneal transplantation is rarely required, but superficial lamellar keratectomy or photo-therapeutic (excimer laser) keratectomy (PTK) may be necessary.

ARCUS SENILIS

Arcus senilis is an extremely common, bilateral, benign peripheral corneal degeneration. Its prevalence is strongly associated with age. It is also associated with hypercholesterolemia and hypertriglyceridemia. Blood lipid studies should be performed in affected individuals under age 50.

Pathologically, lipid droplets involve the entire corneal thickness but are more concentrated in the superficial and deep layers, being relatively sparse in the corneal stroma.

There are no symptoms. Clinically, arcus senilis appears as a hazy gray ring about 2 mm in width and with a clear space between it and the limbus (Figure 6–17). No treatment is necessary, and there are no complications.

HEREDITARY CORNEAL DYSTROPHIES

This is a group of rare hereditary disorders of the cornea of unknown cause characterized by bilateral abnormal deposition of substances and associated with alteration in the normal corneal architecture that may or may not interfere with vision. These corneal dystrophies usually manifest themselves during the first or second decade but sometimes later. They may be stationary or slowly progressive throughout life. Corneal transplantation, when indicated, improves vision in most patients with hereditary corneal dystrophy.

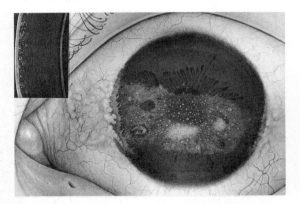
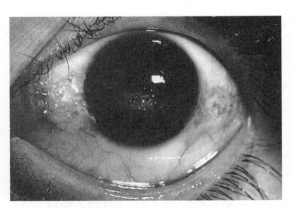

▲ **Figure 6-16.** Two photos showing climatic droplet (Labrador) keratodystrophy. Inset at left shows slitlamp view. (Photo at left courtesy of A Ahmad.)

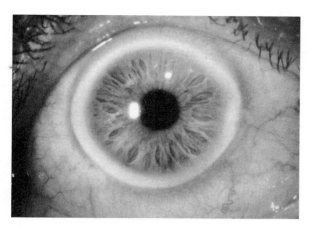

▲ **Figure 6–17.** Arcus senilis.

Anatomically, corneal dystrophies may be classified as epithelial, stromal, or posterior-limiting membrane dystrophies.

▶ Epithelial Corneal Dystrophies
A. Meesmann Dystrophy

This slowly progressive disorder is characterized by microcystic areas in the epithelium. The onset is in early childhood (first 1–2 years of life). The main symptom is slight irritation, and vision is slightly affected. The inheritance is autosomal dominant.

B. Epithelial Basement (Anterior) Membrane Dystrophy

Microcysts, dots, or map or fingerprint patterns, hence the older names Cogan's microcystic dystrophy and map-dot-fingerprint dystrophy, are seen at the level of the epithelial basement membrane. Confocal microscopy demonstrates abnormal epithelial basement membrane protruding into the epithelium, as well as epithelial cell abnormalities and microcysts. Recurrent erosion is common. Vision usually is not significantly affected.

C. Others

Reis–Bückler dystrophy is a dominantly inherited dystrophy affecting primarily Bowman's layer. The disease begins within the first decade of life with symptoms of recurrent erosion. Opacification of Bowman's layer gradually occurs, and the epithelium is irregular. No vascularization is usually noted. Vision may be markedly reduced.

Vortex dystrophy, or cornea verticillata, is characterized by pigmented lines or whorls occurring in Bowman's layer or the underlying stroma and spreading over the entire corneal surface. Visual acuity is not markedly affected. Such a pattern

of radiating pigmented lines may also be seen in patients treated with chlorpromazine, chloroquine, indomethacin, or amiodarone as well as in Fabry's disease.

▶ Stromal Corneal Dystrophies

There are three primary types of stromal corneal dystrophies.

A. Granular Dystrophy

This usually asymptomatic, slowly progressive corneal dystrophy most often begins in early childhood. The lesions consist of central, fine, whitish "granular" lesions in the stroma of the cornea. The epithelium and Bowman's layer may be affected late in the disease. Visual acuity is slightly reduced. Histologically, the cornea shows uniform deposition of hyaline material. Corneal transplantation is not needed except in very severe and late cases. The inheritance is autosomal dominant.

B. Macular Dystrophy

This type of stromal corneal dystrophy is manifested by a dense gray central opacity that starts in Bowman's layer. The opacity tends to spread toward the periphery and later involves the deeper stromal layers. Recurrent corneal erosion may occur, and vision is severely impaired. Histologic examination shows deposition of acid mucopolysaccharide in the stroma and degeneration of Bowman's layer. Penetrating or deep keratoplasty is often required. The inheritance is autosomal recessive.

C. Lattice Dystrophy

Lattice dystrophy starts as fine, branching linear opacities in Bowman's layer in the central area and spreads to the periphery. The deep stroma may become involved, but the process does not reach Descemet's membrane. Recurrent erosion often occurs. Histologic examination reveals amyloid deposits in the collagen fibers. Corneal transplantation, usually penetrating keratoplasty but possibly deep lamellar keratoplasty, is common, as is recurrence of the dystrophy in the graft. The hereditary pattern for lattice dystrophy is autosomal dominant.

▶ Posterior Corneal Dystrophies
A. Fuchs' Dystrophy

This disorder begins in the third or fourth decade and is slowly progressive throughout life. Women are more commonly affected than men. There are central wart-like deposits on Descemet's membrane, thickening of Descemet's membrane, and defects of size and shape of the endothelial cells. Decompensation of the endothelium may occur, particularly after cataract surgery, and leads to edema of the corneal stroma and epithelium, causing blurring of vision. Corneal haze is slowly progressive. Histologic examination of the cornea reveals the wart-like excrescences, which are secreted by the endothelial cells, over Descemet's membrane. Thinning and pigmentation of the endothelium and thickening of Descemet's membrane are characteristics. Penetrating keratoplasty, generally combined with cataract surgery if this has not been performed previously, was the standard treatment once corneal decompensation has developed, but overall has become required less frequently with improvements in cataract surgery and is largely being replaced by deep lamellar endothelial keratoplasty (DLEK), in which the endothelium with only a thin layer of stroma is transplanted.

B. Posterior Polymorphous Dystrophy

This is a common disorder with onset in early childhood. Polymorphous plaques of calcium crystals are observed in the deep stromal layers. Vesicular lesions may be seen in the endothelium. Edema occurs in the deep stroma. The condition is asymptomatic in most cases, but in severe cases, epithelial and total stromal edema may occur. The inheritance is autosomal dominant.

MISCELLANEOUS CORNEAL DISORDERS

THYGESON'S SUPERFICIAL PUNCTATE KERATITIS

Superficial punctate keratitis is an uncommon chronic and recurrent bilateral disorder more common in females. It is characterized by discrete and elevated oval epithelial opacities that show punctate staining with fluorescein, mainly in the pupillary area. The opacities are not visible grossly but can be easily seen with the slitlamp or loupe. Subepithelial opacities underlying the epithelial lesions (ghosts) are often observed as the epithelial disease resolves.

No causative organism has been identified, but a virus is suspected. A varicella-zoster virus has been isolated from the corneal scrapings of one case.

Mild irritation, slight blurring of vision and photophobia are the only symptoms. The conjunctiva is not involved.

Epithelial keratitis secondary to staphylococcal blepharoconjunctivitis is differentiated from superficial punctate keratitis by its involvement of the lower third of the cornea and lack of subepithelial opacities. Epithelial keratitis in trachoma is ruled out by its location in the upper third of the cornea and the presence of pannus. Many other forms of keratitis involving the superficial cornea are unilateral or are eliminated by their histories.

Short-term instillation of corticosteroid drops will often cause disappearance of the opacities and subjective improvement, but recurrences are the rule. The ultimate prognosis is good since there is no scarring or vascularization of the cornea. Untreated, the disease runs a protracted course of 1–3 years. Long-term treatment with topical corticosteroids may prolong the course of the disease for many years and lead to steroid-induced cataract and glaucoma. Therapeutic soft contact lenses have been used to control symptoms in especially bothersome cases. Cyclosporine topical drops, 1% or 2%, have been effective as a substitute for corticosteroids.

RECURRENT CORNEAL EROSION

This is a fairly common and serious mechanical corneal disorder that presents some classic signs and symptoms but may be easily missed if it is not looked for specifically. The patient is usually awakened during the early morning hours by a pain in the affected eye. The pain is continuous, and the eye becomes red, irritated, and photophobic. When the patient attempts to open the eyes in the morning, the lid pulls off the loose epithelium, resulting in pain and redness.

Three types of recurrent corneal erosions can be recognized:

1. **Acquired recurrent erosion (traumatic):** The patient usually gives a history of previous corneal injury. It is unilateral, it occurs with equal frequency in men and women, and the family history is negative. The recurrent erosion occurs most frequently in the center below the pupil regardless of the location of the previous injury.

2. **Recurrent erosion associated with corneal disease:** After corneal ulceration heals, the epithelium may break down in a recurrent fashion (as in HSV "metaherpetic" ulcer).

3. **Recurrent erosion associated with corneal dystrophies:** Recurrent erosions of the cornea may be observed in patients with epithelial basement membrane dystrophy, lattice dystrophy, and ReisBückler's corneal dystrophy.

Recurrent corneal erosion is due to a defect in anchoring of the corneal epithelium between the epithelial basement membrane and Bowman's layer, due to faulty hemidesmosome connections. The epithelium is loose and vulnerable to separation.

Instillation of a local anesthetic relieves the symptoms immediately, and fluorescein staining will show the eroded area, typically a small area in the lower central cornea. Healed erosions often exhibit subepithelial debris.

Treatment consists of a pressure bandage on the eye to promote healing. Mechanical denuding of the loose corneal epithelium may be necessary. The other eye should be kept closed most of the time to minimize movement of the lid over the affected eye. Bed rest is desirable for 24 hours. The cornea usually heals in 2–3 days. To reduce the risk of and promote continued healing, a bland ophthalmic ointment at bedtime is used for several months. In more severe cases, artificial tears are instilled during the day. The use of hypertonic ointment (glucose 40% or sodium chloride 5%) drops is often of value. Therapeutic soft contact lenses, needle micropuncture of Bowman's layer, and PTK have been useful in cases that do not respond to more conservative management.

INTERSTITIAL KERATITIS DUE TO CONGENITAL SYPHILIS

This self-limited inflammatory disease of the cornea, also known as immune stromal keratitis, characteristically is a late manifestation of congenital syphilis, but overall other causes are now more prevalent (see below), partly because of the reduction in incidence of congenital syphilis. Interstitial keratitis rarely occurs in acquired syphilis, of which the incidence has increased markedly in association with HIV infection.

Interstitial keratitis due to congenital syphilis occasionally starts unilaterally, but almost always becomes bilateral weeks to months later. It affects all races and is more common in female than male patients. Symptoms appear between the ages of 5 and 20. Pathologic findings include edema, lymphocytic infiltration, and vascularization of the corneal stroma. It is probably a delayed immune response to stromal antigen retained from passage of *Treponema pallidum* organisms through the cornea before or at birth, because the organisms are not found in the cornea during the acute phase.

▶ Clinical Findings

A. Symptoms and Signs

Hutchinson's triad comprises interstitial keratitis, deafness, and notched upper central incisors. Saddle nose is another sign of congenital syphilis. The patient complains of pain, photophobia, and blurring of vision. Physical signs include conjunctival injection, corneal edema, vascularization of the deeper corneal layers, and miosis. There is an associated severe anterior granulomatous uveitis and blepharospasm due to photophobia. The grayish-pink appearance of the cornea (due to edema and vascularization) that occurs in the acute phase is sometimes referred to as a "salmon patch."

B. Laboratory Findings

Serologic tests for syphilis are positive.

▶ Complications & Sequelae

Corneal scarring and vascularization occur if the process has been particularly severe and prolonged. Secondary glaucoma may result from the uveitis.

▶ Treatment

Topical cycloplegic/mydriatic agents to dilate the pupils are important to prevent formation of posterior synechiae. Corticosteroid drops often relieve the symptoms dramatically but must be continued for long periods to prevent recurrence of symptoms. Dark glasses and a darkened room may be necessary if photophobia is severe. Treatment should be given for systemic syphilis, even though this usually has little effect on the ocular condition. Corneal scarring may necessitate corneal transplant, and glaucoma, if present, may be difficult to control.

▶ Course & Prognosis

The severity of corneal disease is not affected by treatment, which is aimed at prevention of complications. The inflammatory phase lasts 3 or 4 weeks. The corneas then gradually clear, leaving ghost vessels and scars in the corneal stroma.

INTERSTITIAL KERATITIS DUE TO OTHER CAUSES

In the United States, unilateral interstitial (immune stromal) keratitis is usually due to herpes simplex virus and occasionally due to varicella-zoster virus. Commonly no cause is found for active bilateral interstitial keratitis, but congenital syphilis remains the most commonly identified cause of inactive bilateral disease. Tuberculosis, leprosy, cytomegalovirus, measles virus, mumps virus, and Lyme disease are rare causes of interstitial keratitis. Treatment is usually symptomatic, but it is important to establish the cause whenever possible.

Cogan syndrome is a rare disorder generally believed to be a vascular hypersensitivity reaction of unknown origin. It is a disease of young adults and is characterized by non-syphilitic interstitial keratitis and a vestibuloauditory disturbance, usually sudden hearing loss. Corticosteroids are reputed to be of value, but some degree of visual impairment and complete nerve deafness usually supervene. Rarely patients die due to vasculitis, such as aortitis.

CORNEAL PIGMENTATION

Pigmentation of the cornea may occur with or without ocular or systemic disease. There are several distinct varieties.

▶ Krukenberg Spindle

In pigment dispersion syndrome, brown uveal pigment is deposited bilaterally upon the central endothelial surface in a vertical spindle-shaped fashion (Krukenberg spindle). It occurs in a small percentage of people over age 20, usually in myopic women. It can be seen grossly in severe cases, but is best observed with the slitlamp. The visual acuity is only slightly affected, and the progression is extremely slow. Pigmentary glaucoma must be ruled out by regular examination of both intraocular pressures and optic discs.

▶ Blood Staining

This disorder occurs occasionally as a complication of traumatic hyphema with secondary glaucoma and is due to hemosiderin in the corneal stroma. The cornea is golden brown, and vision is decreased. In most cases the cornea gradually clears in 1–2 years.

▶ Kayser–Fleischer Ring

This is a bilateral pigmented ring whose color varies widely from ruby red to bright green, blue, yellow, or brown. Composed of fine granular deposits of copper, each ring is 1–3 mm in diameter and located just inside the limbus at the level of Decemet's membrane. In exceptional cases, there is a second ring.

Kayser–Fleischer rings are almost always due to Wilson's disease (hepatolenticular degeneration) and are an important clinical finding as their presence may obviate the need for liver biopsy in patients with suggestive clinical features and abnormal copper studies. They have been described in chronic liver disease not due to Wilson's disease. In Wilson's disease, the intensity of the pigmentation can be reduced by treatment of the abnormal copper metabolism, such that the corneal signs may be an indicator of response to treatment.

▶ Iron Lines (Hudson–Stähli Line, Fleischer's Ring, Stocker's Line, Ferry's Line)

Localized deposits of iron within the corneal epithelium may occur in sufficient quantity to become visible clinically. The Hudson–Stähli line is a horizontal line at the junction of the middle and lower thirds of the cornea, corresponding to the line of lid closure, in otherwise normal elderly patients. Fleischer's ring surrounds the base of the cone in keratoconus. Stocker's line is a vertical line associated with pterygia, and Ferry's line develops adjacent to limbal filtering blebs. Similar iron deposits are seen at the site of corneal scars.

▼ CONTACT LENSES

Glass contact lenses were first described in 1888 by Adolf Fick and were then used for the treatment of keratoconus by Eugene Kalt. Poor results were achieved until 1945, when Kevin Tuohy of Los Angeles produced a plastic precorneal lens with a diameter of 11 mm. Since that time, advances in contact lens technology have produced several different varieties of lenses, which are broadly divided into two types: rigid and soft lenses. The basic requirement for success of contact lenses is to overcome the effect on oxygen supply to the cornea from wearing an occlusive lens. The optical features of contact lenses are discussed in Chapter 21.

▶ Rigid Lenses
A. Standard Hard Lenses

These direct descendants of Tuohy's lens are made of polymethylmethacrylate (PMMA; Perspex). They are impervious to oxygen and thus rely on pumping of tears into the space between the lens and the cornea during blinking to provide oxygen to the cornea. They are smaller than the corneal diameter. Always for daily wear, these lenses are easy to care for, are relatively inexpensive, and correct vision efficiently, particularly if there is significant astigmatism. Unfortunately, many persons cannot tolerate them. Corneal edema due to corneal hypoxia and spectacle blur (poor vision with spectacle correction after a period of contact lens wear) are common complaints, and they are now rarely used.

B. Rigid Gas-Permeable Lenses

These are rigid lenses made from cellulose acetate butyrate, silicone acrylate, or silicone combined with polymethylmethacrylate. They have the advantage of high oxygen permeability, thus improving corneal metabolism, and greater comfort while retaining the optical properties of rigid lenses, although they are not as easy to tolerate as soft lenses. They are generally used on a daily-wear basis but can be used on an extended-wear (24-hour) basis in exceptional circumstances. Gas-permeable lenses are particularly suitable for correction of keratoconus and astigmatism and when bifocal or multifocal lenses are required.

Orthokeratology is the overnight wear of rigid gas-permeable lenses to correct myopia or astigmatism by reshaping the cornea. It is advocated as a safer, less expensive alternative to refractive surgery, but there is risk of corneal infection. Most ophthalmologists recommend not wearing any type of refractive contact lens through the night.

▶ Soft Lenses
A. Cosmetic Soft Lenses

Hydrogel lenses, based on hydroxymethyl methacrylate (HEMA) or silicone, of which the latter provides greater oxygen permeability, are considerably more comfortable than rigid lenses but are flexible and thus conform to the surface of the cornea. Regular astigmatism can be partially corrected by incorporating cylinder into the soft lens; irregular astigmatism is poorly corrected. They are cheaper to purchase but are less durable and complications are more common than with rigid lenses, including ulcerative keratitis (particularly if the lenses are worn overnight), immune corneal reactions to deposits on the lenses, giant papillary conjunctivitis, reactions to lens-care solutions (especially those containing the preservative thimerosal), corneal edema, and corneal vascularization.

Cosmetic soft contact lenses are usually removed each day, to be cleaned, disinfected, and then stored overnight in solution. With care, a pair of such lenses will last for 1 year but then should be discarded. **Disposable soft contact lenses** for daily wear are readily available, but are more expensive. Soft lenses replaced every 2 to 4 weeks, if properly worn and cared for, are quite safe. Disposable soft contact lenses for overnight (extended) wear, usually to be worn for 1 week and then replaced but potentially to be worn for up to 30 days, are strongly promoted by contact lens manufacturers but generally are not recommended by ophthalmologists because of the increased risk of corneal infection. For aphakic correction, it is occasionally necessary to resort to extended wear because of difficulties with insertion, removal, and care of the lenses.

B. Therapeutic Soft Lenses

The use of therapeutic soft contact lenses has become an indispensable part of the ophthalmologist's management of external eye disease. The lenses form a soft barrier over the cornea, providing protection against trichiasis and exposure. Lenses with high water content can act as a "stent" for epithelial healing, such as in the treatment of recurrent erosions. Patients with pain due to epithelial disease, such as in bullous keratopathy, particularly benefit from therapeutic soft contact lenses. Lenses with low water content can be used to seal small corneal perforations or wound leaks. In all cases of therapeutic contact lens wear, infection can occur. Antimicrobial coverage may be indicated if there is an epithelial defect.

▶ Contact Lens Care

It is essential that all contact lens wearers be made aware of the risks associated with contact lens wear—particularly those patients choosing the high-risk varieties such as extended-wear lenses for cosmetic optical correction purely on the grounds of convenience. All wearers must be under the regular care of a contact lens practitioner. Many of the chronic complications of contact lens wear are asymptomatic in their early and easily treated stages. Any contact lens should be removed immediately if the eye becomes uncomfortable or inflamed, and ophthalmic attention must be sought immediately if symptoms do not rapidly resolve.

Except for daily disposables, contact lenses require regular cleaning and disinfecting, and particularly in the case of soft lenses, removal of protein deposits is required. Disinfection regimens include heat, chemical soaking, and hydrogen peroxide systems. All are effective if used according to the manufacturer's instructions, but some seem to be insufficiently effective against resistant organisms such as *Acanthamoeba* and *Fusarium*.

For contact lens wearers who have developed hypersensitivity reactions to preservatives in their contact lens solutions, there are contact lens care systems that do not contain preservatives. It is important that such individuals are aware of the ability of organisms such as *Pseudomonas* and *Acanthamoeba* to survive in nonpreserved saline solutions. The use of nonpreserved contact lens solutions requires much greater vigilance in the regular disinfection of lenses and lens storage cases. Even with standard contact lens care systems, deposits in contact lens storage cases may prevent effective disinfection. Tap water, which may harbor organisms such as *Acanthamoeba*, should not be used for rinsing contact lenses or contact lens storage cases. Contact lenses should not be worn when bathing in a hot tub or swimming.

CORNEAL TRANSPLANTATION

Corneal transplantation (keratoplasty) is indicated for a number of serious corneal conditions, for example, scarring, edema, thinning, and distortion. **Penetrating keratoplasty** (PK) means full-thickness corneal replacement. **Lamellar keratoplasty** is a partial-thickness procedure to replace the anterior cornea with a variable amount of stroma, extending to **deep lamellar** keratoplasty (DLK), in which almost the entire cornea except the endothelium is replaced. The reverse procedure is **deep lamellar endothelial keratoplasty** (DLEK), of which there are a number of variants such as Descemet's stripping automated endothelial keratoplasty (DSAEK), in which the endothelium with only a thin layer of stroma is transplanted.

Younger donors are preferred for penetrating and deep lamellar endothelial keratoplasties, because there is a direct relationship between age and the health and number of the endothelial cells, but older corneas (50–65 years) are acceptable if the endothelial cell count is adequate. Because of the rapid endothelial cell death rate, the eyes should be enucleated soon after death and refrigerated immediately. Whole eyes should be used within 48 hours, preferably within 24 hours. Modern storage media allow for longer storage. Corneoscleral caps stored in nutrient media may be used up to 6 days after donor death, and preservation in tissue culture media allows storage for as long as 6 weeks.

For lamellar and deep lamellar keratoplasty, corneas can be frozen, dehydrated, or refrigerated for several weeks; the endothelial cells are not important in these partial-thickness procedures involving the anterior cornea.

Diseases, like chemical injuries (see Chapter 19), in which loss of limbal stem cells leads to failure of corneal epithelialization, may benefit from limbal stem cell transplants, from the fellow eye or a donor eye, or amniotic membrane transplants, particularly in preparation for corneal transplantation. For severe corneal disease unsuitable for corneal transplantation, various artificial corneas (keratoprostheses) have been attempted with increasing success.

▶ Techniques

For penetrating or lamellar keratoplasty, the recipient eye is prepared by a partial-thickness cutting of a circle of diseased cornea, such as with a suction trephine (cookie-cutter action), and full-thickness removal with scissors or partial-thickness removal with dissection. For deep lamellar endothelial keratoplasty, the recipient endothelium is removed using instruments inserted into the anterior chamber.

For penetrating keratoplasty, the donor corneoscleral cap is placed endothelium up on a suction Teflon block; the trephine (Figure 6–18) is pressed down into the cornea, and a full-thickness button is punched out. For lamellar, deep lamellar, and deep lamellar endothelial keratoplasty, the process is adapted, using mechanical or possibly laser-cutting devices, to remove the required portion of cornea from a corneoscleral cap or whole globe. Precut tissue for endothelial keratoplasty is now available from eye banks in developed countries.

Developments in sutures (Figure 6–19), instruments, and microscopes, as well as changes in surgical techniques, have significantly improved the prognosis in all patients requiring corneal transplants. Reducing and managing postoperative astigmatism and corneal graft rejection continue to be major problems, particularly after penetrating keratoplasty (see Chapter 16). The use of an intraoperative hand-held keratometer and early suture removal guided by topographical mapping has proved useful in trying to minimize post-graft astigmatism. A large and lengthy multi-institutional study has revealed that the only antigens identified with transplant rejection are those of the ABO blood-type group. For this reason, some surgeons are matching donor and recipient

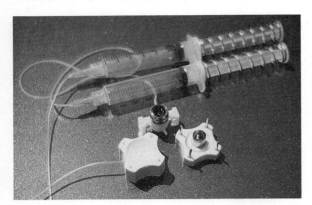

▲ **Figure 6–18.** A popular vacuum corneal punch and trephine. (Manufactured by Barron-Katena.)

ABO types before surgery, especial in high-risk patients (prior rejection, vascularized corneas, etc).

REFRACTIVE SURGERY

The inconvenience of spectacles to many wearers and the complications associated with contact lenses have resulted in a search for surgical solutions to the problem of refractive error.

▶ Radial Keratotomy

Developed initially by Sato of Japan and later by Fyodorov of the USSR, the central cornea is flattened by almost full-thickness radial incisions. The procedure is now rarely performed.

▶ Keratomileusis

In 1961, Barraquer of Colombia reported on the technique of myopic keratomileusis in which a lamellar corneal autograft is removed, shaped with a cryolathe (flattened), and sutured back into position. The procedure, also now rarely performed, was a precursor to laser in situ keratomileousis (LASIK).

▶ Procedures to Correct Astigmatism

Astigmatism continues to be a problem following most corneal operations, especially penetrating keratoplasty, and after cataract surgery. Astigmatism after keratoplasty may be improved by various surgical procedures, including relaxing incisions, compression sutures, and wedge resections. Laser procedures, such as LASIK or surface ablation techniques (LASEK, PRK, epi-LASIK) (see below), may be helpful. Refinements of incision, including adjustment of location according to preoperative corneal astigmatism, are useful in preventing postoperative astigmatism after cataract surgery.

▶ Alloplastic Corneal Implants

Various plastic discs and rings (eg, Intacs) have been placed in the corneal stroma to correct refractive errors but with limited success.

▶ Clear Lens Removal & Phakic Lens Implants

Removal of the crystalline lens (clear lens removal) is widely advocated for treatment of high myopia and presbyopia, but there are significant risks, notably retinal detachment in highly myopic eyes. Insertion of an intraocular lens without removal of the crystalline lens (phakic lens implant) is also undertaken, but corneal endothelial damage and development of cataract are worrisome.

▶ Lasers

An advanced approach to refractive corneal surgery involves the use of lasers (see Chapter 23). The excimer laser has received the most publicity, but the femtosecond laser is also proving useful.

In LASIK, a motorized microkeratome or the femtosecond laser is used to cut a thin lamellar corneal disk, which is folded back. Laser of the stromal bed produces the desired carefully programmed reshaping of the cornea, and then the flap is repositioned. The surface ablation techniques are photorefractive keratectomy (PRK), laser epithelial keratectomy (LASEK), and epi-LASIK. In PRK, only the corneal epithelium is removed prior to the laser treatment. In LASEK and epi-LASIK, the epithelium is removed, with dilute alcohol and a microkeratome respectively, and replaced after the laser treatment. When necessary, the laser delivery in all these techniques can be further refined by wavefront guided technology to take account of the optical aberrations of individual eyes.

Laser refractive surgery is mostly used for myopia, but can also treat astigmatism or hyperopia. Long-term visual results are about the same for the various techniques, but each has its

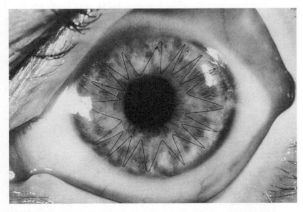

▲ **Figure 6–19.** Penetrating keratoplasty with 10–0 nylon running suture, 3 months after operation.

advantages and disadvantages. Surface ablation (PRK, LASEK) and LASIK now are being used for up to 10 diopters (or more) of myopia with good results. In large ablations, especially with LASIK, the threat of ectasia must be considered. LASIK produces the most rapid recovery, both visually and in terms of discomfort, but surface ablation has become much less uncomfortable, mostly due to effective nonsteroidal anti-inflammatory drugs. Surface haze also is less of a problem than before due to proper cooling of the corneal surface both during and immediately after ablation. The surface ablation techniques are particularly indicated for thin corneas and patients at risk of corneal trauma. Complications of laser refractive corneal surgery include unexpected refractive outcome, fluctuating refraction, irregular astigmatism, regression, epithelial, flap, or interface problems, stromal haze, corneal ectasia, and infection. Previous laser refractive corneal surgery results in particular difficulties when determining intraocular lens power for cataract surgery.

▶ Other Refractive Techniques

Conductive keratoplasty (CK) shows promise along with safety in the treatment of hypermetropia and possibly presbyopia. Laser thermokeratoplasty (LTK) is also being studied for the treatment of low hyperopia.

REFERENCES

Al-Badriyeh D et al: Successful use of topical voriconazole 1% alone as first-line antifungal therapy against Candida albicans keratitis. Ann Pharmacother 2009;43:2103. [PMID: 19861430]

Binder PS, Trattler WB: Evaluation of a risk factor scoring system for corneal ectasia after LASIK. J Refract Surg 2010 Feb 25:1. [Epub ahead of print] [PMID: 20166627]

Bullock JD: Root cause analysis of the fusarium keratitis epidemic of 2004–2006 and prescriptions for preventing future epidemics. Trans Am Ophthalmol Soc 2009;107:194. [PMID: 20126495]

Constantinou M et al: Clinical review of corneal ulcers resulting in evisceration and enucleation in elderly population. Graefes Arch Clin Exp Ophthalmol 2009;247:1389. [PMID: 19475415]

Dart JK et al: Risk factors for microbial keratitis with contemporary contact lenses: a case-control study. Ophthalmology 2008;115:1647. [PMID: 18597850]

Dart JK, Saw VP, Kilvington S: Acanthamoeba keratitis: diagnosis and treatment update 2009. Am J Ophthalmol 2009;148:487. [PMID: 19660733]

Eghrari AO, Daoud YJ, Gottsch JD: Cataract surgery in Fuchs corneal dystrophy. Curr Opin Ophthalmol 2010;21:15. [PMID: 19910792]

Ghosheh FR et al: Trends in penetrating keratoplasty in the United States 1980–2005. Int Ophthalmol 2008;28:147. [PMID: 18084724]

Huang D et al: Phakic intraocular lens implantation for the correction of myopia: a report by the American Academy of Ophthalmology. Ophthalmology 2009;116:2244. [PMID: 19883852]

Jhanji V et al: Microbiological and clinical profiles of patients with microbial keratitis residing in nursing homes. Br J Ophthalmol 2009;93:1639. [PMID: 19574240]

Jurkunas U, Behlau I, Colby K: Fungal keratitis: changing pathogens and risk factors. Cornea 2009;28:638. [PMID: 19512908]

Klintworth GK: Corneal dystrophies, Orphanet J Rare Dis 2009;4:7. [PMID: 19236704]

Knickelbein JE, Hendricks RL, Charukamnoetkanok P: Management of herpes simplex virus stromal keratitis: an evidence-based review. Surv Ophthalmol 2009;54:226. [PMID: 19298901]

Lee Wb et al: Descemet's stripping endothelial keratoplasty: safety and outcomes: a report by the American Academy of Ophthalmology. Ophthalmology 2009;116:1818. [PMID: 19643492]

Llovet F et al: Infectious keratitis in 204 586 LASIK procedures. Ophthalmology 2010;117:232. [PMID: 20006909]

Loh AR et al: Practice patterns in the management of fungal corneal ulcers. Cornea 2009;28:856. [PMID: 19654533]

Najjar DM et al: EDTA chelation for calcific band keratopathy: results and long-term follow-up. Am J Ophthalmol 2004;137:1056. [PMID: 15183790]

Naseri A, McLeod SD: Cataract surgery after refractive surgery. Curr Opin Ophthalmol 2010;21:35. [PMID: 19996749]

Patel A, Hammersmith K: Contact lens-related microbial keratitis: recent outbreaks. Curr Opin Ophthalmol 2008;19:302. [PMID: 18545011]

Patel DV, McGhee CN: Acanthamoeba keratitis: a comprehensive photographic reference of common and uncommon signs. Clin Experiment Ophthalmol 2009;37:232. [PMID: 19723132]

Pleyer U, Schlickeiser S: The taming of the shrew? The immunology of corneal transplantation. Acta Ophthalmol 2009;87:488. [PMID: 19664109]

Poulaki V, Colby K: Genetics of anterior and stromal corneal dystrophies. Semin Ophthalmol 2008;23:9. [PMID: 18214787]

Price MO, Price FW: Descemet's stripping endothelial keratoplasty. Curr Opin Ophthalmol 2007;18:290. [PMID: 17568204]

Price MO et al: Descemet's membrane endothelial keratoplasty: prospective multicenter study of visual and refractive outcomes and endothelial survival. Ophthalmology 2009;116:2361. [PMID: 19875170]

Rabinowitz YS: Intacs for keratoconus. Curr Opin Ophthalmol 2007;18:279. [PMID: 17568203]

Rose L, Kelliher C, Jun AS: Endothelial keratoplasty: historical perspectives, current techniques, future directions. Can J Ophthalmol 2009;44:401. [PMID: 19606160]

Saeed A et al: Risk factors, microbiological findings, and clinical outcomes in cases of microbial keratitis admitted to a tertiary referral center in Ireland. Cornea 2009;28:285. [PMID: 19387229]

Schallhorn SC et al: Wavefront-guided LASIK for the correction of primary myopia and astigmatism: a report by the American Academy of Ophthalmology. Ophthalmology 2008;115:1249. [PMID: 18598819]

Schallhorn SC et al: Comparison of night driving performance after wavefront-guided and conventional LASIK for moderate myopia. Ophthalmology 2009;116:702. [PMID: 19344822]

Settas G et al: Photorefractive keratectomy (PRK) versus laser assisted in situ keratomileusis (LASIK) for hyperopia correction. Cochrane Database Syst Rev 2009;2:DC007112. [PMID: 19370672]

Siganos CS et al: Changing indications for penetrating keratoplasty in Greece, 1982–2006: a multicenter study. Cornea 2010 Feb 15. [Epub ahead of print] [PMID: 20164748]

Stasi K, Chuck RS: Update on phototherapeutic keratectomy. Curr Opin Ophthalmol 2009;20:272. [PMID: 19381088]

Szczotka-Flynn LB, Pearlman E, Ghannoum M: Microbial contamination of contact lenses, lens care solutions, and their accessories: a literature review. Eye Contact Lens 2010;36:116. [PMID: 20168237]

Terry MA et al: Endothelial keratoplasty for Fuchs' dystrophy with cataract: complications and clinical results with the new triple procedure. Ophthalmology 2009;116:631. [PMMID: 19201480]

Verani JR et al: National outbreak of Acanthamoeba keratitis associated with use of a contact lens solution, United States. Emerg Infect Dis 2009;15:1236. [PMID: 19751585]

Wang L et al: Spectrum of fungal keratitis in central China. Clin Experiment Ophthalmol 2009;37:763. [PMID: 19878220]

Wilhelmus KR: Therapeutic interventions for herpes simplex virus epithelial keratitis. Cochrane Database Syst Rev 2008;1:CD002898. [PMID: 18254009]

Wilhelmus KR, Jones DB: Adult-onset syphilitic stromal keratitis. Am J Ophthalmol 2006;141:319. [PMID: 16458687]

Xie L et al: Major shifts in corneal transplantation procedures in north China: 5316 eyes over 12 years. Br J Ophthalmol 2009;93:1291. [PMID: 19556213]

Zhang C et al: Distribution of bacterial keratitis and emerging resistance to antibiotics in China from 2001 to 2004. Clin Ophthalmol 2008;2:575. [PMID: 19668756]

Uveal Tract & Sclera

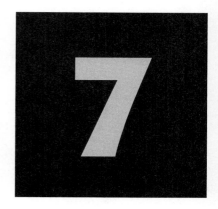

Emmett T. Cunningham, Jr., MD, PhD, MPH,
James J. Augsburger, MD, Zélia M. Corrêa, MD, PhD, and
Carlos Pavesio, MD, FRCOphth

7.1. Uveitis
Emmett T. Cunningham, Jr., MD, PhD, MPH

▼ UVEITIS

The uveal tract consists of the choroid, ciliary body, and iris (Figure 7–1). The term "uveitis" denotes inflammation of the iris (iritis, iridocyclitis), ciliary body (intermediate uveitis, cyclitis, peripheral uveitis, or pars planitis), or choroid (choroiditis). Common usage, however, includes inflammation of the retina (retinitis), retinal vasculature (retinal vasculitis), and intraocular optic nerve (papillitis). Uveitis may also occur secondary to inflammation of the cornea (keratitis), sclera (scleritis), or both (sclerokeratitis). Uveitis usually affects people 20–50 years of age and accounts for 10%–20% of cases of legal blindness in developed countries. Uveitis is more common in the developing world than in the developed countries, due in large part to the greater prevalence of infections that can affect the eye, such as toxoplasmosis and tuberculosis.

▶ Clinical Findings
A. Symptoms and Signs (Table 7–1)

Inflammation of the uveal tract has many causes and may involve one or more regions of the eye simultaneously. Anatomically, intraocular inflammation can be classified as anterior uveitis, intermediate uveitis, posterior uveitis, or diffuse or panuveitis (Figure 7–2).

Anterior uveitis is most common and is usually unilateral and acute in onset. Typical symptoms include pain, photophobia, and blurred vision. Examination usually reveals circumcorneal redness with minimal injection of the palpebral conjunctiva or discharge. The pupil may be small (miosis) or irregular due to the formation of posterior synechiae.

Inflammation limited to the anterior chamber is called "iritis," whereas inflammation involving both the anterior chamber and the anterior vitreous is often referred to as "iridocyclitis." Corneal sensation and intraocular pressure should be checked in every patient with uveitis. Decreased sensation occurs in patients with herpetic uveitis due to simplex or varicella-zoster virus infection or leprosy (see Chapter 15), whereas increased intraocular pressure can occur with herpes simplex virus, varicella-zoster virus, cytomegalovirus, toxoplasmosis, syphilis, sarcoidosis, or an uncommon form of iridocyclitis called glaucomatocyclitic crisis, also known as the Posner–Schlossman syndrome. Clumps of white cells and inflammatory debris termed keratic precipitates are usually evident on the corneal endothelium in patients with active inflammation. Keratic precipitates may be large so-called "mutton fat" or "granulomatous" (Figure 7–3), small and nongranulomatous, or stellate. Granulomatous or nongranulomatous keratic precipitates are usually located inferiorly in a wedge-shaped region known as Arlt's triangle. Stellate keratic precipitates, in contrast, are usually distributed evenly over the entire corneal endothelium and may be seen in uveitis due to herpes simplex virus, varicella-zoster virus, cytomegalovirus, toxoplasmosis, Fuchs' heterochromic iridocyclitis, and sarcoidosis. Keratic precipitates may also be localized to an area of prior or active keritits, most frequently in herpetic keratouveitis. Iris nodules may be present at the iris margin (Koeppe nodules), within the iris stroma (Busacca nodules), or in the anterior chamber angle (Berlin's nodules). Evidence for granulomatous disease, such as mutton fat keratic precipitates or iris nodules, may indicate an infectious cause of uveitis or one of a relatively limited number of noninfectious causes, including sarcoidosis, Vogt–Koyanagi–Harada

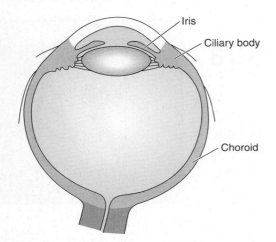

▲ **Figure 7–1.** The uveal tract consists of the iris, the ciliary body, and the choroid.

Table 7–1. Differentiation of Granulomatous and Nongranulomatous Uveitis

	Nongranulomatous	Granulomatous
Onset	Acute	Insidious
Pain	Marked	None or minimal
Photophobia	Marked	Slight
Blurred vision	Moderate	Marked
Circumcorneal flush	Marked	Slight
Keratic precipitates	Small white	Large gray ("mutton fat")
Pupil	Small and irregular	Small and irregular (variable)
Posterior synechiae	Sometimes	Sometimes
Iris nodules	None	Sometimes
Site	Anterior	Anterior, posterior, or diffuse
Course	Acute	Chronic
Recurrence	Common	Sometimes

disease, sympathetic ophthalmia, or lens-induced uveitis. Particularly severe anterior chamber inflammation may result in layering of inflammatory cells in the inferior angle (hypopyon). The most common cause of hypopyon uveitis in North America and Europe is HLA-B27–associated uveitis, whereas the most common cause of hypopyon uveitis in Asia is Behçet's disease. The iris should be examined carefully for evidence of atrophy or transillumination, which can occur in a sectoral or patchy pattern in the setting of herpetic uveitis, or diffusely with Fuchs' heterochromic iridocyclitis, also known as Fuchs uveitis syndrome. The presence of anterior (Figure 7–4) or posterior (Figures 7–5 and 7–6) synechiae should also be noted, as this can predispose the patient to ocular hypertension or glaucoma.

Intermediate uveitis, also called cyclitis, peripheral uveitis, or pars planitis, is the second most common type of intraocular inflammation. The hallmark of intermediate uveitis is vitreous inflammation. Intermediate uveitis is typically bilateral and tends to affect patients in their late teens or early adult years. Men and women are affected equally. Typical symptoms include floaters and blurred vision. Pain, photophobia, and redness are usually absent or minimal, although these symptoms may be more prominent at onset. The most striking finding on examination is vitritis, often accompanied by vitreous condensates, either free-floating as "snowballs" or layered over the pars plana and ciliary body as "snow-banking." Mild anterior chamber inflammation may be present, but if significant, the inflammation is more appropriately termed diffuse uveitis or panuveitis (see later in the chapter). The cause of intermediate uveitis is unknown in the vast majority of patients, although sarcoidosis and

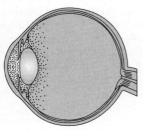
Anterior uveitis
(Iritis, iridocyclitis)

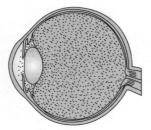
Intermediate uveitis
(Pars planitis, cyclitis)

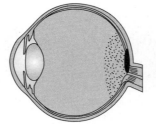
Posterior uveitis
(Retinitis, choroiditis, papillitis)

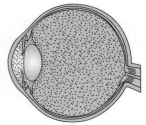
Panveitis
(Diffuse uveitis)

▲ **Figure 7–2.** Anatomic classification of uveitis, including anterior uveitis, intermediate uveitis, posterior uveitis and diffuse, or panuveitis. [Modified after Cunningham ET Jr. Diagnosis and management of acute anterior uveitis. American Academy of Ophthalmology, Focal Points 2002, Volume XX, Number 1 (Section 1 of 3).]

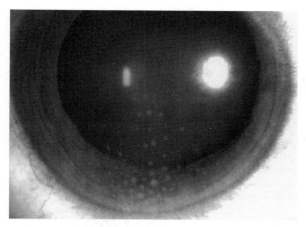

▲ **Figure 7–3.** Granulomatous keratic precipitates located on the inferior corneal endothelium in Arlt's triangle.

multiple sclerosis account for 10%–20% of cases. Syphilis and tuberculosis, although uncommon, should be excluded in all patients. The most common complications of intermediate uveitis include cystoid macular edema, retinal vasculitis, and neovascularization of the optic disk and retina.

Posterior uveitis includes retinitis, choroiditis, retinal vasculitis, and papillitis, which may occur alone or in combination. Symptoms typically include floaters, loss of visual field or scotomas, or decreased vision, which can be severe. Retinal detachment, although infrequent, occurs most commonly in posterior uveitis and may be tractional, rhegmatogenous, or exudative in nature.

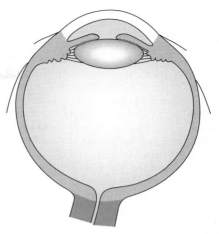

▲ **Figure 7–5.** Posterior synechiae. The iris adheres to the lens. Iris seclusion, iris bombé, ocular hypertension, and glaucoma may result.

B. Laboratory Testing

Laboratory testing is usually not required for patients with mild uveitis and a recent history of trauma or surgery—or with clear evidence of herpes simplex or herpes zoster virus infection, such as a concurrent vesicular dermatitis, dendritic or disciform keratitis, or sectoral iris atrophy. Laboratory testing can also be deferred for otherwise healthy and asymptomatic young to middle-aged patients with a first episode of mild to moderately severe acute, unilateral, nongranulomatous iritis or iridocyclitis that responds promptly to treatment with topical corticosteroids and cycloplegic/mydriatic agents. Patients with recurrent, severe, bilateral, granulomatous, intermediate, posterior, or panuveitis should

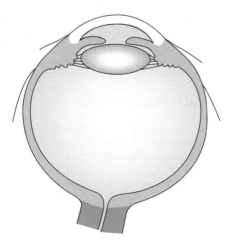

▲ **Figure 7–4.** Anterior synechiae (adhesions). The peripheral iris adheres to the cornea. Ocular hypertension or glaucoma may result.

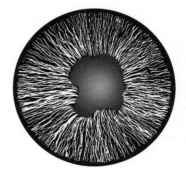

▲ **Figure 7–6.** Posterior synechiae (anterior view). The iris is adherent to the lens in several places as a result of previous inflammation, causing an irregular, fixed pupil. Appropriate treatment with corticosteroids and cycloplegic/mydriatic agents can often prevent such synechiae.

be tested, however, as should any patient whose uveitis fails to respond promptly to standard therapy. Testing for syphilis should include both a Venereal Disease Research Laboratory (VDRL) or rapid plasma reagin (RPR) test and a more specific test for anti-*Treponema pallidum* antibodies, such as the FTA-ABS or MHA-TP assays. Sarcoidosis should be excluded by chest x-ray and serum angiotensin-converting enzyme (ACE) or lysozyme level testing. Tuberculosis should be excluded by the same chest x-ray, and by either skin testing using both purified protein derivative (PPD) or by an interferon-γ release assay (IGRA), such as the QuantiFERON-TB Gold or T-SPOT.TB tests. While the IRGAs provide markedly increased specificity for patients with prior BCG vaccination, a remote history of BCG vaccination should not preclude PPD skin testing in areas where IRGAs are not available, since the PPD test should become negative (<5 mm induration) within 5 years following BCG vaccination. Testing other than for syphilis, tuberculosis, and sarcoidosis should be tailored to findings elicited on history or identified on physical examination. Examples might include an antinuclear antibody (ANA) titer for a young child with chronic iridocyclitis and arthritis suspected of having juvenile idiopathic arthritis (JIA); an HLA-B27 histocompatibility antigen test for patients with arthritis, psoriasis, urethritis, or symptoms consistent with inflammatory bowel disease; or toxoplasmosis IgG and IgM titers for a patient with unilateral panuveitis and focal retinochoroiditis.

► Differential Diagnosis

The differential diagnosis for eye redness and decreased vision is extensive and somewhat beyond the scope of this brief overview. However, entities commonly confused with uveitis include conjunctivitis, distinguished by the presence of discharge and redness involving both the palpebral and bulbar conjunctiva; keratitis, distinguished by the presence of epithelial staining or defects or by stromal thickening or infiltrate; and acute angle closure glaucoma, associated with markedly elevated intraocular pressure, corneal haziness and edema, and a narrow anterior chamber angle, often best visualized in the uninvolved fellow eye. (see Inside Front Cover.)

► Complications & Sequelae

Anterior uveitis can produce both anterior (Figure 7–4) and posterior synechiae (Figures 7–5 and 7–6)). Anterior synechiae can impede aqueous outflow at the chamber angle and cause ocular hypertension or glaucoma. Posterior synechiae, when extensive, can cause secondary angle closure glaucoma by producing pupillary seclusion and forward bulging of the iris (iris bombé). Early and aggressive use of corticosteroids and cycloplegic/mydriatic agents lessens the likelihood of these complications.

Both anterior and posterior chamber inflammation promote lens thickening and opacification. Early in the course,

this can cause a simple shift in refractive error, usually toward myopia. With time, however, cataract progression often limits best-corrected vision. Treatment involves removal of the cataract, but should be done only when the intraocular inflammation is well controlled for at least 6 months, since the risk of intraoperative and postoperative complications is greater in patients with active uveitis. Aggressive use of local and systemic corticosteroids is usually necessary before, during, and after cataract surgery in these patients.

Cystoid macular edema is a common cause of visual loss in patients with uveitis and may be observed in the setting of severe anterior or intermediate uveitis. Longstanding or recurrent macular edema can cause permanent loss of vision due to cystoid degeneration. Both fluorescein angiography and optical coherence tomography can be used to diagnose cystoid macular edema and to monitor its response to therapy.

Retinal detachments, including tractional, rhegmatogenous, and exudative forms, occur infrequently in patients with posterior, intermediate, or panuveitis. Exudative retinal detachment suggests significant choroidal inflammation and occurs most commonly in association with Vogt-Koyanagi-Harada disease, sympathetic ophthalmia, and posterior scleritis or in association with severe retinitis or retinal vasculitis.

► Treatment

Corticosteroids and cycloplegic/mydriatic agents are the mainstays of therapy for uveitis. Care should be taken to rule out an epithelial defect and ruptured globe when a history of trauma is elicited and to check corneal sensation and intraocular pressure to rule out herpes virus infection. Aggressive topical therapy with a potent corticosteroid, such as 1% prednisolone acetate, one or two drops in the affected eye every 1 or 2 hours while awake, usually provides good control of anterior inflammation. Prednisolone acetate is a suspension and needs to be shaken vigorously prior to each use. A cycloplegic/mydriatic agent, such as homatropine 2 or 5%, used two to four times daily, helps prevent synechia formation and reduces discomfort from ciliary spasm.

Noninfectious intermediate, posterior, and panuveitis responds best to sub-Tenon injections of triamcinolone acetonide, usually 1 mL (40 mg) given superotemporally. Intraocular triamcinolone acetonide, 0.05–0.1 mL (2–4 mg), or oral prednisone, 0.5–1.5 mg/kg/d, can also be effective. Corticosteroid-sparing agents such as methotrexate, azathioprine, mycophenolate mofetil, cyclosporine, tacrolimus, cyclophosphamide, chlorambucil, or the TNF-α inhibitors can be required to treat severe or chronic forms of noninfectious inflammation, particularly when there is systemic involvement. Therapy for selected granulomatous forms of uveitis is outlined in Table 7–2.

► Complications of Treatment

Cataract and glaucoma are the most common complications of corticosteroid therapy. Cycloplegic/mydriatic agents weaken accommodation and can be particularly bothersome

Table 7–2. Treatment of Granulomatous Uveitis

	Anti-infective Chemotherapy	Use of Corticosteroids
Toxoplasmosis	If central vision is threatened, give pyrimethamine, 75 mg orally as a loading dose for 2 days followed by 25–50 mg once daily for 4 weeks, in combination with trisulfapyrimidines (sulfadiazine, sulfamerazine, and sulfamethazine, 0.167 g of each per tablet), 2 g orally as loading dose followed by 0.5–1 g 4 times daily for 4 weeks. If a fall in the white blood cell or platelet count occurs during therapy, give folinic acid (leucovorin), 1 mL IM twice weekly or 3 mg orally twice weekly. Alternative chemotheraputic approach for ocular toxoplasmosis: Clindamycin, 300 mg orally 4 times a day with sulfonamides (as above), or spiramycin 1g 3 times daily, or minocycline, 100 mg orally daily for 3–4 weeks.	If the response is not favorable after 2 weeks, continue the anti-infective therapy and give systemic corticosteroids, eg, prednisone, 0.5 mg/kg/d with tapering over 3–4 weeks. Never stop anti-infective therapy prior to stopping corticosteroids.
Tuberculosis	Isoniazid, 300 mg orally daily, rifampicin, 450–600 mg orally daily, and pyridoxine, 50 mg orally daily, for 6–9 months; with ethambutol, 15 mg/kg orally daily and pyrazinamide 1.5–2 g orally daily for initial 2 months.	If a favorable response does not occur in 6 weeks, continue antimycobacterial therapy and give systemic corticosteroids, eg, prednisone, 0.5–1 mg/kg/d, with tapering as allowed by response.
Sarcoidosis	Treat with local corticosteroids, cycloplegic/mydriatic agents, and, as needed, with systemic corticosteroids such as prednisone, 0.5–1 mg/kg/d, with tapering as allowed by response. The usual contraindications to systemic corticosteroid therapy apply. A corticosteroid sparing agent is occasionally required	
Sympathetic ophthalmia	Treat with local corticosteroids, cycloplegic/mydriatic agents, and with systemic corticosteroids in high doses, eg, prednisone, 1–1.5 mg/kg/d. The usual contradictions to systemic corticosteroid therapy apply, and a corticosteroid sparing agent is often required.	

to patients under 45 years of age. Because oral corticosteroids or noncorticosteroid immunosuppressive agents can cause numerous systemic complications, dosing and monitoring are best done in close collaboration with an internist, rheumatologist, or oncologist.

▶ Course & Prognosis

The course and prognosis of uveitis depends to a large extent on the severity, location, and cause of the inflammation. In general, severe inflammation takes longer to treat and is more likely to cause intraocular damage and loss of vision than mild or moderate inflammation. Moreover, anterior uveitis tends to respond more promptly than intermediate, posterior, or panuveitis. Retinal, choroidal, or optic nerve involvement tends to be associated with a poorer prognosis.

ANTERIOR UVEITIS (TABLE 7–3)

1. UVEITIS ASSOCIATED WITH JOINT DISEASE

About 20% of children with the pauciarticular form of JIA (formerly known as juvenile rheumatoid arthritis [JRA] in the United States and juvenile chronic arthritis [JCA] in the United Kingdom) develop a chronic bilateral nongranulomatous iridocyclitis. Girls are affected four to five times more commonly than boys. JIA-associated uveitis is usually

detected at 5–6 years of age following the insidious onset of cataract (leukocoria), a difference in color of the two eyes (heterochromia), a difference in the size or shape of the pupil (anisocoria), or ocular misalignment (strabismus). Often these findings are first noted at a screening vision test performed at school. There is no correlation between the onset of the arthritis and that of the uveitis, which may precede the onset of arthritis by up to 10 years. The knee is the most commonly involved joint. The cardinal signs of the disease are cells and flare in the anterior chamber, small- to medium-sized white keratic precipitates with or without flecks of fibrin on the endothelium, posterior synechiae formation, often progressing to seclusion of the pupil, and cataract. Band keratopathy (Figure 7–7), secondary ocular hypertension or glaucoma, and cystoid macular edema can also be present and cause loss of vision. Patients suspected of having JIA should be evaluated by a rheumatologist and tested for a positive ANA titer.

Treatment of JIA-associated uveitis is challenging. Topical corticosteroids, nonsteroidal anti-inflammatory agents, and cycloplegic/mydriatic agents are all of value. In resistant cases, systemic immunosuppression with non-corticosteroid immunosuppressive agents such as methotrexate, mycophenolate mofetil, or TNF-α inhibitors may be required to control the disease. Cataract surgery is associated with a relatively high risk of postoperative exacerbations, and intraocular lens implantation is usually contraindicated.

Table 7–3. Causes of Anterior Uveitis

Autoimmune
Juvenile idiopathic arthritis
Ankylosing spondylitis
Reiter's syndrome (reactive arthritis)
Inflammatory bowel disease (ulcerative colitis, Crohn's disease)
Lens-induced uveitis
Sarcoidosis
Psoriatic arthritis

Infections
Syphilis
Tuberculosis
Leprosy (Hansen's disease)
Herpes simplex virus
Varicella-zoster virus
Cytomegalovirus
Onchocerciasis
Leptospirosis

Malignancy
Masquerade syndrome
Retinoblastoma
Leukemia
Lymphoma
Malignant melanoma

Other
Idiopathic
Traumatic uveitis, including penetrating injuries
Retinal detachment
Fuchs' heterochromic iridocyclitis (Fuchs' uveitis syndrome)
Glaucomatocyclitic crisis (Posner-Schlossman syndrome)

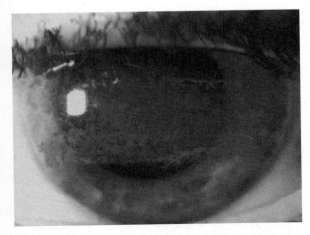

▲ **Figure 7–7.** Extensive band keratopathy in a young girl with juvenile idiopathic arthritis (JIA).

Up to 50% of patients with **ankylosing spondylitis** develop anterior uveitis. There is a marked preponderance for men. The uveitis can vary in severity from mild to severe and often produces pain, photophobia, and blurred vision. Limbal injection is usually present. Keratic precipitates, though usually present, are rarely granulomatous, and iris nodules do not occur. Posterior synechiae, peripheral anterior synechiae, cataracts, and glaucoma are common complications following severe, recurrent, or poorly controlled bouts of inflammation. Macular edema is uncommon, but can occur when the inflammation is severe and spills over to involve the vitreous. Recurrence is the rule and may involve either eye, although bilateral simultaneous involvement is atypical. The HLA-B27 histocompatibility antigen is present in approximately 50% of patients with acute nongranulomatous iritis or iridocyclitis seen in tertiary referral centers, but may be as high as 90% in community practice. Of those patients with anterior uveitis who are HLA-B27 positive, roughly half will experience a nonocular complication of their disease—most commonly ankylosing spondylitis, but Reiter's syndrome (reactive arthritis), inflammatory bowel disease, and psoriatic arthritis may also occur. Imaging and colonoscopy can occasionally confirm diagnoses suspected on clinical grounds.

2. FUCHS' HETEROCHROMIC IRIDOCYCLITIS (FUCHS' UVEITIS SYNDROME)

Fuchs' heterochromic iridocyclitis is uncommon, accounting for less than 5% of all cases of uveitis. The onset is typically insidious during the third or fourth decade of life. Redness, pain, and photophobia tend to be minimal. Patients usually complain of blurred vision due to cataract. Iris heterochromia, best appreciated with natural lighting, can be subtle and is often most obvious over the iris sphincter muscle. Keratic precipitates are often small and stellate and scattered over the entire endothelium. Abnormal blood vessels may be seen in the chamber angle on gonioscopy. Posterior synechiae are uncommon, although they may occur in some patients following cataract surgery. A vitreous reaction may be present in 10% of patients. While loss of stromal pigment tends to make heavily pigmented eyes look hypochromic, stromal atrophy affecting lightly colored irides can actually reveal underlying pigment epithelium on the posterior surface of the iris, causing paradoxic hyperchromia. Pathologically, the iris and ciliary body show moderate atrophy with patchy depigmentation and diffuse infiltration of lymphocytes and plasma cells.

Cataract eventually develops in most patients, whereas glaucoma occurs in 10%–15% of cases. The prognosis is generally good. Cataract surgery can usually be performed without complication, and most patients with glaucoma can be managed with topical medications alone.

3. LENS-INDUCED UVEITIS

Lens-induced (phacogenic) uveitis is an autoimmune disease directed against lens antigens. There are no data at present to substantiate the suggestion that lens material per se is toxic, so the term "phacotoxic uveitis" should be avoided. The classic case occurs when the lens develops a hypermature cataract and the lens capsule leaks lens material into the posterior and anterior chambers. This material elicits an inflammatory reaction characterized by accumulation of plasma cells, mononuclear phagocytes, and a few polymorphonu-clear cells. Typical anterior uveitis symptoms of pain, photophobia, and blurred vision are common. Lens-induced uveitis may also occur following lens trauma or cataract surgery with retained lens material. Phacolytic glaucoma is a common complication. Definitive treatment requires removal of the lens material. Concurrent treatment with corticosteroids, cycloplegic/mydriatic agents, and intraocular pressure–lowering medications is often necessary.

INTERMEDIATE UVEITIS (CYCLITIS, PERIPHERAL UVEITIS, PARS PLANITIS)

Intermediate uveitis affects mainly the intermediate zone of the eye—ciliary body, principally the pars plana, peripheral retina, and vitreous. The cause is unknown in most cases, although syphilis, tuberculosis, and sarcoidosis should be ruled out with appropriate laboratory and ancillary testing. Multiple sclerosis should also be considered, particularly when supportive signs or symptoms are present. Intermediate uveitis is seen mainly among young adults, affects men and women equally, and is bilateral in up to 80% of cases. Common complaints include floaters and blurred vision. Pain, redness, and photophobia are unusual but can accompany a severe first attack. Adequate examination of the ciliary body, pars plana, and peripheral retina requires use of an indirect ophthalmoscope and scleral depression, which often reveals vitreous condensations in the form of snowballs and snowbanking. Adjacent retinal vasculitis is common. Anterior chamber inflammation is invariably mild, and posterior synechiae are uncommon. Posterior subcapsular cataract and cystoid macular edema are the most common causes of decreased vision. In severe cases, cyclitic membranes and retinal detachments may occur. Secondary glaucoma is rare. Corticosteroids are used mainly to treat cystoid macular edema or retinal neovascularization. Topical corticosteroids should be tried for 3–4 weeks to identify patients predisposed to development of corticosteroid-induced ocular hypertension. If no improvement is noted and ocular hypertension does not develop, a posterior sub-Tenon or intraocular injection of triamcinolone acetonide, 40 mg/mL, may be effective. Patients with intermediate uveitis usually do well with cataract surgery.

POSTERIOR UVEITIS (TABLE 7–4)

The retina, choroid, and optic nerve are affected by a variety of infectious and noninfectious disorders, the more common of which are listed in Table 7–4.

Most cases of posterior uveitis are associated with some form of systemic disease. The cause can often be established on the basis of (1) the morphology of the lesions, (2) the

Table 7–4. Causes of Posterior Uveitis

Infectious disorders
Viruses
  Cytomegalovirus, herpes simplex virus, varicella-zoster virus, rubella virus, rubeola virus
Bacteria
  Agents of tuberculosis, brucellosis, sporadic and endemic syphilis; *Borrelia* (Lyme disease); and various hematogenously spread gram-positive and gram-negative pathogens
Fungi
  Candida, Histoplasma, Cryptococcus, Aspergillus
Parasites
  Toxoplasma, Toxocara, Cysticercus, Onchocerca

Noninfectious disorders
Autoimmune disorders
  Behçet's disease
  Vogt–Koyanagi–Harada disease
  Systemic lupus erythematosus
  Wegener's granulomatosis
  Sympathetic ophthalmia
  Retinal vasculitis
Malignancies
  Intraocular lymphoma
  Malignant melanoma
  Leukemia
  Metastatic lesions
Unknown etiology
  Sarcoidosis
  Serpiginous choroiditis
  Acute multifocal placoid pigment epitheliopathy
  Birdshot chorioretinopathy
  Retinal pigment epitheliopathy
  Multiple evanescent white dot syndrome

mode of onset and course of the disease, or (3) the association with systemic symptoms or signs. Other considerations are the age of the patient and whether involvement is unilateral or bilateral. Laboratory and ancillary tests are often helpful.

Lesions of the posterior segment of the eye can be focal, multifocal, geographic, or diffuse. Those that tend to cause clouding of the overlying vitreous should be differentiated from those that give rise to little or no vitreous cells. The type and distribution of vitreous opacities should be described. Inflammatory lesions of the posterior segment are generally insidious in onset, but some may be accompanied by abrupt and profound visual loss.

Worldwide, the most common causes of retinitis in immunocompetent patients are toxoplasmosis, syphilis, and Behçet's disease, whereas the most common causes of choroiditis are sarcoidosis, tuberculosis, and Vogt–Koyanagi–Harada disease. Inflammatory papillitis (optic neuritis) can be caused by any of these diseases, but multiple sclerosis should always be suspected, particularly when associated with eye pain worsened by movement (Chapter 14). Less common causes of posterior uveitis include intraocular lymphoma, acute retinal necrosis (ARN) syndrome, sympathetic ophthalmia, and the "white dot" syndromes such as multiple evanescent white dot syndrome (MEWDS) or acute multifocal posterior placoid epitheliopathy (AMPPE).

▶ Diagnosis & Clinical Features

Diagnostic clues and clinical features of the more commonly encountered posterior uveitis syndromes are described below.

A. Age of the Patient

Posterior uveitis in patients under 3 years of age can be caused by a "masquerade syndrome" such as retinoblastoma or leukemia. Infectious causes of posterior uveitis in this age group include congenital toxoplasmosis, toxocariasis, and perinatal infections due to syphilis, cytomegalovirus, herpes simplex virus, varicella-zoster virus, or rubella virus.

In the age group from 4 to 15 years, the most common causes of posterior uveitis are toxoplasmosis and toxocariasis. Uncommon causes include syphilis, tuberculosis, sarcoidosis, Behçet's syndrome, and Vogt–Koyanagi–Harada disease.

In the age group from 16 to 50 years, the differential diagnosis for posterior uveitis includes syphilis, tuberculosis, sarcoidosis, toxoplasmosis, Behçet's disease, Vogt–Koyanagi–Harada disease, and ARN syndrome.

Patients over age 50 years who present with posterior uveitis may have syphilis, tuberculosis, sarcoidosis, intraocular lymphoma, birdshot chorioretinitis, ARN syndrome, toxoplasmosis, or endogenous endophthalmitis.

B. Laterality

Unilateral posterior uveitis favors a diagnosis of toxoplasmosis, toxocariasis, ARN syndrome, or endogenous bacterial or fungal infection.

C. Symptoms

1. **Reduced vision**—Reduced visual acuity may be present in all types of posterior uveitis but especially in the setting of a macular lesion or retinal detachment. Every patient should be examined for an afferent pupillary defect, which, when present, signifies optic nerve or widespread retinal dysfunction.

2. **Ocular injection**—Eye redness is uncommon in strictly posterior uveitis but can be seen in diffuse uveitis.

3. **Pain**—Pain is atypical in posterior uveitis but can occur in endophthalmitis, posterior scleritis, or optic neuritis, particularly when caused by multiple sclerosis.

D. Signs

Signs important in the diagnosis of posterior uveitis include hypopyon formation, granuloma formation, glaucoma, vitritis, morphology of the lesions, vasculitis, retinal hemorrhages, and scar formation.

1. **Hypopyon**—Disorders of the posterior segment that may be associated with significant anterior inflammation and hypopyon include syphilis, tuberculosis, sarcoidosis, endogenous endophthalmitis, Behçet's disease, and leptospirosis. When this occurs, the uveitis is more appropriately termed diffuse or panuveitis.

2. **Type of uveitis**—Anterior granulomatous uveitis may be associated with conditions that affect the posterior retina and choroid, including syphilis, tuberculosis, sarcoidosis, toxoplasmosis, Vogt–Koyanagi–Harada disease, and sympathetic ophthalmia. On the other hand, nongranulomatous anterior uveitis may be associated with Behçet's disease, ARN syndrome, intraocular lymphoma, or the white dot syndromes.

3. **Glaucoma**—Acute ocular hypertension in association with posterior uveitis can occur with toxoplasmosis, ARN syndrome due to herpes simplex virus or varicella-zoster virus, sarcoidosis, or syphilis.

4. **Vitritis**—Posterior uveitis is often associated with vitritis, usually due to leakage from the inflammatory foci, from retinal vessels, or from the optic nerve head. Severe vitritis tends to occur with infections involving the posterior pole, such as toxoplasmic retinochoroiditis or bacterial endophthalmitis, whereas mild to moderate inflammation usually occurs with primary outer retinal and choroidal inflammatory disorders. Serpiginous choroiditis and presumed ocular histoplasmosis are typically accompanied by little if any vitritis.

5. **Morphology and location of lesions**—

   a. Retina—The retina is the primary target of many types of infectious agents. Toxoplasmosis is the most common cause of retinitis in immunocompetent hosts. The active lesion of toxoplasmosis is generally seen in the company of old, healed scars that may be heavily pigmented. The lesions may appear in a juxtapapillary location and often give rise to retinal vasculitis. The vitreous is generally clouded when large lesions are present. In contrast, retinal infection with herpes viruses, such as cytomegalovirus and varicella-zoster virus, is more common in immunocompromised hosts. Rubella and rubeola virus retinal infections occur primarily in infants, where they tend to produce diffuse pigmentary changes involving the outer retina referred to as "salt and pepper" retinopathy (see Chapter 15).

   b. Choroid—The choroid is the primary target of granulomatous processes such as tuberculosis and sarcoidosis. Patients with tuberculosis and sarcoidosis may present with a focal, multifocal, or geographic choroiditis. Both multifocal and diffuse infiltration of the choroid occur in Vogt–Koyanagi–Harada disease and sympathetic ophthalmia. Birdshot chorioretinopathy and presumed ocular histoplasmosis syndrome, in contrast, almost always produce multifocal choroiditis.

   c. Optic nerve—Primary inflammatory optic neuritis can occur from syphilis, tuberculosis, sarcoidosis, toxoplasmosis, multiple sclerosis, Lyme disease, intraocular lymphoma, or systemic *Bartonella henselae* infection (cat-scratch disease). Peripapillary serous retinal detachment and/or macular star are often present.

E. Trauma

A history of trauma in patients with uveitis raises the possibility of intraocular foreign body or sympathetic ophthalmia. Surgical trauma, including routine operations for cataract and glaucoma, may introduce micro-organisms into the eye and lead to acute or subacute endophthalmitis.

F. Mode of Onset

The onset of posterior uveitis may be acute and sudden or slow and insidious. Diseases of the posterior segment of the eye that tend to present with sudden loss of vision include toxoplasmic retinochoroiditis, ARN syndrome, and bacterial endophthalmitis. Most other causes of posterior uveitis have a more insidious onset.

1. OCULAR TOXOPLASMOSIS

Toxoplasmosis is caused by *Toxoplasma gondii,* an obligate intracellular protozoan. The ocular lesions may be acquired in utero or following systemic infection. Constitutional symptoms may be mild and easily missed. The domestic cat and other feline species serve as definitive hosts for the parasite. Susceptible women who acquire the disease during pregnancy may transmit the infection to the fetus, where it can be fatal. Sources of human infection include oocysts in soil or airborne in dust, undercooked meat containing bradyzoites (encysted forms of the parasite), and tachyzoites (proliferative form) transmitted across the placenta.

▶ Clinical Findings
A. Symptoms and Signs

Patients with toxoplasmic retinochoroiditis present with a history of floaters and blurred vision. In severe cases there may also be pain and photophobia. The ocular lesions consist of fluffy-white areas of focal necrotic retinochoroiditis that may be small or large and single or multiple. Active edematous lesions are often adjacent to healed retinal scars (Figure 7–8). Retinal vasculitis and hemorrhage can be observed. Cystoid macular edema can accompany lesions in or near the macula. Iridocyclitis is frequently seen in patients with severe infections, and intraocular pressure may be elevated.

B. Laboratory Findings

A positive serologic test for *T gondii* with consistent clinical signs is considered diagnostic. An increase in antibody titer is usually not detected during reactivation, but an elevated IgM titer provides strong evidence for recently acquired infection.

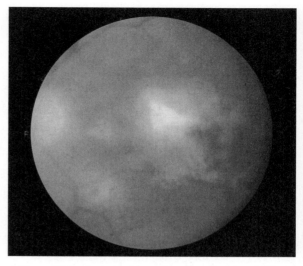

▲ **Figure 7–8.** Recurrent toxoplasmic retinochoroiditis involving the macula, with new fluffy-white lesion adjacent to healed pigmented scar. (Courtesy of S Patel.)

▶ Treatment

Small lesions in the retinal periphery not associated with significant vitritis require no treatment. In contrast, severe or posterior infections are usually treated for 4–6 weeks with pyrimethamine, 25–50 mg daily, and trisulfapyrimidine, 0.5–1 g four times daily. Loading doses of 75 mg of pyrimethamine daily for 2 days and 2 g of trisulfapyrimidine as a single dose should be given at the start of therapy. Patients are usually also given 3 mg of leucovorin calcium twice weekly to prevent bone marrow depression. A complete blood count should be performed weekly during therapy (Table 7–2).

An alternative approach for the treatment of ocular toxoplasmosis consists of administration of clindamycin, 300 mg four times daily, with trisulfapyrimidine, 0.5–1 g four times daily. Clindamycin causes pseudomembranous colitis in 10%–15% of patients. Other antibiotics effective in ocular toxoplasmosis include spiramycin and minocycline. Choroidal neovascularization can be treated with photodynamic therapy (PDT) or intra-vitreal anti-VEGF (vascular endothelial growth factor) injections.

Anterior uveitis associated with ocular toxoplasmosis may be treated with topical corticosteroids and cycloplegic/mydriatic agents. Periocular corticosteroid injections are contraindicated. Topical glaucoma medications are occasionally necessary. Systemic corticosteroids can be used in conjunction with antimicrobial therapy for vision-threatening inflammatory lesions but should never be used for a prolonged period in the absence of antimicrobial coverage.

2. HISTOPLASMOSIS

In some areas of the United States where histoplasmosis is endemic (the Ohio and Mississippi River Valley areas), the diagnosis of choroiditis due to presumed ocular histoplasmosis is common. Patients usually have a positive skin test to histoplasmin and demonstrate "punched-out" spots in the posterior or peripheral fundus. These spots are small, irregularly round or oval, and usually depigmented centrally with a finely pigmented border. Peripapillary atrophy and hyperpigmentation occur frequently. Macular lesions may produce choroidal neovascularization, a complication that should be suspected in every patient with presumed ocular histoplasmosis who presents with decreased vision or evidence of subretinal fluid or hemorrhage. Choroidal neovascularization is effectively treated with corticosteroids, PDT or intravitreal anti-VEGF injections (see Chapter 10).

3. OCULAR TOXOCARIASIS

Toxocariasis results from infection with *Toxocara cati* (an intestinal parasite of cats) or *Toxocara canis* (an intestinal parasite of dogs). Visceral larva migrans is a disseminated systemic infection occurring in a young child (Table 7–5). Ocular involvement rarely occurs in visceral larva migrans.

Ocular toxocariasis may occur without systemic manifestations. Children acquire the disease by close association with pets and by eating dirt (pica) contaminated with toxocara ova. The ingested ova form larvae that penetrate the intestinal mucosa and gain access to the systemic circulation and finally to the eye. The parasite does not infect the intestinal tract of humans.

▶ Clinical Findings
A. Symptoms and Signs

The disease is usually unilateral. *Toxocara* larvae lodge in the retina and die, leading to a marked inflammatory reaction and local production of toxocara antibodies. Children are typically brought to the ophthalmologist because of a red eye, blurred vision, or a whitish pupil (leukocoria).

Three clinical presentations are recognized: (1) a localized posterior granuloma, usually near the optic nerve head or fovea; (2) a peripheral granuloma involving the pars plana, often producing an elevated mass that mimics the snowbank of intermediate uveitis; and (3) chronic endophthalmitis.

B. Laboratory Findings

Characteristic clinical findings and a positive enzyme-linked immunosorbent assay (ELISA) for anti-toxocara antibodies, even at low titer, confirm the diagnosis of ocular toxocariasis. Negative ELISAs are common but do not rule out the possibility of ocular infection. Positive antibody titers of the ocular fluids from patients with suspected ocular toxocariasis have been demonstrated in the setting of a negative serum ELISA, but the test is not routinely available and in any case is seldom necessary.

▶ Treatment

Systemic or periocular injections of corticosteroids should be given when there is evidence of significant intraocular inflammation. Vitrectomy may be necessary in patients with marked vitreous opacity or with significant preretinal traction. Systemic anthelmintic therapy is not indicated for limited ocular disease and in fact may worsen the inflammation by producing more rapid killing of the intraocular parasite.

4. ACQUIRED IMMUNODEFICIENCY SYNDROME

Uveitis is common in patients infected with the human immunodeficiency virus (HIV), particularly in advanced stages of the illness when AIDS develops (see Chapter 15). CD4 T lymphocyte counts are a good predictor of the risk of opportunistic infections, with the majority occurring at counts of less than 100 cells/μL. Uveitis occurs most commonly in the setting of posterior segment infection. Cytomegalovirus retinitis, a geographic retinitis often accompanied by hemorrhage, occurred in 30%–40% of HIV-positive patients at some point in the course of their illness prior to the advent of combination antiretroviral therapy. Other herpesviruses, such as varicella-zoster and herpes simplex, can produce a similar retinitis but are usually distinguished by a very rapid progression. Infections caused by

Table 7–5. Comparison between Visceral and Ocular Larva Migrans

	Visceral Larva Migrans	Ocular Larva Migrans[1]
Average age at onset	2 years	7 years
Fever	+	–
Abdominal symptoms (pain, nausea, diarrhea)	+	–
Nonspecific pulmonary disease	+	–
Hepatosplenomegaly	+	–
Eosinophilia	+	–
Hypergammaglobulinemia	+	–
ELISA (serum anti-*Toxocara* antibodies)	+	±
ELISA (aqueous *Toxocara* antibodies)	–	+
Ocular finding[1]	–	+

[1]Ocular findings of ocular larva migrans; diffuse chronic panuveitis, posterior pole granuloma, or peripheral granuloma.

Table 7–6. Causes of Panuveitis

Sarcoidosis
Tuberculosis
Syphilis
Onchocerciasis
Leptospirosis
Brucellosis
Sympathetic ophthalmia
Behçet's disease
Multiple sclerosis
Cysticercosis
Vogt-Koyanagi-Harada disease
Masquerade syndrome: retinoblastoma, leukemia
Retinal intraocular foreign body

other organisms, such as *T gondii, Treponema pallidum, Cryptococcus neoformans, Mycobacterium tuberculosis, and Mycobacterium avium-intracellulare* occur in less than 5% of HIV-positive patients but should be considered, particularly when there is a history of infection or exposure, when chorioiditis is present, or when the retinitis is atypical in appearance or fails to respond to antiviral therapy. Intraocular lymphoma occurs in less than 1% of HIV-positive patients but should be considered when the retinitis is atypical or is unresponsive to antiviral treatment, especially when neurologic symptoms are present. Diagnosis usually requires vitreous biopsy.

PANUVEITIS (TABLE 7–6)

The term "panuveitis" is used to denote a more or less uniform cellular infiltration of both the anterior and posterior segments. Associated findings, such as retinitis, vasculitis, or choroiditis, can occur and often prompt further diagnostic testing. Tuberculosis, sarcoidosis, and syphilis should always be considered in patients with diffuse uveitis. Less common causes include sympathetic ophthalmia, Vogt–Koyanagi–Harada disease. Behçet's syndrome, birdshot chorioretinopathy, and intraocular lymphoma.

1. TUBERCULOUS UVEITIS

Tuberculosis can cause any type of uveitis but deserves special consideration when granulomatous keratic precipitates or iris or choroidal granulomas are present. Such granulomas, or tubercles, consist of giant and epithelioid cells. Caseating necrosis is characteristic on histopathologic examination. Although the infection is said to be transmitted from a primary focus elsewhere in the body, uveal tuberculosis is uncommon in patients with active pulmonary tuberculosis (see Chapter 15). Evaluation should include a chest x-ray and either skin testing with a PPD or an IRGA. Treatment should involve three or more antituberculous medicines for 6–9 months (Table 7–2).

2. SARCOIDOSIS

Sarcoidosis is a chronic granulomatous disease of unknown cause, usually presenting in the fourth or fifth decade of life. Pulmonary involvement occurs in most patients. Virtually every organ system can be involved, including the skin, bones, liver, spleen, central nervous system, and eyes. The tissue reaction is much less severe than in tuberculous uveitis, and caseation can rarely occur. Anergy on skin testing supports the diagnosis. When the parotid glands are involved, the disease is called uveoparotid fever, or Heerfordt's disease. When the lacrimal glands are involved, the disease is called Mikulicz's syndrome.

Uveitis occurs in approximately 25% of patients with systemic sarcoidosis. As with tuberculosis, any form of uveitis can occur, but sarcoid deserves special consideration when the uveitis is granulomatous or when retinal phlebitis is present, particularly in black patients.

The diagnosis can be supported by an abnormal chest x-ray, especially when hilar adenopathy is present, or by elevated serum ACE, lysozyme, or calcium levels. The strongest evidence comes from histopathologic demonstration of noncaseating granulomas in affected tissues such as lung or conjunctiva. However, biopsies should only be taken when suspicious lesions are clearly evident. A gallium scan of the head, neck, and thorax can provide evidence for subclinical inflammation of the lacrimal, parotid, or salivary glands or of paratracheal or pulmonary lymph nodes.

Corticosteroid therapy given early in the disease may be effective, but recurrences are common. Long-term therapy may require the use of corticosteroid-sparing agents such as methotrexate, azathioprine, or mycophenolate mofetil (Table 7–2).

3. SYPHILIS

Syphilis is an uncommon but treatable cause of uveitis. Intraocular inflammation occurs almost exclusively during the secondary and tertiary stages of infection. All types of uveitis occur. Associated retinitis (Figure 7–9) and papillitis are common. Widespread atrophy and hyperplasia of the retinal pigment epithelium can occur late if untreated. Testing should include one of the commonly used (and less expensive) tests for the production of *T pallidum*–induced anticardiolipin antibodies, such as the VDRL or RPR test, as well as a test for the more specific anti–*T pallidum* antibodies, such as the FTA-ABS or MHA-TP. While the FTA-ABS and MHA-TP tests display high sensitivity and specificity during both secondary and tertiary stages of infection, the VDRL and RPR can be falsely negative in up to 30% of patients with late or latent disease. Falsely positive results can occur in the setting of other spirochetal infections, biliary cirrhosis, or collagen-vascular disease, whereas falsely negative results can occur in severely immunocompromised patients. Patients with uveitis and a positive serologic test for syphilis should undergo examination of the cerebrospinal

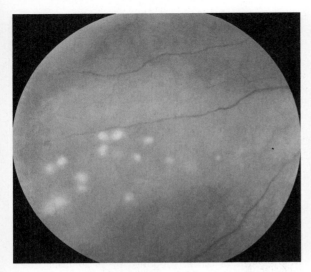

▲ **Figure 7–9.** Characteristic "ground glass" appearance and overlying superficial retinal precipitates in a patient with syphilitic retinitis. (Courtesy of J M Jumper.)

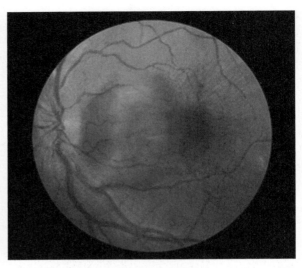

▲ **Figure 7–10.** Serous retinal detachment in a patient with sympathetic ophthalmia. (Courtesy of H R McDonald.)

fluid to rule out neurosyphilis. Treatment consists of aqueous crystalline penicillin G, 2–4 million units, given intravenously every 4 hours for 14 days.

4. SYMPATHETIC OPHTHALMIA

Sympathetic ophthalmia is a rare, but devastating bilateral granulomatous uveitis that comes on 10 days to many years following a perforating eye injury. The vast majority of cases occur within 1 year after injury. The cause is not known, but the disease is probably related to hypersensitivity to some element of the pigment-bearing cells in the uvea. It very rarely occurs following uncomplicated intraocular surgery for cataract or glaucoma and even less commonly following endophthalmitis.

The injured, or exciting, eye becomes inflamed first and the fellow, or sympathizing, eye secondarily. Patients usually complain of photophobia, redness, and blurred vision, although the presence of floaters may be the primary complaint. The uveitis is usually diffuse. Soft yellow-white exudates in the deep layer of the retina (Dalen-Fuchs nodules) are sometimes seen in the posterior segment. Serous retinal detachments can also occur (Figure 7–10).

The recommended treatment of a severely injured sightless eye is enucleation, or possibly evisceration, within 10 days after injury. The sympathizing eye should be treated aggressively with local or systemic corticosteroids. Long term corticosteroid sparing immunosuppressive therapy is often required (Table 7–2). Without treatment, the disease progresses relentlessly to complete bilateral blindness.

UVEITIS IN DEVELOPING COUNTRIES

All forms of uveitis mentioned above also occur in developing countries and some, such as toxoplasmosis and tuberculosis, are relatively common. In addition, more than 95% of all HIV-positive patients live in developing countries, particularly in sub-Saharan Africa and Southeast Asia. In these regions, otherwise opportunistic infections such as cytomegalovirus retinitis are increasing at an alarming rate. A few infectious causes of uveitis deserve special mention, since they occur almost exclusively in patients who either live in or visit developing countries.

1. LEPTOSPIROSIS

Uveitis occurs in up to 10% of patients infected with the spirochete leptospira. Humans are accidental hosts, infected most commonly by contact with or ingestion of infected water supplies. Wild and domestic animals, including rodents, dogs, pigs, and cattle, are the natural hosts and shed large quantities of infectious organisms in their urine. Farmers, veterinarians, and those who work or swim in waters fed by agricultural run off are at particularly high risk.

▶ Clinical Findings
A. Symptoms and Signs

Fever, malaise, and headache are common constitutional symptoms. Renal failure and death can occur in up to 30% of untreated patients. The uveitis may be of any type but is typically diffuse and often associated with hypopyon and retinal vasculitis.

B. Laboratory Findings

Culture of live organisms is only possible early in the infection. Sensitive and specific anti-leptospira antibody tests are available for use on blood or cerebrospinal fluid. A fourfold rise in antibody titer is strong evidence for recent infection.

▶ **Treatment**

Treatment of severe infections includes penicillin, 1.5 million units intravenously every 6 hours for 10 days. Less severe infections can be treated with doxycycline, 100 mg given orally twice daily for 7 days. Topical corticosteroids and cycloplegic/mydriatic agents should be used in conjunction with antibiotic therapy to minimize the complications of anterior uveitis. Posterior sub-Tenon injection of corticosteroids may be necessary for severe intermediate, posterior, or diffuse forms of inflammation.

2. ONCHOCERCIASIS

Onchocerciasis is caused by *Onchocerca volvulus.* The disease afflicts about 15 million people in Africa and Central America and is a major cause of blindness. It is transmitted by *Simulium damnosum,* a black fly that breeds in areas of rapidly flowing streams—thus the term "river blindness." Microfilariae picked up from the skin by the fly mature into larvae that become adult worms in 1 year. The adult parasite produces cutaneous nodules 5–25 mm in diameter on the trunk, thighs, arms, head, and shoulders. Microfilariae cause itching, and healing of skin lesions may lead to loss of skin elasticity and areas of depigmentation.

▶ **Clinical Findings**

A. Symptoms and Signs

Skin nodules may be seen. The cornea reveals nummular keratitis and sclerosing keratitis. Microfilariae swimming actively in the anterior chamber look like silver threads. Death of the microfilariae causes an intense inflammatory reaction and severe uveitis, vitritis, and retinitis. Focal retinochoroiditis may be seen. Optic atrophy may develop secondary to glaucoma.

B. Laboratory Findings

The diagnosis of onchocerciasis is made by skin biopsy and microscopic examination looking for live microfilariae.

▶ **Treatment**

The preferred treatment for onchocerciasis is with nodulectomy and ivermectin. Diethylcarbamazine and suramin have significant toxicity and should be used only when ivermectin is not available.

The great advantage of ivermectin over diethylcarbamazine is that a single oral dose of 100 or 200 µg/kg reduces the worm burden in the skin and anterior chamber more slowly

and therefore with a significant reduction in systemic and ocular reactions. The reduction also persists longer.

The minimum effective dose remains to be determined. A dose of 100 µg/kg may be as effective as 200 µg/kg and is associated with fewer of the mild and transient side effects: fever, headache, etc. Treatment is repeated at 6 or 12 months.

Topical therapy with corticosteroids and cycloplegic/mydriatic agents is helpful for uveitis.

3. CYSTICERCOSIS

Cysticercosis is an uncommon cause of serious ocular morbidity. The disease is endemic in Mexico, Central and South America, and parts of Africa and Asia , with ocular involvement occurring in about one-third of affected patients. Ocular cysticercosis is caused either by the ingestion of eggs of *Taenia solium* or by reverse peristalsis in cases of intestinal obstruction caused by adult tapeworms. Eggs mature and embryos penetrate intestinal mucosa, thus gaining access to the circulation. The larvae (*Cysticercus cellulosae*) is the most common tapeworm that invades the human eye.

▶ **Clinical Findings**

The larvae may reach the subretinal space, producing acute retinitis with retinal edema and subretinal exudates, or the vitreous cavity (Figure 7–11), where a translucent cyst with a dense white spot formed by the invaginated scolex develops. Larvae may live in the eye for as long as 2 years. Death of the larvae inside the eye leads to a severe inflammatory reaction.

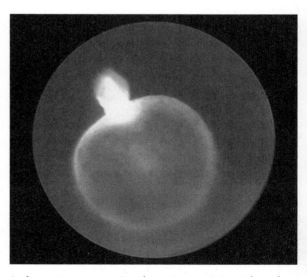

▲ **Figure 7–11.** Intravitreal cyst in a patient with ocular cysticercosis. (Courtesy of G R O'Connor.)

Movements of larvae within the ocular tissue may stimulate a chronic inflammatory reaction and fibrosis. In rare instances, the larva may be seen in the anterior chamber. Involvement of the brain can cause seizures. Focal calcification may be seen in the subcutaneous tissues by x-ray.

▶ **Treatment**

Treatment of intraocular cysticercosis is by surgical removal, usually by pars plana vitrectomy.

7.2. Uveal Tumors
James J. Augsburger, MD, and Zélia M. Corrêa, MD, PhD

This section presents an overview of the most common and most important neoplasms, hamartomas, and choristomas of the uveal tract. Neoplastic lesions of the ciliary body epithelium (Chapter 10), and non-neoplastic disorders (eg, subretinal and suprachoroidal hematomas, nodular posterior scleritis, and fibrovascular disciform lesion due to neovascular age-related macular degeneration) that can simulate uveal tract tumors are discussed in other parts of this book.

BENIGN UVEAL TUMORS

Benign neoplasms are acquired tumors of cells that are atypical but not sufficient to be classified as malignant. They may enlarge slowly, but have little or no invasive potential and no metastatic capability. **Hamartomas** are congenital tumors composed of normal or near-normal cells and tissues for the anatomic site but in excessive amounts. **Choristomas** are congenital cellular tumors consisting of normal cells and tissue elements but not occurring normally at the anatomic site.

▶ Melanocytic Uveal Nevus

A melanocytic uveal nevus is a benign acquired neoplasm composed of mildly abnormal uveal melanocytes. It can develop within any portion of the uvea (iris, ciliary body, or choroid), but the choroid is most frequently involved clinically, with the choroidal nevus being the most commonly encountered discrete intraocular tumor in Caucasians. Epidemiologic studies have shown uveal nevi to be rare in infants and children, uncommon in teenagers and young adults, but relatively frequent in older individuals. Cross-sectional clinical and autopsy studies generally have found melanocytic nevi in 2% to 10% of eyes of Caucasians over the age of 50 years. They are thought to occur with similar frequency in non-Caucasians, but they are much more likely to be overlooked clinically because of the more pronounced melanotic pigmentation of the choroid that obscures the lesion in such individuals.

A typical melanocytic uveal nevus appears as a dark brown to tan lesion regardless of where in the uvea it develops. Most uveal nevi are small (less than 3 mm in maximal basal diameter and less than 0.5 mm in maximal thickness) when first identified, and only about 5% ever achieve a size greater than 5 mm in diameter and/or greater than 1 mm in thickness. Because of their readily visible nature, being noted by the patient as a cosmetic lesion or detected on routine eye examination, melanocytic nevi of the iris are usually detected when they are quite small (Figure 7–12), Melanocytic nevi of the choroid (Figure 7–13) and ciliary body are usually noted either incidentally on routine examination or detected on ocular evaluation prompted by visual symptoms. Iris nevi generally appear quite bland without prominent intrinsic vascularity on slitlamp biomicroscopy; however, they can be associated with peaking of the pupil toward the lesion and localized eversion of the pupil margin (ectropion iridis). Melanocytic choroidal nevi typically appear as thin gray to brown choroidal lesions with feathered margins that blend imperceptibly into the surrounding normal choroid. Drusen are frequently present on the surface of such lesions. Melanocytic choroidal nevi occasionally exhibit prominent clumps of orange pigment (lipofuscin) on their surface and give rise to overlying and surrounding serous subretinal fluid. Rarely, choroidal neovascularization with subretinal

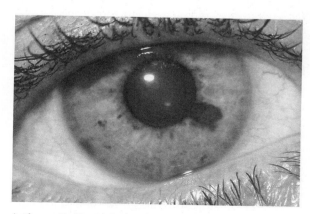

▲ **Figure 7–12.** Typical iris nevus involving pupillary margin. Note also the multiple tiny iris freckles.

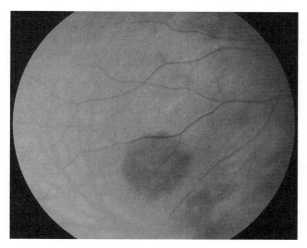

▲ **Figure 7–13.** Typical melanocytic choroidal nevus underlying retinal blood vessels and only about 0.25 mm thick by ultrasonography.

bleeding and/or exudation develops over a melanocytic choroidal nevus.

A particular variant of uveal nevus is the **melanocytoma (magnacellular nevus) of the optic disc**. This typically appears as a dark brown to almost black intrapapillary mass (Figure 7–14). Fundus biomicroscopy frequently shows darkly melanotic tumor cells invading the retinal nerve fiber

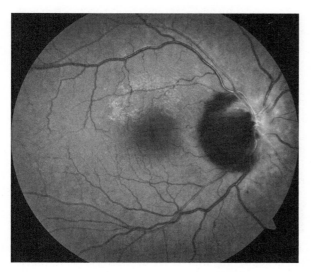

▲ **Figure 7–14.** Melanocytoma (magnacellular nevus) of the optic disc, with typical black color of lesion and replacement of retinal nerve fibers by tumor tissue.

layer at the disc and frequently there is an associated classic juxtapapillary choroidal nevus. Optic disc melanocytoma can cause progressive retinal nerve fiber damage with resultant visual field loss.

Many melanocytic uveal tumors (especially ones that are already relatively large when first detected or which are found in relatively young persons) exhibit limited growth during subsequent follow-up and this should not be regarded as unequivocal evidence that the tumor is malignant or that a nevus is transforming into a malignant melanoma. Because uveal nevi occur so much more frequently than do uveal melanomas, there is considerable overlap of size between larger uveal nevi and small uveal melanomas. Also, melanocytic choroidal and ciliary body nevi that achieve a size substantially greater than 5 mm in diameter and 1 mm in thickness are frequently impossible to distinguish clinically from small choroidal melanomas.

Melanocytic uveal nevi generally require no treatment. However, if there is concern that a melanoctyic iris tumor in the large nevus versus small melanoma category is really a melanoma and not a nevus, fine-needle aspiration biopsy, incisional biopsy, or iridectomy excision of the lesion is probably appropriate. Extramacular melanocytic choroidal nevi that are associated with serous subretinal fluid involving the macula and causing visual blurring and distortion may be treated by focal laser therapy to sites of leakage identified on fluorescein angiography, and choroidal neovascularization associated with a choroidal nevus may be treated by intravitreal anti-VEGF therapy, photodynamic therapy, laser hyperthermia to the entire melanocytic choroidal tumor, or focal photocoagulation depending on its location and extent. A melanocytic choroidal or ciliary body tumor in the large nevus versus small melanoma category may warrant diagnostic transscleral or transvitreal fine-needle aspiration biopsy to establish a pathologic diagnosis.

Uveal melanocytic nevi should be distinguished not only from uveal melanomas (see later) but also from clusters of normal uveal melanocytes—localized flat congenital collections of normal uveal melanocytes, frequently referred to as uveal freckles that frequently darken (and therefore become more apparent) during the later first decade to early second decade of life—and diffuse or sectoral hypermelanotic thickening of portions of the uvea attributable to generalized or limited forms of congenital ocular melanocytosis.

▶ Circumscribed Choroidal Hemangioma

Circumscribed choroidal hemangioma is a benign neoplasm, although regarded by some authorities as a hamartoma even though it is rarely if ever detected at birth or identified in the neonatal period, composed of a localized overgrowth of choroidal blood vessels. It is almost exclusively a unilateral unifocal intraocular tumor. There is no recognized familial hereditary tendency. The average age at detection in most larger reported series is the late 30s to early 40s. Clinically, it appears as a localized, round to oval, dome-shaped,

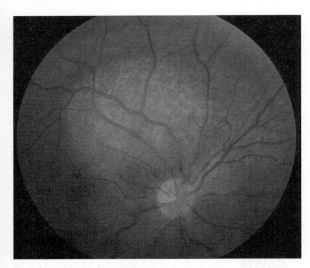

▲ **Figure 7–15.** Circumscribed choroidal hemangioma just superior to optic disc and fovea, with shallow serous subretinal fluid involving the central macula.

reddish-orange mass that is centered posterior to the ocular equator (Figure 7–15). Almost all circumscribed choroidal hemangiomas extend to within about 3 mm from the optic disc or foveola. Most are less than 10 mm in diameter and less than 3.5 mm in thickness when first detected, although tumors larger than 15 mm in basal diameter and more than 5 mm in thickness are encountered occasionally. If the tumor develops in the macula, it frequently causes progressive cystic degeneration of the overlying retina with reduced vision. Juxtapapillary but extramacular circumscribed choroidal hemangiomas are frequently associated with progressive accumulation of serous subretinal fluid that will cause substantial visual blurring and distortion if the central macula is affected. Circumscribed choroidal hemangiomas tend to enlarge slowly during long-term follow-up. Rapid profound enlargement has not been documented.

Fluorescein angiography typically shows rapid filling of the relatively large caliber blood vessels comprising the tumor. Indocyanine green angiography (ICGA) is generally regarded as the more appropriate angiographic study. It typically shows well-defined diffuse early hyperfluorescence of the entire lesion and late washout of its central portion, typically not evident until 20 to 30 minutes after the dye injection. B-scan ocular ultrasonography shows the fusiform to dome-like cross sectional shape of the tumor, which characteristically exhibits internal reflectivity similar to that of orbital fat. This feature can make it difficult to identify the precise interface between the outer surface of the tumor and the inner surface of the overlying sclera.

The most commonly employed initial treatment for small to medium visually symptomatic circumscribed choroidal hemangiomas is photodynamic laser therapy, which generally

results in pronounced flattening of the hemangioma and prompt, sustained resolution of associated serous subretinal fluid and cystoid retinal thickening. Large circumscribed choroidal hemangiomas associated with bullous total serous retinal detachment and/or prominent white fibrous metaplasia of the overlying retinal pigment epithelium may require plaque radiation therapy or some method of external beam radiation therapy (conventional fractionated linear accelerator therapy, stereotactic radiotherapy/gamma knife radiotherapy, or proton beam irradiation) to stabilize and/or shrink the tumor and eliminate the associated retinal detachment. Factors adversely influencing the visual outcome include larger size, subfoveal location, extensive retinal detachment, and worse visual acuity prior to treatment.

▶ Diffuse Choroidal Hemangioma

Diffuse choroidal hemangioma is not a discrete intraocular tumor but rather a diffuse congenital overgrowth (malformation) of relatively normal appearing choroidal blood vessels. It typically occurs in conjunction with an ipsilateral congenital cutaneous facial nevus flammeus affecting the eyelids and periorbital skin of the cheek, forehead, and temple (one of the characteristic lesions of Sturge–Weber syndrome). It is usually unilateral but bilateral involvement has been reported. There is no recognized familial inheritance pattern.

Diffuse choroidal hemangioma appears as reddish-orange thickening of the choroid that tends to be most pronounced around the optic disc and in the macula (Figure 7–16). The optic disc cup on frequently appears large and deep because

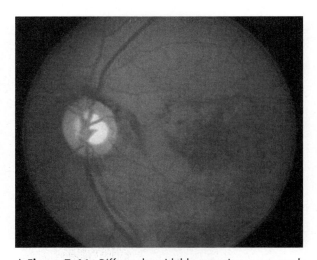

▲ **Figure 7–16.** Diffuse choroidal hemangioma surrounding the optic disc, with its cup appearing large and deep because of the pronounced circumpapillary choroidal vascular thickening. There is clumping of the retinal pigment epithelium in the central macula. See color insert.

of the circumpapillary choroidal thickening. Visual loss occurs because of progressive cystic degeneration of the macula, chronic secondary serous retinal detachment, and/or associated secondary glaucoma.

Photodynamic therapy or plaque radiotherapy to particular areas of choroidal vascular thickening may eliminate secondary subretinal fluid in the macula, but low-dose radiation therapy to the posterior ocular segment is sometimes necessary to stabilize the diffuse choroidal hemangioma and eliminate any associated serous retinal detachment.

▶ Choroidal Osteoma

Choroidal osteoma is a benign choroidal bone tissue neoplasm, although regarded by some authorities as a choristoma even though it is not present at birth or detected in the neonatal period in most affected individuals. It affects women predominantly (9:1 female to male ratio). It is bilateral in approximately 20% of cases, but is always unifocal in affected eyes. There is no generally recognized hereditary tendency. The tumor is usually first detected during the second or third decade of life. It characteristically appears as a rather well-defined gold to off-white juxtapapillary or circumpapillary choroidal plate-like lesion with smooth margins but pseudopod-like protrusions (Figure 7–17). It tends to enlarge slowly following initial detection, but remains plate-like in cross sectional shape. The retinal pigment epithelium is frequently disrupted and clumped over the tumor, and the sensory retina may be thinned or cystic. Choroidal neovascularization frequently develops from the surface and leads to further visual loss on the basis of accumulation of serous and/or hemorrhagic subretinal fluid and exudates and eventual subretinal fibrosis. If the tumor involves the central macula, profound

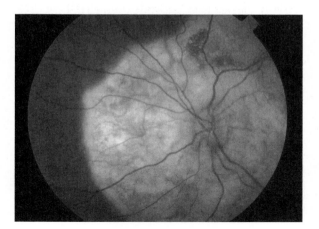

▲ **Figure 7–17.** Choroidal osteoma in typical circumpapillary location. The tumor has a pale color with well-defined smooth margins. There are small caliber blood vessels on its surface and localized subretinal blood superiorly.

visual loss in the eye is the rule. If choroidal neovascularization associated with an extramacular choroidal osteoma occurs and causes visual symptoms, it can be treated by intravitreal anti-VEGF agents, photodynamic laser therapy, or laser photocoagulation. Regression (or at least decalcification) of some choroidal osteomas has been reported. Because the tumor has no recognized malignant potential, no destructive treatment for the tumor is indicated.

UVEAL TUMORS INTERMEDIATE BETWEEN BENIGN AND MALIGNANT

These tumors are categorized as neoplasms of borderline malignancy because clinically they cannot be categorized reliably as either benign or malignant. If a biopsy is performed, pathologic studies may reveal benign cells, malignant cells, or cells deemed to be borderline even by cytologic criteria.

▶ Melanocytic Uveal Neoplasm in Nevus versus Melanoma Category ("Nevoma")

There is considerable size overlap between larger melanocytic uveal nevi (see above) and small uveal melanomas. Although approximately 95% of uveal nevi never exceed 5 mm in maximal basal diameter and 1 mm in thickness, the remaining 5% can achieve substantially larger dimensions. Because uveal nevi are substantially more common than uveal melanomas, there is considerable overlap between melanocytic uveal tumors in the 5 to 10 mm basal diameter and 1 to 3.5 mm thickness ranges. Melanocytic uveal neoplasms in this size range that do not exhibit clearly invasive clinical features are sometimes referred to as "nevomas" or "indeterminate pigmented uveal tumors." An iris melanocytic tumor that might be categorized in this way would be larger (especially in thickness) than the typical iris nevus (Figure 7–12) and associated with peaking of the pupil toward the lesion, eversion of the pupil margin (ectropion iridis), and possibly even abnormally prominent intralesional blood vessels (Figure 7–18) but would not exhibit seeding onto the adjacent iris, implantation tumors on the trabecular meshwork, or full thickness iris replacement (demonstrable by ultrasound biomicroscopy). A choroidal or ciliary body tumor that might be categorized in this way would also be larger (especially in thickness) than the typical choroidal nevus (Figure 7–15), but would exhibit clinical features of dormancy, such as prominent clumps of black retinal pigment epithelial pigment and drusen on its surface, or at least show no apical eruption through Bruch's membrane, retinal invasion, or scleral invasion/transscleral extension (demonstrable by B-scan ultrasonography) (Figure 7–19). In the absence of a tumor specimen that has been evaluated pathologically, one can never be certain which of these tumors is benign (nevus) and which is malignant (melanoma). Although some authorities regard documented growth of a tumor that clinically was classified initially as a nevus as evidence of malignant transformation, it is equally if not more likely that

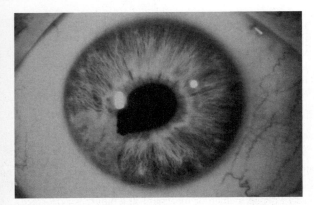

▲ **Figure 7–18.** Amelanotic melanocytic iris neoplasm in nevus versus melanoma category (iris nevoma). Note peaking of the pupil, limited ectropion iridis, and intralesional blood vessels. Histopathologic study of the excised tumor showed it to be a spindle A melanocytic tumor (ie, a nevus).

the tumor is still benign but enlarging or the initial diagnosis was incorrect. There have been no reports of a small melanocytic uveal tumor, initially biopsied and classified pathologically as a nevus then observed to enlarge and reclassified

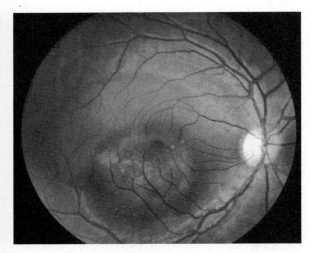

▲ **Figure 7–19.** Melanocytic subfoveal choroidal tumor in nevus versus melanoma category (choroidal nevoma). This visually symptomatic tumor was 2 mm thick. It exhibits a prominent ring of subretinal orange pigment (lipofuscin) on its surface and an associated blister of overlying and surrounding serous subretinal fluid. It was left untreated, spontaneously flattening slightly with disappearance of the orange pigment and subretinal fluid. Follow-up for over 25 years has shown no reactivation.

pathologically as melanoma following repeat biopsy, resection or enucleation. Although transformation of benign uveal nevi into malignant uveal melanomas almost certainly does occur, reported estimates of its frequency are likely to be gross overestimates. Any melanocytic uveal tumor for which treatment is being recommended warrants fine-needle aspiration biopsy or other method of biopsy for confirmation of the diagnosis. In the absence of pathologic confirmation of the diagnosis, the effectiveness of any treatment undertaken is likely to be overestimated, because patients with a nevus who are misdiagnosed clinically as having a melanoma have virtually no risk of local tumor relapse or metastasis following treatment, and underestimate the unnecessary costs and inappropriate concerns borne by patients who have nevi misdiagnosed as melanomas.

▶ Atypical Lymphoid Hyperplasia of the Uvea

Atypical lymphoid hyperplasia of the uvea, previously usually termed benign reactive lymphoid hyperplasia, is focal or diffuse infiltration of the uvea by activated but benign-appearing lymphoid cells. Pathologically, the lymphoid cells are frequently organized into germinal centers that are evident on low to high power microscopy. Immunohistochemically, the lymphoid cells comprising the infiltrates are usually of B-cell lineage but frequently exhibit polyclonal features. Clinically, these lesions appear as tan to creamy focal to diffuse infiltrates in the iris or choroid. B-scan ultrasonography shows generalized choroidal thickening (sometimes with locally accentuated prominence) in diffuse cases, and ultrasound biomicroscopy confirms the solid soft tissue character of iris and iridociliary infiltrates. The retina usually remains attached or shows limited shallow detachment in areas of choroidal infiltration, but progressive disruption of the RPE overlying the infiltrates develops in many cases. Focal or diffuse pink anterior epibulbar masses reminiscent of primary conjunctival lymphoma, occur in some case, and others have posterior peribulbar extraocular soft tissue masses that may only be evident on B-scan ultrasonography. Treatment usually consists of relatively low-dose fractionated external beam radiation therapy, typically resulting in prompt, sustained clinical regression of the lymphoid infiltrates and tumors. If vision is severely compromised prior to treatment, it may not recover even if all of the uveal infiltrates regress completely. Because occasional patients with atypical lymphoid hyperplasia of the uvea eventually develop evidence of systemic lymphoma, all affected patients should probably be monitored periodically.

MALIGNANT UVEAL TUMORS

The component cells of malignant uveal tumor and the tissue they form are clearly abnormal morphologically. Invasive features are generally evident clinically and pathologically, and regional and distant metastases may occur.

▶ Primary Uveal Melanoma

Primary uveal melanoma is an acquired malignant neoplasm that arises from uveal melanocytes. It is almost always unilateral and unifocal. Although characteristic chromosomal abnormalities are present within individual tumor cells, primary uveal melanoma does not usually exhibit any familial hereditary pattern. Uveal melanomas are extremely rare in persons under the age of 20 years but become progressively more frequent with advancing age. The average age at diagnosis of iris melanoma is in the range of 40 to 45 years, while that of patients with choroidal or ciliary body melanoma is between 55 and 60 years. Primary uveal melanoma affects both men and women. The cumulative lifetime incidence of primary uveal melanoma in whites is in the range of 1 in 2000 to 1 in 2500 persons. The average annual incidence in whites is approximately 7 to 8 per million persons per year. An iris melanoma is frequently recognized by the patient as a newly appearing or changing spot on the iris. Choroidal melanomas and most ciliary body melanomas are not evident cosmetically but are detected either on fundus examination prompted by visual symptoms or on routine eye examination. Important risk factors for occurrence of primary uveal melanoma include ocular and oculodermal melanocytosis, cutaneous dysplastic nevus syndrome (familial atypical multiple mole—melanoma [FAMM] syndrome), lighter iris color, white race, and older patient age.

Typical iris melanoma appears as a dark brown to tan nodular iris mass that replaces the normal iris stroma (Figure 7–20). It frequently has prominent intralesional blood vessels and routinely causes peaking and/or splinting of the pupil and eversion of the pupil margin (ectropion iridis). Loss of cohesiveness of the tumor cells frequently results in satellite tumors on the adjacent iris and on the trabecular meshwork, commonly being associated with secondary glaucoma.

Typical ciliary body melanoma appears as a dark nodular peripheral fundus mass (Figure 7–21) associated with prominent

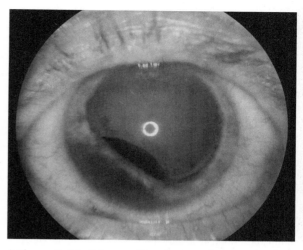

▲ **Figure 7–21.** Primary ciliary body melanoma that has invaded the peripheral iris, the main portion of the darkly melanotic tumor lying posterior to the iris and indenting the lens.

localized dilation of blood vessels in the overlying sclera (sentinel blood vessels). The tumor sometimes extends into the peripheral iris, where it may be evident on slitlamp biomicroscopy and gonioscopy. If thick enough, it may indent and even displace the crystalline lens and cause progressive astigmatism. The tumor occasionally invades the overlying sclera and extends to the external surface of the eye, where it appears as a dark brown flat to nodular vascularized episcleral mass.

Typical choroidal melanoma appears as a dark brown to pale gold subretinal mass (Figure 7–22) that is usually at least

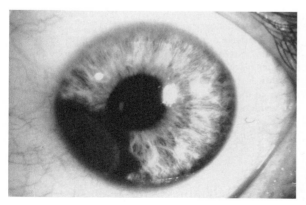

▲ **Figure 7–20.** Darkly melanotic iris melanoma, filling the anterior chamber angle inferonasally and approximately 3 mm thick. Histopathologic study of the excised tumor confirmed it to be a melanoma.

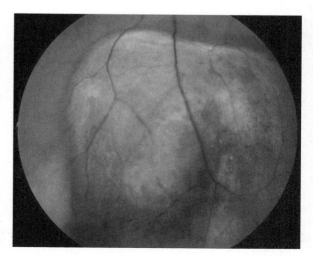

▲ **Figure 7–22.** Primary non-uniformly melanotic choroidal melanoma with a dome-shaped configuration.

7 mm in largest basal diameter, more than 3 mm in thickness, or both when first detected. The average largest basal diameter of choroidal melanomas in most series is in the range of 12 to 13 mm, and the average thickness is in the range of 6 to 6.5 mm. The most common tumor shape is the round to oval-based dome, while the most distinctive tumor shape is the mushroom-like nodule with nodular apical eruption through Bruch's membrane. Occasional choroidal melanomas exhibit a geographic multinodular or diffuse shape.

Ultrasound biomicroscopy is useful for determining the size, shape, and margins of iris and iridociliary body melanomas prior to planned treatment, and for following them after treatment to monitor for regression or relapse. B-scan ultrasonography is appropriate for determining the size, shape, and intraocular location of choroidal and ciliary body melanomas, identifying scleral invasion and transscleral extension to the orbit, and showing (on dynamic imaging) vascular pulsations within the tumor. It is also useful for monitoring after eye preserving therapies, such as I-125 plaque radiotherapy and proton beam irradiation, for regression or relapse.

Patients with primary uveal melanoma have a well-documented propensity to develop metastasis, especially to the liver, regardless of how the primary intraocular tumor is managed. Adverse prognostic factors for eventual metastasis and metastatic death include larger tumor size, ciliary body location, epithelioid melanocytic cell type, complex loops and networks in the vasculogenic mimicry pattern within the tumor, monosomy chromosome 3 status and Class 2 gene expression profile of tumor cells. Iris location, spindle melanocytic cell type, and disomy chromosome 3 status and Class 1 gene expression profile of tumor cells are favorable factors.

Several different treatment options are available for primary uveal melanomas of different sizes, intraocular locations, and associated clinical features. Enucleation is still appropriate for patients with an extremely large intraocular tumor, a tumor surrounding or invading the optic disc, or an eye that is blind and painful due to the tumor. I-125 plaque radiotherapy in the United States, Ru-106 plaque radiotherapy in Europe, and proton beam irradiation are the most commonly employed treatments for small to relatively large choroidal and ciliary body melanomas. These methods are also being used with increasing frequency in some centers as alternatives to iridectomy and iridocyclectomy for many iris and iridociliary melanomas. These radiation therapy methods usually induce long-term tumor shrinkage, but tumor regression is frequently associated with delayed onset radiation-induced cataract, retinopathy and optic neuropathy, and may result in radiation-induced iris neovascularization, neovascular glaucoma, and profound visual loss. Transscleral tumor resection is employed in a few centers for some ciliary body and choroidal melanomas, almost always in conjunction with preoperative proton beam irradiation or post-resection plaque radiotherapy. Transvitreal endoresection, using vitrectomy instruments, of post-equatorial choroidal melanomas is also employed in a few centers, almost always in conjunction with preoperative plaque or proton beam radiation therapy. No prospective comparative clinical trials of resection versus enucleation or plaque radiotherapy have ever been reported. Transpupillary infrared laser hyperthermia (transpupillary thermotherapy—TTT) has been used extensively in some centers to treat small posterior melanocytic choroidal tumors believed to be melanomas, but TTT as single therapy has largely been abandoned, as was laser photocoagulation before it, because of unacceptably high rates of eventual local tumor relapse and even transscleral tumor extension into the orbit. TTT and laser photocoagulation are still used as a supplement to plaque radiotherapy in some centers, mainly for juxtapapillary and macular choroidal melanomas. Most iris and iridociliary melanomas are treated by surgical excision (iridectomy, iridocyclectomy) or plaque radiotherapy.

At present, there is no compelling scientific evidence that any method of treatment of primary uveal melanomas improves survival prognosis. There are no accumulated natural history data documenting the survival of untreated patients with melanocytic uveal tumors encompassing the entire spectrum of such lesions, from extremely small asymptomatic lesions of uncertain pathologic nature to frankly malignant tumors filling much or all of the eye. In the absence of such information, there is no valid standard against which to judge the true effectiveness of treatment. It has been suggested that the longer survival of patients with smaller tumors at the time of treatment (see above) demonstrates that treatment is effective if provided early enough, but there are no comparative clinical trials comparing the survival of treated (any method) and untreated patients with primary uveal melanomas of any defined size category. The Collaborative Ocular Melanoma Study (COMS) in the United States and a number of retrospective comparative survival studies have shown that enucleation and I-125 plaque radiotherapy of medium to relatively large choroidal melanomas provide equivalent post-treatment rates of metastasis and mortality. COMS also showed that low-dose fractionated external beam radiation therapy prior to enucleation did not improve survival prognosis compared with enucleation alone in patients with large choroidal melanomas.

If metastasis from uveal melanoma develops, long-term survival is extremely poor. Although mean survival is longer in patients with limited metastasis identified by pre-symptomatic surveillance than in patients with symptomatic, advanced metastasis at detection, there is no currently available evidence that aggressive treatments, such as surgical resection of metastases or hepatic artery infusion chemotherapy, provide any clinically significant improvement in survival. Furthermore, no adjuvant therapy has been shown to prevent or delay metastasis.

▶ Non-Ophthalmic Primary Cancer Metastatic to the Uvea

Some non-ophthalmic primary cancers metastasize hematogenously to the uvea. Clinically apparent metastatic uveal tumors typically appear as off-white to pink to gold (most

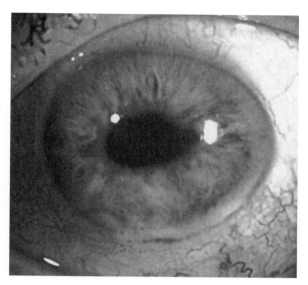

▲ **Figure 7–23.** Multinodular metastasis to the iris and inferior anterior chamber angle from primary lung cancer, causing distortion of the pupil.

carcinomas) or dark brown (skin melanomas). A metastatic tumor that develops in the iris typically appears as a progressively enlarging mass (Figure 7–23) that may be associated with variable blurred vision, ocular pain, signs of intraocular inflammation, and elevated intraocular pressure. A metastatic tumor that develops in the choroid typically appears as a round to oval dome-shaped mass (Figure 7–24) that is frequently associated with overlying and surrounding serous subretinal fluid out of proportion to the size of the tumor.

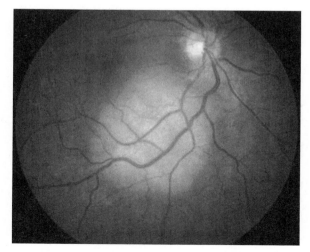

▲ **Figure 7–24.** Unifocal homogeneously creamy colored metastasis to the choroid from primary breast cancer.

Although the most frequent situation is a solitary metastatic tumor in one eye (80% of cases), about 20% of patients will have two or more discrete metastatic tumors in one or both eyes. If left untreated, most metastatic tumors to the uvea enlarge measurably within days to a few weeks.

Different types of non-ophthalmic primary cancers are associated with different frequencies and patterns of uveal metastasis The most common primary cancer types that give rise to clinically detected metastatic uveal tumors are breast cancer in women, lung cancer in men, and colon cancer in both groups.

Metastatic non-ophthalmic primary cancer to the uvea is generally believed to be the most common malignant intraocular neoplasm. In the United States, approximately 25% of all deaths are attributable to cancer. Of these deaths, about 50% are attributable to the effects of metastatic tumors on vital organs such as the liver or brain. At autopsy, approximately 90% of patients dying of metastatic cancer have at least microscopically evident metastatic cancer cells within ocular blood vessels and/or other intraocular tissues. Of these patients with pathologically evident intraocular metastatic cancer cells, only about 10% have uveal tumors that an ophthalmologist might be expected to detect if the patient was examined clinically. Of course, many of these patients are likely to have developed their clinically detectable metastatic uveal tumors while they are obtunded during the final phase of their illness. Only about 50% of these patients are believed to experience clinically symptomatic uveal tumors that prompt clinical evaluation resulting in detection of the intraocular tumor(s).

Since embryologically the eye is essentially an outgrowth of the brain, a metastatic tumor to the eye should be regarded as a metastasis to the brain. About 20% of patients with a metastatic tumor in one or both eyes will have a concurrent metastatic tumor in the brain detectable by CT or MRI. The median survival time following detection of a metastatic uveal tumor is only about 6 months, ranging from about 12 months for patients with metastatic breast cancer to about 3 months for patients with metastatic skin melanoma. Treatment for symptomatic lesions usually consists of palliative external beam radiation therapy, chemotherapy appropriate to the type of cancer, or both.

▶ **Primary Uveal Lymphoma**

Primary uveal lymphoma is a relatively uncommon but important variety of **primary intraocular lymphoma.** Whereas most cases of primary intraocular (vitreoretinal) lymphoma are characterized by accumulation of malignant lymphoid cells beneath the retinal pigment epithelium and within the sensory retina and vitreous (usually bilaterally) and are associated with antecedent, concurrent, or subsequent foci of primary central nervous system lymphoma (see Chapter 10), primary uveal lymphoma is characterized by focal or diffuse infiltrative tumors composed of malignant lymphocytes within the uvea (almost always unilaterally) and occasional subsequent development of systemic (non-CNS) lymphoma. This form of lymphoma bears more similarity to primary conjunctival lymphoma (see Chapter 5) than it does to primary vitreoretinal lymphoma.

Pathologically, the lymphoid cells infiltrating the uvea in this condition tend to be more abnormal in morphological appearance on high power microscopy than those associated with atypical lymphoid hyperplasia (see ealier). Germinal centers within the uvea are unlikely, and immunohistochemical staining and flow cytometry tend to show a more monoclonal character to the cells. As in the vitreoretinal form of primary intraocular lymphoma, the lymphoid cells comprising the infiltrates are usually of B-cell lineage. Clinically, the uveal infiltrates of primary uveal lymphoma appear as tan to creamy focal to diffuse infiltrates in the iris or choroid (Figure 7–25). B-scan ultrasonography shows generalized choroidal thickening (sometimes with locally accentuated prominence) in diffuse cases, and ultrasound biomicroscopy confirms the solid soft tissue character of iris and iridociliary infiltrates. The retina usually remains attached or shows limited shallow detachment in areas of choroidal infiltration, but progressive disruption of the RPE overlying the infiltrates develops in many cases. Less often than in atypical lymphoid hyperplasia, some patients have focal or diffuse pink anterior epibulbar masses reminiscent of primary conjunctival lymphoma, and others exhibit posterior peribulbar extraocular soft tissue masses that may only be evident on B-scan ultrasonography.

Treatment usually consists of fractionated external beam radiation therapy, typically resulting in prompt, sustained clinical regression of the lymphoid infiltrates and tumors. If

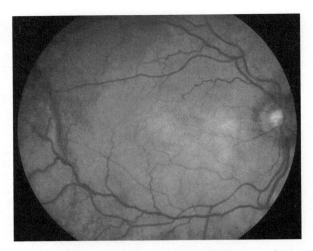

▲ **Figure 7–25.** Diffuse uveal lymphoid infiltration of primary uveal lymphoma, with focal accentuation temporally. See color insert.

vision is severely compromised prior to treatment, it may not recover even if all of the uveal infiltrates regress completely. In aggressive, neglected or misdiagnosed cases, the eye can become blind and painful with congestive features and diffuse intraocular bleeding that can necessitate enucleation. Because about 20% of patients with primary uveal lymphoma eventually develop systemic lymphoma, all affected patients should be monitored periodically.

7.3. Sclera
Carlos Pavesio, MD, FRCOphth

The human sclera consists almost entirely of collagen and comprises five-sixths of the outer tunic of the eye, extending from the cornea anteriorly to the optic foramen posteriorly.

The shape is, in part, maintained by the presence of the intraocular contents and the intraocular pressure. However, the sclera must be rigid enough to provide relatively constant conditions for the intraocular pressure so that, when the eyeball is moved, the intraocular pressure does not fluctuate. In addition, the opacity of the sclera ensures that internal light scattering does not affect the retinal image and the sclera must protect the intraocular contents from injury. Conditions which lead to alterations of these properties may result in changes to vision and eventually, in very severe cases, destruction of the globe with significant or total loss of vision.

Apart from potentially being affected by local factors, the sclera may also be involved in systemic conditions and may be

the first manifestation of such problems. This makes the role of the ophthalmologist very important in their recognition.

INFLAMMATORY CONDITIONS

1. EPISCLERITIS

This is probably a more common condition than realized because the majority of episcleral disease is unrecognized or unreported. The inflammation is localized to the episclera, the vascularized connective tissue overlying the sclera, and Tenon's capsule. It tends to affect young people, typically in the third and fourth decades of life, and is more prevalent in women. The condition is benign, tends to be recurrent and is typically self-limiting. It is unilateral in about two-thirds of cases. Although usually lasting for 1–2 weeks, the duration of episcleritis varies widely between individuals but tends to have the same pattern with each recurrence in a specific individual. In the majority of patients, recurrences occur over a period of 3–6 years, but a few individuals will have recurrences over a longer period of time.

The onset is almost always sudden, with the eye becoming red and uncomfortable within an hour of the start of the attack. Patients may also report heat, ocular surface discomfort and irritation, and tenderness. In nodular cases, one or more nodules can develop, and the redness tends to progress over a few days, but is always confined to the nodules, which may also become quite tender.

On examination the inflammation will be limited to the episclera and may be diffuse, involving one or more quadrants as in simple episcleritis (Figure 7–26), or it may be localized in to a small area, which is swollen producing a nodular episcleritis (Figure 7–27). There is no involvement of the underlying sclera, and keratitis and uveitis are uncommon.

In most cases the cause is unknown, but an association with a local or systemic disorder, such as gout, ocular rosacea, atopy, infection or collagen-vascular disease can be found in up to one-third of the patients.

Even though episcleritis can cause great distress and is unsightly and uncomfortable, there are no long-term complications in simple disease, and in nodular disease complications are rare and confined to changes in the adjacent cornea and sclera after multiple attacks at the same location.

Many patients become aware of warning symptoms prior to the onset of disease, and in such cases the frequent use of topical corticosteroids may be beneficial. In the

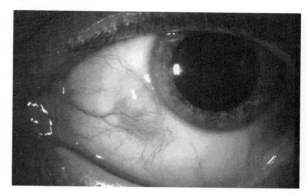

▲ **Figure 7–27.** Nodular episcleritis.

absence of a known etiology, treatment can include the use of chilled artificial tears and eventually topical corticosteroids in more intense cases. Topical nonsteroidal anti-inflammatory drugs (NSAIDs) tend not to be effective. In the presence of a local or systemic disorder, the treatment becomes specific and directed to the underlying condition. In some more resistant cases, the use of oral NSAIDs may be beneficial. The use of systemic corticosteroids is usually restricted to cases associated with an underlying collagen-vascular disease.

2. SCLERITIS

In contrast to episcleritis, scleritis is a much more severe condition, not only because of the intense symptoms, especially pain, but also because it may result in structural damage to the globe and carries a much stronger association with an underlying condition.

Scleritis is uncommon, accounting for less than a quarter of all scleral disease. The average age of onset is 48 years with a range of 11–87 years. Patients over the age of 60 years, have a greater likelihood of more severe disease and to develop complications including visual loss.

Most often the inflammatory process is driven primarily by an immunologic response and less commonly it can be precipitated by local factors such as trauma or infections (Table 7–7). The association with an underlying systemic disease is much stronger than with episcleritis and occurs in up to two-thirds of patients.

Scleritis is one of the very few severely painful eye diseases. However, it is important to remember that even though pain is usually a predominant feature, it may be absent in patients with posterior scleritis and in patients with a unique form of scleral thinning without overt inflammatory features, known as scleromalacia perforans, which usually occurs in association with rheumatoid arthritis. The pain of scleritis is described typically as a deep, boring pain, affecting the periocular bones and often referred to the face, cheek, and jaw as a consequence of involvement of the 5th cranial

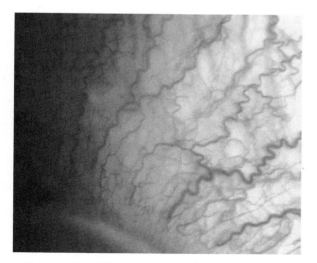

▲ **Figure 7–26.** Diffuse episcleritis. (Reproduced with permission from Watson PG, Hazleman B, Pavesio CE, Green WR, eds. *The Sclera and Systemic Disorders.* 2nd ed. London, England: Butterworth–Heinemann: 2004.)

Table 7–7. Causes of Scleritis

Autoimmune diseases
   Rheumatoid arthritis
   Wegener's granulomatosis
   Relapsing polychondritis
   Polyarteritis nodosa
   Systemic lupus erythematosus
   Ulcerative colitis
   Psoriatic arthritis
   IgA nephropathy

Granulomatous and infectious diseases
   Tuberculosis
   Syphilis
   Sarcoidosis
   Leprosy
   Herpes simplex
   Herpes zoster
   Pseudomonas infection
   Staphylococcal infection
   Streptococcal infection

Others
   Physical agents (irradiation, thermal burns)
   Chemical agents (alkali or acid burns)
   Mechanical causes (trauma, surgery)
   Lymphoma
   Rosacea
   Gout

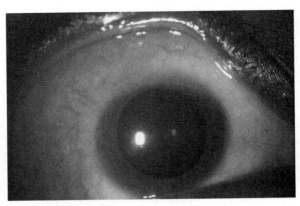

▲ **Figure 7–28.** Anterior diffuse scleritis. (Reproduced with permission from Pavesio C. Scleritis. In: Gupta A, Gupta V, Herbort CP, Khairallah M. *Uveitis Text and Imaging.* New Delhi, India: Jaypee Brothers Medical Publishers (P) Ltd: 2009.) See color insert.

Complications of anterior scleritis include increased transparency of the sclera, staphyloma formation, corneal thinning and vascularization, uveitis, and elevation of intraocular pressure. All are more common in the necrotizing forms of the disease. Visual loss may occur as a consequence of direct corneal involvement, astigmatism due to the loss of scleral support, cataract, uveitis, or glaucoma.

Posterior Scleritis, which involves the non-visible portion of the sclera, is a serious, potentially blinding condition, which tends to be under diagnosed and often treated late.

nerve. The pain typically worsens at night, often waking the patient in the early morning hours, and common analgesics typically offer little symptomatic relief. Other symptoms can include photophobia and reduction of vision.

Anterior Scleritis, which involves the visible portion of the sclera, may show different degrees of severity. A key clinical sign is deep violaceous discoloration of the globe due to dilation of the deep episcleral plexus, which can be diffuse or nodular. Diffuse (Figure 7–28) and nodular (Figure 7–29) disease are less severe in terms of response to therapy and complications and also tend to occur in younger individuals. Necrotizing disease is much more aggressive. It tends to occur in older patients and may present with typical inflammatory features, when it is known as necrotizing scleritis, or without any overt clinical features of inflammation (scleromalacia perforans) (Figure 7–30). Up to two-thirds of patients with the necrotizing scleritis have an underlying systemic disease, and either form may result in staphyloma formation (Figure 7–31). Surgically induced necrotizing scleritis (SINS) is a type of necrotizing scleritis triggered by surgical procedures, especially those involving scleral intervention or the use of anti metabolites (Figure 7–32).

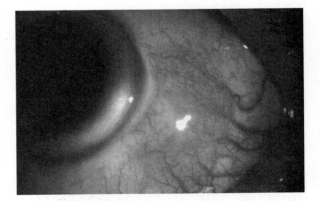

▲ **Figure 7–29.** Anterior nodular scleritis. (Reproduced with permission from Pavesio C. Scleritis. In: Gupta A, Gupta V, Herbort CP, Khairallah M. *Uveitis Text and Imaging.* New Delhi, India: Jaypee Brothers Medical Publishers (P) Ltd: 2009.)

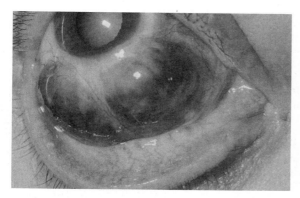

▲ **Figure 7–30.** Scleromalacia perforans in an elderly woman with rheumatoid arthritis.

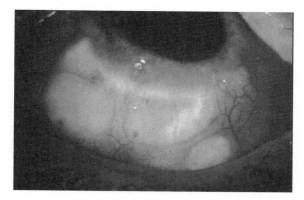

▲ **Figure 7–31.** Necrotizing scleritis resulting in staphyloma. (Reproduced with permission from Pavesio C. Scleritis. In: Gupta A, Gupta V, Herbort CP, Khairallah M. *Uveitis Text and Imaging.* New Delhi, India: Jaypee Brothers Medical Publishers (P) Ltd: 2009.)

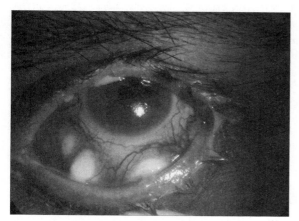

▲ **Figure 7–32.** Necrotizing scleritis following pars plana vitrectomy.

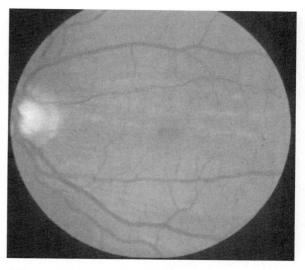

▲ **Figure 7–33.** Choroidal folds due to posterior scleritis. (Reproduced with permission from Watson PG, Hazleman B, Pavesio CE, Green WR, eds. *The Sclera and Systemic Disorders.* 2nd ed. Butterworth Heinemann: 2004.)

The manifestations include pain, but this is not always present, visual disturbance in the form of blurring or distortion, sometimes due to induced myopia, and hypertropia and/or diplopia due to involvement of extraocular muscles. There may be severe visual loss due to macular or optic nerve involvement, but it is not possible to predict in which cases such progression will occur.

Posterior scleritis can be very difficult to diagnose clinically, and small clues such as localized areas of hyperemia hidden in the fornices can be important. Possible other more obvious manifestations include proptosis, choroidal folds (Figure 7–33), fundus mass, serous retinal detachment and optic disk swelling (Figure 7–34). The diagnosis can be confirmed, or in some cases first suggested, by the detection of thickening of the posterior coats of the eye by ultrasonography or computed tomography. Posterior scleritis needs to be differentiated from other causes of choroidal thickening. The presence of fluid in sub-Tenon's space is usually quite helpful (Figure 7–35).

The most frequent causes of scleritis are listed in Table 7–7. Infectious causes of scleritis are much less common and most cases are associated with trauma or surgical procedures, especially retinal detachment surgery with scleral buckle placement, or in patients with an active systemic infection. Investigations are usually guided by the medical history.

Management decisions depend on the type of presentation and risk of complications. Anterior diffuse and nodular scleritis are treated with a systemic NSAID, and options include indomethacin, 75 mg daily, ibuprofen 600 mg daily

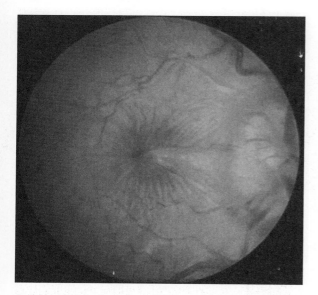

▲ Figure 7–34. Posterior scleritis with optic disk swelling and retinal folds involving the macula. (Reproduced with permission from Watson PG, Hazleman B, Pavesio CE, Green WR, eds. *The Sclera and Systemic Disorders.* 2nd ed. Butterworth Heinemann: 2004.)

or flurbiprofen 300 mg daily. In most cases pain will respond quite quickly, which is a good indication that the treatment is effective. In cases where there is no response after 2 weeks of therapy, then treatment can be increased to the use of systemic corticosteroids. Topical corticosteroids can be used

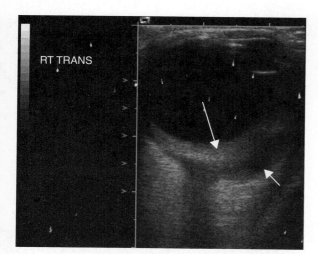

▲ Figure 7–35. B-scan ultrasonography demonstrating scleral thickening (arrow) and fluid in the posterior sub-Tenon's space (arrowhead).

mainly to improve control of symptoms, or to treat associated anterior uveitis, but they have little effect on the course of the scleral inflammation.

In cases of necrotizing disease, initial treatment should be oral corticosteroids, usually prednisolone 1 mg/kg/d. Very frequently an additional immunosuppressive agent becomes necessary. Intravenous methylprednisolone, 1 g per day for three consecutive days, is occasionally needed in very severe cases. Cyclophosphamide is a very useful agent in necrotizing disease, especially cases associated with Wegener's granulomatosis, and may induce disease remission. Other useful agents include azathioprine, mycophenolate mofetil and less frequently cyclosporine A. The treatment of posterior scleritis follows the same principles of treatment as for severe anterior scleritis.

In cases of infectious scleritis, specific antimicrobial therapy needs to be initiated as quickly as possible.

Surgical intervention should be reserved for cases of scleral or corneal perforation to preserve integrity of the globe.

OTHER AFFECTIONS OF THE SCLERA

1. SCLERAL HYALINE PLAQUES

These are common, asymptomatic, small, round, translucent gray areas, usually 2–3 mm in diameter, that occur in the interpalpebral region close to the insertion of the rectus muscles, in patients over the age of 60 years. They are not related to inflammatory events. They probably represent degeneration of scleral collagen at the site of maximal tension of the horizontal muscles.

2. NON-INFLAMMATORY THINNING OF THE SCLERA

The sclera may be thinned as a result of dysgenesis or disease. Ectasia is when the sclera alone becomes stretched, whereas involvement of both the sclera and the underlying uveal tissue is more properly termed a staphyloma.

A. Congenital Anomalies

Colobomas of the sclera are rare, but occasionally the sclera fuses incompletely during development leaving a large ectatic area inferior to the disc, invariably accompanied by uveal tract and retinal colobomas. In peripapillary ectasia, the entire area around the disk bulges outwards. Ectasia of the anterior sclera is rare.

B. Acquired Ectasia

Prolonged elevation of intraocular pressure early in infancy, as may occur with congenital glaucoma, can lead to stretching and thinning of the sclera. Buphthalmos is the term used to describe these very large eyes.

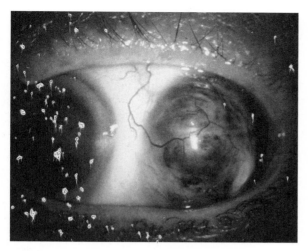

▲ **Figure 7–36.** Large temporal staphyloma following scleritis.

C. Staphyloma

This is the term used for ectatic sclera which has become attached to the underlying uvea. Staphylomas may occur following severe scleritis or uveitis (Figure 7–36), and may be anterior, equatorial or posterior. Anterior staphylomas, located anterior to the equator, are termed calary when they are over the ciliary body (Figure 7–37) and intercalary when they are between the ciliary body and the limbus. They most probably result from a combination of inflammation and high intraocular pressure. They can also develop following surgery, such as trabeculectomy. The majority of posterior staphyloma develop as a result of pathological myopia, but they can also result from congenital, infective, and inflammatory disorders.

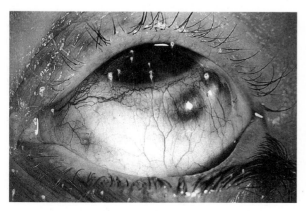

▲ **Figure 7–37.** Ciliary staphyloma. (Courtesy of P Thygeson)

3. NON-INFLAMMATORY THICKENING OF THE SCLERA

A. Nanophthalmos

This happens when the eye develops normally until the embryonic fissure has closed, but then grows very slowly in all dimensions, resulting in a very small eye and consequently high hypermetropia. With age these individuals are prone to develop acute angle closure, because the crystalline lens has a normal size and continues to grow normally.

B. Idiopathic

Abnormal thickening of the posterior coats of the eye can be demonstrated by ultrasonography in some patients without any evidence of inflammation and without resulting in visual loss.

REFERENCES

Uveitis

Albini TA, Karakousis PC, Rao NA: Interferon-gamma release assays in the diagnosis of tuberculous uveitis. Am J Ophthalmol 2008;146:486. [PMID: 18804561]

Ali A, Samson CM: Seronegative spondyloarthropathies and the eye. Curr Opin Ophthalmol 2007;18:476. [PMID: 18162999]

Ament CS, Young LH: Ocular manifestations of helminthic infections: onchocersiasis, cysticercosis, toxocariasis, and diffuse unilateral subacute neuroretinitis. Int Ophthalmol Clin 2006;46:1. [PMID: 16770150]

Atmaca-Sonmez P, Atmaca LS, Aydintug OT. Update on ocular Behcet's disease. Expert Rev Ophthalmol 2007;2:957.

Bonfioli AA, Damico FM, Curi AL, Orefice F: Intermediate uveitis. Semin Ophthalmol 2005;20:147. [PMID: 16282148]

Bonfioli AA, Orefice F: Sarcoidosis. Semin Ophthalmol 2005;20:177. [PMID: 16282152]

Castiblanco CP, Adelman RA: Sympathetic ophthalmia. Graefes Arch Clin Exp Ophthalmol 2009;247:289. [PMID: 18795315]

Chan SM, Gan KD, Weis E: Characteristics and predictors of recurrence of anterior and intermediate uveitis in a Canadian referral centre. Can J Ophthalmol 2010;45:144. [PMID: 20379299]

Chan WM, Lim TH, Pece A, Silva R, Yoshimura N: Verteporfin PDT for non-standard indications—a review of current literature. Graefes Arch Clin Exp Ophthalmol 2010;248:613. [PMID: 20162298]

Chang JH, McCluskey PJ, Wakefield D: Acute anterior uveitis and HLA-B27. Surv Ophthalmol 2005;50:364. [PMID: 15967191]

Chao JR, Khurana RN, Fawzi AA, Reddy HS, Rao NA: Syphilis: reemergence of an old adversary. Ophthalmology 2006;113:2074. [PMID: 16935333]

Cunningham ET Jr: A rationale approach to diagnosing uveitis. Review of Ophthalmology 1999;January:46.

Cunningham ET Jr: Diagnosis and management of acute anterior uveitis. American Academy of Ophthalmology, Focal Points 2002, Volume XX, Number 1 (Section 1 of 3).

Cunningham ET Jr, Baglivo E: Fuchs heterochromic iridocyclitis—syndrome, disease, or both? Am J Ophthalmol 2009;148:479. [PMID: 19782794]

Deuter CME, Kötter I, Wallace GR, et al: Behcet's disease: Ocular effects and treatment. Prog Retin Eye Res 2008;27:111. [PMID: 18035584]

Ehrlich R, Ciulla TA, Maturi R, et al: Intravitreal bevacizumab for choroidal neovascularization secondary to presumed ocular histoplasmosis syndrome. Retina 2009;29:1418. [PMID: 19898179]

Fang W, Yang P: Vogt-Koyanagi-Harada disease. Curr Eye Res 2008;33:517. [PMID: 18600484]

Lee FF, Foster CS: Pharmacotherapy of uveitis. Expert Opin Pharmacother 2010;11:1135. [PMID: 20367272]

Lustig MJ, Cunningham ET Jr: Use of immunosuppressive agents in uveitis. Curr Opin Ophthalmol 2003;14:399. [PMID: 14615647]

Galor A, Davis JL, Flynn HW Jr, et al: Symphathetic Ophthalmia: incidence of ocular complications and vision loss in the sympathizing eye. Am J Ophthalmol 2009;148:704. [PMID: 19665105]

Gaudio PA: Update on ocular syphilis. Curr Opin Ophthalmol 2006;17:562. [PMID: 17065926]

Hemmati HD, Dunn JP: Biologic therapy for uveitis. Expert Rev Ophthalmol 2010;5:225.

Hooper C, McCluskey P: Intraocular inflammation: its causes and investigations. Curr Allergy Asthma Rep 2008;8:331. [PMID: 18606087]

London NJ, Shukla D, Heiden D, et al: HIV/AIDS in the developing world. Int Ophthalmol Clin 2010;50:201. [PMID: 20375872]

Mackensen F, Billing H: Tubulointerstitial nephritis and uveitis syndrome. Curr Opin Ophthalmol 2009;20:525. [PMID: 19752730]

Matsumoto Y, Haen SP, Spaide RF: The white dot syndromes. Comp Ophthalmol Update 2007;8:179. [PMID: 17999832]

Mohamed Q, Zamir E: Update on Fuchs' uveitis syndrome. Curr Opin Ophthalmol 2005;16:356. [PMID: 16264346]

Moorthy RS: Recognizing the 'white dot syndromes'—Part 1. Review of Ophthalmology 2009;16:14340.

Moorthy RS: Recognizing the 'white dot syndromes'—Part 2. Review of Ophthalmology 2009;16:14403.

Prasad AG, Van Gelder RN: Presumed ocular histoplasmosis syndrome. Curr Opin Ophthalmol 2005;16:364. [PMID: 16264347]

Quillen DA, Davis JB, Gottlieb JL, et al: The white dot syndromes. Am J Ophthalmol 2004;137:538. [PMID: 15013878]

Rathinam SR: Ocular manifestations of leptospirosis. J Postgrad Med 2005;51:189. [PMID: 16333191]

Read RW, Holland GN, Rao NA, et al: Revised diagnostic criteria for Vogt-Koyanagi-Harada disease: report of an international committee on nomenclature. Am J Ophthalmol 2001;131:647. [PMID: 11336942]

Read RW, Rao NA, Cunningham ET Jr: Vogt-Koyanagi-Harada disease. Curr Opin Ophthalmol 2000;11:437. [PMID: 11141638]

Read RW, Zamir E, Rao NA: Neoplastic masquerade syndromes. Surv Ophthalmol 2002;47:81. [PMID: 11918892]

Rosenbaum JT, Wernick R: The utility of routine screening of patients with uveitis for systemic lupus erythematosus and tuberculosis. A Bayesian analysis. Arch Ophthalmol 1990;108:1291. [PMID: 2205185]

Rothova A, Ooijman F, Kerkhoff F, Van Der Lelij A, Lokhorst HM: Uveitis masquerade syndromes. Ophthalmology 2001;108:386. [PMID: 11158819]

Sabrosa NA, Zajdenweber M: Nematode infections of the eye: toxocariasis, onchocerciasis, diffuse unilateral subacute neuroretinitis, and cysticercosis. Ophthalmol Clin North Am 2002;15:351. [PMID: 12434484]

Smith JA, Mackensen F, Sne HN, et al: Epidemiology and course of disease in childhood uveitis. Ophthalmology 2009;116:1544. [PMID: 19651312]

Sridharan S, Biswas J: Ocular tuberculosis: an update. Expert Rev Ophthalmol 2007;2:845.

Stewart JM, Cubillan LDP, Cunningham ET Jr: Prevalence, clinical features, and causes of vision loss among patients with ocular toxocariasis. Retina 2005;25:1005. [PMID: 16340531]

Tabbara KF: Tuberculosis. Curr Opin Ophthalmol 2007;18:493. [PMID: 18163002]

Tsai T, O'Brien JM: Masquerade syndromes: malignancies mimicking inflammation in the eye. Int Ophthalmol Clin 2002;42:115. [PMID: 12189607]

Van Gelder RN, Leveque TK: Cataract surgery in the setting of uveitis. Curr Opin Ophthalmol 2009;20:42. [PMID: 19077828]

Wender JD, Eliott D, Jumper JM, Cunningham ET Jr: How to recognize ocular syphilis. Review of Ophthalmology 2008;15:14083.

Zelefsky JR, Cunningham ET Jr: Evaluation and management of elevated IOP in patients with uveitis. American Academy of Ophthalmology, Focal Points 2010, Volume XXVIII, Number 6 (Section 3 of 3).

Uveal Tumors

Aaberg TM Jr, Bergstrom CS, Hickner ZJ, Lynn MJ: Long-term results of primary transpupillary thermal therapy for the treatment of choroidal malignant melanoma. Br J Ophthalmol 2008;92:741. [PMID: 18296506]

Arevalo JF, Shields CL, Shields JA, et al: Circumscribed choroidal hemangioma: characteristic features with indocyanine green videoangiography. Ophthalmology 2000;107:344. [PMID: 10690837]

Augsburger JJ, Corrêa ZM, Schneider S, et al: Diagnostic transvitreal fine-needle aspiration biopsy of small melanocytic choroidal tumors in nevus versus melanoma category. Trans Am Ophthalmol Soc 2002;100:225. [PMID: 12545696]

Augsburger JJ, Corrêa ZM, Shaikh A: Effectiveness of treatments for metastatic uveal melanoma. Am J Ophthalmol 2009;148:119. [PMID: 19375060]

Augsburger JJ, Corrêa ZM, Trichopoulos N: An alternative hypothesis for observed mortality rates due to metastasis after treatment of choroidal melanomas of different sizes. Trans Am Ophthalmol Soc 2007;105:54. [PMID: 18427594]

Augsburger JJ, Corrêa ZM, Trichopoulos N, Shaikh A: Size overlap between benign melanocytic choroidal nevi and choroidal malignant melanomas. Invest Ophthalmol Vis Sci 2008;49:2823. [PMID: 18408179]

Augsburger JJ, Schroeder RP, Territo C, et al: Clinical parameters predictive of enlargement of melanocytic choroidal lesions. Br J Ophthalmol 1989;73:911. [PMID: 2605146]

Bartlema YM, Oosterhuis JA, Journée-De Korver JG, et al: Combined plaque radiotherapy and transpupillary thermotherapy in choroidal melanoma: 5 years' experience. Br J Ophthalmol 2003;87:1370. [PMID: 14609837]

Boixadera A, Garcia-Arumi J, Martinez-Castillo V, et al: Prospective clinical trial evaluating the efficacy of photodynamic therapy for symptomatic circumscribed choroidal hemangioma. Ophthalmology 2009;116:100. [PMID: 18973950]

Butler P, Char DH, Zarbin M, Kroll S: Natural history of indeterminate pigmented choroidal tumors. Ophthalmology 1994;101:710. [PMID: 8152767]

Ciulla TA, Bains RA, Jakobiec FA, et al: Uveal lymphoid neoplasia: a clinical-pathologic correlation and review of the early form. Surv Ophthalmol 1997;41:467. [PMID: 9220569]

Cockerham GC, Hidayat AA, Bijwaard KE, Sheng ZM: Re-evaluation of "reactive lymphoid hyperplasia of the uvea": an immunohistochemical and molecular analysis of 10 cases. Ophthalmology 2000;107:151. [PMID: 10647734]

Collaborative Ocular Melanoma Study Group: The COMS randomized trial of iodine 125 brachytherapy for choroidal melanoma: V. Twelve-year mortality rates and prognostic factors: COMS report No. 28. Arch Ophthalmol 2006;124:1684. [PMID: 17159027]

Conway RM, Chew T, Golchet P, et al: Ultrasound biomicroscopy: role in diagnosis and management in 130 consecutive patients evaluated for anterior segment tumours. Br J Ophthlamol 2005;89:950. [PMID: 16024841]

Coupland SE, Damato B: Understanding intraocular lymphomas. Clin Experiment Ophthalmol 2008;36:564. [PMID: 18954321]

Damato B, Groenewald C, McGalliard J, Wong D: Endoresection of choroidal melanoma. Br J Ophthalmol 1998;82:213. [PMID: 9602614]

Damato BE, Paul J, Foulds WS: Risk factors for residual and recurrent uveal melanoma after trans-scleral local resection. Br J Ophthalmol 1996;80:102. [PMID: 8814738]

Damato BE, Paul J, Foulds WS: Risk factors for metastatic uveal melanoma after trans-scleral local resection. Br J Ophthalmol 1996;80:109. [PMID: 8814739]

Fahmy P, Heegaard S, Jensen OA, Prause JU: Metastases in the ophthalmic region in Denmark 1969–98. A histopathological study. Acta Ophthalmol Scand 2003;81:47. [PMID: 12631019]

Fernandes BF, Krema H, Fulda E, et al: Management of iris melanomas with [125]Iodine plaque radiotherapy. Am J Ophthalmol 2010;149:70. [PMID: 19892312]

Hawkins BS, Collaborative Ocular Melanoma Study Group: The Collaborative Ocular Melanoma Study (COMS) randomized trial of pre-enucleation radiation of large choroidal melanoma: IV. Ten-year mortality findings and prognostic factors. COMS report number 24. Am J Ophthalmol 2004;138:936. [PMID: 15629284]

Höcht S, Wachtlin J, Bechrakis NE, et al: Proton or photon irradiation for hemangiomas of the choroid? A retrospective comparison. Int J Radiat Oncol Biol Phys 2006;66:345. [PMID: 16887287]

Jakobiec FA, Silbert G: Are most iris "melanomas" really nevi? A clinicopathologic study of 189 lesions. Arch Ophthamo 1981;99:2117. [PMID: 7305709]

Khadem JJ, Weiter JJ: Melanocytomas of the optic nerve and uvea. Int Ophthalmol Clin 1997;37:149.

Madreperla SA, Hungerford JL, Plowman PN, et al: Choroidal hemangiomas: visual and anatomic results of treatment by photocoagulation or radiation therapy. Ophthalmology 1997;104:1773. [PMID: 9373106]

Medlock RD, Augsburger JJ, Wilkinson CP, et al: Enlargement of circumscribed choroidal hemangiomas. Retina 1991;11:385. [PMID: 1813953]

Shields CL, Furata M, Berman EL, et al: Choroidal nevus transformation into melanoma: analysis of 2514 consecutive cases. Arch Ophthalmol 2009;127:981. [PMID: 19667334]

Shields CL, Furuta M, Mashayekhi A, et al: Clinical spectrum of choroidal nevi based on age at presentation in 3422 consecutive eyes. Ophthalmology 2008;115:546. [PMID: 18067966]

Shields CL, Honavar SG, Shields JA, et al: Circumscribed choroidal hemangioma: clinical manifestations and factors predictive of visual outcome in 200 consecutive cases. Ophthalmology 2001;108:2237. [PMID: 11733265]

Shields CL, Shields JA, Gross NE, et al: Survey of 520 eyes with uveal metastases. Ophthalmology 1997;104:1265. [PMID: 9261313]

Shields CL, Sun H, Demirci H, Shields JA: Factors predictive of tumor growth, tumor decalcification, choroidal neovascularization, and visual outcome in 74 eyes with choroidal osteoma. Arch Ophthalmol 2005;123:1658. [PMID: 16344436]

Shields JA, Shields CL, Kiratli H, de Potter P: Metastatic tumors to the iris in 40 patients. Am J Ophthalmol 1995;119:422. [PMID: 7709967]

Sclera

Bhat PV, Jakobiec FA, Kurbanyan K, Zhao T, Foster CS: Chronic herpes simplex scleritis: characterization of 9 cases of an underrecognized clinical entity. Am J Ophthalmol 2009;148:779. [PMID: 19674728]

Daniel E, Thorne JE, Newcomb CW, et al: Mycophenolate mofetil for ocular inflammation. Am J Ophthalmol 2010;149:423. [PMID: 20042178]

Doctor P, Sultan A, Syed S. et al: Infliximab for the treatment of refractory scleritis. Br J Ophthalmol 2010;94:579. [PMID: 19955205]

Erkanli L, Akova YA, Guney-Tefekli E, Tugal-Tutkun I: Clinical features, prognosis, and treatment results of patients with scleritis from 2 tertiary eye care centers in Turkey. Cornea 2010;29:26. [PMID: 19907295]

Gangaputra S, Newcomb CW, Liesegang TL et al: Methotrexate for ocular inflammatory diseases. Ophthalmology 2009;116:2188. [PMID: 19748676]

Kacmaz RO, Kempen JH, Newcomb C, et al: Cyclosporine for ocular inflammatory diseases. Ophthalmology 2010;117:576. [PMID: 20031223]

Kim SJ, Flach AJ, Jampol LM: Nonsteroidal anti-inflammatory drugs in ophthalmology. Surv Ophthalmol 2010;55:104. [PMID: 20159228]

Michalova K, Lim L: Biologic agents in the management of inflammatory eye diseases. Curr Allergy Astham Rep 2008;8:339. [PMID: 18606088]

Morley AM, Paesio C: Surgically induced necrotizing scleritis following three-port pars plana vitrectomy without sclera buckling: a series of three cases. Eye 2008;22:162. [PMID: 17304259]

Pasadhika S, Kempen JH, Newcomb CW, et al: Azathioprine for ocular inflammatory diseases. Am J Ophthalmol 2009;148:500. [PMID: 19570522]

Pavesio CE, Meier FM: Systemic disorders associated with episcleritis and scleritis. Curr Opin Ophthalmol 2001;12:471. [PMID: 11734688]

Pujari SS, Kempen JH, Newcomb CW, et al: Cyclophosphamide for ocular inflammatory diseases. Ophthalmology 2010;117:356. [PMID: 19969366]

Raiji VR, Palestine AG, Parver DL: Scleritis and systemic disease association in a community-based referral practice. Am J Ophthalmol 2009;148:946. [PMMID: 19837380]

Sen HN, Sangrave A, Hammel K, Levy-Clarke G, Nussennblatt RB: Infliximab for the treatment of active scleritis. Can J Ophthalmol 2009;44:e9. [PMID: 19506593]

Smith JR, Mackensen F, Rosenbaum JT: Therapy insight: scleritis and its relationship to systemic autoimmune disease. Nat Clin Pract Rheumatol 2007;3:219. [PMID: 17396107]

Watson PG, Hazleman BL, Pavesio CE, et al. The Sclera and Systemic Disorders. 2nd edn, London, Butterworth & Heinemann: 2004.

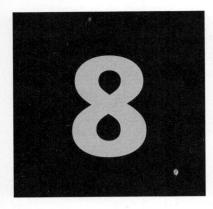

Lens

Richard A. Harper, MD, and John P. Shock, MD

The crystalline lens is a remarkable structure that contributes to focusing of images on the retina. It is positioned just posterior to the iris and is supported by **zonular fibers** arising from the ciliary body and inserting onto the equatorial region of the lens capsule (see Figure 1–12). The lens capsule is a basement membrane that surrounds the lens substance. Epithelial cells near the lens equator divide throughout life and continually differentiate into new lens fibers, so that older lens fibers are compressed into a central **nucleus;** younger, less-compact fibers around the nucleus make up the **cortex.** Because the lens is avascular and has no innervation, it must derive nutrients from the aqueous humor. Lens metabolism is primarily anaerobic owing to the low level of oxygen dissolved in the aqueous.

The eye is able to adjust its focus from distance to near objects because of the ability of the lens to change shape, a phenomenon known as **accommodation.** The inherent elasticity of the lens allows it to become more or less spherical depending on the amount of tension exerted by the zonular fibers on the lens capsule. Zonular tension is controlled by the action of the ciliary muscle, which, when contracted, relaxes zonular tension. The lens then assumes a more spherical shape, resulting in increased dioptric power to bring nearer objects into focus. Ciliary muscle relaxation reverses this sequence of events, allowing the lens to flatten and thus bringing more distant objects into view. As the lens ages, its accommodative power is gradually reduced as lens elasticity decreases.

PHYSIOLOGY OF SYMPTOMS

Symptoms associated with lens disorders are primarily visual. **Presbyopic symptoms** are due to decreased accommodative ability with age and result in diminished ability to perform near tasks. Loss of lens transparency (cataract) results in blurred vision (without pain) for both near and distance. If the lens is partially dislocated (subluxation) due to congenital, developmental, or acquired causes, visual blur can be due to a change in refractive error. Complete dislocation

of the lens from the visual axis results in an **aphakic refractive state;** severely blurred vision results from loss of over one-third of the eye's refractive power, the majority still being provided by the curvature of the cornea.

The lens is best examined with the pupil dilated. A magnified view of the lens can be obtained with a slitlamp or by using the direct ophthalmoscope with a high plus (+10) setting.

CATARACT

A cataract is any opacity in the lens. Aging is the most common cause, but many other factors can be involved, including trauma, toxins, systemic disease (such as diabetes), smoking, and heredity. Age-related cataract is a common cause of visual impairment. Cross-sectional studies place the prevalence of cataracts at 50% in individuals aged 65–74; the prevalence increases to about 70% for those over 75.

The pathogenesis of cataracts is not completely understood. However, cataractous lenses are characterized by protein aggregates that scatter light rays and reduce transparency. Other protein alterations result in yellow or brown discoloration. Additional findings may include vesicles between lens fibers or migration and aberrant enlargement of epithelial cells. Factors thought to contribute to cataract formation include oxidative damage (from free radical reactions), ultraviolet light damage, and malnutrition. No medical treatment has been found that will retard or reverse the underlying chemical changes that occur in cataract formation. However, some recent evidence suggests a protective effect from dietary carotenoids (lutein), but studies evaluating the protective effect of multivitamins have yielded conflicting results.

A **mature cataract** is one in which all of the lens substance is opaque; the **immature cataract** has some transparent regions. . If the lens takes up water, it may become **intumescent.** In the **hypermature cataract,** cortical proteins have become liquid. This liquid may escape through the intact capsule, leaving a shrunken lens with a wrinkled capsule.

A hypermature cataract in which the lens nucleus floats freely in the capsular bag is called a **morgagnian cataract** (Figure 8–1).

Most cataracts are not visible to the casual observer until they become dense enough to cause severe vision loss. The ocular fundus becomes increasingly more difficult to visualize as the lens opacity becomes denser, until the fundus reflection is completely absent. At this stage, the cataract is usually mature, and the pupil may be white.

The clinical degree of cataract formation, assuming that no other eye disease is present, is judged primarily by the patient's symptoms and the visual acuity. Generally speaking, the decrease in visual acuity is directly proportionate to the density of the cataract. However, some individuals who have clinically significant cataracts when examined with the ophthalmoscope or slitlamp see well enough to carry on with normal activities. Others have a decrease in visual acuity out of proportion to the degree of lens opacification. This is due to distortion of the image by the partially opaque lens. The Cataract Management Guideline Panel recommends reliance on clinical judgment combined with visual acuity as the best guide to the appropriateness of surgery but recognizes the need for flexibility, with due regard to a patient's particular functional and visual needs, the environment, and other risks, all of which may vary widely.

AGE-RELATED CATARACT (FIGURES 8–1 AND 8–2)

The normal condensation process in the lens nucleus results in **nuclear sclerosis** after middle age. The earliest symptom may be improved near vision without glasses ("second sight"). This occurs from an increase in the refractive power of the central lens, creating a myopic (nearsighted) shift in refraction. Other symptoms may include poor hue discrimination or monocular diplopia. Most nuclear cataracts are bilateral but may be asymmetric.

Cortical cataracts are opacities in the lens cortex. Changes in the hydration of lens fibers create clefts in a radial pattern around the equatorial region. They also tend to be bilateral, but they are often asymmetric. Visual function is variably affected, depending on how near the opacities are to the visual axis.

Posterior subcapsular cataracts are located in the cortex adjacent to the posterior capsule. They tend to cause visual symptoms earlier in their development owing to involvement of the visual axis. Common symptoms include glare and reduced vision under bright lighting conditions. This lens opacity can also result from trauma, corticosteroid use (topical or systemic), inflammation, or exposure to ionizing radiation.

Age-related cataract is usually slowly progressive over years, and death may occur before surgery becomes necessary. If surgery is indicated, lens extraction improves visual acuity in over 90% of cases. The remainder of patients either has preexisting retinal damage or, in rare cases, develop serious postsurgical complications that prevent significant visual improvement, for example, glaucoma, retinal detachment, intraocular hemorrhage, or infection.

CHILDHOOD CATARACT (FIGURES 8–3 AND 8–4)

Childhood cataracts are divided into two groups: **congenital (infantile) cataracts,** which are present at birth or appear shortly thereafter, and **acquired cataracts,** which occur later and are usually related to a specific cause. Either type may be unilateral or bilateral.

About one-third of childhood cataracts are hereditary, while another third are secondary to metabolic or infectious diseases or associated with a variety of syndromes. The final one-third results from undetermined causes. Acquired cataracts arise most commonly from trauma, either blunt or penetrating. Other causes include uveitis, acquired ocular infections, diabetes, and drugs.

▶ Clinical Findings

A. Congenital Cataract

Congenital lens opacities are common and often visually insignificant (see also Chapter 17). A partial opacification or one out of the visual axis—or not dense enough to interfere significantly with light transmission—requires no treatment other than observation for progression. Dense central congenital cataracts require surgery.

Congenital cataracts that cause significant visual loss must be detected early, preferably in the newborn nursery by the pediatrician or family physician. Large, dense white cataracts may present as leukocoria (white pupil), noticeable by the parents, but many dense cataracts cannot be seen by the parents. Unilateral infantile cataracts that are dense, central, and larger than 2 mm in diameter will cause permanent deprivation amblyopia if not treated within the first 2 months of life and thus require surgical management on an urgent basis. Even then there must be careful attention to avoidance of amblyopia (see also Chapter 17) related to postoperative anisometropia. Symmetric (equally dense) bilateral cataracts may require less-urgent management, although bilateral deprivation amblyopia can result from unwarranted delay. When surgery is undertaken, there must be as short an interval as is reasonably possible between surgeries on the two eyes.

B. Acquired Cataract

Acquired cataracts often do not require the same urgent care (aimed at preventing amblyopia) as infantile cataracts because the children are usually older and the visual system more mature. Surgical assessment is based on the location, size, and density of the cataract, but a period of observation along with subjective visual acuity testing can be part of the decision-making process. Because unilateral cataract in children

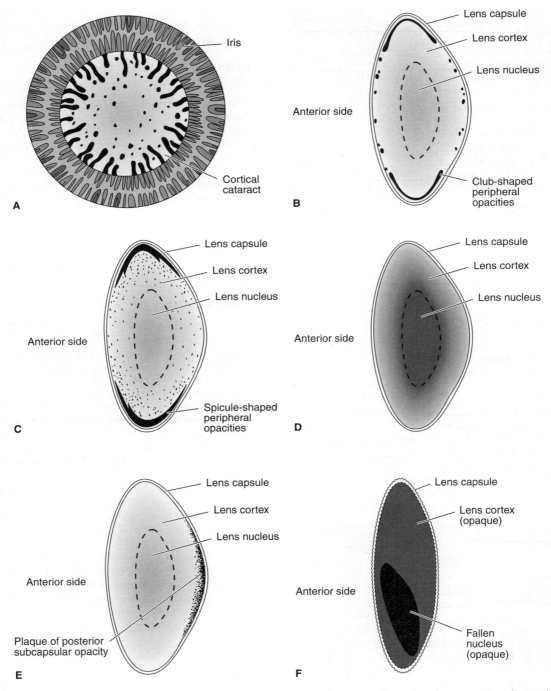

▲ **Figure 8–1.** Age-related cataract. **A** and **B:** "Coronary" type cortical cataract (frontal and cross-sectional views): club-shaped peripheral opacities with clear central lens; slowly progressive. **C:** "Cuneiform" type cortical cataract: peripheral spicules and central clear lens; slowly progressive. **D:** Nuclear sclerotic cataract: diffuse opacity principally affecting nucleus; slowly progressive. **E:** Posterior subcapsular cataract: plaque of granular opacity on posterior capsule; may be rapidly progressive. **F:** "Morgagnian" type (hypermature lens): the entire lens is opaque, and the lens nucleus has fallen inferiorly.

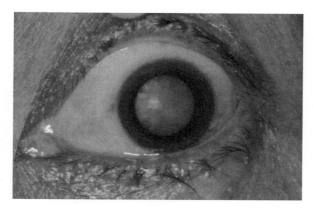

▲ **Figure 8–2.** Mature age-related cataract viewed through a dilated pupil.

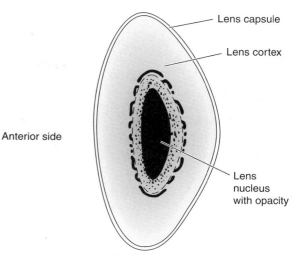

▲ **Figure 8–4.** Congenital cataract, zonular type. One zone of lens involved. The cortex is relatively clear.

will not produce any symptoms or signs parents would routinely notice, screening programs are important for case finding.

TRAUMATIC CATARACT

Traumatic cataract (Figures 8–5 to 8–7) is most commonly due to a foreign body injury to the lens or blunt trauma to the eyeball. Air rifle pellets and fireworks are a frequent cause; less-frequent causes include arrows, rocks, contusions, overexposure to heat ("glassblower's cataract"), and ionizing radiation. Most traumatic cataracts are preventable. In industry, the best safety measure is a good pair of safety goggles.

The lens becomes white soon after the entry of a foreign body, since interruption of the lens capsule allows aqueous and sometimes vitreous to penetrate into the lens structure. The patient is often an industrial worker who gives a history of striking metal upon metal. A minute fragment of a steel

hammer, for example, may pass through the cornea and lens at a tremendous rate of speed and lodge in the vitreous or retina.

CATARACT SECONDARY TO INTRAOCULAR DISEASE ("COMPLICATED CATARACT")

Cataract may develop as a direct effect of intraocular disease upon the physiology of the lens (eg, severe recurrent uveitis). The cataract usually begins in the posterior subcapsular area

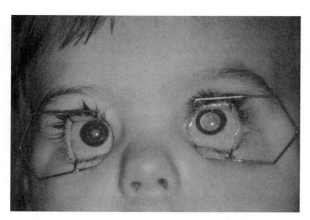

▲ **Figure 8–3.** Congenital cataract (right eye) with dilated pupils. See color insert.

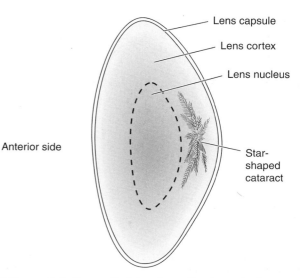

▲ **Figure 8–5.** Traumatic "star-shaped" cataract in the posterior lens. This is usually due to ocular contusion and is only detectable through a well-dilated pupil.

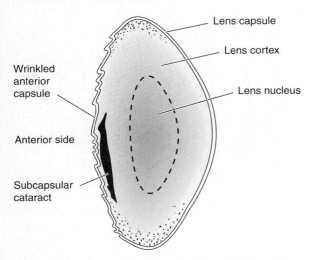

▲ **Figure 8–6.** Traumatic cataract with wrinkled anterior capsule.

and eventually involves the entire lens structure. Intraocular diseases commonly associated with the development of cataracts are chronic or recurrent uveitis, glaucoma, retinitis pigmentosa, and retinal detachment. These cataracts are usually unilateral. The visual prognosis is not as good as in ordinary age-related cataract.

CATARACT ASSOCIATED WITH SYSTEMIC DISEASE

Bilateral cataracts occur in many systemic disorders including diabetes mellitus (Figure 8–8), hypocalcemia (of any

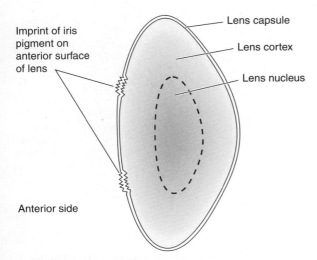

▲ **Figure 8–7.** Imprint of iris pigment on anterior surface of lens.

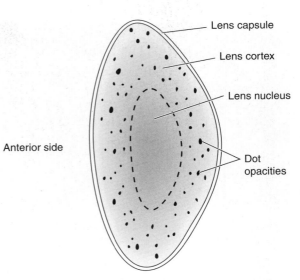

▲ **Figure 8–8.** Punctate dot cataract. This type of cataract is sometimes seen as an ocular complication of diabetes mellitus. It may also be congenital.

cause), myotonic dystrophy, atopic dermatitis, galactosemia, and Down, Lowe (oculo-cerebro-renal), and Werner syndromes (see Chapters 15 and 18).

DRUG-INDUCED CATARACT

Corticosteroids administered over a long period of time, either systemically or in drop form, can cause lens opacities. Other drugs associated with cataract include phenothiazines, amiodarone, and strong miotic drops such as phospholine iodide.

CATARACT SURGERY

Cataract surgery has undergone dramatic change during the past 30 years with the introduction of the operating microscope and microsurgical instruments, the development of intraocular lenses, and alterations in techniques for local anesthesia. Further refinements continue to occur, with automated instrumentation and modifications of intraocular lenses allowing surgery through small incisions.

The generally preferred method of cataract surgery in **adults and older children** preserves the posterior portion of the lens capsule and thus is known as **extracapsular cataract extraction.** An incision is made at the limbus or in the peripheral cornea, either superiorly or temporally. An opening is formed in the anterior capsule (anterior capsulorhexis), and the nucleus and cortex of the lens are removed. An intraocular lens can then be placed in the empty "capsular bag," supported by the intact posterior capsule.

The technique of **phacoemulsification** is now the most common form of extracapsular cataract extraction in developed countries. It utilizes a handheld ultrasonic vibrator to disintegrate the hard nucleus such that the nuclear material and cortex can be aspirated through a small incision of approximately 3 mm. This same incision size is then adequate for insertion of foldable intraocular lenses. If a rigid intraocular lens is used, the wound needs to be extended to approximately 5 mm. In developing countries, particularly rural areas, the instruments for phacoemulsification are not available. **Manual sutureless small incision cataract surgery** (MSICS) is based on the traditional nuclear expression form of extracapsular cataract extraction, in which the nucleus is removed intact, but utilizing a small incision. The cortex is removed by manual aspiration. MSICS may be indicated for dense cataracts unsuitable for phacoemulsification.

The advantages of small-incision surgery, either phacoemulsification or MSICS, are: more controlled operating conditions, avoidance of suturing, rapid wound healing with lesser degrees of corneal distortion, and reduced postoperative intraocular inflammation—all contributing to more rapid visual rehabilitation. The main intraoperative complication of extracapsular surgery is posterior capsular tear, for which the main predisposing factors include previous trauma, dense cataract, unstable lens, and small pupil, possibly leading to displacement of nuclear material into the vitreous ("dropped nucleus") that generally necessitates complex vitreoretinal surgery. Postoperatively there may be secondary opacification of the posterior capsule that requires discission using the neodymium:YAG laser (see Posterior Capsule Opacification later in the chapter).

Pars plana lensectomy or phacofragmentation, in which the lens is removed via the pars plana in conjunction with posterior vitrectomy using automated lens and vitreous cutters, may be performed to facilitate vitreo-retinal surgery, although conventional phacoemulsification surgery is now more commonly undertaken under such circumstances, or to remove a completely dislocated lens or a partially dislocated lens that is not amenable to phacoemulsification (see later in the chapter). Whether phacofragmentation is required depends upon the severity of cataract.

Intracapsular cataract extraction, consisting of removal of the entire lens together with its capsule, is rarely performed today. The incidence of postoperative retinal detachment and cystoid macular edema is significantly higher than after extracapsular surgery, but intracapsular surgery is still a useful procedure when facilities for extracapsular surgery are not available and occasionally for treatment of a dislocated lens.

▶ Intraocular Lenses

There are many styles of intraocular lenses, but most designs consist of a central biconvex optic and two legs (or **haptics**) to maintain the optic in position. The optimal intraocular lens position is within the capsular bag following an extracapsular procedure. This is associated with the lowest incidence of postoperative complications, such as pseudophakic bullous keratopathy, glaucoma, iris damage, hyphema, and lens decentration. The newest posterior chamber lenses are made of flexible materials such as silicone and acrylic polymers. This flexibility allows the lens implant to be folded, thus decreasing the required incision size. Lens designs that incorporate **multifocal optics** or partially restore accommodation, have also been produced. The goal of these designs is to provide the patient with good vision for both near and distance without glasses, which current monofocal designs are less likely to do.

After intracapsular surgery—or if there is inadvertent damage to the posterior capsule during extracapsular surgery—intraocular lenses can be placed in the anterior chamber or sometimes fixated in the ciliary sulcus.

Methods of calculating the correct dioptric power of an intraocular lens are discussed in Chapter 21. If an intraocular lens cannot be safely placed or is contraindicated, postoperative refractive correction generally requires a contact lens or aphakic spectacles.

▶ Postoperative Care

If a small-incision technique is used, the postoperative recovery period is usually shortened. The patient is usually ambulatory on the day of surgery but is advised to move cautiously and avoid straining or heavy lifting for about a month. The eye may be patched on the day of surgery. Protection at night by a metal shield is often suggested for several days after surgery. Temporary glasses can be used a few days after surgery, but in most cases the patient sees well enough through the intraocular lens to wait for permanent glasses (usually provided 4–8 weeks after surgery).

▶ Complications of Adult Cataract Surgery

Cataract surgery in adults has a very low rate (2%–5%) of complications that result in permanent impairment of vision. The rarest, but also most serious complications include intraocular infection (endophthalmitis, 0.1%) and intraocular hemorrhage (less than 0.5%), either of which can result in severe visual loss. Suspicion of endophthalmitis requires vitreous tap for microscopy and culture, and intravitreal injection of antibiotics (see Table 22–1). Vitrectomy is sometimes indicated (see Chapter 9). Other complications include retinal detachment, cystoid macular edema, glaucoma, corneal edema, and ptosis. The most common complication is posterior capsule opacification but this is amenable to treatment.

▶ Posterior Capsule Opacification

In the past, up to 50% of eyes developed opacification of the posterior capsule ("after-cataract") (Figure 8–9) after uncomplicated adult extracapsular cataract extraction. Improved surgical techniques and new intraocular lens designs, particularly sharp posterior edges on the optics, have significantly reduced the incidence. About 10% of eyes require

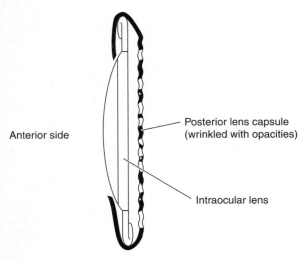

▲ Figure 8–9. Posterior capsule opacification ("after-cataract").

Anterior side

Posterior lens capsule (wrinkled with opacities)

Intraocular lens

treatment for posterior capsule opacification following uncomplicated phacoemulsification surgery but the recorded incidence depends upon duration of follow-up.

Persistent subcapsular lens epithelium favors regeneration of lens fibers, giving the posterior capsule a "fish egg" appearance (Elschnig's pearls). The proliferating epithelium may produce multiple layers, leading to frank opacification. These cells may also undergo myofibroblastic differentiation. Their contraction produces numerous tiny wrinkles in the posterior capsule, resulting in visual distortion. All of these factors may lead to reduced visual acuity.

The neodymium:YAG laser provides a noninvasive method for discission of the posterior capsule (see Chapter 23). Pulses of laser energy cause small "explosions" in target tissue, creating an opening in the posterior capsule in the pupillary axis. Complications of this technique include a transient rise in intraocular pressure, damage to the intraocular lens, and rupture of the anterior hyaloid face with forward displacement of vitreous into the anterior chamber, potentially leading to rhegmatogenous retinal detachment or cystoid macular edema. The rise in intraocular pressure is usually detectable within 3 hours after treatment and resolves within a few days with treatment. Rarely the pressure does not return to normal for several weeks. Small pits or cracks may occur on the intraocular lens but usually have no effect on visual acuity. No significant damage seems to be done to corneal endothelium with the neodymium:YAG laser.

▶ Childhood Cataract Surgery

Cataract surgery in young children is hindered by more difficult anterior capsulorhexis, as well as the need to make an opening in the posterior capsule (posterior capsulorhexis)

and to remove part of the vitreous (anterior vitrectomy) to reduce the incidence of posterior capsule opacification, which is much higher than after adult cataract surgery. The cataracts are less dense than in adults and can usually be removed by an irrigation–aspiration technique, without the need for phacoemulsification.

Optical correction can consist of spectacles in older bilaterally aphakic children, but most childhood cataract operations are followed by contact lens correction, with adjustment of power as the refractive status of the eye changes with growth. Intraocular lenses are being used. They avoid the difficulties associated with contact lens wear, but there are difficulties calculating the appropriate power.

▶ Prognosis

The visual prognosis for childhood cataract patients requiring surgery is not as good as that for patients with age-related cataract. The associated amblyopia and occasional anomalies of the optic nerve or retina limit the degree of useful vision that can be achieved in this group of patients. The prognosis for improvement of visual acuity is worst following surgery for unilateral congenital cataracts and best for incomplete bilateral congenital cataracts that are slowly progressive. Glaucoma is a common long-term complication.

DISLOCATED LENS (ECTOPIA LENTIS)

Partial or complete lens dislocation (subluxation) (Figure 8–10) may be hereditary or may result from trauma.

▶ Hereditary Lens Dislocation

Hereditary lens dislocation is usually bilateral and may be an isolated familial anomaly or due to inherited connective tissue disorder such as homocystinuria, Marfan's syndrome or Weill-Marcehsani syndrome (Chapter 15). The vision is blurred, particularly if the lens is dislocated out of the line of vision. If dislocation is partial, the edge of the lens and the zonular fibers holding it in place can be seen in the pupil. If the lens is completely dislocated into the vitreous, it can be seen with the ophthalmoscope.

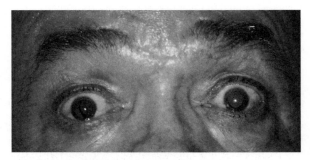

▲ Figure 8–10. Partially dislocated (subluxed) lens. (right eye) with dilated pupils. See color insert.

A partially dislocated lens is often complicated by cataract formation. If that is the case, the cataract may have to be removed, but this procedure should be delayed as long as possible because there is a significant risk of vitreous loss, predisposing to retinal detachment. If the lens is free in the vitreous, it may lead in later life to the development of glaucoma of a type that responds poorly to treatment. If dislocation is partial and the lens is clear, the visual prognosis is good.

▶ Traumatic Lens Dislocation

Partial or complete traumatic lens dislocation may occur following a contusion injury such as a blow to the eye with a fist. If the dislocation is partial, there may be no symptoms; but if the lens is floating in the vitreous, the patient has blurred vision and usually a red eye. Iridodonesis, a quivering of the iris when the patient moves the eye, is a common sign of lens dislocation and is due to the lack of lens support. This is present both in partially and in completely dislocated lenses but is more marked in the latter.

Uveitis and glaucoma are common complications of dislocated lens, particularly if dislocation is complete. If there are no complications, dislocated lenses are best if left untreated. If uveitis or uncontrollable glaucoma occurs, lens extraction must be done despite the poor results possible from this operation. For completely dislocated lenses, the technique of choice is pars plana lensectomy or phacofragmentation, depending upon the density of cataract. Some partially dislocated (subluxed) lenses are amenable to phacoemulsification with various adaptations, such as capsular tension rings or support hooks.

REFERENCES

Age-Related Eye Disease Study Research Group: Risk factors associated with age-related nuclear and cortical cataract: a case control study in the Age-Related Eye Disease Study, AREDS report no. 5. Ophthalmology 2001;108:1400. [PMID: 114700690]

Alio JL et al: Crystalline lens optical dysfunction through aging. Ophthalmology 2005;112:2022. [PMID: 16183126]

Ang GS, Wheelan S, Green FD: Manual small incision cataract surgery in a United Kingdom university teaching hospital setting. Int Ophthalmol 2010;30:23. [PMID: 19129974]

Aravind S et al: Cataract surgery and intraocular lens manufacturing in India. Curr Opin Ophthalmol 2008;19:60. [PMID: 18090900]

Artzén D et al: Capsule complication during cataract surgery: case-control study of preoperative and intraoperative risk factors: Swedish Capsule Rupture Study Group report 2. J Cataract Refract Surg 2009;35:1688. [PMID: 19781460]

Ashwin PT, Shah S, Wolffsohn JS: Advances in cataract surgery. Clin Exp Optom 2009;92:333. [PMID: 19570151]

Awasthi N, Guo S, Wagner BJ: Posterior capsular opacification: a problem reduced but not yet eradicated. Arch Ophthalmol 2009;127:555. [PMID: 19365040]

Blecher MH, Kirk MR: Surgical strategies for the management of zonular compromise. Curr Opin Ophthalmol 2008;19:31. [PMID: 18090895]

Buznego C, Trattler WB: Presbyopia-correcting intraocular lenses. Curr Opin Ophthalmol 2009;20:13. [PMID: 19077824]

Cataract Management Guideline Panel: Cataract in adults: management of functional impairment. Clinical Practice Guideline, Number 4. Rockville, MD. US Department of Health and Human Services, Public Health Service, Agency for Health Care Policy and Research. AHCPR Pub. No. 93-0542. Cataract in the Adult Eye. Preferred Practice Pattern. San Francisco: American Academy of Ophthalmology; 2001.

Congdon N et al: Causes and prevalence of visual impairment among adults in the United States. Arch Ophthalmol 2004;122:477. [PMID: 15078664]

Dureau P: Pathophysiology of zonular diseases. Curr Opin Ophthalmol 2008;19:27. [PMID: 18090894]

Fernandez MM, Afshari NA: Nutrition and the prevention of cataracts. Curr Opin Ophthalmol 2008;19:66. [PMID: 18090901]

Findl O et al: Interventions for preventing posterior capsule opacification. Cochrane Database Syst Rev 2010 Feb 17;2:CD003738. [PMID: 20166069]

Gogate PM: Small incision cataract surgery: complications and mini-review. Indian J Ophthalmol 2009;57:45, [PMID: 19075410]

Ho LY et al: Clinical predictors and outcomes of pars plana vitrectomy for retained lens material after cataract extraction. Am J Ophthalmol 2009;147:587. [PMID: 19195636]

Infant Aphakia Treatment Study Group: The infant aphakia treatment study: design and clinical measures at enrolment. Arch Ophthalmol 2010;128:21. [PMID: 20065212]

Jakobsson G et al: Capsule complication during cataract surgery: retinal detachment after cataract surgery with capsule complication: Swedish Capsule Rupture Study Group report 4. J Cataract Refract Surg 2009;35:1699. [PMID: 19781462]

Johansson B et al: Capsule complication during cataract surgery: long-term outcomes: Swedish Capsule Rupture Study Group report 3. J Cataract Refract Surg 2009;35:1694. [PMID: 19781461]

Kim SY et al: Long-term results of lensectomy in children with ectopia lentis. J Pediatr Ophthalmol Strabismus 2008;45:13. [PMID: 18286957]

Knudtson MD et al: Age-related eye disease, quality of life and functional activity. Arch Ophthalmol 2005;123:807. [PMID: 15955982]

Lin AA, Buckley EG: Update on pediatric cataract surgery and intraocular lens implantation. Curr Opin Ophthalmol 2010;21:55. [PMID: 19855277]

Lloyd IC, Ashworth J, Biswas S, Abadi RV: Advances in the management of congenital and infantile cataract. Eye 2007;21:1301. [PMID: 17914433]

Lu Y et al: Visual results and complications of primary intraocular lens implantation in infants aged 6 to 12 months. Graefes Arch Clin Exp Ophthalmol 2010 Feb 17. [Epub ahead of print] [PMID: 20162296]

Lundström M et al: Endopohthalmitis after cataract surgery: a nationwide prospective study evaluating incidence in relation to incision type and location. Ophthalmology 2007;114:866. [PMID: 17324467]

Malik A et al: Local anesthesia for cataract surgery. J Cataract Refract Surg 2010;36:133. [PMID: 20117717]

Narendran N et al: The Cataract National Database electronic multicentre audit of 55,567 operations: risk stratification for posterior capsule rupture and vitreous loss. Eye 2009;23:31. [PMID: 18327164]

Nordlund ML et al: Techniques for managing common complications of cataract surgery. Curr Opin Ophthalmol 2003;14:7. [PMID: 12544804]

Pepose JS: Maximizing satisfaction with prebyopia-correcting intraocular lenses: the missing links. Am J Ophthalmol 2008;146:641. [PMID: 18789794]

Richter GM et al. Prevalence of visually significant cataract and factors associated with unmet need for cataract surgery: Los Angeles Latino Eye Study. Ophthalmology 2009;116:2327. [PMID: 19815276]

Strenk SA, Strenk LM, Guo S: Magnetic resonance imaging of the anterioposterior position and thickness of the aging, accommodating, phakic, and pseudophakic ciliary muscle. J Cataract Refract Surg 2010;36:235. [PMID: 20152603]

Tabin G, Chen M, Espandar L: Cataract surgery for the developing world. Curr Opin Ophthalmol 2008;19:55. [PMID: 18090899]

von Lany H et al: Displacement of nuclear fragments into the vitreous complicating phacoemulsification surgery in the UK: clinical features, outcomes and management. Br J Ophthalmol 2008;92:493. [PMID: 17962391]

Vrensen GF. Early cortical opacities: a short overview. Acta Ophthalmol 2009;87:602. [PMID: 19719805]

Zetterström C, Kugelberg M: Paediatric cataract surgery. Acta Ophthalmol Scand 2007;85:698. [PMID: 17944624]

Vitreous

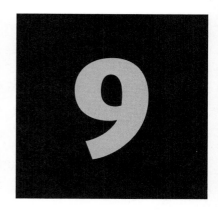

Steve Charles, MD

INTRODUCTION

The last three decades of the twentieth century saw an explosion of interest in the vitreous because of the development of vitreoretinal surgery. Prior to this period, large numbers of patients were blinded by inoperable vitreoretinal diseases. One goal of this chapter is to help the medical student, intern, resident, general ophthalmologist and optometrist become aware of the indications for vitreoretinal surgery, many of which are time sensitive. Many vitreoretinal conditions have implications for the family medical practitioner, internist, and emergency physician.

VITREOUS ANATOMY AND ITS RELEVANCE TO PATHOLOGY

The vitreous fills the space between the lens and the retina and consists of a three-dimensional collagen fiber matrix and a hyaluronan gel (Figure 9–1). (The older term, "vitreous humor" is less commonly used today.) The outer surface of the vitreous, known as the cortex, is in contact with the lens (anterior vitreous cortex) and adherent in varying degrees to the surface of the retina (posterior vitreous cortex) (Figure 9–2).

Aging, hemorrhage, inflammation, trauma, myopia, and other processes often cause hypocellular contraction of the vitreous collagen matrix. The posterior vitreous cortex then separates from areas of low adherence to the retina and may produce traction on areas of greater adherence. The vitreous base extends from the equator anteriorly and is a zone of great adherence. The vitreous virtually never detaches from the vitreous base. The vitreous is also adherent to the optic nerve and, to a lesser extent, the macula and retinal vessels. Adherence to the macular region is a significant factor in the pathogenesis of epimacular membrane, macular hole, and vitreomacular traction syndrome.

Previously it was taught that the vitreous developed cavities from a process known as syneresis, ultimately resulting in "collapse" of the vitreous. It is now believed that collagen cross-linking and selective loss of retinal adherence rather than cavity formation are the primary events. Even though the vitreous may migrate inferiorly when separated from the retina, this process causes less force at the zones of vitreoretinal adherence than the traction caused by saccadic eye motion. Saccadically induced, dynamic forces play a significant role in the development of retinal breaks (tears), damage to the retinal surface, and bleeding from torn vessels (Figure 9–3). Further contraction of the vitreous caused by invasion of retinal pigment epithelial, glial, or inflammatory cells may result in sufficient static traction to detach the retina without retinal tears.

Prior to vitreoretinal surgery, vitreous "bands" were thought to cause traction on the retina, and largely unsuccessful attempts were made to cut them with scissors. The visualization provided by vitreoretinal endoillumination systems has contributed to our knowledge of anatomy and demonstrated that these bands are contiguous with the transparent posterior vitreous cortex that is also responsible for substantial traction. Traction bands virtually only exist when penetrating trauma creates a path through the vitreous or from severe necrosis, usually due to toxocariasis. Even these bands are usually contiguous with the posterior vitreous cortex.

EXAMINATION OF THE VITREOUS AND VITREORETINAL INTERFACE

Normal vitreous is essentially transparent, yet it is capable of producing substantial force on the retina. Vitreoretinal traction can often be inferred by the configuration of the retinal surface (Figure 9–4). Transparent vitreous can best be seen by using a narrow, off-axis, slitbeam, a three-mirror contact lens, and a stereo biomicroscope (Figure 9–5). Visualization is significantly enhanced by dark adaptation of the observer. A biomicroscope with a broad, on-axis, slitbeam or a direct ophthalmoscope is usually not suitable for observing the vitreous.

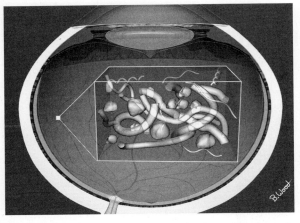

▲ **Figure 9–1.** The vitreous consists of a three-dimensional matrix of collagen fibers and a hyaluronan gel.

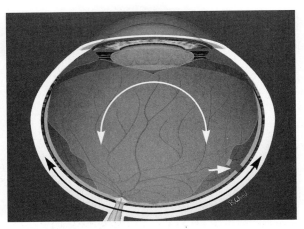

▲ **Figure 9–3.** Motion of partially detached vitreous **(white arrow),** induced by saccades **(black arrow)** and resulting in a retinal break **(arrowhead).**

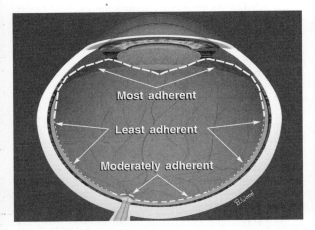

▲ **Figure 9–2.** The vitreous cortex is adherent to the lens and especially to the retinal surface to varying degrees.

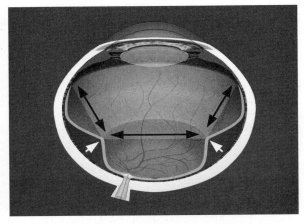

▲ **Figure 9–4.** Abnormal retinal configuration **(white arrows)** indicating vitreoretinal traction **(black arrows).**

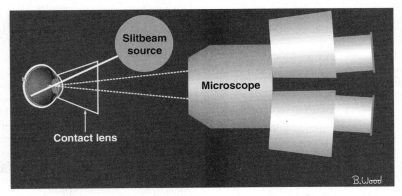

▲ **Figure 9–5.** A narrow, off-axis slitbeam, contact lens, and biomicroscope offer the best view of transparent vitreous.

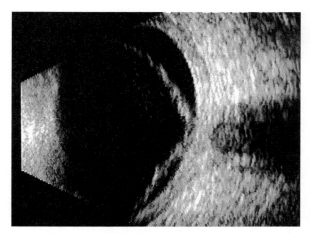

▲ **Figure 9–6.** B-scan.

Indirect ophthalmoscopes provide a large field of view, are capable of looking "around" some lenticular and vitreous opacities, and provide a stereoscopic view. Many observers only attempt to look "through" the vitreous, ignoring the opportunity to look "at" the vitreous, especially if it is abnormal. Visualization of vitreoretinal traction is enhanced rather than adversely affected by eye motion. In addition, mobility of the vitreous is an excellent gauge of the extent of vitreoretinal traction. It is often possible to see some portion of the retina in eyes with substantial vitreous hemorrhages by looking at the periphery first to establish a plane of focus, but the viewing path though semi-opaque vitreous is much less in the periphery than when attempting to visualize the optic nerve. The vitreous is often clearer superiorly. Sitting the patient up for a period of time may cause blood to migrate inferiorly, enabling a better view of the retina.

If the vitreous is too opaque to see the retina, B-scan ultrasonography should be used to determine if the retina is attached or a tumor, foreign body, dislocated lens, dislocated intraocular lens, or choroidal detachment is present (Figure 9–6).

Optical coherence tomography (OCT) utilizes light to construct a 3-D model of the macula and posterior retina from a series of optical B-scan images (see Chapter 2). Spectral domain OCT with tracking produces much better resolution than time domain OCT. The resolution is approximately 5 microns. OCT is ideal for visualization of vitreomacular traction, epimacular membranes, macular holes, macular cysts, macular edema, subretinal fluid, pigment epithelial detachments and choroidal neovascular membranes.

▼ SYMPTOMS OF VITREORETINAL DISEASE

FLOATERS

Most people experience "floaters" at some point during their life. These may be described as strings, spider webs, small saucer-like objects, or a transparent ring. Posterior vitreous detachment occurs in at least 70% of the population and causes the majority of floater complaints. Fortunately, most floaters prove to be clinically insignificant after examination of the retina fails to reveal any retinal breaks or other pathology. Careful, timely, peripheral retina examination using an indirect ophthalmoscope through a widely dilated pupil is essential any time a patient complains of the onset of floaters. Any change in the nature of floaters is also an indication for peripheral retinal examination within a few days. Floaters secondary to posterior vitreous separation are better termed vitreous condensations, emphasizing their origin from pre-existing vitreous collagen fibers and surfaces. Erythrocytes and, on occasion, inflammatory cells can result in the patient seeing floaters, often described as saucer-like. A ring-like floater is usually a result of visualizing the zone of posterior vitreous cortex previously adherent to the optic nerve. Vitreous hemorrhage (Figure 9–7) is an indication for careful examination to determine if a vascular disease such as diabetic retinopathy, venous occlusive disease, hemoglobinopathy, or leukemia is present. The presence of inflammatory cells demands a workup for sarcoidosis, candida, lymphomas, and other systemic disorders. Although floaters are common, it is crucial that careful retinal examination be done before a patient is reassured that only posterior vitreous separation has occurred.

Small, uniform, spherical, golden objects known as asteroid hyalosis frequently occur in the vitreous (Figure 9–8). Although they have an impressive appearance, they almost never interfere with vision and need no treatment. It was once taught that asteroid hyalosis is associated with diabetes, but this was subsequently disproved.

Vitrectomy is very rarely indicated for floaters. Many patients overreact to floaters and need counseling rather

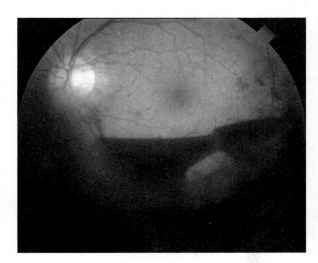

▲ **Figure 9–7.** Vitreous hemorrhage.

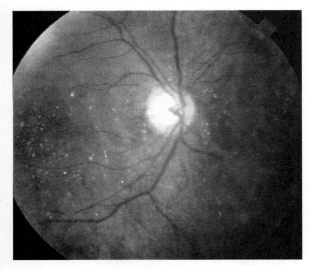

▲ **Figure 9–8.** Asteroid hyalosis.

than surgery with the associated risk of retinal detachment and cataract. Although some ophthalmologists perform YAG laser vitreolysis for floaters, this is rarely effective and has risk of retinal detachment and cataract.

LIGHT FLASHES (PHOTOPSIA)

Light flashes—better termed "photopsia"—are caused by mechanical stimulation of the retina, usually secondary to the vitreous separating from the retina. Jagged, lightning-like, bilateral scintillating scotomas secondary to migraine (50% are not accompanied by a headache) are often mistakenly confused with photopsia. The majority of patients experiencing posterior vitreous separation will experience light flashes, especially during saccades, until separation has stabilized. Posterior vitreous separation is never "complete" as the vitreous always remains attached to the peripheral vitreous base. Any patient with the recent onset of photopsia must have a timely, careful examination of the retinal periphery with a dilated pupil and indirect ophthalmoscope.

▼ VITREORETINAL DISEASES

VITREOMACULAR DISEASE

Until the development of optical coherence tomography (OCT), a plano contact lens was the optimal way to study vitreomacular disease. OCT, especially spectral domain OCT, is superior to clinical examination and an essential adjunct.

Epimacular membranes (EMM) are usually caused by posterior vitreous separation. It is thought that excessive adherence of the posterior vitreous cortex to the retinal surface results in a partial thickness retinal defect when the posterior vitreous separate. Glial cells migrate through the defect onto the retinal surface and cause hypocellular contraction. EMM is treated by vitrectomy and membrane peeling, best performed with end-opening forceps although other tools are used as well. Peeling the internal limiting membrane (ILM) after peeling the epimacular membrane eliminates striae and hastens visual recovery. Patients with EMM complain of metamorphopsia and reduced vision, experiencing dramatic improvement in symptoms after the EMM and ILM are removed.

Vitreomacular traction syndrome (VMT) was thought to be rare until advent of OCT. It is thought to be caused by excessive adherence of the posterior vitreous cortex to the retinal surface coupled with hypocellular vitreous contraction. In some cases separation of the posterior vitreous cortex from the retina is incomplete with a layer remaining attached and then contracting. More typically, the taut posterior vitreous cortex adherent to the macula creates macular elevation, distortion, and reduced vision. Vitrectomy usually with ILM peeling is extremely effective in managing these cases.

Macular holes development is related to posterior vitreous separation but the exact mechanism is unknown. The Gass classification, which categorizes macular holes according to clinical findings, does not influence management decisions. The core issue is to determine if the hole is partial or full thickness on OCT. Symptomatic partial thickness holes require vitrectomy with ILM peeling and SF6 gas. If asymptomatic, they can be observed. Full thickness holes require vitrectomy with ILM peeling and SF6 gas, which results in a 90% rate of closure of the hole and significant visual improvement.

RETINAL BREAKS & RHEGMATOGENOUS RETINAL DETACHMENT

As described above, posterior vitreous separation in eyes with abnormal vitreoretinal adherence can result in retina tears (breaks). Retina breaks occur more commonly in patients with myopia as they may have lattice degeneration, which is genetically linked to myopia. Symptomatic retinal breaks are said to be more significant than asymptomatic, although patients vary widely in their reporting of symptoms. Large tears are more significant than small tears. Small round holes, especially those inside lattice degeneration, seldom cause retinal detachment. Operculated holes or round atrophic holes are far less likely to cause retinal detachment than flap (horseshoe) tears (Figure 9–9).

DIABETIC RETINOPATHY

Patients with proliferative diabetic retinopathy may bleed into the vitreous from retinal neovascularization. These patients must be managed aggressively with laser panretinal photocoagulation, often combined with anti-VEGF therapy using intravitreal injections of bevacizumab (Avastin) or similar agents. If the blood prevents visualization of the

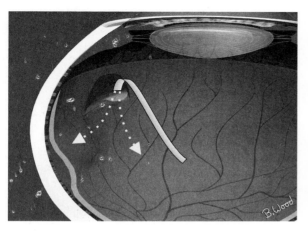

▲ **Figure 9–9.** Passage of liquid vitreous through horseshoe retinal tear leading to retinal detachment.

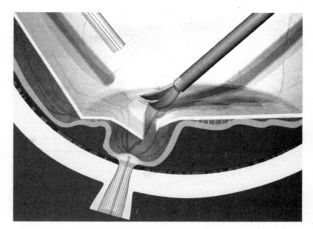

▲ **Figure 9–11.** Scissors segmentation of epiretinal membrane to release tangential traction.

retina, ultrasound examination must be performed to rule out traction retinal detachment. Vitrectomy can be done to improve vision and apply endolaser panretinal photocoagulation (Figure 9–10).

Diabetic traction retinal detachments are managed using vitreoretinal surgery, incorporating techniques such as scissors segmentation (Figure 9–11) and delamination (Figure 9–12) of epiretinal membranes. Coagulation of transected neovascularization is accomplished using endolaser or bipolar diathermy probes (Figure 9–13).

COMPLICATIONS OF CATARACT SURGERY

Approximately 0.5%–1% of cataract surgery patients ultimately develop rhegmatogenous retinal detachment,

presumably related to alterations in the vitreous during or after surgery. These patients present with light flashes, photopsia, loss of peripheral vision, and loss of central vision once the macula is detached. Vitreous loss is usually said to occur after 1% of cataract surgeries, but recent evidence suggests that the incidence may be closer to 5%. Retinal detachment is more common after capsule rupture, vitreous loss, and anterior vitrectomy (Figure 9–14).

Capsule rupture during cataract surgery may result in displacement of lens material or occasionally the entire lens into the vitreous. Inflammation and phacolytic glaucoma usually develop unless only a small amount of cortex is dislocated. Vitrectomy plus fragmentation is very effective in removing posterior dislocated lens material (Figure 9–15).

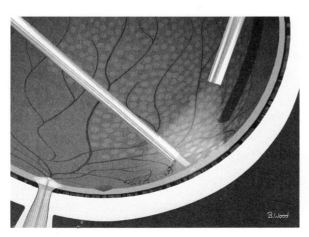

▲ **Figure 9–10.** Endolaser retinal photocoagulation.

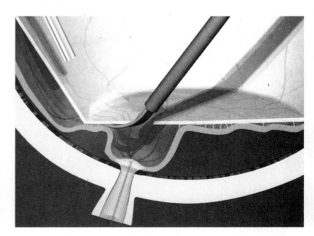

▲ **Figure 9–12.** Scissors delamination to remove adherent epiretinal membrane.

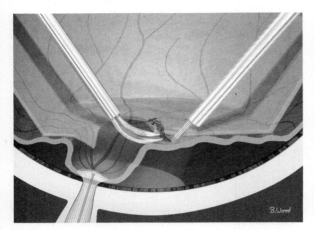

▲ **Figure 9–13.** Coagulation of transected vessels with bipolar endoilluminator during segmentation or delamination.

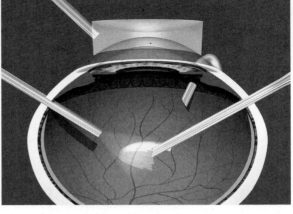

▲ **Figure 9–15.** Vitrectomy with contact lens and endoillumination to allow fragmentation and removal of posterior dislocated lens material.

Endophthalmitis may occur within a few days after cataract surgery and can rapidly result in loss of the eye unless recognized and treated very rapidly. Most cases are best treated by performing a vitreous tap for culture and sensitivity and injecting intravitreal antibiotics. Severe cases in which the retina can still be seen on clinical examination may be treated with vitrectomy as well. Eyes infected with aggressive organisms are often lost, even with prompt diagnosis and appropriate treatment. Any patient with pain, decreased vision, or increasing inflammation should be seen immediately to determine if endophthalmitis is present. Endophthalmitis can also result from a leaking filtering bleb, trauma, or endogenous sources such as an intravenous line or indwelling catheter.

TRAUMA

Penetrating ocular trauma often results in a vitreous hemorrhage, which may be accompanied by significant retinal damage. Vitreous mobility as judged by indirect ophthalmoscopy and ultrasonography helps determine the timing of vitrectomy after penetrating trauma without a foreign body. Mobile vitreous, even if completely opaque from hemorrhage, can be observed if ultrasound demonstrates the retina to be attached and no foreign body is present. Vitrectomy is typically performed 7–10 days after initial wound repair after posterior vitreous separation occurs, active bleeding subsides, and the cornea is clearer. If early vitreous contraction

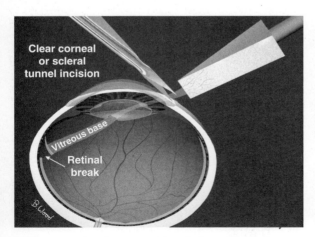

▲ **Figure 9–14.** Vitreous traction during and after cataract surgery can lead to retinal breaks and detachment.

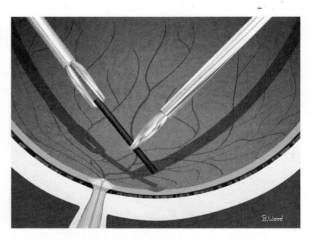

▲ **Figure 9–16.** Removal of intraocular foreign body with diamond-coated forceps.

is indicated by decreased mobility, vitrectomy should be performed before fibrosis and secondary traction retinal detachment occur.

If a metallic (ferrous or copper), toxic, or potentially infectious intraocular foreign body is present, prompt vitrectomy and forceps removal of the foreign body is indicated (Figure 9–16) (see Chapter 19). Occasionally a plastic or glass foreign body or a shotgun pellet can be observed without surgery or until vitreoretinal traction occurs.

SUMMARY

Study of vitreoretinal diseases is fascinating and can have major impact on visual outcomes. New technologies and techniques are being developed at an explosive pace, producing great improvement in the outcomes after vitreoretinal surgery. Many eyes formerly untreatable have experienced restored vision in recent years. Advances in biotechnology are likely to produce phenomenal advances in the future.

REFERENCES

Bajaire B et al: Vitreoretinal surgery of the posterior segment for explosive trauma in terrorist warfare. Graefes Arch Clin Exp Ophthalmol 2006;244:991. [PMID: 16440208]

Chaudhry IA et al: Incidence and visual outcome of endophthalmitis associated with intraocular foreign bodies. Graefes Arch Clin Exp Ophthalmol 2008;246:181. [PMID: 17468878]

Dhingra N et al: Early vitrectomy for fundus obscuring dense vitreous haemorrhage from presumptive retinal tears. Graefes Arch Clin Exp Ophthalmol 2007;245:301. [PMID: 16802133]

Ehlers JP et al: Metallic intraocular foreign bodies: characteristics, interventions, and prognostic factors for visual outcome and globe survival. Am J Ophthalmol 2008;146:427. [PMID: 18614135]

Gonzales CR, Singh S, Schwartz SD: 25-Gauge vitrectomy for pediatric vitreoretinal conditions. Br J Ophthalmol 2009;93:787. [PMID: 19211601]

Hollands H et al: Acute-onset floaters and flashes: is this patient at risk for retinal detachment? JAMA 2009;302:2243. [PMID: 19934426]

Jakobsson G et al: Capsule complication during cataract surgery: retinal detachment after cataract surgery with capsule complication: Swedish Capsule Rupture Study Group report 4. J Cataract Refract Surg 2009;35:1699. [PMID: 19781462]

Koizumi H et al. Three-dimensional evaluation of vitreomacular traction and epiretinal membrane using spectral-domain optic coherence tomography. Am J Ophthalmol 2008;145:509. [PMID: 18191099]

Krause L et al: Incidence and outcome of endophthalmitis over a 13-year period. Can J Ophthalmol 2009;44:88. [PMID: 19169320]

Kumagai K et al: Long-term follow-up of vitrectomy for diffuse nontractional diabetic macular edema. Retina 2009;29:464. [PMID: 19289987]

Nam Y et al: Comparison of 25- and 23-gauge sutureless microincision vitrectomy surgery in the treatment of various vitreoretinal diseases. Eye 2009 Aug 14. [Epub ahead of print] [PMID: 19680275]

Narendran N et al: The Cataract National Database electronic multicentre audit of 55,567 operations: risk stratification for posterior capsule rupture and vitreous loss. Eye 2009;23:31. [PMID: 18327164]

Newman DK: Surgical management of the late complications of proliferative diabetic retinopathy. Eye 2010 Feb 5. [Epub ahead of print] [PMID: 20139916]

Ng JQ et al: Management and outcomes of postoperative endophthalmitis since the endophthalmitis vitrectomy study: The Endophthalmitis Population Study of Western Australia (EPSWA)'s fifth report. Ophthalmology 2005;112:1199. [PMID: 15921759]

Salehi-Had H et al: Visual outcomes of vitreoretinal surgery in eyes with severe open-globe injury presenting with no-light-perception vision. Graefes Arch Clin Exp Ophthalmol 2009;247:477. [PMID: 19172288]

Shah SP et al: Factors predicting outcome of vitrectomy for diabetic macular oedema: results of a prospective study. Br J Ophthalmol 2006;90:33. [PMID: 16361663]

Sheard RM et al: Vitreoretinal surgery after childhood ocular trauma. Eye 2007;21:793. [PMID: 16601744]

Sonmez K et al: Vitreomacular traction syndrome: impact of anatomical configuration on anatomical and visual outcomes. Retina 2008;28:1207. [PMID: 19430388]

Tammewar AM et al: Imaging vitreomacular interface abnormalities in the coronal plane by simultaneous combined scanning laser and optical coherence tomography. Br J Ophthalmol 2009;93:366. [PMID: 19019945]

Wickham L et al: Outcomes of surgery for posterior segment intraocular foreign bodies—a retrospective review of 17 years of clinical experience. Graefes Arch Clin Exp Ophthalmol 2006; Jun 21 [Epub ahead of print]. [PMID: 16788826]

Yeh S, Colyer MH, Weichel ED: Current trends in the management of intraocular foreign bodies. Curr Opin Ophthalmol 2008;19:225. [PMID: 18408498]

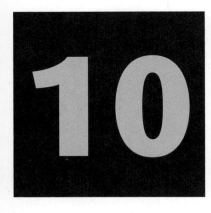

Retina

Emily C. Fletcher, MBChB, MRCOphth,

N. Victor Chong, MD, FRCS, FRCOphth,

James J. Augsburger, MD, and Zélia M. Corrêa, MD, PhD

10.1. Retina & Retinal Disorders

Emily C. Fletcher, MBChB, MRCOphth, and N. Victor Chong, MD, FRCS, FRCOphth

▼ RETINA

The human retina is the most complex of the ocular tissues with a highly organized structure. It receives the visual image, produced by the optical system of the eye, and converts the light energy into an electrical signal, which undergoes initial processing and is then transmitted through the optic nerve to the visual cortex, where the structural (form, color, and contrast) and spatial (position, depth, and motion) attributes are perceived. The anatomy of the retina is described in Chapter 1, Figure 1–17 showing its layers. Function and functional disturbance in the retina often can be localized to a single layer or a single cell type.

PHYSIOLOGY

Rod and cone cells in the photoreceptor layer are responsible for the initial transformation, by the process of phototransduction, of light stimuli into the nerve impulses that are conducted through the visual pathways to the visual cortex. These photoreceptors are arranged such that there is an increased density of cones in the center of the macula (fovea), decreasing to the periphery, and a higher density of rods in the periphery. In the foveola, there is a nearly 1:1 relationship between each cone photoreceptor, its ganglion cell, and the emerging nerve fiber, whereas in the peripheral retina, many photoreceptors connect to the same ganglion cell. The fovea is responsible for good spatial resolution (visual acuity) and color vision, both requiring high ambient light (photopic vision) and being best at the foveola, while the remaining retina is utilized primarily for motion, contrast, and night (scotopic) vision.

The rod and cone photoreceptors are located in the avascular outermost layer of the sensory retina. Each rod photoreceptor cell contains rhodopsin, a photosensitive visual pigment embedded in the double-membrane disks of the photoreceptor outer segment. It is made up of two components, an opsin protein combined with a chromophore. The opsin in rhodopsin is scotopsin, which is formed of seven transmembrane helices. It surrounds the chromophore, retinal, which is derived from vitamin A. When rhodopsin absorbs a photon of light, 11-cis retinal is isomerized to all-trans retinal and eventually to all-trans retinol. The resulting configurational change initiates a secondary messenger cascade. Peak light absorption by rhodopsin occurs at approximately 500 nm, which is the blue-green region of the light spectrum. Spectral sensitivity studies of cone photopigments have shown peak wavelength absorption at 430, 540, and 575 nm for blue-, green-, and red-sensitive cones, respectively. The cone photopigments are composed of 11-cis retinal bound to other opsin proteins than scotopsin.

Night (scotopic) vision is mediated entirely by rod photoreceptors. With this dark-adapted form of vision, varying shades of gray are seen, but colors cannot be distinguished. As the retina becomes fully light-adapted, the spectral sensitivity of the retina shifts from a rhodopsin-dominated peak of 500 nm to approximately 560 nm, and color sensation becomes evident. An object takes on color when it selectively reflects or transmits certain wavelengths of light within the visible spectrum (400–700 nm). Daylight (photopic) vision is mediated primarily by cone photoreceptors, and twilight (mesopic) vision by a combination of cones and rods.

The photoreceptors are maintained by the retinal pigment epithelium, which plays an important role in the visual process. It is responsible for phagocytosis of the outer segments of the photoreceptors, transport of vitamins, and reduction of light scatter, as well as providing a selective barrier between the choroid and retina. The basement membrane of the retinal pigment epithelial cells forms the inner layer of Bruch's membrane, which is otherwise composed of a specialized extracellular matrix and the basement membrane of the choriocapillaris as its outer layer. Retinal pigment epithelial cells have little capacity for regeneration.

EXAMINATION

Examination of the retina is described in Chapter 2 and depicted in Figures 2–11 to 2–17. The retina can be examined with a direct or indirect ophthalmoscope or with a slitlamp (biomicroscope) and handheld or contact biomicroscopy lens. This allows identification of the type, level, and extent of retinal disease. Retinal imaging techniques (Figures 2–26 to 2–30) are useful adjuncts to clinical examination, enabling identification of anatomical, vascular (both retinal and choroidal), and functional abnormalities. They include fundus photography, fluorescein angiography, optical coherence tomography (OCT), indocyanine green angiography, and autofluorescence. The clinical application of visual electrophysiologic and psychophysical tests is described in Chapter 2.

AGE-RELATED MACULAR DEGENERATION

Age-related macular degeneration (AMD) affects people aged over 55 and is the leading cause of irreversible blindness in the developed world. It is a complex multifactorial progressive disease. Current evidence suggests genetic susceptibility involving the complement pathway and environmental risk factors, including increasing age, white race, and smoking. Among whites aged over 55, the 10-year risk of developing AMD is approximately 11.5% for early and 1.5% for late disease.

▶ Pathogenesis

The pathogenesis is still poorly understood; however, degeneration of the retinal pigment epithelium, linked to oxidative stress, seems to be a crucial component. Changes in the adjacent extracellular matrix of Bruch's membrane and the formation of subretinal deposits are central to disease progression. Progressive diffuse thickening of Bruch's membrane reduces the ability of oxygen to diffuse through to the retinal pigment epithelium and photoreceptors. The resulting hypoxia results in release of growth factors and cytokines, which stimulate growth of choroidal new vessels. Development of single or multiple areas of weakness in Bruch's membrane allows the new vessels to grow through into the subretinal space, between the retinal pigment epithelium and the retina, to form a choroidal neovascular membrane. The new vessels leak serous fluid and/or blood, resulting in distortion and reduction of clarity of central vision. Alternatively, visual loss results from progression of the degenerative process to cell death and atrophy of the retinal pigment epithelium.

▶ Genetic Factors

Twin studies and linkage analysis have identified multiple loci for genes related to AMD. The two most important loci are at 1q25–31 (complement factor H–CFH) and 10q26 (age-related maculopathy susceptibility 2-ARMS2/HTRA serine peptidase 1-HTRA1). The genes can be divided into those which have an influence on structural (HTRA1), inflammatory (CFH, C3, C2, and Factor B), and lipid (APOE) pathways. HTRA1 is a heat shock protein that is involved in the degradation of extracellular proteins such as that found in Bruch's membrane. Polymorphisms in its promoter gene have been found to be associated with a 10-fold increased risk of AMD. CFH is involved in the alternative complement pathway, thereby identifying an inflammatory component to the pathogenesis of AMD. Its Y402H polymorphism is associated with an increased risk of AMD. C3 mutations confer a 3-fold increased risk, whereas C2 and Factor B appear to have a protective effect. The function of the LOC387715 gene, which is found within the ARMS2 locus next to HTRA1, is unknown but a polymorphism is associated with a 2–3-fold increased risk of AMD, with an additive effect from the CFH polymorphism.

Individuals with genetic predisposition are even more likely to develop the disease if they smoke or have a low intake of antioxidants.

▶ Classification

AMD can be classified simply into early and late, the latter being subdivided into geographic atrophy and neovascular disease. The Age-Related Eye Disease Study (AREDS) devised a grading system based on fundal features, of which a simplified form is also useful clinically.

1. EARLY AMD

Early AMD is characterized by limited drusen, pigmentary change, or retinal pigment epithelial atrophy. The level of associated visual impairment is variable and may be minimal. Fluorescein angiography demonstrates irregular patterns of retinal pigment epithelial hyperplasia and atrophy.

Drusen are visualized clinically as yellow deposits, which are situated within Bruch's membrane. They vary in size and shape. They may be discrete or confluent (Figure 10–1). Histopathologically, drusen may also be detected as diffuse subretinal deposits, either basal laminar deposits, formed mainly of collagen-based material and situated between the plasma and basement membranes of the retinal pigment

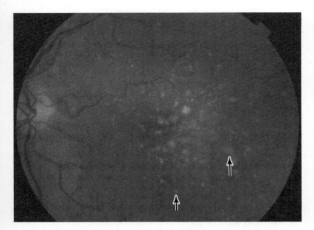

▲ **Figure 10–1.** AMD with discrete (small arrow) and large confluent (large arrow) macular drusen. See color insert.

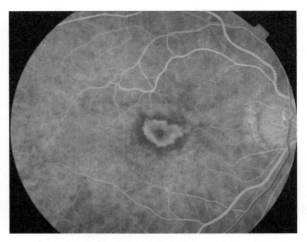

▲ **Figure 10–2.** Flourescein angiogram of classic choroidal neovascularization showing well-circumscribed, lacy pattern.

epithelium, or basal linear deposits, consisting of granular lipid-rich material located within Bruch's membrane.

Pigmentary change may be due to focal clumps of pigmented cells in the subretinal space and outer retina, or attenuated areas of hypopigmented retinal pigment epithelium progressing to atrophy.

2. LATE AMD

Geographic atrophy ("dry AMD") is responsible for up to 20% of legal blindness attributable to AMD. It manifests as well-demarcated areas, larger than two disk diameters, of atrophy of the retinal pigment epithelium and photoreceptor cells, allowing direct visualization of the underlying choroidal vessels. Accumulation of lipofuscin in the retinal pigment epithelium is thought to contribute to the atrophic changes. Visual loss occurs once the fovea is affected. Geographic atrophy is best monitored with autofluorescence imaging, different patterns of abnormality possibly providing clarification of disease progression.

Neovascular ("wet") AMD is characterized by the development of choroidal neovascularization or serous retinal pigment epithelial detachment. Choroidal new vessels may grow in a flat cartwheel or sea-fan configuration away from their site of entry into the subretinal space to form a choroidal neovascular membrane. Hemorrhagic detachment of the retina may undergo fibrous metaplasia, resulting in an elevated subretinal mass called a disciform scar. Permanent loss of central vision ensues. OCT imaging identifies both subretinal and intraretinal fluid, along with the choroidal neovascular membrane. Fluorescein angiography should be performed on all patients with AMD with new onset of reduced vision or distortion, as the most sensitive method for detection of choroidal neovascularization. It can also guide treatment options. Choroidal

neovascularization can be classified angiographically into either classic or occult, depending on the pattern of new vessel growth. Classic is characterized by early hyperfluorescence, which is usually well circumscribed and may have a lacy pattern (Figure 10–2). Occult is characterized by ill-defined and late hyperfluorescence. For research studies, choroidal neovascularization has been subdivided into predominantly classic, in which more than 50% of the lesion has the characteristics of classic choroidal neovascularization; minimally classic, in which less than 50% of the lesion has the characteristics of classic choroidal neovascularization; and pure occult, in which no classic component can be identified.

Retinal pigment epithelial detachment is included in the category of neovascular AMD because of its strong, although not absolute, association with choroidal neovascularization, to the extent that choroidal neovascularization should be assumed to be present until investigations or natural history has excluded it. Serous retinal pigment epithelial detachment may develop from influx of proteinaceous material through a plane of cleavage at the site of drusen. Focal retinal pigment epithelial detachment may also develop from leak of serous fluid from the choroid through small defects in Bruch's membrane. Retinal pigment epithelial detachments may spontaneously flatten, with variable visual results, but usually leaving an area of geographic atrophy.

It is uncertain whether retinal angiomatous proliferation (RAP) is a manifestation of AMD, but it usually presents in the same clinical setting. The cause is unknown. It manifests as superficial (inner retinal) hemorrhage with retinal pigment epithelial detachment and extensive exudation (Figure 10–3) and is characterized by anastomosis between the retinal and choroidal circulations (Figure 10–4).

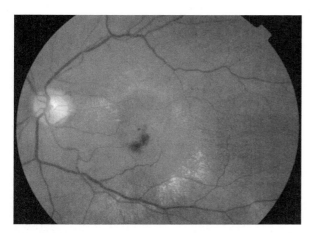

▲ **Figure 10–3.** RAP with superficial hemorrhage, retinal pigment epithelial detachment, and extensive exudation. See color insert.

Risk of Progression to Late AMD

The AREDS, which includes an interventional longitudinal study of progression of AMD, has identified pigmentary changes and large drusen (>250 microns) to be the most important fundal features predictive of progression to late AMD, from which a simple clinical scoring system to predict risk of progression has been devised. Points are assigned according to whether pigmentary changes or large drusen can be identified on fundoscopy. For patients with no late disease, 1 point is assigned for each eye with large drusen, for each eye with pigmentary abnormalities, and if neither eye

has large drusen for intermediate-size drusen present in both eyes. For patients with late disease in one eye, 2 points are assigned for the eye with late disease and 1 point for each of large drusen or pigmentary abnormalities in the fellow eye. The 5-year risk of progression to late AMD is 0.5%, 3.0%, 12.0%, 25%, and 50%, respectively, as the cumulative score rises from 0 to 4.

Prophylactic Therapy

Treatment with oral **vitamins and antioxidants,** comprising vitamin C (500 g), vitamin E (400 IU), betacarotene (15 mg), and zinc (80 mg) and copper (2 mg) daily, was found in the AREDS to reduce the 5-year risk of progression to late AMD from 28% to 20% in patients with cumulative scores of 3 or 4 on the risk prediction score (see above) but did not show any benefit for those with lower cumulative scores. In a separate study, smokers taking betacarotene have been shown to have an increased risk of development of lung cancer. Therefore, smokers and ex-smokers are advised to omit the betacarotene.

Smoking is a proven risk factor for development of all forms of macular degeneration. Cessation of smoking is thought to reduce the rate of progression, although further trials are required to establish the extent of its effect. It is recommended that smoking be discontinued, together with change in lifestyle to incorporate gentle daily exercise, which lowers the risk of AMD. It takes about 20 years of smoking cessation to reduce the level of risk of development of AMD to that of a non smoker.

Retinal laser photocoagulation reduces the extent of drusen but increases the rate of choroidal neovascularization and is not recommended outside a clinical trial.

Treatment of Neovascular AMD

Vascular endothelial growth factor (VEGF) plays a crucial role in the expansion of choroidal neovascular membranes. It induces both angiogenesis and increased permeability. Blocking VEGF (**anti-VEGF therapy**) has become the preferred treatment for neovascular AMD.

Ranibizumab (Lucentis, Genentech) is a humanized Fab fragment of a murine monoclonal anti-VEGF antibody, which is able to bind all isoforms of VEGF. It is able to penetrate through all layers of the retina and is administered by intravitreal injection. The MARINA trial showed stabilization of vision in 94% of eyes with minimally classic or occult lesions and improvement in 34%. The ANCHOR trial showed similar results, with significant benefit over photodynamic therapy (PDT) (see later in the chapter) for predominantly classic lesions.

Currently, ranibizumab is the treatment of choice for all forms of neovascular AMD. Repeated intravitreal injections are well tolerated with minimal side effects, but the ideal treatment regimen is still under investigation. Long-term monthly injections, which are a significant burden to patients and health care systems, may not be needed, but a

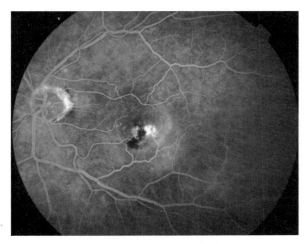

▲ **Figure 10–4.** Mid-venous phase of fluorescein angiogram of RAP showing the retino-choroidal anastomosis and early filling of the pigment epithelial detachment.

loading phase of three injections at monthly intervals followed by a maintenance phase of injection frequency being determined by disease activity is probably required. The small PrONTO trial suggested that monthly monitoring with treatment according to results of OCT provides near-equivalent visual outcome to monthly dosing, but this was not confirmed in a larger study using the original retreatment criteria. More rigorous treatment criteria are being investigated to optimize outcome without having to rely upon monthly injections.

The oligonucleotide aptamer (chemically synthesized single-stranded nucleic acid), **pegaptanib** (Macugen, Eyetech), binds the major pathogenic isoform of VEGF, VEGF165. It is administered by intravitreal injection. Stabilization of vision has been demonstrated in 71% of patients, with improvement occurring in 6% (VISION trial).

Bevacizumab (Avastin, Genentech) is a humanized full-length monoclonal antibody to VEGF. Initially it was thought not to be able to pass through the retina, but it has been widely used with good results. Several (CATT, IVAN, VIBERA and GEFAL) trials are currently being undertaken in the United States and Europe to evaluate its efficacy and safety compared to ranibizumab.

Conventional **retinal laser photocoagulation** can achieve direct destruction of a choroidal neovascular membrane. It requires confluent high-energy burns over and around the whole membrane. The overlying retina is also destroyed, the laser scar may expand, leading to visual loss, and the rate of recurrence of the neovascular membrane is high. Laser photocoagulation is only used for choroidal neovascular membranes that are more than 200 microns from the center of the foveal avascular zone (extrafoveal).

Photodynamic therapy (PDT) requires an intravenous infusion of a photosensitive dye, verteporfin (Visudyne, Novartis), which is activated by a low-energy visible laser (689 nm). However, this treatment has now largely been replaced by anti-VEGF treatments.

Combining anti-VEGF therapy with PDT steroids, or other agents continues to be investigated. The Mont Blanc study showed that PDT with ranibizumab is no better than ranibizumab alone. Other agents being investigated include the VEGF trap, a designer molecule that binds to VEGF to prevent it binding to its receptor, and RNA interference (RNAi) technology to prevent transcription of VEGF or its receptors.

Surgery for late AMD continues to be studied with mixed results. Options include surgical removal of the choroidal neovascular membrane, macular translocation, and retinal pigment epithelial transplantation. Surgery is recommended only as part of a clinical trial.

MYOPIC MACULAR DEGENERATION

Pathologic myopia is one of the leading causes of blindness in the United States and is much more common in the Far East and Japan. It is characterized by progressive elongation

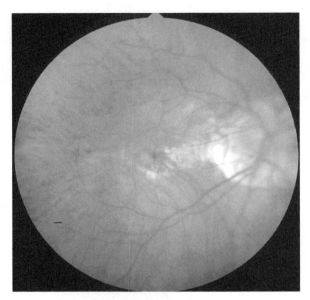

▲ **Figure 10–5.** Myopic macular degeneration with choroidal vessels visible through atrophic retinal pigment epithelium and peripapillary atrophy. See color insert.

of the eye with subsequent thinning and atrophy of the choroid and retinal pigment epithelium in the macula. Usually there is at least 6 diopters myopia. Peripapillary chorioretinal atrophy and linear breaks in Bruch's membrane ("lacquer cracks") are characteristic findings on fundoscopy (Figure 10–5). Degenerative changes of the macular pigment epithelium resemble those found in older patients with AMD. A characteristic lesion of pathologic myopia is a raised, circular, pigmented macular lesion called a Fuchs spot. Most patients are in the fifth decade when the degenerative macular changes cause a slowly progressive loss of vision; rapid loss of visual acuity is usually caused by serous and hemorrhagic macular detachment overlying a choroidal neovascular membrane, which occurs in 5%–10% of patients.

Fluorescein angiography shows delayed filling of choroidal and retinal blood vessel and is helpful in identifying and locating the site of choroidal neovascularization in eyes with serous or hemorrhagic detachment of the macula. Anti-VEGF therapy has become the treatment of choice for sub- or juxta-foveal choroidal neovascularization.

The chorioretinal changes of pathologic myopia predispose to retinal breaks and thus to retinal detachment. Peripheral retinal findings may include paving-stone degeneration, pigmentary degeneration, and lattice degeneration. Retinal breaks usually occur in areas involved with chorioretinal lesions, but they also arise in areas of apparently normal retina. Some of these breaks, particularly those of the "horseshoe" and round retinal tear type, will progress to rhegmatogenous retinal detachment.

RETINAL VASCULAR DISEASES

DIABETIC RETINOPATHY

Diabetic retinopathy is one of the leading causes of blindness in the Western world, particularly among individuals of working age. Chronic hyperglycemia, hypertension, hypercholesterolemia, and smoking are all risk factors for development and progression of retinopathy. Young people with type I (insulin-dependent) diabetes do not develop retinopathy for at least 3–5 years after the onset of the systemic disease. Type II (non-insulin-dependent) diabetics may have retinopathy at the time of diagnosis, and it may be the presenting manifestation.

▶ Screening

Early detection and treatment of diabetic retinopathy is essential. Readily detectable changes occur before vision is affected. Their identification and appropriate treatment will usually prevent permanent visual loss. Screening for diabetic retinopathy should be performed within 3 years from diagnosis in type I diabetes, on diagnosis in type II diabetes, and annually thereafter in both types. Digital fundal photography has been proven to be an effective and sensitive method for screening. Seven-field photography is the gold standard, but two 45° fields, one centered on the macula and the other centered on the disk, are becoming the method of choice in most screening programs. Mydriasis is necessary for best quality photographs, especially if there is cataract.

Diabetic retinopathy can progress rapidly during pregnancy. Every pregnant diabetic woman should be examined by an ophthalmologist or digital fundal photography in the first trimester and at least every 3 months until delivery.

▶ Classification

Diabetic retinopathy can be classified into nonproliferative retinopathy, maculopathy, and proliferative retinopathy.

▶ Nonproliferative Retinopathy

Diabetic retinopathy is a progressive microangiopathy characterized by small-vessel damage and occlusion. The earliest pathologic changes are thickening of the capillary endothelial basement membrane and reduction of the number of pericytes. The capillaries develop tiny dot-like outpouchings called microaneurysms. Flame-shaped hemorrhages are so shaped because of their location within the horizontally oriented nerve fiber layer.

Mild nonproliferative retinopathy is characterized by at least one microaneurysm. In moderate nonproliferative retinopathy, there are extensive microaneurysms, intraretinal hemorrhages, venous beading, and/or cotton wool spots

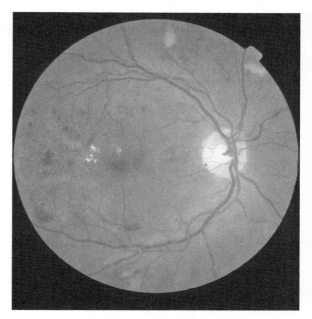

▲ **Figure 10–6.** Moderate nonproliferative diabetic retinopathy showing microaneurysms, deep hemorrhages, flame-shaped hemorrhage, exudates, and cotton wool spots. See color insert.

(Figure 10–6). Severe nonproliferative retinopathy is characterized by cotton-wool spots, venous beading, and intraretinal microvascular abnormalities (IRMA). It can be diagnosed when there are intraretinal hemorrhages in four quadrants, venous beading in two quadrants, or severe IRMA in one quadrant.

▶ Maculopathy

Diabetic maculopathy manifests as focal or diffuse retinal thickening or edema, caused primarily by a breakdown of the inner blood–retinal barrier at the level of the retinal capillary endothelium, which allows leakage of fluid and plasma constituents into the surrounding retina. It is more common in type II diabetes and requires treatment once it becomes clinically significant (Figure 10–7), which is defined as any retinal thickening within 500 microns of the fovea, hard exudates within 500 microns of the fovea associated with retinal thickening, or retinal thickening greater than one disc diameter in size, of which any part lies within one disc diameter of the fovea.

Maculopathy can also be due to ischemia, which is characterized by macular edema, deep hemorrhages, and little exudation. Fluorescein angiography shows loss of retinal capillaries with enlargement of the foveal avascular zone (Figure 10–8).

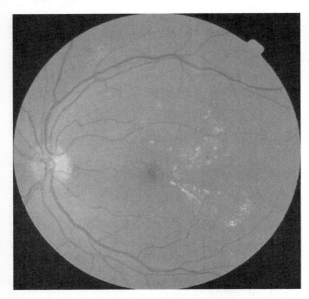

▲ **Figure 10–7.** Clinically significant macular edema with two circinate rings of exudates. See color insert.

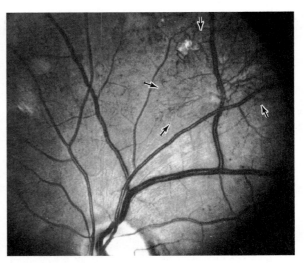

▲ **Figure 10–9.** Frond of neovascular tissue **(arrows)** arising from the superotemporal vascular arcade in proliferative diabetic retinopathy.

▶ Proliferative Retinopathy

The most severe ocular complications of diabetes mellitus are due to proliferative diabetic retinopathy. Progressive retinal ischemia eventually stimulates the formation of delicate new vessels that leak serum proteins (and fluorescein) profusely (Figures 10–9 and 10–10). Early proliferative diabetic retinopathy is characterized by the presence of any new vessels on the optic disk (NVD) or elsewhere in the retina (NVE). High-risk characteristics are defined as new vessels

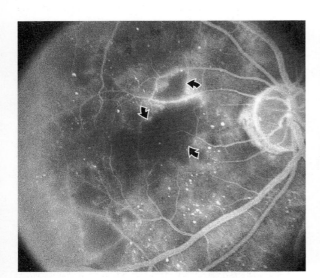

▲ **Figure 10–8.** Fluorescein angiogram shows hypofluorescence from capillary nonperfusion **(arrows)**, with enlargement of the foveal avascular zone, typical of ischemic diabetic maculopathy.

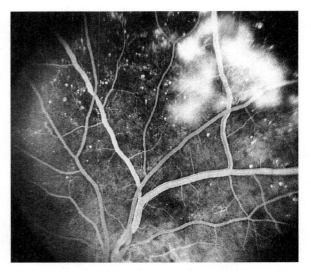

▲ **Figure 10–10.** Fluorescein angiogram of proliferative diabetic retinopathy shows leakage from the neovascular tissue. The pinpoint areas of hyperfluorescence are microaneurysms.

on the optic disk extending more than one-third disk diameter, any new vessels on the optic disk with associated vitreous hemorrhage, or new vessels elsewhere in the retina extending more than one-half disk diameter with associated vitreous hemorrhage.

The fragile new vessels proliferate onto the posterior face of the vitreous and become elevated once the vitreous starts to contract away from the retina. If the vessels bleed, massive vitreous hemorrhage may cause sudden visual loss (Figure 10–11). There is a risk of developing neovascularization and vitreous hemorrhage once a complete posterior vitreous detachment has developed. In eyes with proliferative diabetic retinopathy and persistent vitreoretinal adhesions, elevated neovascular fronds may undergo fibrous change and form tight fibrovascular bands, which cause vitreoretinal traction. This can lead to either progressive traction retinal detachment or, if a retinal tear is produced, rhegmatogenous retinal detachment. The retinal detachment may be heralded or concealed by vitreous hemorrhage. When vitreous contraction is complete in these eyes, proliferative retinopathy tends to enter the burned-out or "involutional" stage. Advanced diabetic eye disease may also be complicated by iris neovascularization (rubeosis iridis) and neovascular glaucoma.

Proliferative retinopathy develops in 50% of type I diabetics within 15 years of onset of their systemic disease. It is less prevalent in type II diabetics, but as there are more patients with type II diabetes, more patients with proliferative retinopathy have type II than type I diabetes.

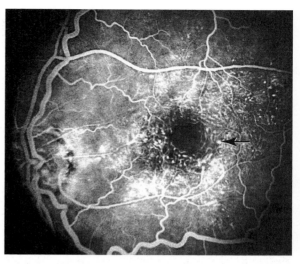

▲ **Figure 10–12.** Fluorescein angiogram in nonproliferative diabetic retinopathy shows microaneurysms **(arrow)** and perifoveal retinal vascular changes.

▶ Imaging

OCT is invaluable in the identification and monitoring of macular edema as well as identification of structural changes within the retina. The development of spectral domain OCT, with increased scan speed and resolution and eye tracking with improved reproducibility, has further enhanced disease assessment and monitoring.

Fluorescein angiography is useful for identifying microvascular abnormalities in diabetic retinopathy (Figure 10–12). Large filling defects of capillary beds—"capillary nonperfusion"—show the extent of retinal ischemia (Figure 10–8) and are usually most prominent in the midperiphery. The fluorescein leakage associated with retinal edema may assume the petaloid configuration of cystoid macular edema (CME) or may be diffuse (Figure 10–13). This can help determine prognosis as well as extent and placement of laser treatment. Eyes with macular edema and significant ischemia have a poorer visual prognosis, with or without laser treatment, than eyes with edema and relatively good perfusion.

▶ Treatment

The mainstay of prevention of progression of retinopathy is good control of hyperglycemia, systemic hypertension, and hypercholesterolemia.

Ocular treatment depends on the location and severity of the retinopathy. Eyes with diabetic macular edema that is not clinically significant should usually be monitored closely without laser treatment. Clinically significant macular edema requires focal laser if focal and grid laser if diffuse. Argon

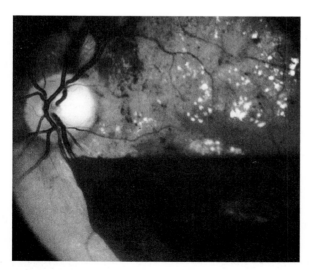

▲ **Figure 10–11.** Proliferative diabetic retinopathy with preretinal hemorrhage obscuring the inferior macula. Macular exudates, microaneurysms, and intraretinal hemorrhages are also present.

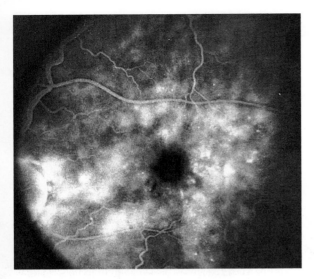

▲ **Figure 10–13.** Late-phase fluorescein angiogram shows hyperfluorescence typical of diffuse (noncystoid) diabetic macular edema.

laser to the macula should be sufficient to produce only light burns, as laser scars can expand and affect vision. Subthreshold treatment, in which no retinal burn is visualized at the time of treatment, and micropulse laser have been shown to be just as effective with less scarring. Intravitreal injections of triamcinolone or anti-VEGF agents are also effective.

By inducing regression of new vessels, pan-retinal laser photocoagulation (PRP) reduces the incidence of severe visual loss from proliferative diabetic retinopathy by 50%. Several thousand regularly spaced laser burns are applied throughout the retina to reduce the angiogenic stimulus from ischemic areas. The central region bordered by the disk and the major temporal vascular arcades is spared (Chapter 23). Patients at greatest risk of visual loss are those with high risk characteristics. If treatment is delayed until high risk characteristics have developed, it is essential that adequate PRP is achieved without delay. Treatment of severe nonproliferative retinopathy has not been shown to alter the visual outcome; however, if the patient has type II diabetes, poor glycemic control, or cannot be monitored sufficiently carefully, treatment before proliferative disease has developed may be justified.

Vitrectomy is able to clear vitreous hemorrhage and relieve vitreoretinal traction. Once extensive vitreous hemorrhage occurs, 20% of eyes will progress to no perception of light vision within 2 years. Early vitrectomy is indicated for type I diabetics with extensive vitreous hemorrhage and severe, active proliferation and whenever vision in the fellow eye is poor. Otherwise, vitrectomy can be delayed for up to a year as vitreous hemorrhage will clear spontaneously in 20% of eyes. Intravitreal anti-VEGF therapy a few days

preoperatively is associated with a reduced re-bleed rate and better visual outcome post operatively. Vitrectomy for proliferative diabetic retinopathy with only mild vitreous hemorrhage is only useful in eyes that have already undergone PRP and have extensive new vessels that have started to fibrose. Tractional retinal detachment does not require vitrectomy until the detachment has involved the fovea. Rhegmatogenous detachment complicating proliferative diabetic retinopathy requires urgent vitrectomy.

Complications following vitrectomy are more common in the type I diabetics undergoing delayed vitrectomy and type II diabetics undergoing early vitrectomy. They include phthisis bulbi, raised intraocular pressure with corneal edema, retinal detachment, and infection.

RETINAL VEIN OCCLUSION

Retinal vein occlusion is a common and easily diagnosed retinal vascular disorder with potentially blinding complications. The patient presents with sudden painless loss of vision. The clinical appearance varies from a few small scattered retinal hemorrhages and cotton-wool spots to a marked hemorrhagic appearance with both deep and superficial retinal hemorrhage (Figure 10–14), which rarely may break through into the vitreous cavity.

In **central retinal vein occlusion** the retinal abnormalities involve all four quadrants of the fundus. In **branch retinal vein occlusion** typically they are confined to one quadrant because the occlusion usually occurs at the site of an arteriovenous crossing (Figure 10–15), but they may involve the upper or lower half (hemispheric branch retinal vein occlusion), or just the macula (macular branch retinal vein occlusion).

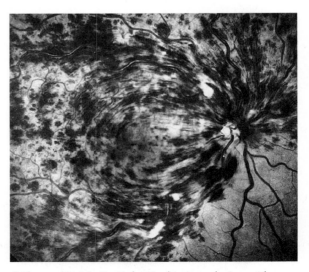

▲ **Figure 10–14.** Central retinal vein occlusion with extensive superficial retinal hemorrhage obscuring macular and optic nerve detail.

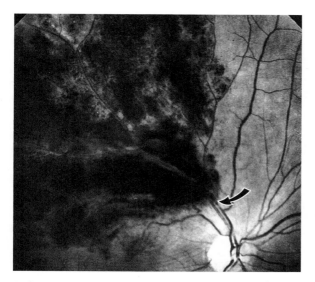

▲ **Figure 10–15.** Branch retinal vein occlusion involves the superotemporal vein. The point of obstruction **(arrow)** is at an arteriovenous crossing.

Patients are usually over 50 years of age, and more than 50% have associated cardiovascular disease. Predisposing factors and investigations are discussed in Chapter 15. Chronic open-angle glaucoma should always be excluded (see Chapter 11). The major complications associated with retinal vein occlusion are reduced vision from macular edema, neovascular glaucoma secondary to iris neovascularization, and retinal neovascularization.

1. MACULAR EDEMA IN RETINAL VEIN OCCLUSION

Macular dysfunction occurs in almost all eyes with central retinal vein occlusion. Although some will show spontaneous improvement, most will have persistent decreased central vision as a result of chronic macular edema, which is also the main cause of persisting impairment of visual acuity in branch retinal vein occlusion.

Macular edema due to central retinal vein occlusion does not respond to laser treatment. In branch retinal vein occlusion, grid-pattern macular argon laser photocoagulation may be indicated when vision loss due to macular edema persists for several months without any spontaneous improvement.

Intravitreal injection of anti-VEGF agents or steroids may be useful. The BRAVO and CRUISE studies, both large multicenter trials, have shown benefit from monthly ranibizumab injections for macular edema secondary to branch and central retinal vein occlusion, respectively. The SCORE study has shown that intravitreal preservative-free triamcinolone provides no benefit compared to laser in branch retinal vein

occlusion, but improved outcome compared to observation in central retinal vein occlusion, although it is uncertain whether the optimal dose is 1 mg or 4 mg. Ozurdex (Allergan), an intravitreal implant containing 0.7 mg dexamethasone in a solid polymer drug delivery system, which can be injected into the vitreous using a 22 gauge needle and dissolves completely, has been shown to accelerate improvement in visual acuity compared to placebo in macular edema due to branch or central retinal vein occlusion. The most commonly reported adverse events during the first 6 months after treatment included increased intraocular pressure, but for which only 0.7% of patients required laser or surgical procedures.

2. IRIS AND RETINAL NEOVASCULARIZATION IN RETINAL VEIN OCCLUSION

Nearly one-third of central retinal vein occlusions are ischemic with significant retinal capillary nonperfusion seen on fluorescein angiography; one-half of these will develop neovascular glaucoma. The standard treatment for iris neovascularization is PRP, although it may also be controlled with intravitreal anti-VEGF agents.

In branch retinal vein occlusion, retinal neovascularization may develop if retinal capillary nonperfusion exceeds five disk diameters in area. Sectoral retinal laser photocoagulation to the area of ischemic retina reduces the risk of vitreous hemorrhage by one-half.

Clinical trials continue to investigate the role of vitrectomy, with or without arteriovenous sheathotomy, to facilitate reperfusion of the retina and reduction of macular edema.

RETINAL ARTERY OCCLUSION

Central retinal artery occlusion causes painless catastrophic visual loss occurring over a period of seconds; antecedent transient visual loss (amaurosis fugax) may be reported. Visual acuity ranges between counting fingers and light perception in 90% of eyes at initial examination. Twenty-five percent of eyes have cilioretinal arteries that continue to perfuse the macula, potentially preserving central vision. An afferent pupillary defect can appear within seconds, preceding any fundus abnormalities, which include opacification of the superficial retina due to infarction, and reduced blood flow in the retinal vessels, possibly manifesting as segmentation of the blood column in the retinal arterioles. A foveal cherry-red spot (Figure 10–16) develops due to preservation of the relatively normal appearance of the choroidal pigment and retinal pigment epithelium through the extremely thin retina overlying the foveola, surrounded by the pale swollen retina of the rest of the macula. The fundal abnormalities resolve within 4–6 weeks, leaving a pale optic disk as the major ocular finding. In older patients, giant cell arteritis must be excluded and if necessary treated immediately with high-dose systemic corticosteroids. Other causes of central retinal artery occlusion are arteriosclerosis and emboli from carotid or cardiac sources. These are discussed further in Chapter 15.

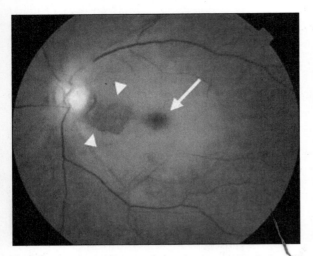

▲ **Figure 10–16.** Acute central retinal artery occlusion with cherry-red spot **(arrow)** and preserved retina due to cilioretinal arterial supply **(arrowheads)**. See color insert. (Courtesy of Esther Posner.)

Branch retinal artery occlusion also causes sudden painless visual loss but usually manifesting as impairment of visual field. Visual acuity is only reduced if there is foveal involvement. The extent of the fundal abnormalities, primarily retinal opacification as in central retinal artery occlusion but sometimes accompanied by cotton-wool spots along its border, is determined by the extent of retinal infarction. The cause is often embolic disease, for which clinical evaluation and investigations need to be undertaken (see Chapter 15).

▶ **Treatment**

Irreversible retinal damage occurs within a few hours of complete central retinal artery occlusion. Sudden decrease in intraocular pressure resulting in increased retinal perfusion can be achieved with anterior chamber paracentesis and intravenous acetazolamide. This is particularly indicated in embolic central retinal artery occlusion. Inhaled oxygen–carbon dioxide mixture induces retinal vasodilation and increases the Po2 at the retinal surface. Thrombolytic therapy, infused directly into the ophthalmic artery or administered systemically, has been shown to be beneficial but patients rarely present sufficiently early to warrant treatment. Systemic anticoagulants are generally not employed unless necessitated by an embolic cause, such as atrial fibrillation.

RETINAL ARTERIAL MACROANEURYSM

Retinal macroaneurysms are fusiform or round dilations of retinal arterioles occurring within the first three orders of arteriolar bifurcation. Most cases are unilateral, involving the

superotemporal artery. Two-thirds of patients have associated systemic hypertension.

Macroaneurysms may result in retinal edema, exudation, or hemorrhage typically with an "hourglass" configuration due to bleeding deep and superficial to the retina. Hemorrhage is usually followed by fibrosis of the macroaneurysm such that no treatment is required. If edema threatens the macula, the macroaneurysm can be treated by confluent laser photocoagulation followed by a direct hit. There is a risk that this direct hit will result in hemorrhage, but this usually settles with fibrosis of the macroaneurysm.

RETINOPATHY OF PREMATURITY

Retinopathy of prematurity (ROP) is a vasoproliferative retinopathy that affects premature and low-birth-weight infants. The etiology, classification (Table 10–1), screening regime, and treatment are also discussed in Chapter 17.

▶ **Treatment**

All babies younger than 30 weeks gestational age, or a birth weight of 1500 g or less, and those that receive prolonged supplemental oxygen therapy should undergo repeated screening from 2–4 weeks after birth until the retina is fully vascularized, the retinal changes have undergone spontaneous resolution, or appropriate treatment has been given. Treatment with peripheral retinal laser is recommended once there is stage 2 disease with venous dilation and arterial tortuosity in the posterior segment ("plus" disease), the latter now being the main indication for treatment. Vitreoretinal surgery may be appropriate for eyes with stage 4 or 5 disease but is only recommended when such disease occurs in the better eye as the visual prognosis continues to be poor.

A significant number of infants with ROP undergo spontaneous regression. Peripheral retinal changes of regressed ROP include avascular retina, peripheral folds, and retinal breaks; associated changes in the posterior pole may include straightening of the temporal vessels, temporal stretching of the macula, and retinal tissue that appears to be dragged over the disk (Figure 10–17). Other ocular findings of regressed ROP include myopia (which may be asymmetric), strabismus, cataract, and angle-closure glaucoma.

Table 10–1. Stages of Retinopathy of Prematurity

Stage	Clinical Findings
1	Demarcation line
2	Intraretinal ridge
3	Ridge with extraretinal fibrovascular proliferation
4	Subtotal retinal detachment
5	Total retinal detachment

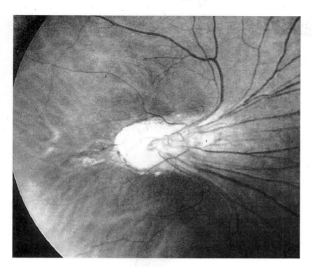

▲ **Figure 10–17.** ROP with stretching of the macula and straightening of retinal vessels.

RETINAL DETACHMENT AND RELATED RETINAL DEGENERATIONS

Retinal detachment is the separation of the sensory retina, ie, the photoreceptors and inner retinal layers, from the underlying retinal pigment epithelium. There are three main types: rhegmatogenous, traction, and serous or hemorrhagic detachment.

1. RHEGMATOGENOUS RETINAL DETACHMENT

The most common type of retinal detachment, rhegmatogenous retinal detachment is characterized by a full-thickness break (a "rhegma") in the sensory retina, variable degrees of vitreous traction, and passage of liquefied vitreous through the break into the subretinal space. A spontaneous rhegmatogenous retinal detachment is usually preceded or accompanied by a posterior vitreous detachment and is associated with myopia, aphakia, lattice degeneration, and ocular trauma. Binocular indirect ophthalmoscopy with scleral depression (Figures 2–15 and 2–17), or slitlamp examination with a handheld or contact biomicroscopy lens, reveals elevation of the translucent detached sensory retina with one or more full-thickness sensory retinal breaks, such as a horseshoe tear, round atrophic hole, or anterior circumferential tear (retinal dialysis). The location of retinal breaks varies according to type; horseshoe tears are most common in the superotemporal quadrant, atrophic holes in the temporal quadrants, and retinal dialysis in the inferotemporal quadrant. When multiple retinal breaks are present, they are usually within 90° of one another.

▶ Treatment

The principal aims of detachment surgery are to find and treat all the retinal breaks, cryotherapy or laser being applied to create an adhesion between the retinal pigment epithelium and the sensory retina, thus preventing any further influx of fluid into the subretinal space, to drain subretinal fluid, internally or externally, and relieve vitreoretinal traction. Various surgical techniques are employed.

In **pneumatic retinopexy** air or expandable gas is injected into the vitreous to maintain the retina in position, while the chorioretinal adhesion induced by laser or cryotherapy achieves permanent closure of the retinal break. It has a lower success rate than other methods and is used only when there is a small accessible single retinal break, minimal subretinal fluid, and no vitreoretinal traction.

Scleral buckling maintains the retina in position, while the chorioretinal adhesion forms, by indenting the sclera with a sutured explant in the region of the retinal break. This also relieves vitreo-retinal traction and displaces subretinal fluid away from the retinal break. The success rate is 92%–94% in suitably selected cases. Complications include change in refractive error, diplopia due to fibrosis or involvement of extraocular muscles in the explant, extrusion of the explant, and possibly increased risk of proliferative vitreoretinopathy.

Pars plana vitrectomy allows relief of vitreo-retinal traction, internal drainage of subretinal fluid, if necessary by injection of perfluorocarbons or heavy liquids, and injection of air or expandable gas to maintain the retina in position, or injection of oil if longer-term tamponade or the retina is required. It is used if there are superior, posterior, or multiple retinal breaks, when visualization of the retina is inhibited, such as by vitreous hemorrhage, and if there is significant proliferative vitreoretinopathy. The introduction of 23 and 25 rather than 20 gauge vitrectomy instruments has made possible sutureless surgery, with the advantages of reduced operating time, less anterior segment inflammation, improved patient comfort, and more rapid recovery of vision, but greater risks of postoperative hypotony and endophthalmitis. The 25 gauge system is mainly recommended for macular surgery as there are reports of worse outcome with the 23 gauge system. Vitrectomy frequently induces or accelerates cataract formation and postoperative posturing may be required.

The visual results of surgery for rhegmatogenous retinal detachment primarily depend on the preoperative status of the macula. If the macula has been detached, recovery of central vision is usually incomplete. Thus, surgery should be performed urgently if the macula is still attached. Once the macula is detached, delay in surgery for up to 1 week does not adversely influence visual outcome.

2. TRACTION RETINAL DETACHMENT

Traction retinal detachment is most commonly due to proliferative diabetic retinopathy. It can also be associated with proliferative vitreoretinopathy, ROP, or ocular trauma. In comparison to rhegmatogenous retinal detachment, traction retinal detachment has a more concave surface and is likely to be more localized, usually not extending to the ora serrata. The tractional forces actively pull the sensory retina away from the underlying pigment epithelium toward the vitreous base. Traction is due to formation of vitreal, epiretinal, or subretinal membranes consisting of fibroblasts and glial and retinal pigment epithelial cells. Initially the detachment may be localized along the vascular arcades, but progression may spread to involve the midperipheral retina and the macula. Focal traction from cellular membranes can produce a retinal tear and lead to combined traction-rhegmatogenous retinal detachment.

Proliferative vitreoretinopathy is a complication of rhegmatogenous retinal detachment and is the most common cause of treatment failure.

▶ Treatment

Pars plana vitrectomy allows removal of the tractional elements followed by removal of the fibrotic membranes. Retinotomy and/or injection of perfluorocarbons or heavy liquids may be required to flatten the retina. Gas tamponade, silicone oil, or scleral buckling may be used.

3. SEROUS & HEMORRHAGIC RETINAL DETACHMENT

Serous and hemorrhagic retinal detachment occurs in the absence of either retinal break or vitreoretinal traction. They form as a result of accumulation of fluid beneath the sensory retina and are caused primarily by diseases of the retinal pigment epithelium and choroid. Degenerative, inflammatory, and infectious diseases, including the multiple causes of subretinal neovascularization, may be associated with serous retinal detachment and are described in an earlier section of this chapter. This type of detachment may also be associated with systemic vascular or inflammatory disease, or intraocular tumors (see Chapters 7 and 15).

▶ Lattice Degeneration

Lattice degeneration is the most common vitreoretinal degeneration. The estimated incidence in the general population is 6%–10%, of which up to 50% have bilateral disease. It is more commonly found in myopic eyes with some familial tendency. It produces localized round, oval, or linear areas of retinal thinning, with pigmentation, branching white lines, and whitish-yellow flecks, and firm vitreoretinal adhesions at its margins. Lattice degeneration results in retinal detachment in only a small percentage of affected eyes, but 20%–30% of eyes with retinal detachment have lattice degeneration. Strong family history of retinal detachment, retinal detachment in the fellow eye, high myopia, and aphakia require the patient to be informed of the risks of retinal detachment and the relevant symptoms but rarely warrant prophylactic treatment with cryosurgery or laser photocoagulation.

▶ Peripheral Chorioretinal Atrophy

Peripheral chorioretinal atrophy (paving stone degeneration) is a common benign chorioretinal degeneration found in nearly one-third of adult eyes. It is thought to be due to choroidal vascular insufficiency and is associated with peripheral vascular disease. The lesions appear as isolated or grouped, small, discrete, yellow-white areas with prominent underlying choroidal vessels and pigmented borders.

RETINOSCHISIS

Degenerative retinoschisis is a common acquired peripheral retinal disorder that is believed to develop from coalescence of preexisting peripheral cystoid degeneration. The cystic elevation is most commonly found in the inferotemporal quadrant, followed by the superotemporal quadrant. It develops into one of two forms, typical or reticular, although clinically the two are difficult to differentiate.

Typical degenerative retinoschisis forms a round or ovoid area of retinal splitting in the outer plexiform layer. Posterior extension and hole formation in the outer layer is uncommon and therefore poses low risk of progression to retinal detachment.

Reticular degenerative retinoschisis is characterized by round or oval areas of retinal splitting in the nerve fiber layer forming a bullous elevation of an extremely thin inner layer. Retinal holes occur in 23%, and posterior extension or progression to rhegmatogenous retinal detachment may occur and requires treatment.

▶ Natural History

Degenerative retinoschisis is present in about 4% of the population and is bilateral in approximately 30% of affected individuals. Spontaneous regression occurs in up to 9% of cases. Progression to retinal detachment occurs in up to 2%, with increased risk for those with a family history of retinal detachment. Whether cataract extraction increases the risk of retinal detachment is uncertain. Retinal detachment occurs in one of two ways. A hole in the outer but not the inner retinal layer allows the cystic fluid through the defect. This type is usually not or is only slowly progressive, and therefore a demarcation line forms. It rarely requires treatment. In the second type, holes form in both the inner and the outer layers. This causes collapse of the schisis and full thickness retinal detachment forms. Progression is quick, and treatment is required by pneumatic retinopexy, scleral buckle, or vitrectomy, depending on the size and position of the retinal holes and whether there is any proliferative vitreoretinopathy.

▶ Differentiation from Retinal Detachment

Retinoschisis causes an absolute scotoma in the visual field, whereas retinal detachment causes a relative scotoma. The cystic elevation of retinoschisis is usually smooth with no associated vitreous pigment cells. The surface of retinal detachment is usually corrugated with pigment cells in the vitreous ("tobacco dust"). Longstanding retinal detachment produces atrophy of the underlying retinal pigment epithelium, resulting in a pigmented demarcation line. As the retinal pigment epithelium is healthy in retinoschisis, there is no demarcation line. If argon laser photocoagulation to the outer retinal layer, aimed through an inner layer break, creates an equal gray response as in an adjacent area of normal retina, this is thought to be diagnostic of retinoschisis.

MACULAR HOLE

Macular hole is a full-thickness absence of the sensory retina in the macula. This disorder occurs most often in elderly patients and is typically unilateral. Biomicroscopy of the symptomatic eye reveals a full-thickness, round or oval, sharply defined hole measuring one-third disk diameter in the center of the macula, which may be surrounded by a ring detachment of the sensory retina (Figures 10–18 and 10–19). Visual acuity is impaired, and metamorphopsia and a central scotoma are present on Amsler grid testing. The Watzke-Allen slit beam test correlates well with the presence of a full-thickness macular hole. A slit beam of light positioned across the macular hole is described by the patient as being either thinned or broken.

Macular hole results from tangential traction in the epiretinal vitreous cortex. Its development is divided into four stages. In stage 1, occult hole, there is a yellow spot at the foveola with loss of the foveal reflex. This stage is reversible if a posterior vitreous detachment occurs. In stage 2, there is enlargement with a deep perifoveal yellow ring. In stage 3, the well-circumscribed full-thickness macular hole is surrounded by a cuff of subretinal fluid. In stage 4, the full-thickness hole is associated with a posterior vitreous detachment (see Chapter 9).

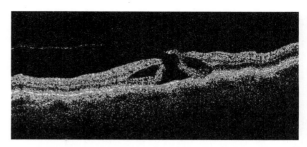

▲ **Figure 10–19.** OCT of macular hole showing edema as well as detachment of the surrounding cuff of retina.

OCT is the best method of diagnosis and assessment before and after surgery. Treatment to reattach the retina of the cuff surrounding the macular hole involves vitrectomy, separation of the posterior hyaloid, removal (peeling) of the retinal internal limiting membrane, and intravitreal injection of gas, which provides a scaffold for glial call repair. For a few days, patients may need to undertake face down posturing and to avoid sleeping on their back. Cataract due to the intraocular gas develops in most cases, but cataract surgery is often performed at the time of the macular hole surgery, if it has not been performed previously. Use of stains improves visualization of the internal limiting and has greatly improved the rate of closure of macular holes, but the potential toxicity of the stains is debated.

Anatomic closure of macular holes can be achieved in up to 90% of cases but does not always correlate with improvement of function. Twenty to twenty-five percent of patients with anatomically closed macular holes fail to achieve vision greater than 20/50, particularly in traumatic and chronic holes.

EPIMACULAR MEMBRANES

Fibrocellular membranes may proliferate on the retinal surface of the macula or peripheral retina. Contraction of these epimacular membranes (EMM) causes varying degrees of visual distortion, intraretinal edema, and degeneration of the underlying retina. Biomicroscopy usually shows wrinkling (striae) of the retina and distortion of retinal vessels (Figure 10–20). Rarely there may be retinal hemorrhages, cotton-wool spots, serous retinal detachment, and macular changes that simulate a macular `hole (pseudo-macular hole). Posterior vitreous detachment is nearly always present. OCT is valuable in the identification of EMM and to monitor for development of macular edema. Disorders associated with EMM include retinal tears with or without rhegmatogenous retinal detachment, vitreous inflammatory diseases, trauma, and a variety of retinal vascular diseases.

Visual acuity usually remains stable, suggesting that contraction of EMM is a short-lived and self-limited process. Surgical peeling of severe EMM can be performed to treat visual distortion, but recurrence occurs in some cases (see Chapter 9).

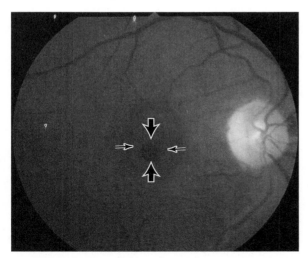

▲ **Figure 10–18.** Macular hole **(large arrows)** with surrounding sensory retinal detachment **(small arrows)**. See Figure 19–10.

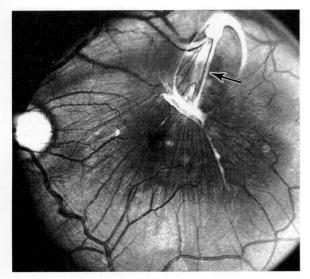

▲ **Figure 10–20.** EMM elevates retinal vessels **(arrow)** and produces retinal striae.

TRAUMATIC AND RELATED MACULOPATHIES

Blunt trauma to the anterior segment of the eye may cause a contrecoup injury to the retina, **commotio retinae.** The retinal whitening in the macular area usually clears completely; however, it may result in a pigmented retinal scar or macular hole with permanent impairment of central vision. Traumatic **choroidal rupture** (Figure 10–21) also may result in permanent visual loss.

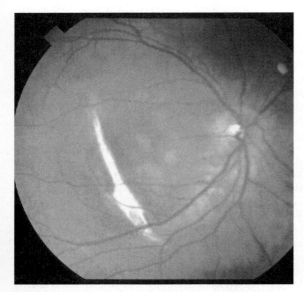

▲ **Figure 10–21.** White sclera visible through a choroidal rupture.

Purtscher retinopathy, characterized by bilateral, multiple patches of superficial retinal whitening and hemorrhages, occurs after severe compression injury to the head or trunk. **Terson syndrome,** manifesting as retinal, preretinal, or vitreous hemorrhage, occurs in approximately 20% of patients with intracranial hemorrhage and elevated intracranial pressure, particularly being associated with subarachnoid hemorrhage due to rupture of intracranial aneurysm. **Solar retinopathy,** manifesting as bilateral sharply demarcated and often irregularly shaped partial-thickness hole or depression in the center of the fovea, occurs after sun-gazing.

CENTRAL SEROUS CHORIORETINOPATHY

Central serous chorioretinopathy (CSR) is characterized by serous detachment of the sensory retina due to multi-focal areas of hyperpermeability of the choroidal vessels and alteration in the pumping function of the retinal pigment epithelium. It affects young to middle-aged men and is associated with type A personality, chronic steroid use, and stress. Presentation is with sudden onset of blurred vision, micropsia, metamorphopsia, and central scotoma. Visual acuity is often only moderately decreased and may be improved to near-normal with a small hyperopic correction.

Fundal examination reveals a round or oval area of retinal elevation, variable in size and position, but usually in the macula (Figure 10–22). There may be central yellowish-gray spots representing subretinal exudates. Occasionally there is a serous retinal pigment epithelial detachment in the superior portion. There may be evidence of previous episodes in the form of mild atrophic retinal pigment epithelial lesions. Diagnosis is most easily confirmed on OCT. Approximately 80% of eyes with CSR undergo spontaneous resorption and recovery of normal visual acuity within 6 months after the onset of symptoms. However, despite normal acuity, many patients have a mild permanent visual defect, such as a

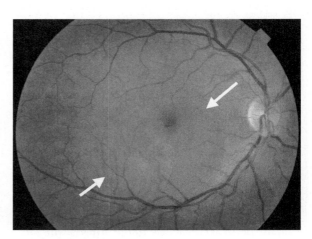

▲ **Figure 10–22.** CSR showing a circular central retinal elevation **(arrows)**.

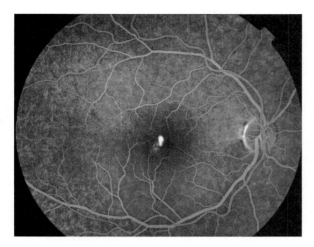

▲ **Figure 10-23.** Early fluorescein angiogram showing a smokestack configuration of dye leakage in CSR.

decrease in color sensitivity, micropsia, or relative scotoma. Twenty to thirty percent of patients will have one or more recurrence of the disease. Complications, including subretinal neovascularization and chronic CME, have been described in patients with frequent and prolonged serous detachments.

Various patterns of abnormality are seen on fluorescein angiography, of which the most characteristic is a "smokestack" configuration of fluorescein dye leaking from the choriocapillaris followed by accumulation below the retinal pigment epithelium or sensory retina (Figures 10–23 and 10–24). Argon laser photocoagulation to the site of leak

significantly shortens the duration of the sensory detachment with quicker recovery of central vision, but there is no evidence that prompt photocoagulation improves final visual outcome. It is not recommended for lesions close to central fixation because scar formation may cause permanent impairment of vision. For such lesions, PDT, including a low dose (fluence) technique, and micropulse laser have produced encouraging results without the scarring associated with conventional laser treatment. Treatment outcomes are less favorable for any CSR accompanied by retinal pigment epithelial detachment. In all cases, the duration and location of disease, the condition of the fellow eye, and occupational visual requirements are important considerations in determining treatment recommendations.

MACULAR EDEMA

Retinal edema involving the macula may be due to intraocular inflammatory disease, retinal vascular disease, epimacular membrane, intraocular surgery, inherited or acquired retinal degeneration, or drug therapy, or it may be idiopathic. It may be diffuse when nonlocalized intraretinal fluid results in thickening of the macula. Focal macular edema, due to fluid accumulation in honeycomb-like spaces of the outer plexiform and inner nuclear layers, is known as **cystoid macular edema (CME).** It has a characteristic appearance on OCT, which is a good noninvasive method of monitoring response to treatment (Figure 10–25). On fluorescein angiography, fluorescein dye leaks from the perifoveal retinal capillaries and peripapillary region, accumulating in a flower-petal pattern around the fovea (Figure 10–26).

The most frequent cause of CME is cataract surgery, especially if the surgery was complicated or prolonged. Complete posterior vitreous detachment seems to provide some protection against its development. After routine phacoemulsification surgery, CME is detectable on fluorescein angiography in approximately 25% of eyes and on clinical examination in about 2%. It usually manifests at 4–12 weeks postoperatively, but in some instances its onset may be delayed for months or years. Many patients with CME of less than 6 months' duration have self-limited leakage that resolves without treatment. Topical steroid and/or nonsteroidal anti-inflammatory therapy may accelerate improvement in visual acuity in patients

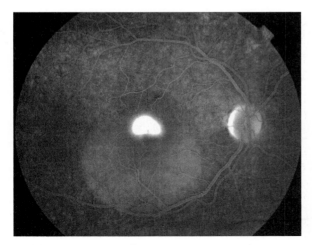

▲ **Figure 10-24.** Late fluorescein angiogram showing accumulation of dye in the serous detachment of CSR.

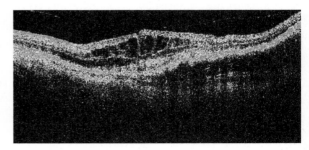

▲ **Figure 10-25.** OCT of CME.

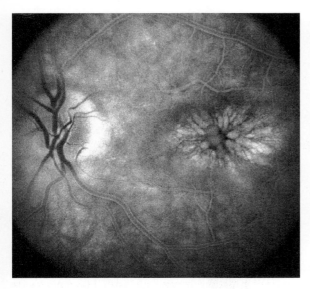

▲ **Figure 10–26.** Flower-petal pattern of fluorescein dye in a patient with CME after cataract surgery.

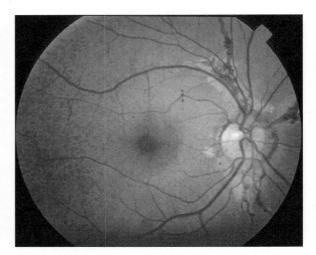

▲ **Figure 10–27.** Multiple angioid streaks extending from the optic nerve.

with chronic postoperative macular edema. In resistant cases, treatment with orbital floor or intravitreal triamcinolone may be beneficial. If there is vitreous traction, early YAG laser vitreolysis (see Chapter 23) or vitrectomy should be considered. If an intraocular lens implant is the cause of postoperative macular edema, due to its design, positioning, or inadequate fixation, removal of the lens implant should be considered.

ANGIOID STREAKS

Angioid streaks appear as irregular, jagged tapering lines that radiate from the peripapillary retina into the macula and peripheral fundus (Figure 10–27). The streaks represent linear, crack-like dehiscence in Bruch's membrane. The lesions are rarely noted in children and probably develop in the second or third decade of life. Early in the disease, the streaks are sharply outlined and red-orange or brown. Subsequent fibrovascular tissue growth may partially or totally obscure the streak margins.

Nearly 50% of patients with angioid streaks have an associated systemic disease, including pseudoxanthoma elasticum due to mutations in the recessive ABCC6 gene, Paget disease of bone, Ehlers–Danlos syndrome, hemoglobinopathy, or a hemolytic disorder. Complications that can result in significant visual impairment include direct involvement of the fovea, choroidal neovascularization, and traumatic choroidal rupture. Patients with angioid streaks should be warned of the potential risk of choroidal rupture from even relatively mild eye trauma.

Angioid streaks should be suspected in any patient who presents with choroidal neovascularization and no or few drusen in the fellow eye.

▶ Treatment

Retinal laser photocoagulation may be used on extrafoveal neovascular membranes, but recurrence is frequent and likely to occur on the foveal side of the resultant scar. PDT is unable to prevent the progression of the disease in most patients, and prophylactic treatment of angioid streaks before subretinal neovascularization develops is not recommended. Anti-VEGF therapy shows promising results, but information is limited to case reports.

INFLAMMATORY DISEASES AFFECTING THE RETINA, RETINAL PIGMENT EPITHELIUM, AND CHOROID

▶ Presumed Ocular Histoplasmosis Syndrome (POHS)

POHS is characterized by serous and hemorrhagic detachments of the macula due to subretinal neovascularization, associated with multiple peripheral atrophic chorioretinal scars (histo spots) and peripapillary chorioretinal scarring (see Chapter 7) in the absence of vitreal inflammation. It usually occurs in healthy patients between the third and sixth decades of life, and the scars are probably caused by an antecedent subclinical systemic infection with *Histoplasma capsulatum*. However, only 3% of people with histoplasmosis develop histo spots, which usually remain quiescent, and only 5% of people with histo spots develop choroidal neovascularization. The visual prognosis depends on the proximity of the neovascular membrane to the center of the fovea. If it extends inside the foveal avascular zone, only 15% of eyes will retain 20/40 vision. There is a significant risk of choroidal neovascularization in the fellow eye, and patients should be instructed in the frequent use of an Amsler grid and the importance of prompt examination when abnormalities are detected.

▶ Treatment

Treatment options are similar to those for choroidal neovascularization due to AMD. Intravitreal injections have additional risks in younger patients because their posterior vitreous has not detached, but intravitreal bevacizumab produces significant improvement in vision at 1 year. Surgical removal of subfoveal membranes has been disappointing, with stabilization of vision occurring only in those with preoperative visual acuity worse than 20/100.

▶ Acute Multifocal Posterior Placoid Pigment Epitheliopathy (AMPPPE)

AMPPPE typically affects healthy young patients who develop rapidly progressive bilateral vision loss in association with multifocal flat gray-white subretinal lesions involving the pigment epithelium (Figure 10–28). The cause is unknown, but it is associated with a preceding viral illness. The characteristic feature of the disease is the rapid resolution of the fundus lesions and a delayed return of visual acuity to near-normal levels. Although the prognosis for visual recovery in this acute self-limited disease is good, many patients will identify small residual paracentral scotomas when carefully tested. The prognosis in atypical cases, such as unilateral disease or older presentation, is more guarded. Extensive pigmentary changes resulting from

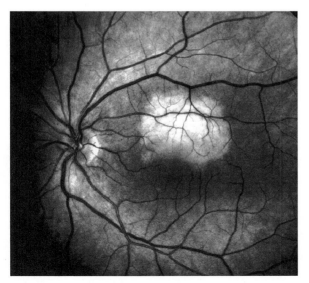

▲ **Figure 10–28.** Macular lesion of acute multifocal posterior placoid pigment epitheliopathy.

AMPPPE may mimic widespread retinal degeneration, but the clinical history and normal electro-physiologic findings should lead to the correct diagnosis. Treatments include immunosuppressants, either local or systemic, the latter for severe cases including the rare cases associated with central nervous system disease, PDT, and anti-VEGF therapy.

▶ Serpiginous (Geographic Helicoid Peripapillary) Choroidopathy

This is a chronic progressive and recurrent inflammatory disease of the retinal pigment epithelium, choriocapillaris, and choroid. It characteristically involves the juxtapapillary retina and extends radially to involve the macula and peripheral retina. Unlike AMPPPE, the affected areas are contiguous. Recurrence is the norm. Patients tend to be older than those of AMPPPE. The active stage manifests itself as sharply demarcated gray-yellow lesions with irregular borders that appear to involve the pigment epithelium and choriocapillaris. Vitritis, anterior uveitis, and choroidal neovascularization may occur. Involvement is usually bilateral, and the cause is unknown. The natural history of this indolent inflammatory disease is variable and may correlate with the presence of disease in the fellow eye. Local, including intravitreal, or systemic corticosteroid treatment may be of benefit when active inflammation is present. Determination of optimal treatment of choroidal neovascularization is hampered by the rarity of cases.

▶ Birdshot Retinochoroidopathy (Vitiliginous Chorioretinitis)

This is a syndrome characterized by diffuse cream-colored patches at the level of the pigment epithelium and choroid, retinal vasculitis associated with CME, and vitritis. Strong association with a subtype of HLA-A29 and other features suggest that genetic predisposition and retinal autoimmunity play a role in its manifestations. The course of the disease is that of exacerbation and remission with variable visual outcomes. Visual loss may be due to chronic CME, optic atrophy, macular scarring, or choroidal neovascularization. Electroretinography is useful for diagnosis and monitoring disease progression and response to treatment. Treatment with corticosteroids alone does not seem to be effective. Other immunosuppressants may be beneficial.

▶ Acute Macular Neuroretinopathy (AMN)

AMN is characterized by the acute onset of paracentral scotomas and mild visual acuity loss accompanied by wedge-shaped parafoveal retinal lesions in the deep sensory retina of one or both eyes. The macular lesions are subtle, reddish-brown, and best seen with a red-free light. The patients are usually young adults with a history of acute viral illness. While the retinal lesions may fade, the scotomas tend to persist and remain symptomatic.

▶ Multiple Evanescent White Dot Syndrome (MEWDS)

MEWDS is an acute and self-limited unilateral disease that affects mainly young women and is characterized clinically by multiple white dots at the level of the pigment epithelium, vitreous cells, and transient electroretinographic abnormalities. The cause is unknown. There is no evidence of associated systemic disease. The retinal lesions gradually regress in a matter of weeks, leaving only minor retinal pigment epithelial defects. Occasionally it progresses to become **acute zonal occult outer retinopathy (AZOOR),** with positive visual phenomena, symptomatic visual field impairment, typically manifesting as enlarged blind spots, that may be progressive, and angiographic, autofluorescence, and electrophysiological evidence of retinal dysfunction.

There seems to be overlap between AZOOR, MEWDS, AMN, birdshot chorioretinopathy, serpiginous choroidopathy, AMPPE, and the entities of multifocal choroiditis (MFC), diffuse subretinal fibrosis syndrome, and punctate inner choroidopathy (PIC), each being a different manifestation of similar pathophysiological processes, such that the umbrella term **white dot syndromes** has been suggested. The treatment options for all of them include immunosuppressants, either topical or systemic, and PDT or anti-VEGF therapy if there is choroidal neovascularization.

MACULAR DYSTROPHIES

Macular dystrophies are genetically determined although not necessarily evident at birth. They are not necessarily associated with systemic disease. Usually the disorder is restricted to the macula with symmetrical involvement. In the early stages of some macular dystrophies, visual acuity is reduced but the macular changes are subtle or not visible clinically, such that the patient's symptoms may be dismissed as spurious. Conversely, in other macular dystrophies, the fundoscopic changes are very striking when the patient is still asymptomatic. One method of classifying the more common macular dystrophies is according to which layers of the retina are presumed to be involved (Table 10–2).

Table 10–2. Anatomic Classification of Macular Dystrophies

Inner retina
X-linked juvenile retinoschisis
Photoreceptors
Cone-rod dystrophy
Retinal pigment epithelium
Stargardt disease
Best disease

▶ X-Linked Juvenile Retinoschisis

This X-linked recessively inherited disease affects young males and is characterized by a macular lesion called "foveal schisis." On slitlamp examination, foveal schisis appears as small superficial retinal cysts arranged in a stellate pattern accompanied by radial striae centered in the foveal area (Figure 10–29). The disorder is slowly progressive. Visual acuity begins to fall during the middle of the teenage years, reducing to between 20/40 and 20/200 as the disease progresses. Fifty percent of patients have peripheral retinoschisis with peripheral visual field abnormalities. The posterior pole appears normal on fluorescein angiography, assisting differentiation from CME. X-linked retinoschisis is thought to be due to Muller cell dysfunction. There is a negative electroretinogram (ERG) (normal a-wave amplitude with reduced b-wave amplitude), which is typical of disorders affecting the inner retina leaving the photoreceptor cells intact. Female carriers have normal ERGs.

The main differential diagnosis for foveal schisis is enhanced S-Cone (Goldmann-Favre) syndrome, which is an autosomal recessive condition with extinguished ERG and typical peripheral disk-like pigmentation (Figure 10–30).

The genetic abnormality in X-linked juvenile retinoschisis is a mutation in the RS1 gene, which codes for a retina-specific extracellular protein (retinoschisin), secreted by photoreceptors but involved in cell–cell interactions and cellular adhesion in the inner retina. Carriers can be identified by DNA analysis.

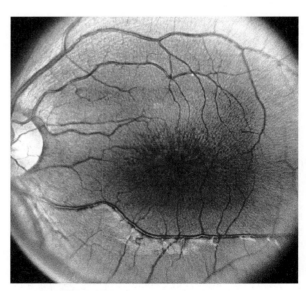

▲ **Figure 10–29.** X-linked juvenile retinoschisis with typical superficial retinal cysts in the fovea.

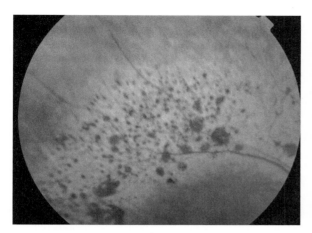

▲ **Figure 10–30.** Enhanced S-cone syndrome showing typical disk-like pigmentation around the vascular arcades.

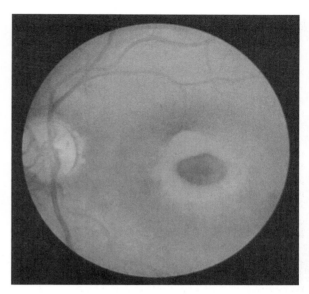

▲ **Figure 10–31.** Cone dystrophy with bull's-eye pattern of macular depigmentation.

▶ Cone-Rod Dystrophies

The cone-rod dystrophies constitute a relatively rare group of disorders that may be regarded as a single entity showing variable expressivity. Most cases are recessive, with mutation of the ABCA4 gene being the most common known cause, but autosomal dominant inheritance has also been recorded. There is predominant involvement of cone photoreceptors, with progressive color vision defects and loss of visual acuity. Photophobia is a common early symptom.

Fundal appearance varies greatly. In many patients, it is normal at initial presentation. There may be optic nerve pallor with no obvious macular changes, leading to misdiagnosis of optic nerve disease. The characteristic bilateral, symmetric bull's-eye pattern of macular depigmentation, visualized on fluorescein angiography as a zone of hyperfluorescence surrounding a central nonfluorescent spot, is relatively uncommon (Figure 10–31). If it occurs, chloroquine retinopathy has to be excluded. Fundus autofluorescence is becoming the preferred method of retinal imaging for both diagnosis and monitoring. Electroretinography shows marked loss of cone function and slight to moderate loss of rod function. It is essential for diagnosis and prognosis.

▶ Stargardt Disease/Fundus Flavimaculatus

Stargardt disease is by far the most common macular dystrophy. It is an autosomal recessive disorder with mutations in the ABCA4 (retina-specific ATP-binding cassette transporter) gene, which are also the most common known cause of cone-rod dystrophies (see above).

Stargardt disease is associated with fundus flavimaculatus, which is characterized by multiple yellow-white fleck lesions of variable size and shape, confined to the retinal pigment epithelium (Figure 10–32). The different phenotypes can be partly explained by different mutations in the same genes.

Severely pathogenic mutations tend to cause cone-rod dystrophies, moderately pathogenic mutations fundus flavimaculatus, and mildly pathogenic mutations Stargardt disease. The carrier rate for ABCA4 gene mutations is about 1 in 100.

Stargardt disease typically presents before age 15 with reduced central vision. About one-third of patients presents in the first decade of life, one-third in the second decade of life, and one-third over 20 years of age. Initially there is no macular abnormality clinically, but subsequently there develops a bronze metal appearance together with mid-peripheral

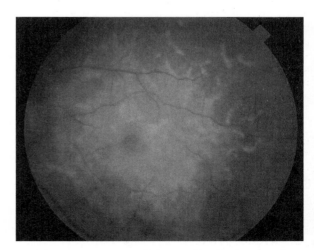

▲ **Figure 10–32.** Stargardt disease/fundus flavimaculatus with multiple irregular fleck lesions involving the macula.

retinal flecks, like those seen in fundus flavimaculatus. Fundus autofluorescence shows a range of abnormalities. Pattern ERG is completely extinguished, even when central vision is good. The full-field ERG is usually normal. Once visual acuity has dropped to 20/40, it will decline to 20/200 in 5 years. Gene mutations can be detected in 50%–75% of patients.

There is a dominant form of Stargardt disease, which is rare and has a genetic mutation in ELOVL4 gene.

Patients with fundus flavimaculatus present later than patients with Stargardt disease. They have retinal flecks distributed over the whole of the posterior pole of each eye. Central vision tends to be preserved until after 40 years of age, but full-field ERG changes are more common and are important for predicting prognosis.

▶ Best Disease (Juvenile-Onset Vitelliform Dystrophy)

Best disease is an autosomal dominant disorder with variable penetrance and expressivity. Onset is usually in childhood. The fundoscopic appearance is variable and ranges from a mild pigmentary disturbance within the fovea to the typical vitelliform or "egg yoke" lesion located in the central macula (Figure 10–33). This characteristic cyst-like lesion is gener-

ally quite round and well demarcated and contains homogeneous opaque yellow material lying at the apparent level of the retinal pigment epithelium. The "egg yoke" may degenerate and be associated with subretinal neovascularization, subretinal hemorrhage, and extensive macular scarring. Visual acuity often remains good, and the ERG is normal. An abnormal electro-oculogram (EOG) is the hallmark of the disease. The genetic abnormality is a mutation in the BEST1 (VMD2) gene, which encodes a transmembrane calcium-sensitive chloride channel (bestrophin) expressed in retinal pigment epithelium.

HEREDITARY RETINAL DEGENERATIONS

▶ Retinitis Pigmentosa

Retinitis pigmentosa is a group of heterogeneous hereditary retinal degenerations characterized by progressive dysfunction of the photoreceptors, associated with progressive cell loss and eventual atrophy of several retinal layers. Inheritance of the typical form can be autosomal recessive, autosomal dominant, or X-linked recessive. Digenic and mitochondrial inheritance may also be responsible.

The hallmark symptoms of retinitis pigmentosa are night blindness (nyctalopia) and gradually progressive peripheral visual field loss as a result of increasing and coalescing ring scotomas. The most characteristic fundoscopic findings are attenuated retinal arterioles, waxy pale optic disk, mottling of the retinal pigment epithelium, and peripheral retinal pigment clumping, referred to as "bone-spicule formation" (Figure 10–34). Although retinitis

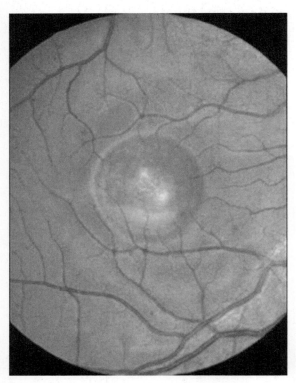

▲ **Figure 10–33.** Best disease with a well-demarcated cyst-like macular lesion.

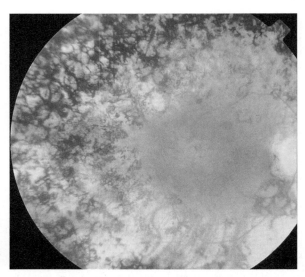

▲ **Figure 10–34.** Retinitis pigmentosa with arteriolar narrowing and peripheral retinal pigment clumping.

pigmentosa is a generalized photoreceptor disorder, in most cases rod function is more severely affected, predominantly leading to poor scotopic vision. The ERG usually shows either markedly reduced or absent retinal function. The EOG lacks the usual light rise.

There has been rapid progress in identification of mutations in retinitis pigmentosa. Relevant genes identified so far can be found on the Retnet website (http://www.sph.uth.tmc.edu/Retnet/). Patients should be referred to specialized centers for genetic counseling and selective mutation analysis. Genetic analysis is useful to identify female carriers in families with X-linked disease and to diagnose dominant disease. In recessive disease, specific features are needed for genetic analysis to be worthwhile.

Fundus Albipunctatus/Retinitis Punctata Albescens

Fundus albipunctatus is an autosomal recessive nonprogressive dystrophy characterized by a myriad of discrete small white dots at the level of the pigment epithelium sprinkled about the posterior pole and midperiphery of the retina. Patients are night-blind with normal visual acuity, normal visual fields, and normal color vision. While the ERG and EOG are usually normal, dark adaptation thresholds are markedly elevated. Retinitis punctata albescens is the less common progressive variant of this dystrophy. Both conditions are extremely rare.

Leber Congenital Amaurosis

Leber congenital amaurosis (LCA) is an autosomal recessive disorder of rods and cones. It presents as a triad of severe visual impairment or blindness beginning in the first year of life, nystagmus, and generalized retinal dystrophy. The fundoscopic findings are variable; most patients show either a normal appearance or only subtle retinal pigment epithelial granularity and mild vessel attenuation. A markedly reduced or absent ERG indicates generalized photoreceptor dysfunction, and in infants this is the only method by which an absolute diagnosis can be made.

There may be ocular manifestations only (pure LCA), or there may be nonocular abnormalities, including mental retardation, oculodigital reflex (eye poking), seizures, and renal or muscular abnormalities. The division between these entities is unclear, and they are best classified on a genetic basis. Nine causal genes have been identified, accounting for 65% of cases. The RPE65 gene mutation has been extensively investigated, including successful gene therapy in dogs, the most famous of which is Lancelot, suggesting that subretinal delivery of the RPE65 vector in human subjects is feasible. Project 3000 aims to identify and perform genetic testing on all cases of LCA in the United States. Human clinical trials of gene therapy have started in England and the United States.

Gyrate Atrophy

Gyrate atrophy is an autosomal recessive disorder due to reduced activity of ornithine aminotransferase (OAT), a mitochondrial matrix enzyme that catalyzes several amino acid pathways, resulting in raised serum ornithine. The OAT gene has been mapped to chromosome 10. The incidence of this disorder is relatively high in Finland, and the ophthalmologic features are the most prominent manifestations of the disease. Patients initially present with myopia and then develop nyctalopia within the first decade of life, followed by progressive loss of peripheral visual field. Characteristic sharply demarcated circular areas of chorioretinal atrophy develop in the midperiphery of the fundus during the teenage years and become confluent with macular involvement late in the course of the disease. The ERG is decreased or absent, and the EOG is reduced.

Reduction in dietary intake of arginine has been shown to slow progression of the disease. It is most effective when commenced during childhood. Other treatments include pyridoxine supplementation and supplemental dietary lysine.

COLOR VISION DEFECTS

Cone photoreceptors are responsible for color vision, visual pigments (opsins) in their outer segments absorbing light of wavelengths between 400 and 700 nm. Spectral sensitivity studies have identified blue, green, and red cone photoreceptors. A minimal requirement for color (hue) discrimination is the presence of at least two kinds of cone photopigment (opsin), and normal color vision requires the presence of all three (trichromacy). The red and green cone opsins are encoded by adjacent genes on the X-chromosome. The blue cone opsin is encoded on chromosome 7. Color vision testing is described in Chapter 2.

Color vision defects are either congenital (inherited) or acquired. Acquired color vision defects vary in type and severity, depending on the location and source of the ocular pathology, and frequently affect one eye more than the other. Males and females are equally affected.

Congenital color vision defects are constant in type and severity throughout life and affect both eyes equally. They are more common in men than women. The most common congenital color vision defect, red-green color deficiency, is a form of dichromacy, with only two out of three cone opsins functioning normally. It results from mutation in the gene encoding for either the red (**protanopia**) or green (**deuteranopia**) cone opsin. It is X-linked recessive and affects 8% of males and 0.5% of females. Although color discrimination is abnormal, visual acuity is normal. The third type of dichromacy, **tritanopia,** in which there is loss of blue-yellow discrimination due to defect in the blue cone opsin, is a rare autosomal dominant condition resulting from a mutation on chromosome 7.

There are two forms of monochromacy. Although both leave the affected individual completely without color discrimination (achromatopsia), they are two quite separate entities. In the less common **cone monochromacy** (1 in 100,000), visual acuity is normal but there is no hue discrimination. Only one type of cone photoreceptor is present. It is usually due to **blue cone monochromacy,** an X-linked recessive condition resulting from mutations in the genes encoding for both red and green cone opsins. In **rod monochromacy** (1 in 30,000), an autosomal recessive condition caused by mutations in genes encoding proteins of the photoreceptor cation channel or cone transducin, there are no functioning cones, resulting in achromatic vision, low visual acuity, photophobia, and nystagmus.

10.2. Retinal Tumors
James J. Augsburger, MD, and Zélia M. Corrêa, MD, PhD

This section presents an overview of the most common and most important neoplasms, hamartomas, and choristomas of the retina and ciliary body epithelia. Neoplastic lesions of the ciliary body as a component of the uveal tract (see Chapter 7), and non-neoplastic disorders (eg, persistent hyperplastic primary vitreous, ocular toxocariasis, and pars planitis) that can simulate retinoblastoma and other retinal tumors are discussed in other parts of this book.

BENIGN RETINAL TUMORS

Benign neoplasms are acquired tumors of cells that are atypical but not sufficient to be classified as malignant. They may enlarge slowly but have little or no invasive potential and no metastatic capability. **Hamartomas** are congenital tumors composed of normal or near normal cells and tissues for the anatomic site but in excessive amounts. **Choristomas** are congenital tumors consisting of normal cells and tissue elements but not occurring normally at the anatomic site.

▶ Retinal Astrocytoma

Retinal astrocytoma (sometimes termed "retinal astrocytic hamartoma" despite the lesion being rarely present at birth or identified in the neonatal period) is an acquired benign neoplasm that arises from the astrocytes within the retinal nerve fiber layer. It may be part of an inheritable syndrome, usually tuberous sclerosis, or a non-inherited isolated entity. Frequently in tuberous sclerosis there are multifocal and bilateral lesions, whereas non-syndromic retinal astrocytomas are almost exclusively unilateral and unifocal.

Retinal astrocytomas usually become manifested during the first or second decade of life. When small, they appear as ill-defined translucent lesions of the inner retina (opalescent patches). Slightly larger lesions appear as discrete, opaque white nodules of the inner retina (Figure 10–35). Occasional larger, more mature lesions exhibit an irregular nodular character that has been likened to a "white mulberry". Retinal astrocytomas identified early in life typically enlarge slightly

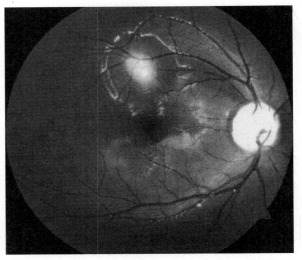

▲ **Figure 10–35.** Solitary retinal astrocytoma superior to right fovea in an 11-year-old boy with tuberous sclerosis.

during follow-up, but most lesions in individuals over the age of 25 years remain stable. Rarely, a retinal astrocytoma of either the syndromic or isolated variety undergoes substantial progressive enlargement associated with malignant transformation. Generally, no treatment is indicated unless substantial enlargement is documented.

▶ Retinal Capillary Hemangioma (von Hippel tumor)

Retinal capillary hemangioma is an acquired benign neoplasm of the retina, composed of neural retinal cells transformed into poorly differentiated small cells with prominent nuclei and little cytoplasm by a mutation of both alleles of the VHL gene, which is located on the short arm of chromosome 3 (p25.5 region). It may be part of a syndrome (von Hippel–Lindau disease, VHL), when there are likely to be multifocal and bilateral lesions, or an isolated entity, when

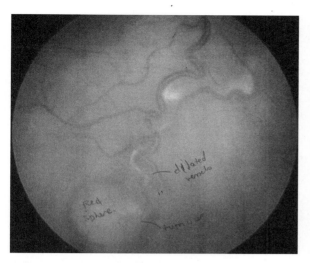

▲ **Figure 10–36.** Classic retinal capillary hemangioma inferiorly. The tumor is fed and drained by dilated tortuous retinal blood vessels. Note intraretinal and subretinal exudates along the blood vessels. See color insert.

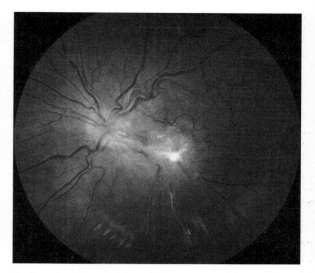

▲ **Figure 10–37.** Combined hamartoma of the retina involving the right macula. Tumor exhibits deep gray color due to retinal pigment epithelial involvement, superficial white color due to retinal gliosis, and angulated retinal blood vessels with the lesion.

there is likely to be a solitary, unilateral lesion. In response to angiogenic factor(s) produced by its cells, the tumor attracts a dense collection of blood vessels that gives it the appearance of an intraretinal red sphere (hence the name "hemangioma") supplied by a dilated, tortuous retinal arteriole and drained by a dilated, tortuous retinal venule (Figure 10–36). The tumor blood vessels tend to be leaky, resulting in accumulation of intraretinal edema and exudates, and subretinal fluid and exudates. As the tumor enlarges, the exudative retinal detachment usually increases in extent and becomes associated with substantial vitreoretinal fibrosis resulting in additional tractional retinal detachment. Tumors of this type occur anywhere in the fundus from the optic disc to the peripheral retina but most frequently in the equatorial or post-equatorial region. They are not present at birth, frequently starting to develop during the teenage years. Treatment of small von Hippel tumors is usually by laser photocoagulation or cryotherapy. Larger lesions frequently require vitreoretinal surgery to address the associated exudative-tractional retinal detachment. Depending on the size and location of the retinal tumors and extent of exudative-tractional retinal detachment when the lesions are first detected, vision in treated eyes can range from excellent to no perception of light.

Combined Hamartoma of the Retina

Combined hamartoma of the retina is a benign congenital malformation composed of overgrown and disorganized normal retinal components with a characteristic clinical appearance. The three typical features are deep gray color due to

involvement of retinal pigment epithelium, superficial white "gliosis", and prominent angulated retinal blood vessels within the lesion (Figure 10–37). The lesion is usually adjacent to or surrounding the optic nerve (juxta- or circumpapillary) and is virtually always unifocal and unilateral. If the macula is involved, usually vision is impaired. Generally no treatment is indicated but there is a frequent association with neurofibromatosis (see Chapter 14), usually type 2 so affected children may need to be screened for vestibular schwannoma.

Congenital Hypertrophy of the Retinal Pigment Epithelium (CHRPE)

CHRPE is a benign focal congenital malformation of the retinal pigment epithelium characterized pathologically by increased size (hypertrophy) and increased number (hyperplasia) of retinal pigment epithelial cells in a localized region of the fundus. The abnormal RPE cells tend to be densely packed with large melanin granules. The lesion is always present at birth but is frequently not identified until late childhood or adulthood. CHRPE occurs in three distinct clinical patterns.

Typical unifocal CHRPE appears as a nummular flat black to dark gray lesion, most frequently in the peripheral fundus (Figure 10–38). It ranges in size from a tiny dot of black pigment to a geographic lesion 5 mm or more in diameter, with well-defined smooth margins and no detachment of the overlying retina. With time the lesion may undergo focal or diffuse depigmentation. Typical unifocal CHRPE

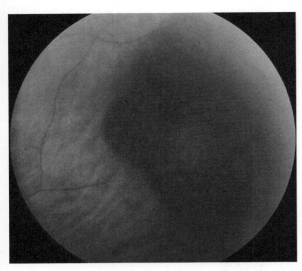

▲ **Figure 10–38.** Typical unifocal peripheral CHRPE. In spite of the appearance of the lesion suggesting considerable thickness, B-scan ultrasonography showed no measurable thickness.

rarely has been noted to give rise to an adenoma or adenocarcinoma of the retinal pigment epithelium, so periodic monitoring for nodular change is advisable.

The **typical multifocal clustered** variety of CHRPE (grouped pigmentation of the retina, retinal "bear tracks"), is characterized by multiple small to intermediate size, oval to cigar-shaped, CHRPE lesions clustered in one region of the fundus of one eye (Figure 10–39). The lesions do not affect

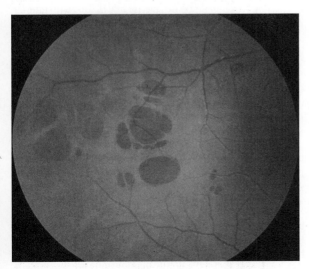

▲ **Figure 10–39.** Typical unilateral clustered CHRPE, commonly referred to as "bear tracks".

vision and do not appear to have any potential to give rise to RPE neoplasms.

The **atypical multifocal bilateral non-clustered** variety of CHRPE tends to occur in individuals with Gardner's syndrome and related familial colonic polyposis–carcinoma disorders. The outline of the individual lesions tends to be angulated, sometimes having areas of depigmentation along its margin. The lesions are scattered across the fundus, not clustered in a single area. The atypical multifocal bilateral non-clustered variety of CHRPE has not been reported to give rise to RPE neoplasms, but affected individuals need to be screened for polyps and cancer of the colon, and possibly be advised to undergo prophylactic colectomy.

▶ Benign Adenoma of the Non-Pigmented Ciliary Epithelium (Fuchs Adenoma)

This is an acquired benign neoplasm of the non-pigmented ciliary body epithelium, essentially a neuroepithelial adenoma. Usually detected in middle aged or older individuals (women more than men), it is unilateral and unifocal in almost all affected persons. It may become large enough to be visible on peripheral fundus examination or during cataract surgery, but in many cases is noted only at autopsy. Once detected, the tumor tends to enlarge very slowly in most cases. If such a lesion is suspected and shows progression during follow-up, transscleral surgical excision can be performed. As tumors of this type clinically cannot be distinguished reliably from ciliary body melanomas, enucleation is still performed occasionally.

RETINAL TUMORS OF INTERMEDIATE CHARACTER

These tumors are categorized as neoplasms of borderline malignancy because clinically they cannot be categorized reliably as benign or malignant. If biopsy is performed, pathologic studies may reveal benign cells, malignant cells, or cells deemed to be borderline even by cytologic criteria.

▶ Retinoma

Retinoma is a benign, spontaneously arrested form of retinoblastoma (see below). Classified pathologically as a "retinocytoma", it consists of benign appearing neuroepithelial cells. Arising within the first few years of life, it may not be detected until older childhood or even adulthood. Usually unilateral and unifocal, bilateral multifocal disease has been reported and retinomas are occasionally encountered on pathological examination of eyes enucleated for active retinoblastoma.

Retinoma appears as an opalescent or off-white retinal tumor of limited size, usually less than 7 mm in diameter and less than 2 mm in thickness (Figure 10–40). The tumor usually exhibits few, if any, fine blood vessels on its surface and is not associated with any dilation or tortuosity of large

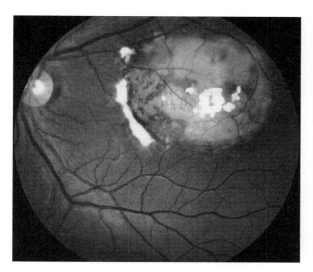

▲ **Figure 10–40.** Macular retinoma in a man whose son had bilateral retinoblastoma. This oval fundus lesion exhibits paracentral calcification, central translucency, extensive clumping of the retinal pigment epithelium, and chorioretinal atrophy along its nasal margin.

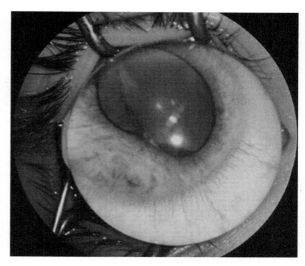

▲ **Figure 10–41.** Congenital medulloepithelioma of the ciliary body and peripheral iris. Note the associated lens coloboma due to the tumor's effect on the zonule in its meridian.

caliber afferent and efferent retinal blood vessels. Limited chorioretinal atrophy is evident along the margins of some lesions, and foci of calcification are frequently present. There is no retinal detachment and the overlying vitreous is normal.

Retinoma has a tendency to transform into active retinoblastoma later in life, so affected individuals probably should be examined at least twice yearly for life for evidence of malignant transformation.

▶ Medulloepithelioma

Medulloepithelioma is a benign to malignant intraocular neoplasm that usually arises from the primitive neuroepithelium of the ciliary body during embryologic development. Rare cases have arisen within the retina and optic disc, but the cells of origin in such cases are uncertain. Intraocular medulloepithelioma is a unilateral, unifocal tumor. Because the tumor arises from immature neuroepithelial cells, the vast majority of cases occur in children less than 10 years old. Typical medulloepithelioma is characterized by cords of primitive neuroepithelial cells and multiple epithelial lined cysts, the fluid within them having the same staining characteristics as vitreous. The tumor cells tend to be rather bland in most cases, and malignancy of such tumors is generally defined by the presence and extent of invasion of adjacent tissues histopathologically. Occasionally medulloepitheliomas have heterotopic elements such as cartilage, glandular tissue, and hair follicles, and are then regarded as "teratoid".

Clinically, typical medulloepithelioma appears as a white to pink ciliary body tumor that not infrequently invades the peripheral iris (Figure 10–41). Intralesional cysts are often a prominent component of the tumor and, together with the full extent of the solid portion, they can be identified by ultrasound biomicroscopy. The tumor is probably present at birth in many cases but is frequently not detected until the child is between 2 and 6 years old. The tumor tends to grow slowly and progressively. Occasionally it stimulates abrupt development of diffuse iris neovascularization with cosmetic iris discoloration, ocular pain due to neovascular glaucoma, and a red congested eye.

Treatment options for ciliary body medulloepithelioma include transscleral tumor resection, plaque radiation therapy, and enucleation. Although a few benign ciliary body medulloepitheliomas have been excised successfully, most if not all malignant tumors of this type have either been resected incompletely or recurred locally following excision that was believed to have been complete. Plaque radiation therapy has been attempted in a number of cases with limited success. Most eyes containing a medulloepithelioma have ultimately come to enucleation. Metastasis from intraocular medullepithelioma is extremely rare.

MALIGNANT RETINAL TUMORS

The component cells of malignant retinal tumor and the tissue they form are clearly abnormal morphologically. Invasive features are generally evident clinically and pathologically, and regional and distant metastases may occur.

▶ Retinoblastoma

Retinoblastoma is a primary malignant intraocular tumor that arises from immature neuroepithelial cells of the developing retina (retinoblasts). Most develop within the first few years of life because retinal neuroepithelial cells tend to lose their tendency to give rise to retinoblastoma as they mature. Some are present at birth, occasionally even being identified by prenatal imaging.

Pathologically retinoblastoma is composed of small round neoplastic cells that invade and replace the normal retina. Individual tumor cells tend to have a large nucleus and disproportionately small amount of cytoplasm. Intralesional necrosis and foci of calcification are usually evident. Clinically disease is either unilateral (usually unifocal) or bilateral (usually multifocal). Most individuals with bilateral and/or multifocal retinoblastoma have a functionally significant mutation or deletion involving one allele of the retinoblastoma gene (a tumor suppressor gene localized to the q14 locus of the long arm of chromosome 13) in most, if not all, of their cells, with the high likelihood of the genetic abnormality being transmitted to any offspring as an autosomal dominant condition with approximately 90% penetrance. In contrast, most individuals with unilateral, unifocal retinoblastoma will not have a germline mutation in the retinoblastoma gene and will not transmit the disease to their offspring. Thus, recognized risk factors for occurrence of retinoblastoma include a positive parental history of bilateral, multifocal, and/or familial retinoblastoma and the presence of chromosome 13q deletion syndrome. The cumulative lifetime incidence of retinoblastoma has been estimated to be about 1 in 15,000 to 1 in 18,000 individuals in most western countries.

The typical small retinoblastoma tumor appears as a translucent to dull white retinal nodule (Figure 10–42). As the tumor gets larger, it gradually attracts dilated tortuous afferent and efferent retinal blood vessels and develops a fine network of capillaries on its surface (Figure 10–43). Larger discrete retinal tumors tend to develop intralesional foci of degenerative calcification, which can usually be detected by B-scan ultrasonography and CT scanning. Serous retinal detachment develops around the tumor, possibly extending to involve most of the retina and become bullous. Eventually tumor cells are shed from the surface of the tumor into the surrounding subretinal fluid and/or overlying vitreous (Figure 10–44). These tumor "seeds" can implant on the undersurface of the detached retina, the inner surface of the retinal pigment epithelium, the inner surface of the pars plana or pars plicata, the zonular fibers, or posterior surface of the iris, and even extend into the anterior chamber to implant on the anterior surface of the iris and the trabecular meshwork. In eyes with extensive retinoblastoma, secondary iris neovascularization and neovascular glaucoma develop frequently. Retinoblastoma has a tendency to invade the optic disc with extraocular extension along the orbital optic nerve, the choroid with transscleral extension via vascular and

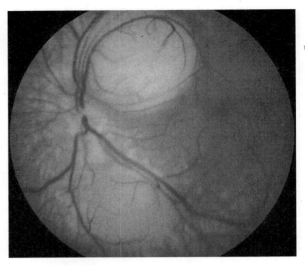

▲ **Figure 10–42.** Two discrete intraretinal retinoblastoma tumors in in the left eye of a child with bilateral retinoblastoma. The slightly larger superior tumor is more opaque while the smaller inferior tumor is more translucent.

neural foramina into the orbit, and the trabecular meshwork with extraocular extension into the anterior orbit or conjunctival lymphatics. Once retinoblastoma extends outside the eye, it tends to grow aggressively in the periocular tissues, extend via the optic nerve to the brain, and rapidly metastasize widely. Untreated, children with metastatic retinoblastoma rarely survive for more than one year.

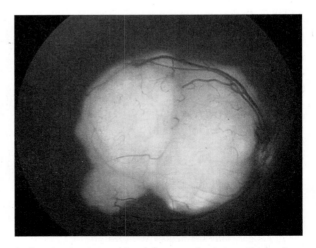

▲ **Figure 10–43.** Multinodular macular intraretinal retinoblastoma tumor formed by coalescence of three distinct tumors. Note the prominent retinal blood vessels on the surface of the tumor.

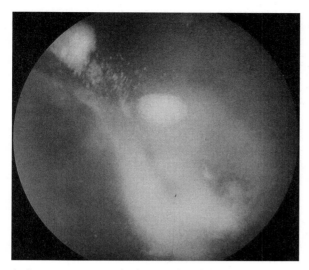

▲ **Figure 10–44.** Finely dispersed and clumped retinoblastoma seeds in vitreous.

Retinoblastoma in children with a positive family history of the disease is frequently identified by screening examinations when the extent of intraocular disease is limited (ie, few tumors, small tumors, and no vitreous seeds). In contrast, retinoblastoma in children with unilateral and/or non-familial retinoblastoma is usually not detected until the parents or pediatrician note a white pupil ("leukocoria", Figure 10–45) due to external light reflecting off the white intraocular tumor, strabismus due to impaired vision in one or both eyes, or discoloration of the iris due to iris neovascularization. In most developed countries, the median age at initial diagnosis is about 12 months for bilateral and about 24 months for unilateral retinoblastoma. In developing countries, the median age at detection tends to be substantially higher in both groups.

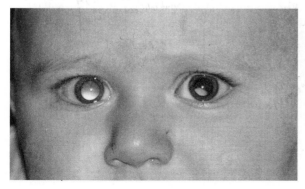

▲ **Figure 10–45.** White pupillary reflection (leukocoria) in each eye, more pronounced in the right, due to bilateral retinoblastoma.

Over the years, a number of classification systems have been developed to categorize affected eyes according to the likelihood of disease eradication in combination with ocular preservation (Reese–Ellsworth classification, Essen prognosis classification, International Classification of Intraocular Retinoblastoma). None was intended to be used as a staging system for patient survival. Nevertheless, because more extensive intraocular disease is likely to be associated with higher probability of extraocular tumor extension and metastasis, patients with more advanced intraocular retinoblastoma according to any of these systems tend to have a worse survival prognosis. Several different staging systems also have been developed that categorize children with retinoblastoma according to probability of cure or death (AJCC-Retinoblastoma, International Staging System for Retinoblastoma).

For a child with retinoblastoma confined within the eye, the recommended initial treatment depends on the number, size, locations, and types (primary intraretinal tumors, tumor seeds, implantation tumors) of intraocular tumors, the visual status and potential of the affected eye(s), whether the disease is unilateral or bilateral, the types and severity of secondary abnormalities of the eye (eg, retinal detachment, iris neovascularization), the general health of the child, and available resources. Because some children with familial and/or bilateral-multifocal retinoblastoma develop an independent retinoblastoma-like malignant neoplasm in the brain (most commonly in the pineal gland, where it is regarded as a pineoblastoma or ectopic intracranial retinoblastoma) and because of the propensity for retinoblastoma to extend extraocularly via the optic nerve and sclera, if possible, MRI of orbits and brain is performed routinely prior to treatment. Children with one or a few small discrete extramacular tumors, without associated tumor seeding or subretinal fluid, are typically managed by focal laser therapy for posterior (post-equatorial) tumors and focal cryotherapy for anterior tumors. Children with a solitary medium size intraretinal tumor in one or both eyes may be managed initially by plaque radiation therapy. Most children with one or more larger tumors, macular or juxtapapillary tumor, extensive non-rhegmatogenous retinal detachment, and/or subretinal and/or intravitreal tumor seeds at baseline are currently treated initially by intravenous chemotherapy using a carboplatin-based drug regimen, supplemented by focal obliterative therapies to the residual tumors once the original tumors have shrunken and the retinal detachment has diminished or resolved. Fractionated external beam radiation therapy (EBRT), once the mainstay of treatment for bilateral retinoblastoma, is now generally reserved for eyes with residual or recurrent retinoblastoma following a complete course of intravenous chemotherapy supplemented by local obliterative therapies. The principal reasons for the switch from EBRT were development of a carboplatin-based chemotherapy regimen consistently effective for intraocular disease and the recognition that EBRT in early childhood in children with bilateral retinoblastoma is associated with a relatively high frequency of subsequent and frequently fatal bony and soft tissue second malignant neoplasms in the field of radiation. If EBRT is employed today, the start of therapy is delayed until after the age of one year whenever possible. A new treatment for moderate to advanced intraocular unilateral or bilateral retinoblastoma is selective catheterization of the orifice of the ophthalmic artery followed by slow pulsed infusion of a chemotherapeutic drug, such as melphalan, under fluoroscopic imaging, but the long-term benefits and risks have yet to be determined. Some eyes with extensive intraocular retinoblastoma, particularly ones that are blind and painful, have neovascular glaucoma, or have extensive intraocular bleeding and/or ocular congestion, and eyes that have failed to respond to eye-preserving therapies must still be managed by enucleation. Any eye enucleated for retinoblastoma must undergo thorough histopathological examination for optic nerve invasion, transscleral tumor extension to the orbit, massive choroidal invasion, and other adverse prognostic factors for subsequent orbital tumor relapse or metastasis that may prompt post-enucleation adjuvant chemotherapy or orbital radiotherapy.

Initial treatment for a child with regional extraocular extension by retinoblastoma at presentation but no evidence of intracranial invasion or metastasis is currently being investigated. The standard treatment is enucleation of the affected eye with intensive chemotherapy and orbital irradiation.

Initial treatment for a potentially salvageable child with extraorbital retinoblastoma or retinoblastoma-associated pineoblastoma at presentation is also under study. In most cases, treatment consists of intensive initial intravenous chemotherapy, surgical debulking of the residual intracranial and/or extracranial tumor(s), focal adjuvant radiation therapy to metastatic sites, and bone-marrow transplantation. Although there have been some lasting cures of children with extracranial metastasis, there have been few, if any, cures of children with intracranial extension or metastasis of retinoblastoma or pineoblastoma.

▶ Non-Ophthalmic Primary Cancer Metastatic to the Retina

Occasionally non-ophthalmic primary cancers give rise to metastases to the retina, optic disk and/or vitreous. Although metastatic lesions to these sites are substantially less common than metastatic tumors to the uvea (see Chapter 7), they represent a distinct subgroup of malignant intraocular lesions that should be recognized by ophthalmologists. They usually occur in middle aged or older individuals with a history or other evidence of a non-ophthalmic primary cancer capable of metastasizing. Metastases to the retina tend to appear as patchy pale infiltrative lesions obscuring the retinal blood vessels (Figure 10–46), except from primary skin melanoma, which not surprisingly usually appear as a dark brown to black infiltrative lesion. Metastatic tumors to the optic disc tend to appear as infiltrates invading and replacing the disc tissue. Metastatic vitreous cells are indistinguishable

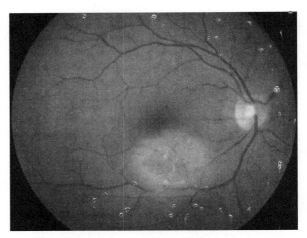

▲ **Figure 10–46.** Retinal metastasis from primary breast cancer to just below the right macula.

from inflammatory vitreous cells and must be suspected on the basis of the systemic clinical history. As with metastatic tumors to the uvea, metastases to the retina, optic disc, and vitreous must be regarded as equivalent to metastases to the brain, with corresponding unfavorable prognostic implications for survival. Treatment options for retinal and optic disc metastases include EBRT and chemotherapy appropriate to the cancer type. Metastatic cancer cells in the vitreous can be removed by posterior vitrectomy, but then the eye must usually be treated by EBRT to prevent reaccumulation.

▶ Primary Vitreoretinal Lymphoma

Primary vitreoretinal lymphoma is a distinct subtype of **primary intraocular lymphoma.** It is characterized by diffuse infiltration of the vitreous by malignant lymphoid cells and geographic accumulations of malignant lymphoid cells beneath the retinal pigment epithelium. Some patients also develop scattered malignant lymphoid infiltrates within the sensory retina (Figure 10–47). Primary vitreoretinal lymphoma is regularly associated with independent (nonmetastatic) foci of lymphoma within the brain and cerebrospinal fluid (primary central nervous system lymphoma) in the absence of systemic lymphoma. The malignant lymphoid cells in this disorder are usually of B-cell lineage, and the CNS and intraocular tumors are typically characterized histopathology as diffuse large cell lymphoma. Older middle aged to elderly individuals are usually affected with involvement of both eyes, simultaneously or sequentially, in 80% of cases.

Primary intraocular lymphoma is frequently misdiagnosed as uveitis and treated unsuccessfully for a number of months before its true nature is recognized. Diagnosis of primary vitreoretinal lymphoma requires cytopathologic and immunocytochemical analysis of the lymphoid cells in a vitreous sample

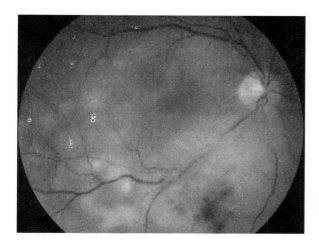

▲ **Figure 10–47.** Primary vitreoretinal lymphoma in right eye. Fundus features include vitreous haze due to intravitreal cells, ill-defined retinal infiltrate of lymphoma cells inferotemporal to the optic disk, an associated patch of intraretinal blood, and scattered yellow subretinal retinal pigment epithelial infiltrates temporally and inferotemporally. See color insert.

obtained by posterior vitrectomy (or in rare cases from discrete geographic subretinal pigment epithelial infiltrates by fine-needle aspiration biopsy or endo-incisional biopsy), or pathologic confirmation of primary CNS lymphoma in the context of characteristic intraocular features in one or both eyes. Ocular treatment depends on whether one or both eyes are affected, whether there is concurrent active primary CNS lymphoma, how and when any prior primary CNS lymphoma had been treated, and the general health and survival prognosis of the patient. If vitreous cells are a prominent feature of the condition, a posterior vitrectomy can be performed (on one or both eyes) for therapeutic purposes. Specific treatment options for the residual primary intraocular lymphoma include intravenous chemotherapy, usually a methotrexate based regimen, EBRT to one or both eyes (and the brain if it is involved clinically), and a series of intravitreal injections of methotrexate. Discrete lymphoid infiltrates in the eye typically regress rapidly in response to these treatments, and long-term remissions frequently but not always occur. Unfortunately, median patient survival following diagnosis of primary vitreoretinal lymphoma is generally about 3 years, with death usually caused by relapse and progression of the CNS lymphoma.

REFERENCES

Retina & Retinal Disorders

Bhatnagar A et al: Diabetic retinopathy in pregnancy. Curr Diabetes Rev 2009;5:151. [PMID: 19689249]

Biousse V et al: Thrombolysis for central retinal artery occlusion. J Neuroophthalmol 2007;27:215. [PMID: 17895823]

Boon CJ et al: Clinical and molecular genetic analysis of Best vitelliform macular dystrophy. Retina 2009;29:835. [PMID: 19357557]

Boon CJ et al: The spectrum of ocular phenotypes caused by mutations in the BEST1 gene. Prog Retin Eye Res 2009;28:187. [PMID: 19375515]

Boyer DS et al: Subgroup analysis of the MARINA study of ranibizumab in neovascular age-related macular degeneration. Ophthalmology 2007;114:246. [PMID: 17270674]

Bressler NM: Antiangiogenic approaches to age-related macular degeneration today. Ophthalmology 2009;116:S15. [PMID: 19800535]

Chakravarthy U, Evans J, Rosenfeld PJ: Age-related macular degeneration. BMJ 2010;340:c981. [PMID: 20189972]

Chan WM et al: Half-dose verteporfin photodynamic therapy for acute central serous chorioretinopathy: one-year results of a randomized controlled trial. Ophthalmology 2008;115:1756. [PMID: 18538401]

Chew EY et al: Summary results and recommendations from the Age-Related Eye Disease Study. Arch Ophthalmol 2009;127:1678. [PMID: 20008727]

Chung DC, Traboulsi EI: Leber congenital amaurosis: clinical correlations with genotypes, gene therapy trials updates, and future directions. J AAPOS 2009;13:587. [PMID: 20006823]

Cohen SY: Anti-VEGF drugs as the 2009 first-line therapy for choroidal neovascularization in pathologic myopia. Retina 2009;29:1062. [PMID 19734760]

DeAngelis MM et al: Cigarette smoking, CFH, APOE, ELOVL4 and risk of neovascular age-related macular degeneration. Arch Ophthalmol 2007;125:49. [PMID: 17210851]

Dhawahir-Scala FE et al: To posture or not to posture after macular holes surgery. Retina 2008;28:60. [PMID: 18185139]

di Lauro R et al: Intravitreal bevacizumab for surgical treatment of severe proliferative diabetic retinopathy. Graefes Arch Clin Exp Ophthalmol 2010 Feb 5. [Epub ahead of print] {PMID: 20135139}

Ding X, Patel M, Chan CC: Molecular pathology of age-related macular degeneration. Prog Retin Eye Res 2009;28:1. [PMID: 19026761]

Do V: Antiangiogenic approaches to age-related macular degeneration in the future. Ophthalmology 2009;116:S24. [PMID: 19800536]

Drack AV, Johnston R, Stone EM: Which Leber congenital amaurosis patients are eligible for gene therapy trials? J AAPOS 2009;13:463. [PMID: 19840725]

Ehrlich R et al: Intravitreal bevacizumab for choroidal neovascularization secondary to presumed ocular histoplasmosis syndrome. Retina 2009;29:1418. [PMID: 19898179]

Farah ME, Maia M, Rodrigues EB: Dyes in ocular surgery: principles for use in chemovitrectomy. Am J Ophthalmol 2009;148:332. [PMID: 19477708]

Fine HF et al: Acute zonal occult outer retinopathy in patients with multiple evanescent white dot syndrome. Arch Ophthalmol 2009;127:66. [PMID: 19139340]

Fiore T el al: Acute posterior multifocal placoid pigment epitheliopathy: outcome and visual prognosis. Retina 2009;29:994. [PMID: 19491729]

Grover D, Li TJ, Chong CC: Intravitreal steroids for macular edema in diabetes. Cochrane Database Syst Rev 2008;1:CD005656.

Holz FG et al: Progression of geographic atrophy and impact of fundus autofluorescence patterns in age-related macular degeneration. Am J Ophthalmol 2007;143:463. [PMID: 17239336].

Hornan D et al: Use of pegaptanib for recurrent and non-clearing vitreous haemorrhage in proliferative diabetic retinopathy. Eye 2010 Mar 12. [Epub ahead of print] [PMID: 20224599]

Inoue R et al: Association between the efficacy of photodynamic therapy and indocyanine green angiography findings for central serous chorioretinopathy. Am J Ophthalmol 2010;149:441. [PMID: 20172070]

Ip MS et al: A randomized trial comparing the efficacy and safety of intravitreal triamcinolone with observation to treat vision loss associated with macular edema secondary to central retinal vein occlusion: the Standard Care vs Corticosteroid for Retinal Vein Occlusion (SCORE) study report 5. Arch Ophthalmol 2009;127:1101. [PMID: 19752419]

Jeganathan VS, Verma N: Safety and efficacy of intravitreal anti-VEGF injections for age-related macular degeneration. Curr Opin Ophthalmol 2009;20:223. [PMID: 19367163]

Kaiser PK et al: Ranibizumab for predominantly classic neovascular age-related macular degeneration: subgroup analysis of first-year ANCHOR results. Am J Ophthalmol 2007;144:850. [PMID: 17949673]

Kilpatrick ES, Rigby AS, Atkin SL: The Diabetes Control and Complications Trial: the gift that keeps giving. Nat Rev Endocrinol 2009;5:537. [PMID: 19763126]

Krishnadev N, Meleth AD, Chew EY: Nutritional supplements for age-related macular degeneration. Curr Opin Ophthalmol 2010 Mar 6. [Epub ahead of print] [PMID: 20216418]

Lalwani GA et al: A variable-dosing regimen with intravitreal ranibizumab for neovascular age-related macular degeneration: year 2 of the PrONTO Study. Am J Ophthalmol 2009;148:43. [PMID: 19376495]

Lindblad AS et al: Change in area of geographic atrophy in the Age-Related Eye Disease Study: AREDS report number 26. Arch Ophthalmol 2009;127:1168. [PMID: 19752426]

Mantagos IS, Vanderveen DK, Smith LE: Emerging treatments for retinopathy of prematurity. Semin Ophthalmol 2009;24:82. [PMID: 19373691]

Matsumoto Y, Haen SP, Spaide RF: The white dot syndromes. Compr Ophthalmol Update 2007;8:179. [PMID: 17999832]

Mitchell P et al: Ranibizumab (Lucentis) in neovascular age-related macular degeneration: evidence from clinical trials. Br J Ophthalmol 2009 May 20 [Epub ahead of print] [PMID: 19443462]

Moore AT: Childhood macular dystrophies. Curr Opin Ophthalmol 2009;20:363. [PMID: 19587597]

Nicholson BP, Schachat AP: A review of clinical trials of anti-VEGF agents for diabetic retinopathy. Graefes Arch Clin Exp Ophthalmol 2010 Feb 20. [Epub ahead of print] [PMID: 20174816]

Nussenblatt RB, Liu B, Li Z: Age-related macular degeneration: an immunologically driven disease. [PMID: 19431076]

Reibaldi M et al: Standard-fluence versus low-fluence photodynamic therapy in chronic central serous chorioretinopathy: a nonrandomized clinical trial. Am J Ophthalmol 2010;149:307. [PMID: 19896635]

Robson AG et al: Functional characteristics of patients with retinal dystrophy that manifest abnormal parafovea annuli of high density fundus autofluorescence; a review and update. Doc Ophthalmol 2008;116:79. [PMID: 17985165]

Robson AG et al: Functional correlates of fundus autofluorescence abnormalities in patients with RPGR or RIMS1 mutations

causing cone or cone rod dystrophy. Br J Ophthalmol 2008;92:95. [PMID: 17962389]

Rudkin AK, Lee AW, Chen CS: Central retinal artery occlusion: timing and mode of presentation. Eur J Neurol 2009;16:674. [PMID: `9374663]

Scott AW, Bressler SB: Retinal angiomatous proliferation or retinal anastomosis to the lesion. Eye 2010;24:491. [PMID: 20019765]

Scott IU et al: A randomized trial comparing the efficacy and safety of intravitreal triamcinolone with standard care to treat vision loss associated with macular edema secondary to branch retinal vein occlusion: the Standard Care versus Corticosteroid for Retinal Vein Occlusion (SCORE) study report 6. Arch Ophthalmol 2009;127:1115. [PMID: 19752420]

Shuler RK et al: Neovasular age-related macular degeneration and its association with LOC387715 and complement factor H polymorphism. Arch Ophthalmol 2007;125:63. [PMID: 17210853]

Vedula SS, Krzystolik MG: Antiangiogenic therapy with anti-vascular endothelial growth factor modalities for neovascular age-related macular degeneration. Cochrane Database syst Rev 2008;2:CD005139. [PMID: 18425911]

Williams GA: 25-, 23-, or 20-gauge instrumentation for vitreous surgery? Eye 2008;22:1263. [PMID: 18292789]

Yilmaz T et al: Intravitreal triamcinolone acetonide injection for treatment of refractory diabetic macular edema: a systematic review. Ophthalmology 2009;116:902. [PMID: 19410949]

Retinal Tumors

Abramson DH, Dunkel IJ, Brodie SE, et al: A phase I/II study of direct intraarterial (ophthalmic artery) chemotherapy with melphalan for intraocular retinoblastoma. Initial results. Ophthalmology 2008;115:1398. [PMID: 18342944]

Arnold AC, Hepler RS, Yee RW, et al: Solitary retinal astrocytoma. Surv Ophthalmol 1985;30:173. [PMID: 4081977]

Brodie SE, Pierre Gobin Y, Dunkel IJ, et al: Persistence of retinal function after selective ophthalmic artery chemotherapy infusion for retinoblastoma. Doc Ophthalmol 2009;119:13. [PMID: 19169884]

Chantada G, Doz F, Antoneli CB, et al: A proposal for an international retinoblastoma staging system. Pediatr Blood Cancer 2006;47:801. [PMID: 16358310]

Cohn AD, Quiram PA, Drenser KA, et al: Surgical outcomes of epiretinal membranes associated with combined hamartoma of the retina and retinal pigment epithelium. Retina 2009;29:825. [PMID: 19276871]

Coupland SE, Damato B: Understanding intraocular lymphomas. Clin Experiment Ophthalmol 2008;36:564. [PMID: 18954321]

Eagle RC, Shields JA, Donoso L, Milner RS: Malignant transformation of spontaneously regressed retinoblastoma, retinoma/retinocytoma variant. Ophthalmology 1989;96:1389. [PMID: 2780006]

Edge SB, Byrd DR, Compton CC, et al: (Eds). AJCC Cancer Staging Manual, 7th edition. Springer; 2009.

Elizalde J, Ubia S, Barraquer RI: Adenoma of the nonpigmented ciliary epithelium. Eur J Ophthalmol 2006;16:630. [PMID: 16952109]

Gallie BL, Ellsworth RM, Abramson DH, Phillips RA: Retinoma: spontaneous regression of retinoblastoma or benign manifestation of the mutation? Br J Cancer 1982;45:513. [PMID: 7073943]

Gallie BL, Phillips RA, Ellsworth RM, et al: Significance of retinoma and phthisis bulbi for retinoblastoma. Ophthalmology 1982;89:1393. [PMID: 7162783]

Holdt M, Jurklies C, Schueler A, et al: Intraocular medulloepithelioma – series of 10 cases and review of the literature. Klin Monbl Augenheilkd 2009;226:1017. [PMID: 20108196]

Hungerford JL, Toma NMG, Plowman PN, Kingston JE: External beam radiotherapy for retinoblastoma. I. Whole eye technique. Br J Ophthalmol 1995;79:109. [PMID: 7696227]

Linn Murphree A: Intraocular retinoblastoma: the case for a new group classification. Ophthalmol Clin North Am 2005;18:41. [PMID: 15763190]

Margo C, Hidayat A, Kopelman J, Zimerman LE: Retinocytoma. A benign variant of retinoblastoma. Arch Ophthalmol 1983;101:1519. [PMID: 6626001]

Meyer CH, Rodrigues EB, Mennel S, et al: Grouped congenital hypertrophy of the retinal pigment epithelium follows developmental patterns of pigmentary mosaicism. Ophthalmology 2005;112:841. [PMID: 15878064]

Murphree AL, Villablanca JG, Deegan WF, et al: Chemotherapy plus local treatment in the management of intraocular retinoblastoma. Arch Ophthalmol 1996;114:1348. [PMID: 8906025]

Pe'er J, Hochberg FH, Foster CS: Clinical review: treatment of vitreoretinal lymphoma. Ocul Immunol Inflamm 2009;17:299. [PMID: 19831557]

Roarty JD, McLean IW, Zimmerman LE: Incidence of second neoplasms in patients with bilateral retinoblastoma. Ophthalmology 1988;95:1583. [PMID: 3211467]

Shields CL, Mashayekhi A, Ho T, et al: Solitary congenital hypertrophy of the retinal pigment epithelium: clinical features and frequency of enlargement in 330 patients. Ophthalmology 2003;110:1968. [PMID: 14522773]

Shields CL, Thangappan A, Hartzell K, et al: Combined hamartoma of the retina and retinal pigment epithelium in 77 consecutive patients. Visual outcome based on macular versus extramacular tumor location. Ophthalmology 2008;115:2246. [PMID: 18995912]

Shields JA, Shields CL, Gündüz K, Eagle RC: Adenoma of the ciliary body epithelium. Arch Ophthalmol 1999;117:592. [PMID: 10326955]

Singh AD, Santos CM, Shields CL, et al: Observations on 17 patients with retinocytoma. Arch Ophthalmol 2000;118:199. [PMID: 10676785]

Smith BJ, O'Brien JM: The genetics of retinoblastoma and current diagnostic testing. J Pediatric Ophthalmol Strabismus 1996;33120. [PMID: 8965236]

Touriño R, Conde-Freire R, Cabezas-Agricola JM, et al: Value of the congenital hypertrophy of the retinal pigment epithelium in the diagnosis of familial adenomatous polyposis. Int Ophthalmol 2004;25:101. [PMID: 15290889]

Trichopoulos N, Augsburger JJ, Schneider S: Adenocarcinoma arising from congenital hypertrophy of the retinal pigment epithelium. Graefes Arch Clin Exp Ophthalmol 2006;244:125. [PMID: 15983818]

Ulbright TM, Fulling KH, Helveston EM: Astrocytic tumors of the retina. Differentiation of sporadic tumor from phakomatosis-associated tumors. Arch Pathol Lab Med 1984;108:160. [PMID: 6421263]

Watkins LM, Rubin PA: Metastatic tumors of the eye and orbit. Int Ophthalmol Clin 1998;38:117. [PMID: 9532476]

Wong WT, Agrón E, Coleman HR, et al: Clinical characterization of retinal capillary hemangioblastomas in a large population of patients with von Hippel–Lindau disease. Ophthalmology 2008;115:181. [PMID: 17543389]

Wong WT, Chew EY: Ocular von Hippel–Lindau disease: clinical update and emerging treatments. Curr Opin Ophthalmol 2008;19:213. [PMID: 18408496]

Wong WT, Liang KJ, Hammel K, et al: Intravitreal ranibizumab therapy for retinal capillary hemangioblastoma related to von Hippel–Lindau disease. Ophthalmology 2008;115:1957. [PMID: 18789534]

Zimmer-Galler IE, Robertson DM: Long-term observations of retinal lesions in tuberous sclerosis. Am J Ophthalmol 1995;119:318. [PMID: 7872393]

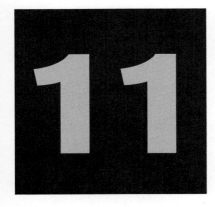

Glaucoma

John F. Salmon, MD, FRCS

Glaucoma is an acquired chronic optic neuropathy characterized by optic disk cupping and visual field loss. It is usually associated with elevated intraocular pressure. There are different types of glaucoma (Table 11–1), which helps to explain, for example, why one patient with glaucoma may have no symptoms, while another experiences sudden pain and inflammation. In the majority of cases, there is no associated ocular disease (primary glaucoma).

About 60 million people have glaucoma. An estimated 3 million Americans are affected, and of these cases, about 50% are undiagnosed. About 6 million people are blind from glaucoma, including approximately 100,000 Americans, making it the leading cause of preventable blindness in the United States. Primary open-angle glaucoma, the most common form among blacks and whites, causes insidious asymptomatic progressive bilateral visual loss that is often not detected until extensive field loss has already occurred. Blacks are at greater risk than whites for early onset, delayed diagnosis, and severe visual loss. Angle-closure glaucoma accounts for 10%–15% of cases in whites. This percentage is much higher in Asians and Inuit. Primary angle-closure glaucoma may account for over 90% of bilateral blindness due to glaucoma in China. Normal-tension glaucoma is the most common type in Japan.

The mechanism of raised intraocular pressure in glaucoma is impaired outflow of aqueous resulting from abnormalities within the drainage system of the anterior chamber angle (open-angle glaucoma) or impaired access of aqueous to the drainage system (angle-closure glaucoma) (Table 11–2). Treatment is directed toward reducing the intraocular pressure and, when possible, correcting the underlying cause. Although in normal-tension glaucoma intraocular pressure is within the normal range, reduction of intraocular pressure may still be beneficial.

Intraocular pressure can be reduced by decreasing aqueous production or increasing aqueous outflow, using medical, laser, or surgical treatments. Medications, usually administered topically, are available to reduce aqueous production or increase aqueous outflow. Surgically bypassing the drainage system is useful in most forms of glaucoma if there is a failure to respond to medical treatment. In recalcitrant cases, laser or cryotherapy can be used to ablate the ciliary body to reduce aqueous production. Improving access of aqueous to the anterior chamber angle in angle-closure glaucoma may be achieved by peripheral laser iridotomy or surgical iridectomy if the cause is pupillary block, miosis if there is angle crowding, or cycloplegia if there is anterior lens displacement. In the secondary glaucomas, consideration must always be given to treating the primary abnormality.

In all patients with glaucoma, the necessity for treatment and its effectiveness are assessed by regular determination of intraocular pressure (tonometry), inspection of optic disks, and measurement of visual fields.

The management of glaucoma is best undertaken by an ophthalmologist, but detection of asymptomatic cases is dependent on the cooperation and assistance of all medical personnel, particularly optometrists. Ophthalmoscopy to detect optic disk cupping and tonometry to measure intraocular pressure should be part of the routine ophthalmologic examination of all patients over 35 years of age. This is especially important in patients with a family history of glaucoma and in high-risk groups such as blacks, who should undergo regular screening every 2 years from age 35 and annually from age 50.

PHYSIOLOGY OF AQUEOUS HUMOR

Intraocular pressure is determined by the rate of aqueous production and the resistance to outflow of aqueous from the eye.

▶ Composition of Aqueous

The aqueous is a clear liquid that fills the anterior and posterior chambers of the eye. Its volume is about 250 μL, and its rate of production, which is subject to diurnal variation, is about 2.5 μL/min. The osmotic pressure is slightly higher

Table 11–1. Glaucoma Classified According to Etiology

A. Primary glaucoma
1. Open-angle glaucoma
   a. Primary open-angle glaucoma (chronic open-angle glaucoma, chronic simple glaucoma)
   b. Normal-tension glaucoma (low-tension glaucoma)
2. Angle-closure glaucoma

B. Congenital glaucoma
1. Primary congenital glaucoma
2. Glaucoma associated with other developmental ocular abnormalities
   a. Anterior chamber cleavage syndromes
      Axenfeld–Rieger syndrome
      Peters' syndrome
   b. Aniridia
3. Glaucoma associated with extraocular developmental abnormalities
   a. Sturge–Weber syndrome
   b. Marfan's syndrome
   c. Neurofibromatosis 1
   d. Lowe's syndrome
   e. Congenital rubella

C. Secondary glaucoma
1. Pigmentary glaucoma
2. Exfoliation syndrome
3. Due to lens changes (phacogenic)
   a. Dislocation
   b. Intumescence
   c. Phacolytic
4. Due to uveal tract changes
   a. Uveitis
   b. Posterior synechiae (seclusio pupillae)
   c. Tumor
   d. Ciliary body swelling
5. Iridocorneoendothelial (ICE) syndrome
6. Trauma
   a. Hyphema
   b. Angle contusion/recession
   c. Peripheral anterior synechiae
7. Postoperative
   a. Ciliary block glaucoma (malignant glaucoma)
   b. Peripheral anterior synechiae
   c. Epithelial downgrowth
   d. Following corneal graft surgery
   e. Following retinal detachment surgery
8. Neovascular glaucoma
   a. Diabetes mellitus
   b. Central retinal vein occlusion
   c. Intraocular tumor
9. Raised episcleral venous pressure
   a. Carotid-cavernous fistula
   b. Sturge–Weber syndrome
10. Steroid-induced

D. Absolute glaucoma: The end result of any uncontrolled glaucoma is a hard, sightless, and often painful eye.

Table 11–2. Glaucoma Classified According to Mechanism of Intraocular Pressure Rise

A. Open-angle glaucoma
1. Pretrabecular membranes: All of these may progress to angle-closure glaucoma due to contraction of the pretrabecular membranes.
   a. Neovascular glaucoma
   b. Epithelial downgrowth
   c. ICE syndrome
2. Trabecular abnormalities
   a. Primary open-angle glaucoma
   b. Congenital glaucoma
   c. Pigmentary glaucoma
   d. Exfoliation syndrome
   e. Steroid-induced glaucoma
   f. Hyphema
   g. Angle contusion or recession
   h. Iridocyclitis (uveitis)
   i. Phacolytic glaucoma
3. Posttrabecular abnormalities
   a. Raised episcleral venous pressure

B. Angle-closure glaucoma
1. Pupillary block (iris bombé)
   a. Primary angle-closure glaucoma
   b. Seclusio pupillae (posterior synechiae)
   c. Intumescent lens
   d. Anterior lens dislocation
   e. Hyphema
2. Anterior lens displacement
   a. Ciliary block glaucoma
   b. Central retinal vein occlusion
   c. Posterior scleritis
   d. Following retinal detachment surgery
3. Angle crowding
   a. Plateau iris
   b. Intumescent lens
   c. Mydriasis for fundal examination
4. Peripheral anterior synechiae
   a. Chronic angle closure
   b. Secondary to flat anterior chamber
   c. Secondary to iris bombé
   d. Contraction of pretrabecular membranes

than that of plasma. The composition of aqueous is similar to that of plasma except for much higher concentrations of ascorbate, pyruvate, and lactate and lower concentrations of protein, urea, and glucose.

▶ Formation & Flow of Aqueous

Aqueous is produced by the ciliary body. An ultrafiltrate of plasma produced in the stroma of the ciliary processes is modified by the barrier function and secretory processes of the ciliary epithelium. Entering the posterior chamber, the aqueous passes through the pupil into the anterior chamber (Figure 11–1) and then to the trabecular meshwork in the

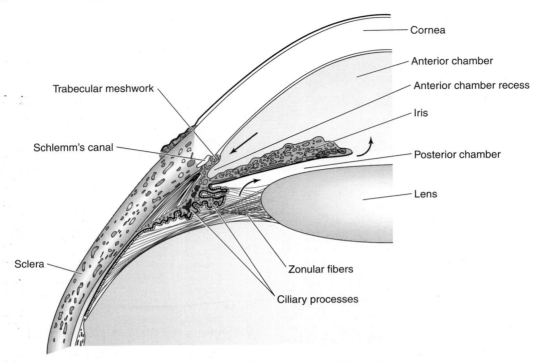

▲ **Figure 11–1.** Anterior segment structures. Arrows indicate direction of flow of aqueous.

anterior chamber angle. During this period, there is some differential exchange of components with the blood in the iris.

Intraocular inflammation or trauma causes an increase in the protein concentration. This is called plasmoid aqueous and closely resembles blood serum.

▶ Outflow of Aqueous

The trabecular meshwork is composed of beams of collagen and elastic tissue covered by trabecular cells that form a filter with a decreasing pore size as the canal of Schlemm is approached. Contraction of the ciliary muscle through its insertion into the trabecular meshwork increases pore size in the meshwork, and hence the rate of aqueous drainage. Passage of aqueous into Schlemm's canal depends on cyclic formation of transcellular channels in the endothelial lining. Efferent channels from Schlemm's canal (about 30 collector channels and 12 aqueous veins) conduct the fluid directly into the venous system. Some aqueous passes between the bundles of the ciliary muscle into the suprachoroidal space and then into the venous system of the ciliary body, choroid, and sclera (uveoscleral flow) (Figure 11–1).

The major resistance to aqueous outflow from the anterior chamber is the juxtacanalicular tissue adjacent to the endothelial lining of Schlemm's canal, rather than the venous system. But the pressure in the episcleral venous network

determines the minimum level of intraocular pressure that can be achieved by medical therapy.

PATHOPHYSIOLOGY OF GLAUCOMA

The major mechanism of visual loss in glaucoma is retinal ganglion cell apoptosis, leading to thinning of the inner nuclear and nerve fiber layers of the retina and axonal loss in the optic nerve. The optic disk becomes atrophic, with enlargement of the optic cup (see later in the chapter).

The pathophysiology of intraocular pressure elevation—whether due to open-angle or to angle-closure mechanisms—will be discussed as each disease entity is considered (see later in the chapter). The effects of raised intraocular pressure are influenced by the time course and magnitude of the rise in intraocular pressure. In acute angle-closure glaucoma, the intraocular pressure reaches 60–80 mm Hg, resulting in acute ischemic damage to the iris with associated corneal edema and optic nerve damage. In primary open-angle glaucoma, the intraocular pressure does not usually rise above 30 mm Hg and retinal ganglion cell damage develops over a prolonged period, often many years. In normal-tension glaucoma, retinal ganglion cells may be susceptible to damage from intraocular pressures in the normal range, or the major mechanism of damage may be optic nerve head ischemia.

CLINICAL ASSESSMENT IN GLAUCOMA

▶ Tonometry

Tonometry is measurement of intraocular pressure. The most widely used instrument is the Goldmann applanation tonometer, which is attached to the slitlamp and measures the force required to flatten a fixed area of the cornea. Corneal thickness influences the accuracy of measurement. Intraocular pressure is overestimated in eyes with thick corneas and underestimated in eyes with thin corneas. This difficulty may be overcome by the Pascal dynamic contour tonometer. Other applanation tonometers are the Perkins tonometer and the Tono-Pen, both of which are portable, and the pneumatotonometer, which can be used with a soft contact lens in place when the cornea has an irregular surface. The Schiotz tonometer is portable and measures the corneal indentation produced by a known weight. (For further discussion of tonometry, see Chapter 2; for tonometer disinfection techniques, see Chapter 20.)

The normal range of intraocular pressure is 11–21 mm Hg (Figure 11–2). The distribution is Gaussian, but with the curve skewed to the right. In the elderly, average intraocular pressure is higher, giving an upper limit of 24 mm Hg. The intraocular pressure is subject to diurnal fluctuation throughout the day. In primary open-angle glaucoma, 32%–50% of affected individuals will have a normal intraocular pressure when first measured. Conversely, isolated raised intraocular pressure does not necessarily mean that the patient has primary open-angle glaucoma, since other evidence in the form of a glaucomatous optic disk or visual field changes is necessary for diagnosis. If the intraocular pressure is consistently

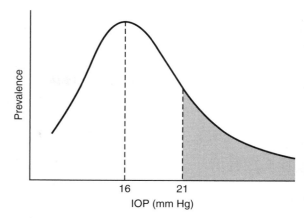

▲ **Figure 11–2.** Distribution of intraocular pressure in individuals over the age of 40 years.

elevated in the presence of normal optic disks and visual fields (ocular hypertension), the patient should be observed periodically as a glaucoma suspect.

▶ Gonioscopy (See Also Chapter 2)

The anterior chamber angle is formed by the junction of the peripheral cornea and the iris, between which lies the trabecular meshwork (Figure 11–3). The configuration of this angle—that is whether it is wide (open), narrow, or closed—has an important bearing on the outflow of aqueous. The anterior chamber angle width can be estimated by oblique illumination with a penlight (Figure 11–4) or by slitlamp

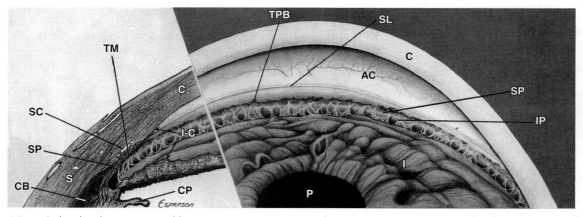

AC = anterior chamber	**I** = iris	**S** = sclera	**TM** = trabecular meshwork
C = cornea	**I-C** = iris-corneal angle	**SC** = Schlemm's canal	**TPB** = trabecular pigment band
CB = ciliary body	**IP** = iris processes	**SL** = Schwalbe's line	
CP = ciliary process	**P** = pupil	**SP** = scleral spur	

▲ **Figure 11–3.** Composite illustration showing anatomic **(left)** and gonioscopic **(right)** view of normal anterior chamber angle. (Courtesy of R Shaffer.)

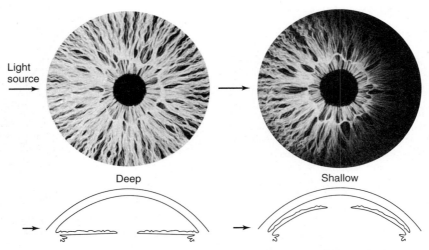

Light
source

Deep   Shallow

▲ **Figure 11-4.** Estimation of depth of anterior chamber by oblique illumination (diagram). (Courtesy of R Shaffer.)

observation of the depth of the peripheral anterior chamber, but it is best determined by gonioscopy, which allows direct visualization of the angle structures (Figure 11–3). If it is possible to visualize the full extent of the trabecular meshwork, the scleral spur, and the iris processes, the angle is open. Being able to see only Schwalbe's line or a small portion of the trabecular meshwork means that the angle is narrow. Being unable to see Schwalbe's line means that the angle is closed.

Large myopic eyes have wide angles, and small hyperopic eyes have narrow angles. Enlargement of the lens with age narrows the angle and accounts for some cases of angle-closure glaucoma.

▶ Optic Disk Assessment

The normal optic disk has a central depression—the physiologic cup—whose size depends on the bulk of the fibers that form the optic nerve relative to the size of the scleral opening through which they must pass. In hyperopic eyes, the scleral opening is small, and thus the optic cup is small; the reverse is true in myopic eyes. Glaucomatous optic atrophy produces specific disk changes characterized chiefly by loss of disk substance—detectable as enlargement of the optic disk cup—associated with disk pallor in the area of cupping. Other forms of optic atrophy cause widespread pallor without increased disk cupping.

In glaucoma, there may be concentric enlargement of the optic cup or preferential superior and inferior cupping with focal notching of the rim of the optic disk (Figure 11–5). The optic cup also increases in depth as the lamina cribrosa is displaced backward. As cupping develops, the retinal vessels on the disk are displaced nasally (Figure 11–6). The end result of glaucomatous cupping is the so-called "bean-pot" cup in which no neural rim tissue is apparent (Figure 11–7).

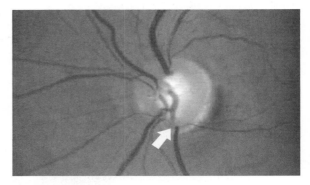

▲ **Figure 11-5.** Early glaucoma showing inferior focal notching of the neuroretinal rim **(arrow)**.

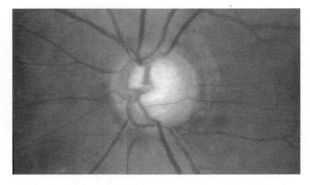

▲ **Figure 11-6.** Typical glaucomatous cupping. Note the nasal displacement of the vessels and hollowed-out appearance of the optic disk except for a thin border.

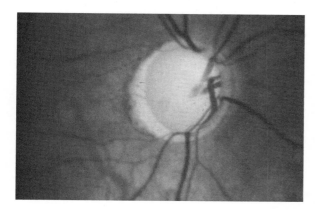

▲ **Figure 11–7.** Glaucomatous ("bean-pot") cupping of the optic disk.

The "cup–disk ratio" is a useful way of recording the size of the optic disk in glaucoma patients. It is the ratio of cup size to disk diameter, for example, a small cup is 0.1 and a large cup 0.9. In the presence of visual field loss or elevated intraocular pressure, a cup–disk ratio greater than 0.5 or significant asymmetry between the two eyes is highly suggestive of glaucomatous atrophy.

Clinical assessment of the optic disk can be performed by direct ophthalmoscopy or by examination with the 78-diopter lens or special corneal contact lenses that give a three-dimensional view (see Chapter 2).

Other clinical evidence of neuronal damage in glaucoma is atrophy of the retinal nerve fiber layer, which precedes the development of optic disk changes. It is detectable by ophthalmoscopy or fundal photography, both aided by using red-free light, optical coherence tomography, scanning laser polarimetry, or scanning laser tomography (see Chapter 2).

▶ Visual Field Examination

Regular visual field examination is essential to the diagnosis and follow-up of glaucoma. Glaucomatous field loss is not in itself specific, since it consists of nerve fiber bundle defects that may be seen in other forms of optic nerve disease; but the pattern of field loss, the nature of its progression, and the correlation with changes in the optic disk are characteristic of the disease.

Glaucomatous field loss involves mainly the central 30° of field (Figure 11–8). Contiguous extension of the blind spot into Bjerrum's area of the visual field—at 15° from fixation—produces a Bjerrum scotoma and then an arcuate scotoma. Focal areas of more pronounced loss within Bjerrum's area are known as Seidel scotomas. Double arcuate scotomas—above and below the horizontal meridian—are often accompanied by a nasal step (of Roenne) because of differences in size of the two arcuate defects. Peripheral field loss tends to start in the nasal periphery as a constriction of the isopters. Subsequently, there may be connection to an arcuate defect, producing peripheral breakthrough. The temporal peripheral field and the central 5°–10° are affected late in the disease. Central visual acuity is not a reliable index of progress of the disease. In end-stage disease, there may be normal central acuity but only 5° of visual field in each eye. The patient may have 20/20 visual acuity but be legally blind.

Various ways of testing the visual fields in glaucoma include the automated perimeter (for example, Humphrey, Octopus, or Henson), the Goldmann perimeter, the Friedman field analyzer, and the tangent screen. (For testing techniques, see Chapter 2.) Conventional automated perimetry, most commonly using the Humphrey perimeter, employs a white stimulus on a white background (white-on-white perimetry). Visual field defects are not detected until there is about 40% retinal ganglion loss. Refinements to detect earlier visual field changes include blue-on-yellow perimetry, also known as short-wavelength automated perimetry (SWAP), frequency-doubling perimetry (FDP), and high-pass resolution perimetry.

TREATMENT OF RAISED INTRAOCULAR PRESSURE

▶ Medical Treatment (Also See Chapter 22)
A. Suppression of Aqueous Production

Topical **beta-adrenergic blocking agents** may be used alone or in combination with other drugs. Timolol maleate 0.25% and 0.5%, betaxolol 0.25% and 0.5%, levobunolol 0.25% and 0.5%, metipranolol 0.3%, and carteolol 1% solutions twice daily and timolol maleate 0.1%, 0.25%, and 0.5% gel once daily in the morning, some formulated without preservatives (preservative-free), are the currently available preparations. The major contraindications to their use are chronic obstructive airway disease—particularly asthma—and cardiac conduction defects. Betaxolol, with its relatively greater selectivity for $\beta1$ receptors, less often produces respiratory side effects, but it is also less effective at reducing intraocular pressure. Depression, confusion, and fatigue may occur with the topical beta-blocking agents. The frequency of systemic effects and the availability of other agents have reduced the popularity of the beta-adrenergic blocking agents.

Apraclonidine (0.5% solution three times daily and 1% solution before and after laser treatment) is an α_2-adrenergic agonist that decreases aqueous humor formation without effect on outflow. It is particularly useful for preventing rise of intraocular pressure after anterior segment laser treatment and can be used on a short-term basis in refractory cases. It is not suitable for long-term use because of tachyphylaxis (loss of therapeutic effect over time) and a high incidence of allergic reactions. **Epinephrine** and **dipivefrin** have some effect on aqueous production but are rarely used these days.

Brimonidine (0.2% solution twice daily) is an α-adrenergic agonist that primarily inhibits aqueous production and

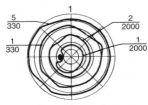

Baring of the blind spot. The earliest nerve fiber bundle defect.

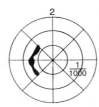

Incipient double nerve fiber bundle defect (Bjerrum scotoma).

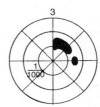

Bjerrum scotoma isolated from blind spot.

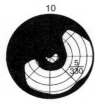

End stages in glaucoma field loss. Remnant of central field still shows nasal step.

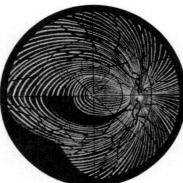

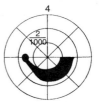

Fully developed nerve fiber bundle defect with nasal step (arcuate scotoma).

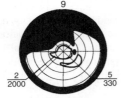

Peripheral depression with double nerve fiber bundle defect. Isolation of central field.

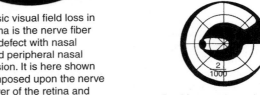

The basic visual field loss in glaucoma is the nerve fiber bundle defect with nasal step and peripheral nasal depression. It is here shown superimposed upon the nerve fiber layer of the retina and the retinal vascular tree. All perimetric changes in glaucoma are variations of these fundamental defects.

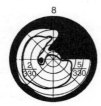

Double arcuate scotoma with peripheral breakthrough and nasal step.

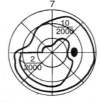

Nasal depression connected with arcuate scotoma. Nasal step of Rönne.

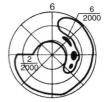

Peripheral breakthrough of large nerve fiber bundle defect with well-developed nasal step.

Seidel scotoma. Islands of greater visual loss within a nerve fiber bundle defect.

▲ **Figure 11–8.** Visual field changes in glaucoma. (Reproduced, with permission, from Harrington DO: The Visual Fields: A Textbook and Atlas of Clinical Perimetry, 5th ed. Mosby, 1981.)

secondarily increases aqueous outflow. It may be used as a first-line or adjunctive agent, but allergic reactions are common. It is available combined with timolol in the same solution.

Dorzolamide hydrochloride 2% solution, including a preservative-free preparation, and **brinzolamide** 1% (two or three times daily) are topical carbonic anhydrase inhibitors that are especially effective when employed adjunctively, although not as effective as systemic carbonic anhydrase inhibitors. The main side-effects are a transient bitter taste and allergic blepharoconjunctivitis. Dorzolamide is also available combined with timolol in the same solution, including a preservative-free preparation. Outside the United States, brinzolamide is available combined with timolol in the same solution.

Systemic **carbonic anhydrase inhibitors**—acetazolamide is the most widely used, but dichlorphenamide and methazolamide are alternatives—are used in chronic glaucoma when topical therapy is insufficient and in acute glaucoma when very high intraocular pressure needs to be controlled quickly. They are capable of suppressing aqueous production by 40%–60%. Acetazolamide can be administered orally in a dosage of 125–250 mg up to four times daily or as Diamox Sequels 500 mg once or twice daily, or it can be given intravenously (500 mg). The carbonic anhydrase inhibitors are associated with major systemic side effects that limit their usefulness for long-term therapy.

Hyperosmotic agents influence aqueous production as well as dehydrate the vitreous body (see below).

B. Facilitation of Aqueous Outflow

The **prostaglandin analogs**—bimatoprost 0.003%, latanoprost 0.005%, travoprost 0.004%, and tafluprost 0.0015% (preservative-free) solutions, each once daily at night, and unoprostone 0.15% solution twice daily—increase uveoscleral outflow of aqueous. They are highly effective first-line or adjunctive agents. In many countries but not the United States, bimatoprost, latanoprost, and travoprost are available combined with timolol 0.5% in the same solution for use once daily. All the prostaglandin analogs may produce conjunctival hyperemia, hyperpigmentation of periorbital skin, eyelash growth, and permanent darkening of the iris (particularly in green-brown and yellow-brown irides). These drugs have also been rarely associated with reactivation of uveitis and herpes keratitis and can cause macular edema in predisposed individuals.

Parasympathomimetic agents increase aqueous outflow by action on the trabecular meshwork through contraction of the ciliary muscle. **Pilocarpine** is not commonly used since the advent of prostaglandin analogs but can be useful in some patients. It is given as 0.5%–6% solution instilled up to four times a day or as 4% gel instilled at bedtime. Carbachol 0.75%–3% is an alternative cholinergic agent. Parasympathomimetic agents produce miosis with dimness of vision, particularly in patients with cataract, and accommodative spasm that may be disabling to younger patients. Retinal detachment is a serious but rare occurrence.

C. Reduction of Vitreous Volume

Hyperosmotic agents render the blood hypertonic, thus drawing water out of the vitreous and causing it to shrink. This is in addition to decreasing aqueous production. Reduction in vitreous volume is helpful in the treatment of acute angle-closure glaucoma and in malignant glaucoma when anterior displacement of the crystalline lens (caused by volume changes in the vitreous or choroid) produces angle closure (secondary angle-closure glaucoma).

Oral **glycerin (glycerol),** 1 mL/kg of body weight in a cold 50% solution mixed with lemon juice, is the most commonly used agent, but it should be used with care in diabetics. Alternatives are oral isosorbide and intravenous mannitol (see Chapter 22 for dosages).

D. Miotics, Mydriatics, and Cycloplegics

Constriction of the pupil is fundamental to the management of primary angle-closure glaucoma and the angle crowding of plateau iris. Pupillary dilation is important in the treatment of angle closure secondary to iris bombé due to posterior synechiae.

When angle closure is secondary to anterior lens displacement, cycloplegic/mydriatic agents (cyclopentolate and atropine) are used to relax the ciliary muscle and thus tighten the zonular apparatus in an attempt to draw the lens backward.

▶ Surgical & Laser Treatment
A. Peripheral Iridotomy, Iridectomy, and Iridoplasty

Pupillary block in angle-closure glaucoma is most satisfactorily overcome by forming a direct communication between the anterior and posterior chambers that removes the pressure difference between them. Laser peripheral iridotomy is best done with the neodymium: YAG laser, although the argon laser may be necessary in dark irides. Surgical peripheral iridectomy is performed if YAG laser iridotomy is ineffective. YAG laser iridotomy is preventive when used in patients with narrow angles before closure attacks occur.

In some cases of acute angle closure when it is not possible to control the intraocular pressure medically or YAG laser iridotomy cannot be performed, argon laser peripheral iridoplasty (ALPI) can be undertaken. A ring of laser burns on the peripheral iris contracts the iris stroma, mechanically pulling open the anterior chamber angle.

B. Laser Trabeculoplasty

Application of laser (either argon or frequency-doubled Q-switched Nd:YAG) burns via a goniolens to the trabecular meshwork facilitates aqueous out-flow by virtue of its effects on the trabecular meshwork and Schlemm's canal or cellular events that enhance the function of the meshwork. The technique is applicable to many forms of open-angle glaucoma, and the results are variable depending on the underlying cause. The pressure reduction usually allows decrease of medical therapy and postponement of glaucoma surgery. Treatments can be repeated (see Chapter 23). Laser trabeculoplasty may be used in the initial treatment of primary open-angle glaucoma. In most cases, the intraocular pressure gradually returns to the pretreatment level 2–5 years later. The outcome of subsequent glaucoma drainage surgery may be adversely affected.

C. Glaucoma Drainage Surgery

The increased effectiveness of medical and laser treatment has reduced the need for glaucoma drainage surgery, but surgery is able to produce a more marked reduction in intraocular pressure.

Trabeculectomy is the procedure most commonly used to bypass the normal drainage channels, allowing direct access from the anterior chamber to the subconjunctival and orbital tissues (Figure 11–9). The major complication is fibrosis in the episcleral tissues, leading to closure of the new drainage pathway. This is most likely to occur in young patients, in blacks, in patients with secondary glaucoma, and in those who have previously undergone glaucoma drainage surgery or other surgery involving the episcleral tissues. Perioperative or postoperative adjunctive treatment with antimetabolites such as 5-fluorouracil and mitomycin C (in low dosage) reduces the risk of bleb failure and is associated with good intraocular pressure control but may lead to bleb-related complications like persistent ocular discomfort, bleb infection, or maculopathy from persistent ocular hypotony. Trabeculectomy markedly accelerates cataract formation.

Implantation of a silicone tube to form a permanent conduit for aqueous flow out of the eye is an alternative procedure for eyes that are unlikely to respond to trabeculectomy.

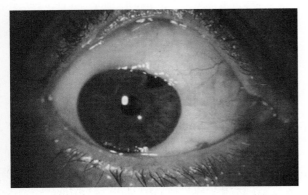

▲ **Figure 11–9.** Trabeculectomy showing an upper nasal "bleb" and peripheral iridectomy. See color insert.

This includes eyes with secondary glaucoma—particularly neovascular glaucoma—and glaucoma following corneal graft surgery.

Viscocanalostomy and **deep sclerectomy with collagen implant** avoid full-thickness incisions into the eye. The intraocular pressure reduction is not as good as that achieved with trabeculectomy, but there is less potential for complications. They are technically difficult to perform.

Goniotomy and **trabeculotomy** are useful techniques in treating primary congenital glaucoma, in which there appears to be an obstruction to aqueous drainage in the internal portion of the trabecular meshwork.

D. Cyclodestructive Procedures

Failure of medical and surgical treatment in advanced glaucoma may lead to consideration of laser or surgical destruction of the ciliary body to control intraocular pressure. Cryotherapy, thermal mode neodymium:YAG laser, or diode laser can all be used to destroy the ciliary body. Treatment is usually applied externally through the sclera, but endoscopic laser application systems are available.

▼ PRIMARY GLAUCOMA

PRIMARY OPEN-ANGLE GLAUCOMA

Primary open-angle glaucoma is the most common form in blacks and whites. In the United States, 1.29%–2% of persons over age 40, rising to 4.7% of persons over age 75, are estimated to have primary open-angle glaucoma. The disease is four times more common and six times more likely to cause blindness in blacks. There is a strong familial tendency in primary open-angle glaucoma, and close relatives of affected individuals should undergo regular screening.

The chief pathologic feature of primary open-angle glaucoma is a degenerative process in the trabecular meshwork, including deposition of extracellular material within the meshwork and beneath the endothelial lining of Schlemm's canal. This differs from the normal aging process. The consequence is a reduction in aqueous drainage leading to a rise in intraocular pressure.

Juvenile-onset open-angle glaucoma (a familial primary open-angle glaucoma with early onset), about 5% of familial cases of primary open-angle glaucoma, and about 3% of nonfamilial cases of primary open-angle glaucoma are associated with mutations in the myocilin gene on chromosome 1.

Raised intraocular pressure precedes optic disk and visual field changes by months to years. Although there is a clear association between the level of intraocular pressure and the severity and rate of progression of visual loss, there is great variability between individuals in the effect on the optic nerve of a given pressure elevation. Some eyes tolerate elevated intraocular pressure without developing disk or field changes (ocular hypertension; see later in the chapter); others develop glaucomatous changes with consistently "normal" intraocular pressure (low-tension glaucoma; see later in the chapter). Nevertheless, higher levels of intraocular pressure are associated with greater field loss at presentation. When there is glaucomatous field loss on first examination, the risk of further progression is much greater. Since intraocular pressure is the only treatable risk factor, it remains the focus of therapy. There is strong evidence that control of intraocular pressure slows disk damage and field loss. For each 1-mm Hg reduction of intraocular pressure, there is an approximately 10% decreased risk of progression of glaucoma.

If there are extensive disk changes or field loss, it is advisable to reduce the intraocular pressure as much as possible, preferably to less than 15 mm Hg. A patient with only a suspicion of disk or field changes may need less vigorous treatment. In all cases, the inconveniences and possible complications of treatment must be considered. Many glaucoma patients are old and frail and may not tolerate vigorous treatment. In order to gain a perspective on the need for treatment, an initial period of observation without treatment may be necessary to determine the rate of progression of disk and field changes. There is no justification for subjecting an elderly patient to extremes of treatment when the likelihood of their developing significant visual loss during their lifetime is small.

▶ Diagnosis

The diagnosis of primary open-angle glaucoma is established when glaucomatous optic disk or field changes are associated with elevated intraocular pressures, a normal-appearing open anterior chamber angle, and no other reason for intraocular pressure elevation. At least one-third of patients with primary open-angle glaucoma have a normal intraocular pressure when first examined, so repeated tonometry can be helpful.

▶ Screening for Glaucoma

The major problem in detection of primary open-angle glaucoma is the absence of symptoms until relatively late in the disease. When patients first notice field loss, substantial optic nerve damage has already occurred. If treatment is to be successful, it must be started early in the disease, and this depends on an active screening program. Unfortunately, glaucoma screening programs are hampered by the unreliability of a single intraocular pressure measurement in the detection of primary open-angle glaucoma and the complexities of relying on optic disk or visual field changes. At present it is necessary to rely for early diagnosis predominantly on regular ophthalmologic assessment of first-degree relatives of affected individuals.

▶ Course & Prognosis

Without treatment, open-angle glaucoma may progress insidiously to complete blindness. If antiglaucoma drops control the intraocular pressure in an eye that has not suffered extensive glaucomatous damage, the prognosis is good (although visual field loss may progress despite normalized intraocular pressure). When the process is detected early, most glaucoma patients can be successfully managed medically. Trabeculectomy is a good option in patients who progress despite medical treatment (Figure 11–9).

NORMAL-TENSION GLAUCOMA (LOW-TENSION GLAUCOMA)

Some patients with glaucomatous optic disk or visual field changes have an intraocular pressure consistently below 21 mm Hg. These patients have normal-tension (low-tension) glaucoma. The pathogenesis may involve an abnormal sensitivity to intraocular pressure because of vascular or mechanical abnormalities at the optic nerve head, or this may be a purely vascular disease. There may be an inherited predisposition, normal-tension glaucoma being particularly common in Japan. A few families with normal tension glaucoma have an abnormality in the optineurin gene on chromosome 10. Some studies have shown an association with vasospasm. Disk hemorrhages are more frequently seen in normal-tension than in primary open-angle glaucoma and often herald progression of field loss.

Before the diagnosis of normal-tension glaucoma can be established, a number of entities must be excluded:

1. Prior episode of raised intraocular pressure, such as caused by anterior uveitis, trauma, or topical steroid therapy.

2. Large diurnal variation in intraocular pressure with significant elevations, usually early in the morning.

3. Postural changes in intraocular pressure with a marked elevation when lying flat.

4. Intermittent elevations of intraocular pressure, such as in subacute angle closure.

5. Underestimation of intraocular pressure due to reduced corneal thickness.

6. Other causes of optic disk and field changes, including congenital disk abnormalities, inherited optic neuropathy, and acquired optic atrophy due to tumors or vascular disease.

Among patients diagnosed with normal-tension glaucoma, approximately 60% have progressive visual field loss, suggesting the possibility of acute ischemic events in the pathogenesis of those without progression. Reduction of intraocular pressure is beneficial in patients with progressive visual field loss, but this may not be achieved with medical therapy. Glaucoma drainage surgery with an anti-metabolite may be required. The possibility of a vascular basis for normal-tension glaucoma has led to the use of systemic calcium channel blockers, but definite benefit from this intervention has yet to be demonstrated.

OCULAR HYPERTENSION

Ocular hypertension is elevated intraocular pressure without disk or field abnormalities and is more common than primary open-angle glaucoma. The rate at which such individuals develop glaucoma is approximately 1%–2% per year. The risk increases with increasing intraocular pressure, increasing age, greater optic disk cupping, a positive family history for glaucoma, and perhaps myopia, diabetes mellitus, and cardiovascular disease. The development of disk hemorrhages in a patient with ocular hypertension also indicates an increased risk for development of glaucoma.

Patients with ocular hypertension are considered glaucoma suspects and should undergo regular monitoring (once or twice a year) of intraocular pressures, optic disks, and visual fields. It is likely that many ocular hypertensives who do not develop glaucoma have relatively thick corneas, producing an overestimation of intraocular pressure. Measurement of central corneal thickness may therefore be useful to determine which patients are at risk of developing glaucoma. Conversely, many individuals with ocular hypertension may have glaucoma, but the retinal ganglion cell damage is not detectable with currently available techniques. Developments in perimetry and retinal nerve fiber layer imaging are addressing this issue.

PRIMARY ANGLE-CLOSURE GLAUCOMA

Primary angle closure occurs in anatomically predisposed eyes without other pathology. Elevation of intraocular pressure is a consequence of obstruction of aqueous outflow by occlusion of the trabecular meshwork by the peripheral iris. The condition may manifest as an ophthalmic emergency or may remain asymptomatic until visual loss occurs. The diagnosis is made by examination of the anterior segment and careful gonioscopy. Primary angle-closure glaucoma is the term that should be used only when primary angle closure has resulted in optic nerve damage and visual field loss. Risk factors include increasing age, female gender, family history of glaucoma, and South-East Asian, Chinese, or Inuit ethnic background.

1. ACUTE ANGLE CLOSURE

Acute angle closure ("acute glaucoma") occurs when sufficient iris bombé develops to cause occlusion of the anterior chamber angle by the peripheral iris. This blocks aqueous outflow, and the intraocular pressure rises rapidly, causing severe pain, redness, and blurring of vision. Angle closure develops in hyperopic eyes with preexisting anatomic narrowing of the anterior chamber angle, usually when it is exacerbated by enlargement of the crystalline lens associated with aging. The acute attack is often precipitated by pupillary dilation. This occurs spontaneously in the evenings, when the level of illumination is reduced. It may be due to medications with anticholinergic or sympathomimetic activity (eg, atropine for preoperative medication, antidepressants,

nebulized bronchodilators, nasal decongestants, or tocolytics). It may occur rarely with pupillary dilation for ophthalmoscopy. If pupillary dilation is necessary in a patient with a shallow anterior chamber (easily detected by oblique illumination with a penlight [Figure 11–4]), it is best to rely on short-acting mydriatics, avoid constricting the pupil with pilocarpine, and advise the patient to seek attention immediately in the event of ocular pain or redness or increasingly blurred vision.

▶ Clinical Findings

Acute angle closure is characterized by sudden onset of visual loss accompanied by excruciating pain, halos, and nausea and vomiting. Patients are occasionally thought to have acute gastrointestinal disease. Other findings include markedly increased intraocular pressure, a shallow anterior chamber, a steamy cornea, a fixed, moderately dilated pupil, and ciliary injection. It is important to perform gonioscopy on the fellow eye to confirm the anatomic predisposition to primary acute angle closure.

▶ Differential Diagnosis (See Inside Front Cover)

Acute iritis causes more photophobia than acute glaucoma. Intraocular pressure is usually not elevated; the pupil is constricted or irregular in shape and the cornea is usually not edematous. Marked flare and cells are present in the anterior chamber, and there is deep ciliary injection.

Acute conjunctivitis is usually bilateral, and there is little or no pain and no visual loss. There is discharge from the eye and an intensely inflamed conjunctiva but no ciliary injection. The pupillary responses and intraocular pressure are normal, and the cornea is clear.

▶ Complications & Sequelae

If treatment is delayed, the peripheral iris may adhere to the trabecular meshwork (anterior synechiae), producing irreversible occlusion of the anterior chamber angle requiring surgery. Optic nerve damage is common.

▶ Treatment

Acute angle closure is an ophthalmic emergency!

Treatment is initially directed at reducing the intraocular pressure. Intravenous and oral acetazolamide—along with topical agents, such as beta-blockers and apraclonidine, and, if necessary, hyperosmotic agents—will usually reduce the intraocular pressure. Pilocarpine 2% should be instilled one-half hour after commencement of treatment, by which time reduction of iris ischemia and lowering of intraocular pressure allow the sphincter pupillae to respond to the drug. Topical steroids may also be used to reduce secondary intraocular inflammation. Once the intraocular pressure is under control, laser peripheral iridotomy should be undertaken to form a permanent connection between the anterior and posterior chambers, thus preventing recurrence of iris bombé. This is most often done with the neodymium:YAG laser (see above). Surgical peripheral iridectomy is the conventional treatment if laser treatment is unsuccessful, but ALPI may be performed. The fellow eye should always undergo prophylactic laser iridotomy.

2. SUBACUTE ANGLE CLOSURE

The same etiologic factors operate in subacute as in acute angle closure except that episodes of elevated intraocular pressure are of short duration and are recurrent. The episodes of angle closure resolve spontaneously, but there is accumulated damage to the anterior chamber angle, with formation of peripheral anterior synechiae. Subacute angle closure will occasionally progress to acute closure.

There are recurrent short episodes of unilateral pain, redness, and blurring of vision associated with halos around lights. Attacks often occur in the evenings and resolve overnight. Examination between attacks may show only a narrow anterior chamber angle with peripheral anterior synechiae. The diagnosis can be confirmed by gonioscopy. Treatment consists of laser peripheral iridotomy.

3. CHRONIC ANGLE-CLOSURE GLAUCOMA

Patients with the anatomic predisposition to anterior-chamber angle closure may never develop episodes of acute rise in intraocular pressure but form increasingly extensive peripheral anterior synechiae accompanied by a gradual rise in intraocular pressure. These patients present in the same way as those with primary open-angle glaucoma, often with extensive visual field loss in both eyes. Occasionally, they have attacks of subacute angle closure.

On examination, there is elevated intraocular pressure, narrow anterior chamber angles with variable amounts of peripheral anterior synechiae, and optic disk and visual field changes.

Laser peripheral iridotomy should always be undertaken as the first step in the management of these patients. Intraocular pressure is then controlled medically if possible, but the extent of peripheral anterior synechia formation and sluggish outflow through the remaining trabecular meshwork make pressure control very difficult, so that drainage surgery is often required. Cataract extraction with intraocular lens implantation can be effective in controlling the intraocular pressure, provided no more than two quadrants of synechial angle closure are present. Epinephrine and strong miotics must not be used unless peripheral iridotomy or iridectomy has been performed because they will accentuate angle closure.

4. PLATEAU IRIS

Plateau iris is an uncommon condition in which the central anterior chamber depth is normal but the anterior chamber angle is very narrow because of an anterior position of the ciliary processes. Such an eye has little pupillary block, but dilation will cause bunching up of the peripheral iris, occluding the angle (angle crowding), even if peripheral iridotomy or iridectomy has been performed. Affected individuals present with acute angle closure at a young age, with recurrences after peripheral laser iridotomy or surgical iridectomy. Long-term miotic therapy or laser iridoplasty is required.

5. CONGENITAL GLAUCOMA

Congenital glaucoma is rare. It can be subdivided into (1) primary congenital glaucoma, in which the developmental abnormalities are restricted to the anterior chamber angle; (2) the anterior segment developmental anomalies—Axenfeld–Rieger syndrome and Peters anomaly, in which iris and corneal development are also abnormal; and (3) a variety of other conditions—including aniridia, Sturge–Weber syndrome, neurofibromatosis-1, Lowe (oculo-cerebro-renal) syndrome, and congenital rubella—in which the developmental anomalies of the angle are associated with other ocular or extraocular abnormalities.

▶ Clinical Findings

Congenital glaucoma is manifest at birth in 50%, diagnosed in the first 6 months in 70%, and diagnosed by the end of the first year in 80% of cases. The earliest and most common symptom is epiphora. Photophobia and decreased corneal luster may be present. Increased intraocular pressure is the cardinal sign. Glaucomatous cupping of the optic disk is a relatively early—and the most important—change. Later findings include increased corneal diameter (above 11.5 mm is considered significant) (Figure 11–10), epithelial edema, tears of Descemet's membrane, and increased depth of the anterior chamber (associated with general enlargement of the anterior segment of the eye), as well as edema and opacity of the corneal stroma.

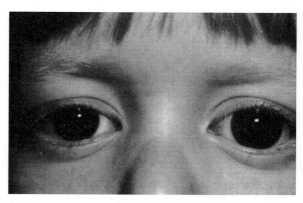

▲ **Figure 11–10.** Congenital glaucoma (buphthalmos).

▶ Differential Diagnosis

Megalocornea, corneal clouding due to congenital dystrophy or mucopolysaccharidoses, and traumatic rupture of Descemet's membrane should be ruled out. Measurement of intraocular pressure, gonioscopy, and evaluation of the optic disk are important in making the differential diagnosis. Assessment generally requires examination under general anesthesia.

▶ Course & Prognosis

In untreated cases, blindness occurs early. The eye undergoes marked stretching and may even rupture with minor trauma. Typical glaucomatous cupping occurs relatively soon, emphasizing the need for early treatment. Treatment is always surgical, and either a goniotomy or trabeculectomy can be undertaken.

ANTERIOR SEGMENT DEVELOPMENTAL ANOMALIES

These rare diseases constitute a spectrum of maldevelopment of the anterior segment, involving the angle, iris, cornea, and occasionally the lens. Usually there is some hypoplasia of the anterior stroma of the iris, with bridging filaments connecting the iris stroma to the cornea. If these bridging filaments occur peripherally and connect to a prominent, axially displaced Schwalbe's line (posterior embryotoxon), the disease is known as **Axenfeld's syndrome.** If there are broader iridocorneal adhesions associated with the disruption of the iris, with polycoria and, in addition, skeletal and dental anomalies, the disorder is called **Rieger's syndrome** (an example of iridotrabecular dysgenesis). If adhesions are between the central iris and the central posterior surface of the cornea, the disease is known as **Peters' anomaly** (an example of iridocorneal trabeculodysgenesis).

These diseases are usually dominantly inherited, although sporadic cases have been reported. Mutations on chromosomes 4, 6, and 13, probably involving homeobox genes, have been identified in pedigrees with Axenfeld–Rieger syndrome. Glaucoma occurs in approximately 50% of such eyes and often does not present until late childhood or early adulthood. Goniotomy has a much lower success rate in these cases, and trabeculotomy or trabeculectomy may be recommended. Many such patients require long-term medical glaucoma therapy, and the prognosis is guarded for long-term retention of good visual function.

ANIRIDIA

The distinguishing feature of aniridia, as the name implies, is the vestigial iris. In many cases, little more than the root of the iris or a thin iris margin is present. Other deformities of the eye may be present, such as congenital cataracts, corneal dystrophy, and foveal hypoplasia. Vision is usually poor.

Glaucoma frequently develops before adolescence and is usually refractory to medical or surgical management.

This rare syndrome is genetically determined. Both autosomal dominant and autosomal recessive inheritance have been reported.

If medical therapy is ineffective, glaucoma drainage surgery should be undertaken.

▼ SECONDARY GLAUCOMA

Increased intraocular pressure occurring as one manifestation of some other eye disease is called secondary glaucoma. These diseases are difficult to classify satisfactorily. Treatment involves controlling intraocular pressure by medical and surgical means but also dealing with the underlying disease if possible.

PIGMENTARY GLAUCOMA

Pigment dispersion syndrome is characterized by abnormal deposition of pigment in the anterior chamber—notably in the trabecular meshwork that presumably impedes outflow of aqueous and on the posterior corneal surface (Krukenberg's spindle)—and iris transillumination defects. Ultrasound studies show a posterior bowing of the iris with contact between the iris and zonules or ciliary processes, suggesting that pigment granules are rubbed off from the back surface of the iris as a result of friction, resulting in the iris transillumination defects. The syndrome occurs most often in myopic males between the ages of 25 and 40 who have a deep anterior chamber with a wide anterior chamber angle.

The pigmentary changes may be present without glaucoma, but such persons must be considered "glaucoma suspects." Up to 10% develop glaucoma within 5 years of presentation and 15% within 15 years (**pigmentary glaucoma**). A number of pedigrees of autosomal dominant inheritance of pigmentary glaucoma have been reported, and a gene for pigment dispersion syndrome has been mapped to chromosome 7.

Both miotic therapy and laser peripheral iridotomy have been shown to reverse the abnormal iris configuration, but whether they have long-term benefit on glaucoma development and progression is not yet clear. (Because the patients are usually young myopes, miotic therapy is poorly tolerated unless administered as pilocarpine once daily, preferably at bedtime.)

Both pigment dispersion syndrome and pigmentary glaucoma are notable for a propensity to episodes of markedly elevated intraocular pressure—characteristically after exercise or pupillary dilation—and pigmentary glaucoma may progress rapidly. An additional problem is the young age at which pigmentary glaucoma usually develops, increasing the chance that glaucoma drainage surgery will be necessary and that antimetabolite therapy will be required. Laser trabeculoplasty is frequently used in this condition but is unlikely to obviate the need for drainage surgery.

PSEUDOEXFOLIATION GLAUCOMA

In **pseudoexfoliation syndrome,** fine white deposits of a fibrillary material are seen on the anterior lens surface (in contrast to the true exfoliation of the lens capsule caused by exposure to infrared radiation, ie, "glassblower's cataract"), ciliary processes, zonule, posterior iris surface, loose in the anterior chamber, and in the trabecular meshwork (along with increased pigmentation). These deposits can also be detected histologically in the conjunctiva, suggesting a more widespread abnormality. The disease usually occurs in patients over age 65 and is reported to be particularly common in Scandinavia, although this may reflect ascertainment bias. The cumulative risk of developing glaucoma is 5% at 5 years and 15% at 10 years. Two polymorphisms in the coding region of the gene lysyl oxidase-like gene (LOXL1, located on chromosome 15q24.1) are associated with pseudo-exfoliation glaucoma. Treatment is as for primary open-angle glaucoma. Eyes with pseudoexfoliation syndrome have a greater incidence of complications during cataract surgery.

GLAUCOMA SECONDARY TO CHANGES IN THE LENS

▶ Lens Dislocation

The crystalline lens may be dislocated as a result of trauma or spontaneously, as in Marfan's syndrome. Anterior dislocation may cause obstruction of the pupillary aperture, leading to iris bombé and angle closure. Posterior dislocation into the vitreous is also associated with glaucoma, although the mechanism is obscure. It may be due to angle damage at the time of traumatic dislocation.

In anterior dislocation, the definitive treatment is lens extraction once the intraocular pressure has been controlled medically. In posterior dislocation, the lens is usually left alone and the glaucoma treated as primary open-angle glaucoma.

▶ Intumescence of the Lens

In this rare condition, the lens may take up fluid during cataractous change, increasing markedly in size. It may then encroach upon the anterior chamber, producing both pupillary block and angle crowding and resulting in acute angle closure. Treatment consists of lens extraction once the intraocular pressure has been controlled medically.

▶ Phacolytic Glaucoma

Some advanced cataracts may develop leakiness of the anterior lens capsule, which allows passage of liquefied lens proteins into the anterior chamber. There is an inflammatory reaction in the anterior chamber, and the trabecular meshwork becomes edematous and obstructed with lens proteins, leading to an acute rise in intraocular pressure. Lens extraction is the definitive treatment once the intraocular pressure has been controlled medically and intensive topical steroid therapy has reduced the intraocular inflammation.

GLAUCOMA SECONDARY TO CHANGES IN THE UVEAL TRACT

▶ Uveitis

The intraocular pressure is usually below normal in uveitis because the inflamed ciliary body is functioning poorly. However, elevation of intraocular pressure may also occur through a number of different mechanisms. The trabecular meshwork may become blocked by inflammatory cells from the anterior chamber, with secondary edema, or may occasionally be involved in an inflammatory process specifically directed at the trabecular cells (trabeculitis). One of the most common causes of raised intraocular pressure in individuals with uveitis is the use of topical steroids. Chronic or recurrent uveitis produces permanent impairment of trabecular function, peripheral anterior synechiae, and occasionally angle neovascularization, all of which increase the chance of secondary glaucoma. Seclusio pupillae due to 360° posterior synechiae produces iris bombé and acute angle-closure glaucoma. The uveitis syndromes that tend to be associated with secondary glaucoma are Fuchs heterochromic cyclitis, HLA-B27–associated acute anterior uveitis, and uveitis due to herpes zoster and herpes simplex.

Treatment is directed chiefly at controlling the uveitis with concomitant medical glaucoma therapy as necessary, avoiding miotics because of the increased chance of posterior synechia formation. Long-term therapy, including surgery, is often required because of irreversible damage to the trabecular meshwork.

Acute angle closure due to seclusion of the pupil may be reversed by intensive mydriasis but often requires laser peripheral iridotomy or surgical iridectomy. Any uveitis with a tendency to posterior synechia formation must be treated with mydriatics whenever the uveitis is active to reduce the risk of pupillary seclusion.

▶ Tumor

Uveal tract melanomas may cause glaucoma by anterior displacement of the ciliary body, causing secondary angle closure, direct involvement of the anterior chamber angle, blockage of the filtration angle by pigment dispersion, and angle neovascularization. Enucleation is usually necessary.

▶ Ciliary Body Swelling

Forward rotation of the ciliary body, resulting in anterior displacement of the lens-iris diaphragm and secondary angle-closure glaucoma, may also occur after vitreoretinal surgery or retinal cryotherapy, in posterior uveitis, and with topiramate therapy.

IRIDOCORNEAL ENDOTHELIAL (ICE) SYNDROME (ESSENTIAL IRIS ATROPHY, CHANDLER SYNDROME, IRIS NEVUS SYNDROME)

This rare idiopathic condition of young adults is usually unilateral and manifested by corneal decompensation, glaucoma, and iris abnormalities (corectopia and polycoria).

GLAUCOMA SECONDARY TO TRAUMA

Contusion injuries of the globe may be associated with an early rise in intraocular pressure due to bleeding into the anterior chamber (hyphema). Free blood blocks the trabecular meshwork, which is also rendered edematous by the injury. Treatment is initially medical, but surgery may be required if the pressure remains elevated, which is particularly likely if there is a second episode of bleeding.

Late effects of contusion injuries on intraocular pressure are due to direct angle damage. The interval between the injury and the development of glaucoma may obscure the association. Clinically, the anterior chamber is seen to be deeper than in the fellow eye, and gonioscopy shows recession of the angle. Medical therapy is usually effective, but drainage surgery may be required.

Laceration or contusional rupture of the anterior segment is associated with loss of the anterior chamber. If the chamber is not reformed soon after the injury—either spontaneously, by iris incarceration into the wound, or surgically—peripheral anterior synechiae will form and result in irreversible angle closure.

GLAUCOMA FOLLOWING OCULAR SURGERY

▶ Ciliary Block Glaucoma (Malignant Glaucoma)

Surgery upon an eye with markedly increased intraocular pressure and a closed or narrow angle can lead to ciliary block glaucoma. Postoperatively, the intraocular pressure is higher than expected and the lens is pushed forward as a result of the collection of aqueous in and behind the vitreous body. Patients initially become aware of blurred distance vision but improved near vision. This is followed by pain and inflammation.

Treatment consists of cycloplegics, mydriatics, aqueous suppressants, and hyperosmotic agents. Hyperosmotic agents are used to shrink the vitreous body and let the lens move backwards.

Posterior sclerotomy, vitrectomy, and even lens extraction may be needed.

▶ Peripheral Anterior Synechiae

Just as with trauma to the anterior segment (see above), surgery that results in a flat anterior chamber will lead to formation of peripheral anterior synechiae. Early surgical reformation of the chamber is required if it does not occur spontaneously.

NEOVASCULAR GLAUCOMA

Neovascularization of the iris (rubeosis iridis) and anterior chamber angle is most often secondary to widespread retinal ischemia such as occurs in advanced diabetic retinopathy and ischemic central retinal vein occlusion. Glaucoma results initially from obstruction of the angle by the fibrovascular membrane, but subsequent contraction of the membrane leads to angle closure.

Treatment of established neovascular glaucoma is difficult and often unsatisfactory. Both the stimulus to neovascularization and the raised intraocular pressure need to be treated. Intravitreal injection of bevacizumab (a monoclonal antibody that inhibits vascular endothelial growth factor) can reverse the iris neovascularization. Topical atropine 1% and intensive topical steroids should be given to reduce inflammation and improve comfort. In many cases, vision is lost and cyclodestructive procedures are necessary to control the intraocular pressure.

GLAUCOMA SECONDARY TO RAISED EPISCLERAL VENOUS PRESSURE

Raised episcleral venous pressure may contribute to glaucoma in Sturge–Weber syndrome, in which a developmental anomaly of the angle is also often present, and carotid-cavernous fistula, which may also cause angle neovascularization due to widespread ocular ischemia. Medical treatment cannot reduce the intraocular pressure below the level of the abnormally elevated episcleral venous pressure, and surgery is associated with a high risk of complications.

STEROID-INDUCED GLAUCOMA

Topical, periocular, and intraocular corticosteroids may produce a type of glaucoma that simulates primary open-angle glaucoma, particularly in individuals with a family history of the disease, and will exaggerate the intraocular pressure elevation in those with established primary open-angle glaucoma. Withdrawal of the medication usually eliminates these effects, but permanent damage can occur if the situation goes unrecognized too long. If topical steroid therapy is absolutely necessary, medical glaucoma therapy will usually control the intraocular pressure. Systemic steroid therapy is less likely to cause a rise in intraocular pressure. It is imperative that patients receiving topical or systemic steroid therapy undergo periodic tonometry and ophthalmoscopy, particularly if there is a family history of glaucoma.

REFERENCES

AGIS (Advanced Glaucoma Intervention Study) Investigators: 7. The relationship between control of intraocular pressure and visual field deterioration. Am J Ophthalmol 2000;130:429. [PMID: 11024415]

Aung T et al: Configuration of the drainage angle, intraocular pressure and optic disc cupping in subjects with chronic angle-closure glaucoma. Ophthalmology 2005;112:28. [PMID: 15629816]

Bengtsson B et al: Fluctuation of intraocular pressure and glaucoma progression in the Early Manifest Glaucoma Trial. Ophthalmology 2007;114:205. [PMID: 17097736]

Bengtsson B, Patella VM, Heijl A: Prediction of glaucomatous visual field loss by extrapolation of linear trends. Arch Ophthalmol 2009;127:1610. [PMID: 20008716]

Broman AT et al: Estimating the rate of progressive visual field damage in those with open-angle glaucoma, from cross-sectional data. Invest Ophthalmol Vis Sci 2008;49:66.[PMID: 18172076]

Budenz DL: A clinician's guide to the assessment and management of nonadherence in glaucoma. Ophthalmology 2009;116:S43. [PMID: 19837260]

Busbee BG: Update on treatment strategies for bleb-associated endophthalmitis. Curr Opin Ophthalmol 2005;16:170. [PMID: 15870574]

Chauhan BC et al: Practical recommendations for measuring rates of visual field change in glaucoma. Br J Ophthalmol 2008;92:569. [PMID: 18211935]

Chen PP et al: Blindness in patients with treated open-angle glaucoma. Ophthalmology 2003;110:726. [PMID: 12689894]

Deva NC et al: Risk factors for first presentation of glaucoma with significant visual field loss. Clin Experiment Ophthalmol 2008;36:217. [PMID: 18412589]

Gedde SJ et al: Three-year follow-up of the Tube versus Trabeculectomy Study. Am J Ophthalmol 2009. [PMID: 19674729]

Gordon MO et al: The Ocular Hypertension Treatment Study: baseline factors that predict the onset of primary open-angle glaucoma. Arch Ophthalmol 2002;120:714. [PMID: 12049575]

Greenfield DS et al: The cupped disc. Who needs neuroimaging? Ophthalmology 1998;105:1866. [PMID: 9787356]

Heijl A et al: Natural history of open-angle glaucoma. Ophthalmology 2009;116:2271. [PMID: 19854514]

Herndon LW: Central corneal thickness as a risk factor for advanced glaucoma damage. Arch Ophthalmol 2004;122:17. [PMID: 14718289]

Hitchings RA: Glaucoma: an area of darkness. Eye 2009; 23:1764. [PMID: 18791552]

Hodge WG et al: The efficacy and harm of prostaglandin analogues for IOP reduction in glaucoma patients compared to dorzolamide and brionidine: a systematic review. Br J Ophthalmol 2008;92:7. [PMID: 18156371]

Hong CH et al: Glaucoma draining devices: a systemic literature review and current controversies. Surv Ophthalmol 2005;50:48. [PMID: 15621077]

Hsieh JW et al: Clinical characteristics and prognostic significance of disc hemorrhage in open-angle and angle-closure glaucoma. J Glaucoma 2009 Oct 22. [Epub ahead of print] [PMID: 19855298]

Hughes E et al: 24-hour monitoring of intraocular pressure in glaucoma management: a retrospective review. J Glaucoma 2003;12:232. [PMID: 12782841]

Jampel HD et al: Perioperative complications of trabeculectomy in the Collaborative Initial Glaucoma Treatment Study (CIGTS). Am J Ophthalmol 2005;140:16. [PMID: 15939389]

Kersey JP, Broadway DC: Corticosteroid-induced glaucoma: a review of the literature. Eye 2006;20:407. [PMID: 15877093]

Konstas AGP et al: Factors associated with long-term progression or stability in exfoliation glaucoma. Arch Ophthalmol 2004;122:29. [PMID: 14718291]

Lama PJ et al: Antifibrotics and wound healing in glaucoma surgery. Surv Ophthalmol 2003;48:314. [PMID: 12745005]

Leske MC et al: Predictors of long-term progression in the Early Manifest Glaucoma Trial. Ophthalmology 2007;114:1965. [PMID: 17628686]

Macdonald E, Mukherjee S, Jay J: The increasingly iatrogenic indications for mitomycin C trabeculectomy over 10 years. Can J Ophthalmol 2009;44:205. [PMID: 19491957]

Martus P et al: Predictive factors for progressive optic nerve damage in various types of chronic open-angle glaucoma. Am J Ophthalmol 2005;139:999. [PMID: 15953429]

Mendicino ME et al: Long-term surgical and visual outcomes in primary congenital glaucoma: 360 degrees trabeculotomy versus goniotomy. J AAPOS 2000;4:205. [PMID: 10951295]

Moraczewski AL et al: Outcomes of treatment of neovascular glaucoma with intravitreal bevacizumab. Br J Ophthalmol 2009;93:589. [PMID: 19074917]

Musch DC et al: Factors associated with intraocular pressure before and during 9 years of treatment in the Collaborative Initial Glaucoma Treatment Study. Ophthalmology 2008;115:927. [17964655]

Niyadurupola N, Broadway DC: Pigment dispersion syndrome and pigmentary glaucoma—a major review. Clin Experiment Ophthalmol 2009;36:868. [PMID: 19278484]

Nouri-Mahdavi K et al: Predictive factors for glaucomatous visual field progression in the Advanced Glaucoma Intervention Study. Ophthalmology 2004;111:1627. [PMID: 15350314]

Papadopoulos M, Khaw PT: Advances in the management of paediatric glaucoma. Eye 2007;21:1319. [PMID: 17914435]

Parrish RK et al: A comparison of latanoprost, bimatoprost, and travoprost in patients with elevated intraocular pressure. A 12-week, randomized, masked-evaluator multicentre study. Am J Ophthalmol 2003;135:688. [PMID: 12719078]

Parrish RK 2nd et al: Five-year follow-up optic disc findings of the Collaborative Initial Glaucoma Treatment Study. Am J Ophthalmol 2009;147:717. [PMID: 19152871]

Rahman MQ, Montgomery DM, Lazaridou MN: Surveillance of glaucoma medical therapy in a Glasgow teaching hospital: 26 years' experience. Br J Ophthalmol 2009;93:1572. [PMID: 19628493]

Ray K, Mookherjee S: Molecular complexity of primary open-angle glaucoma: current concepts. J Genet 2009;88:451. [PMID: 20090207]

Rees G et al: Intentional and unintentional nonadherence to ocular hypotensive treatment in patients with glaucoma. Ophthalmology 2010 Feb 12. [Epub ahead of print] [PMID: 20153902]

Sharan S et al: Late-onset bleb infections: prevalence and risk factors. Can J Ophthalmol 2009;44:279. [PMID: 19491982]

Suominen S et al: The effect of deep sclerectomy on intraocular pressure of normal-tension glaucoma patients: 1-year results. Acta Ophthalmol 2009 Sep 21. [Epub ahead of print] [PMID: 19775310]

Tarongoy P, Ho CL, Walton DS: Angle-closure glaucoma: the role of the lens in the pathogenesis, prevention, and treatment. Surv Ophthalmol 2009;54:211. [PMID: 19298900]

Thorleifsson G et al: Common sequence variants in the LOXL1 gene confer susceptibility to exfoliation glaucoma. Science 2007;317:1397 [PMID: 17690259]

Tsai JC. A comprehensive perspective on patient adherence to topical glaucoma therapy. Ophthalmology 2009;116:S30. [PMID: 19837258]

van der Valk R et al: Intraocular pressure-lowering effects of all commonly used glaucoma drugs: a meta-analysis of randomized clinical trials. Ophthalmology 2005;112:1177. [PMID: 15921747]

Wakabayashi T et al: Intravitreal bevacizumab to treat iris neovascularization and neovascular glaucoma secondary to ischemic retinal diseases in 41 consecutive cases. Ophthalmology 2008;115:1571. [PMID: 18440643]

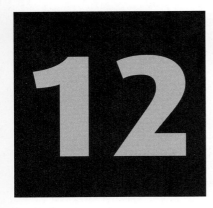

Strabismus

W. Walker Motley, MS, MD, and Taylor Asbury, MD

Under normal binocular viewing conditions, the image of the object of regard falls simultaneously on the fovea of each eye (bifoveal fixation) and the vertical retinal meridians are both upright. Any ocular misalignment, such that only one eye views the object of regard with the correct vertical orientation, is called "strabismus." The misalignment may be in any direction—inward, outward, up, down, or torsional. The amount of deviation is the angle by which the deviating eye is misaligned. Strabismus present under binocular viewing conditions is **manifest strabismus, heterotropia,** or **tropia** (see Box 12.1 for definitions). A deviation present only after binocular vision has been interrupted (eg, by occlusion of one eye) is called **latent strabismus, heterophoria,** or **phoria.**

Strabismus is present in about 4% of children. Treatment should be started as soon as a diagnosis is made in order to ensure the best possible visual acuity and binocular visual function. There is no such thing as "outgrowing" childhood strabismus. Strabismus may also be acquired, due to cranial nerve palsies, orbital masses, orbital fractures, or Graves' ophthalmopathy.

PHYSIOLOGY

1. MOTOR ASPECTS

▶ Individual Muscle Functions (Table 12–1)

Each of the six extraocular muscles plays a role in positioning the eye about three axes of rotation. The primary action of a muscle is the principal effect it has on eye rotation. Lesser effects are called secondary or tertiary actions. The precise action of any muscle depends on the orientation of the eye in the orbit and the influence of the orbital connective tissues, which regulates the direction of action of the extraocular muscles by acting as their functional mechanical origins (the active pulley hypothesis).

The medial and lateral rectus muscles adduct and abduct the eye, respectively, with little effect on elevation or torsion. The vertical rectus and oblique muscles have both vertical and torsional functions. In general terms, the vertical rectus muscles are the main elevators and depressors of the eye, and the obliques are mostly involved with torsional positioning. The vertical effect of the superior and inferior rectus muscles is greater when the eye is abducted. The vertical effect of the obliques is greater when the eye is adducted.

▶ Field of Action

The position of the eye is determined by the equilibrium achieved by the pull of all six extraocular muscles. The eyes are in the **primary position of gaze** when they are looking straight ahead with the head and body erect. To move the eye into another direction of gaze, the agonist muscle contracts to pull the eye in that direction and the antagonist muscle relaxes. The field of action of a muscle is the direction of gaze in which that muscle exerts its greatest contraction force as an agonist, for example, the lateral rectus muscle undergoes the greatest contraction in abducting the eye (Table 12–1).

▶ Synergistic & Antagonistic Muscles (Sherrington's Law)

Synergistic muscles are those that have the same field of action. Thus, for vertical gaze, the superior rectus and inferior oblique muscles are synergists in moving the eye upward. Muscles synergistic for one function may be antagonistic for another. For example, the superior rectus and inferior oblique muscles are antagonists for torsion, the superior rectus causing intorsion and the inferior oblique extorsion. The extraocular muscles, like skeletal muscles, show reciprocal innervation of antagonistic muscles (Sherrington's law). Thus, in dextroversion (right gaze), the right medial and left lateral rectus muscles are inhibited while the right lateral and left medial rectus muscles are stimulated.

BOX 12.1. DEFINITIONS

Angle Kappa: The main angle between the visual axis and the central pupillary line. When the eye is fixing a light, if the corneal reflection is centered on the pupil, the visual axis and the central pupillary line coincide and the angle kappa is zero. Ordinarily, the light reflex is 2°–4° nasal to the pupillary center, giving the appearance of slight exotropia (positive angle kappa). A negative angle kappa gives the false impression of esotropia.

Conjugate movement: Movement of the eyes in the same direction at the same time.

Deviation: Magnitude of ocular misalignment, usually measured in prism diopters (see later in the chapter) but sometimes measured in degrees.

Comitant deviation: Deviation not significantly affected by which eye is fixing or direction of gaze, typically a feature of childhood (nonparetic) strabismus.

Incomitant deviation: Deviation varies according to which eye is fixing and direction of gaze, usually a feature of recent onset extraocular muscle paresis and other types of acquired strabismus.

Primary deviation: Incomitant deviation measured with the normal eye fixing (Figure 12–2).

Secondary deviation: Incomitant deviation measured with the affected eye fixing.

Ductions: (Figure 12–3) Monocular rotations with no consideration of the position of the other eye.

Adduction: Inward rotation.

Abduction: Outward rotation.

Supraduction (elevation): Upward rotation.

Infraduction (depression): Downward rotation.

Fusion: Formation of one image from the two images seen simultaneously by the two eyes. Fusion has two aspects.

Motor fusion: Adjustments made by the brain in innervation of extraocular muscles in order to bring both eyes into bifoveal and torsional alignment.

Sensory fusion: Integration in the visual sensory areas of the brain of images seen with the two eyes into one picture.

Heterophoria (phoria): Latent deviation of the eyes held straight by binocular fusion.

Esophoria: Tendency for one eye to turn inward.

Exophoria: Tendency for one eye to turn outward.

Hyperphoria: Tendency for one eye to deviate upward.

Hypophoria: Tendency for one eye to deviate downward.

(See Hypotropia.)

Heterotropia (tropia):

Strabismus: Manifest deviation of the eyes that cannot be controlled by binocular vision.

Esotropia: Convergent manifest deviation ("crossed eyes").

Exotropia: Divergent manifest deviation ("wall eyes").

Hypertropia: Manifest deviation of one eye upward.

Hypotropia: Manifest deviation of one eye upward. By convention, in the absence of specific causation to account for the lower position of one eye, vertical deviations are designated by the higher eye (eg, right hypertropia, not left hypotropia, when the right eye is higher).

Incyclotropia: Manifest rotation of the 12 o'clock meridian of one eye about its anteroposterior axis toward the midline of the head.

Excyclotropia: Manifest rotation of the 12 o'clock meridian of one eye about its anteroposterior axis away from the midline of the head.

Orthophoria: The absence of any tendency of either eye to deviate when fusion is suspended. This state is rarely seen clinically. A small phoria is normal.

Prism diopter (PD): The unit of angular measurement used to characterize ocular deviations. A 1 diopter prism deflects a ray of light toward the base of the prism by 1 cm at 1 m. One degree of arc equals approximately 1.7 PD.

Secondary deviation: (Figure 12–2) The deviation measured with the paretic eye fixing and the normal eye deviating.

Torsion: Rotation of the eye about its anteroposterior axis (Figure 12–3).

Intorsion (incycloduction): Rotation of the 12 o'clock meridian of the eye toward the midline of the head.

Extorsion (excycloduction): Rotation of the 12 o'clock meridian of the eye away from the midline of the head.

Vergences (disjunctive movements): Movement of the two eyes in opposite directions.

Convergence: The eyes turn inward.

Divergence: The eyes turn outward.

Versions: Binocular rotations of the eyes in qualitatively the same direction.

Table 12–1. Functions of the Ocular Muscles

Muscle	Primary Action	Secondary Actions
Lateral rectus	Abduction	None
Medial rectus	Adduction	None
Superior rectus	Elevation	Adduction, intorsion
Inferior rectus	Depression	Adduction, extorsion
Superior oblique	Intorsion	Depression, abduction
Inferior oblique	Extorsion	Elevation, abduction

▶ Yoke Muscles (Hering's Law)

For movements of both eyes in the same direction, the corresponding agonist muscles receive equal innervation (Hering's law). The pair of agonist muscles with the same primary action is called a yoke pair. The right lateral rectus and the left medial rectus muscles are a yoke pair for right gaze. The right inferior rectus and the left superior oblique muscles are a yoke pair for gaze downward and to the right. Table 12–2 lists the yoke muscle combinations.

▶ Motor Fusion

Motor fusion is the process by which the activity of the extraocular muscles is adjusted to maintain the necessary ocular alignment for sensory fusion (see later in the chapter). It is stimulated by disparity in images received from the two eyes, such as results from the object of regard moving toward or away from the subject.

▶ Development of Binocular Movement

The neuromuscular system of an infant is immature, so that it is not uncommon in the first few months of life for ocular alignment to be unstable. Transient exodeviations are most common and are associated with immaturity of the accommodation-convergence system. Gradually improving visual acuity together with maturation of the ocular motor system allows a more stable ocular alignment by age 2 to 3 months. Any ocular misalignment after this age should be investigated by an ophthalmologist.

Table 12–2. Yoke Muscles in Cardinal Positions of Gaze

Eyes up and right	RSR and LIO
Eyes up and left	LSR and RIO
Eyes right	RLR and LMR
Eyes left	LLR and RMR
Eyes down and right	RIR and LSO
Eyes down and left	LIR and RSO

2. SENSORY ASPECTS

▶ Binocular Vision, Sensory Fusion, & Stereopsis

Binocular vision, the ability to combine the visual information from two eyes viewing the same scene into a single image, provides several advantages, not least the potential for three-dimensional vision (stereopsis). The corresponding disadvantage is that the process is dependent upon maintenance of ocular alignment.

The retinal locations upon which fall the images of a single object in the two eyes are known as **corresponding retinal points.** Since the two eyes are not in precisely the same location, the images on these retinal points are not exactly the same. **Sensory fusion** is the process whereby disparities between the two images at corresponding retinal points are overcome to allow a single image to be perceived. In reality there is not absolute correspondence between the retinal points that can be stimulated to produce a single image. Each point of the retina in each eye is capable of fusing stimuli that strike sufficiently close to the corresponding retinal point in the other eye. The representation in space of this region of fusible points is called **Panum's area.** It is narrowest at fixation and progressively increases in size with increasing eccentricity in the visual field. Sensory fusion is also dependent upon the images in the two eyes being sufficiently similar, equality of size being a particularly important factor.

In contradistinction to sensory fusion, **stereopsis** relies upon recognition of the disparities of images that are being fused, effectively utilizing parallax. It is quantified as the smallest detectable disparity, around 60 seconds of arc being high-grade (fine) stereopsis, which is only possible with bifoveal fixation, and around 1000 seconds of arc being low-grade (gross) stereopsis. Although stereopsis is essential for high-grade depth perception, monocular clues such as apparent size of objects, interposition of objects, and motion parallax can be used to judge depth.

▶ Sensory Phenomena in Strabismus

Strabismus is associated with various sensory phenomena, including diplopia and visual confusion, abnormal (anomalous) retinal correspondence, suppression, amblyopia, and eccentric fixation. The occurrence of these phenomena is related to whether the strabismus is present during the development of the visual system, which occurs up to age 7 or 8.

A. Diplopia and Visual Confusion

In the presence of strabismus, each fovea receives a different image. The image of the object of regard falls on the fovea of the fixing eye and the object is localized straight ahead, whereas the same image falls on an extrafoveal retinal area in the deviating eye and the object is localized in some other direction, so that the object of regard is perceived to be in two places (**diplopia**), with a true image from the fixing eye and a false image from the deviating eye. Correspondingly, the object responsible for the image falling on the fovea of the deviating eye is localized straight ahead, so that it and the object of regard are perceived to be in the same place (**visual confusion**). Whereas diplopia is common in acquired strabismus, awareness of visual confusion is unusual.

B. Abnormal Retinal Correspondence

In the presence of manifest strabismus, an extrafoveal retinal locus may become the preferred point of fixation in the deviating eye, resulting in **abnormal (anomalous) retinal correspondence (ARC)**. There may be exact correlation between the position of this locus and the angle of strabismus (harmonious ARC or ARC with identity) or not (unharmonious ARC or ARC without identity). ARC is present only under binocular viewing conditions, in contrast to eccentric fixation (see below). ARC avoids diplopia and visual confusion because the extrafoveal retinal locus of fixation in the deviating eye is localized straight ahead during binocular viewing. It also facilitates binocular function, possibly resulting in low-grade stereopsis.

C. Suppression

Suppression is a common sensory adaptation in childhood strabismus, avoiding diplopia and visual confusion and, also like ARC, being present only under binocular viewing conditions. The image seen by one eye predominates and that seen by the other eye is suppressed due to the presence in the deviating eye of an area of reduced visual sensitivity within the visual field. This **suppression scotoma** is termed a facultative scotoma because it is not present when the suppressing eye is tested alone, contrasting with amblyopia (see below), which persist when the affected eye is tested alone.

In esotropia, the suppression scotoma is usually approximately horizontally elliptical in shape, extending on the retina from just temporal to the fovea to the point in the nasal extrafoveal retina on which the image of the object of regard falls. In exotropia, the suppression scotoma tends to be larger, usually extending from the fovea to include the entire temporal half of the retina. If there is alternating fixation, the suppression scotoma is present in whichever eye is deviating. Suppression precludes high-grade stereopsis because of the lack of bifoveal fixation, but low-grade stereopsis may still be present due to ARC (see earlier in the chapter). In the absence of strabismus, a blurred image (usually due to anisometropia) in one eye may also lead to suppression.

D. Amblyopia

Prolonged abnormal visual experience in a child under the age of 7 years may lead to **amblyopia** (reduced visual acuity in excess of that explicable by organic disease). The three main causes of amblyopia are strabismus, unequal refractive error (anisometropia), and visual deprivation (eg, congenital cataract, ptosis or optic nerve hypoplasia). Often, more than one etiology is present. Though previously thought to be untreatable after 7 years of age, recent studies show that some forms of amblyopia may be successfully treated in older children.

In strabismus, the eye used habitually for fixation retains normal acuity whereas acuity is persistently reduced in the nonpreferred eye. In esotropia, amblyopia is common and often severe, whereas in exotropia it is uncommon and usually mild. If spontaneous alternation of fixation is present, amblyopia does not develop.

E. Eccentric Fixation

In eyes with severe amblyopia, an extrafoveal retinal area may be used for fixation even under monocular viewing conditions, in contrast to ARC (see earlier in the chapter) when the phenomenon only occurs under binocular viewing conditions. Gross eccentric fixation can be readily identified by occluding the preferred eye and asking the patient to look directly at a light source with the nonpreferred eye. An eye with gross eccentric fixation will appear not to be looking directly at the light source and will have an eccentric corneal light reflection. More subtle degrees of eccentric fixation can be detected by an ophthalmoscope that projects a target, the patient being asked to look directly at its center. If the target is projected onto any area other than the fovea, eccentric fixation is present.

CLINICAL EVALUATION OF STRABISMUS

1. HISTORY

A careful history is important in the diagnosis of strabismus.

- Laterality. Does the deviation only occur in one eye or does it alternate?

- Direction. Is the deviation inward, outward, upward, or downward?

- Duration. When was the deviation first noticed? Was the onset gradual or sudden?

- Frequency. Is the deviation constant or intermittent? If intermittent, how often does it occur? Has the frequency increased, decreased, or remained the same since it was first noticed?

- Modifying factors. Is the deviation worse with fatigue, illness, or alcohol use?

- Associated symptoms. Is there diplopia, asthenopia (eyestrain), visual confusion, or headache?

- Past ocular history—including any history of spectacle wear, ocular trauma, or surgery.

- Past medical history—including any history of prematurity, developmental delay, neurological disorder, or thyroid disease.

- Family history—including any history of strabismus, "squint," "cast", amblyopia, "lazy eye," or other ocular disease in the family?

2. EXAMINATION

▶ Visual Acuity

Visual acuity should be evaluated even if only a rough approximation or comparison of the two eyes is possible. Each eye is evaluated by itself, since binocular testing will not reveal poor vision in one eye. For the very young child, it may only be possible to establish that an eye is able to follow a moving target. The target should be as small as the child's age, interest, and level of alertness allow. Fixation is described as being normal if it is central (foveal) and steady, and maintained while the eye follows a moving object. In a preverbal child with manifest strabismus, a fixation preference for one eye implies amblyopia of the fellow eye. In a preverbal child without obvious manifest strabismus, fixation preference can be tested by holding a 15 prism diopter (PD) (see Box 12.1) vertical prism before each eye to induce a vertical disparity in images (induced tropia test). Placing the prism in front of an eye that was fixing will induce a compensatory vertical movement in both eyes, without any refixational movement if the same eye continues to fix or a refixational movement of both eyes if the fellow takes over fixation. Placing the prism in front of an eye that was not fixing will not result in any movement of either eye. Another technique for quantitatively measuring visual acuity in younger children is forced-choice preferential looking, in which the child's responses are observed to simultaneous presentation of striped gratings of a range of frequencies and an otherwise identical shaped but plain target of the same mean luminance. Threshold of detection (grating acuity) is determined by the highest frequency (cycles per second) of grating that results in consistent preferential looking by the child. It is usually better than recognition acuity, particularly in amblyopic eyes.

By the age of 2½–3 years, it is possible to perform recognition visual acuity testing using Allen pictures. By age 4 years, many children will understand the Snellen tumbling "E" game or the HOTV recognition test. HOTV testing is generally preferred, the tumbling "E" game being prone to reversal errors in young children. By age 5 or 6 years, most children can perform Snellen visual acuity testing. At this age, single optotype Snellen acuity has normally developed fully, but Snellen acuity to a line of multiple optotypes (linear acuity) may not develop fully for another 2 years. In this situation, crowded optotypes may be used to simulate linear acuity test.

▶ Determination of Refractive Error

It is important to determine the cycloplegic refractive error by retinoscopy (see Chapter 21). Cycloplegic refraction is most often performed utilizing cyclopentolate 1% ophthalmic solution. Occasionally, atropine 1% solution or ointment is used to ensure complete cycloplegia, or in children with dark irides that do not cycloplege well in response to weaker agents.

▶ Inspection and Ocular Examination

Inspection alone may show whether strabismus is constant or intermittent, alternating or nonalternating, and whether it is variable. Associated ptosis and abnormal position of the head should be noted. The quality of fixation of each eye separately and of both eyes together should be assessed. Nystagmus indicates unstable fixation and usually reduced visual acuity.

Prominent epicanthal folds that obscure all or part of the nasal sclera may give an appearance of esotropia (pseudostrabismus). Although this entity is confusing to lay persons as well as some physicians, these children have a normal corneal light reflection test. Prominent epicanthal folds gradually disappear by 4 or 5 years of age.

Ocular examination is essential to ensure that strabismus or reduced vision is not due to structural abnormalities. In children esotropia may be the presenting feature of various diseases, including congenital anomalies such as optic nerve hypoplasia, retinoblastoma, and optic nerve glioma.

▶ Determination of Angle of Strabismus (Angle of Deviation)

A. Cover Testing (Figure 12–1)

All four components of cover testing, (1) the cover test, (2) the uncover test, (3) the alternate cover test, and (4) the prism and alternate cover test, require fixation of a target, which may be in any direction of gaze at distance or near.

1. The **cover test** identifies manifest strabismus. As the examiner observes one eye, a cover is placed in front of the fellow eye to block its view of the target. If the observed eye moves to take up fixation, it was not previously fixing the target, and a manifest strabismus is present. The direction of movement reveals the direction of deviation (eg, if the observed eye moves outwards to pick up fixation esotropia is present). The cover test is performed on each eye. Childhood strabismus is usually **comitant**, meaning that the magnitude of the manifest strabismus is not significantly influenced by which eye is fixing, or the direction of gaze. Cranial nerve palsies (paretic strabismus), except when longstanding, and other types of acquired strabismus are usually **incomitant**, the magnitude of the manifest strabismus being less when the unaffected eye is fixing (**primary deviation**) than when the affected eye is fixing (**secondary deviation**) (Figure 12–2), and varying with direction of gaze (see Box 12.1).

2. The **uncover test** provides information on fixation preference if there is manifest strabismus, or identifies latent strabismus if there is no manifest strabismus. As the cover is removed from the eye following the cover test, the eye emerging from under cover is observed. If the position of the uncovered eye changes, either a manifest strabismus is present and the uncovered eye is once again taking up fixation, indicating that it is the preferred eye,

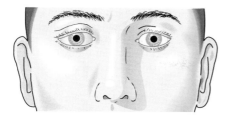

Eyes straight (maintained in position by fusion).

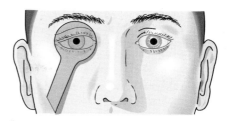

Position of eye under cover in orthophoria (fusion-free position). The right eye under cover has not moved.

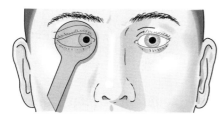

Position of eye under cover in esophoria (fusion-free position). Under cover, the right eye has deviated inward. Upon removal of cover, the right eye will immediately resume its straight-ahead position.

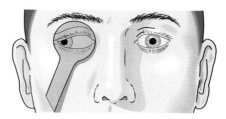

Position of eye under cover in exophoria (fusion-free position). Under cover, the right eye has deviated outward. Upon removal of the cover, the right eye will immediately resume its straight-ahead position.

▲ **Figure 12–1.** Cover testing. The patient is directed to look at a target at eye level 6 m (20 ft) away. Note: In the presence of strabismus, the deviation will remain when the cover is removed.

or interruption of binocular vision has allowed it to deviate, and a latent strabismus is present. In either case, the direction of corrective movement indicates the type of manifest or latent strabismus, with the same pattern as in the cover test (eg, outwards in esotropia or esophoria). In manifest strabismus also there will be a movement of the fellow eye but in the opposite direction (eg, inwards in

esotropia). In latent strabismus there will be no movement of the fellow eye. If the uncover test results in no movement of the uncovered eye, either a manifest strabismus is present but the fellow eye has maintained fixation, indicating alternating fixation, or there is no manifest or latent strabismus (orthophoria), which is rarely seen clinically. The uncover test is also performed on each eye.

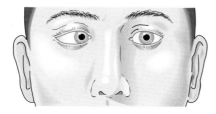

Primary deviation
(left eye fixing)

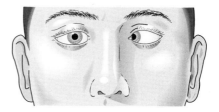

Secondary deviation (right eye fixing;
"overshoot" of sound left eye)

▲ **Figure 12–2.** Paresis of horizontal muscle (right lateral rectus). Secondary deviation is greater than primary deviation because of Hering's law. With the left eye fixing, the right eye is deviated inward because of the paretic right lateral rectus. For the right eye to fix, the paretic right lateral rectus muscle must receive excessive stimulation. The yoke muscle—the left medial rectus—also receives the same excessive stimulation (Hering's law), which causes "overshoot."

3. The **alternate cover (cross-cover) test** reveals the total deviation (manifest plus latent strabismus). The cover is placed alternately in front of one eye and then the other. It should be moved rapidly from one eye to the other to prevent re-fusion of a latent strabismus.

4. The **prism and alternate cover test** quantifies strabismus. Increasing strength of prism is placed in front of one eye until there is neutralization of the movement on alternate cover testing, thus measuring both the manifest and latent components. For example, to measure the full extent of an esodeviation, the cover is alternated while prisms of increasing base-out strength are placed in front of one eye until there is no horizontal refixational movement of the deviated eye. More than the required strength of prism will result in reversal of direction of the refixational movement. Larger deviations may require prisms held before both eyes, but prisms should never be "stacked" in the same direction before one eye.

B. Other Tests of Alignment

The various types of cover test require patient cooperation and some degree of useful vision in both eyes. Two other methods commonly used depend on observing the position of the corneal light reflection, but both are less accurate than cover tests and their results must be adjusted if the angle kappa is abnormal (see Box 12.1).

1. **Hirschberg method.** The patient fixes on a light at a distance of about 33 cm. Decentration of the light reflection is noted in the deviating eye. By allowing 18 PD for each millimeter of decentration, an estimate of the angle of deviation can be made.

2. **Prism reflex method (Krimsky test).** The patient fixes on light at a distance of about 33 cm. A prism is placed before the deviating eye, and the strength of the prism required to center the corneal reflection measures the angle of deviation.

▶ Ductions (Monocular Rotations) (Figure 12–3)

With one eye covered, the other eye follows a moving target in all directions of gaze. Any decrease of rotation indicates limitation in the field of action of the respective muscle due to weakness of contraction or failure of relaxation of its antagonist.

▶ Versions (Conjugate Ocular Movements)

Hering's law states that yoke muscles receive equal stimulation during any conjugate ocular movement. Versions are tested by having the eyes fix a light in the nine cardinal positions: primary—straight ahead; secondary—right, left, up, and down; and tertiary—up and right, down and right, up and left, and down and left (Table 12–2). Difference in

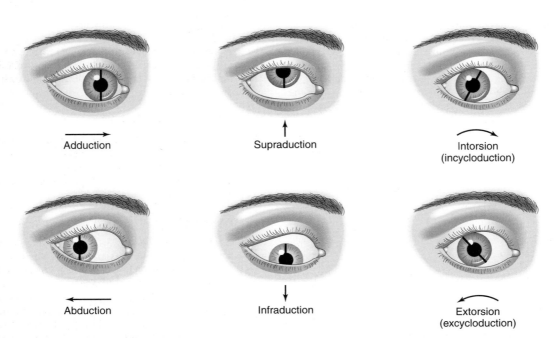

Figure 12–3. Ductions (monocular rotations), right eye. Arrows indicate direction of eye movement from primary position.

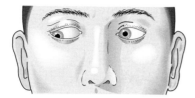 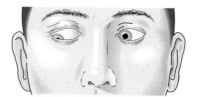

Fixing with normal right eye   Fixing with paretic left eye

▲ **Figure 12–4.** Testing versions. Example of paretic left superior oblique.

rotation of one eye relative to the other is noted as underaction or overaction. By convention, in the tertiary positions, the oblique muscles are said to be underacting or overacting with respect to the yoke rectus muscle. Fixation by the normal eye in the field of action of a paretic muscle results in underaction of the paretic muscle. Conversely, fixation with the eye with the paretic muscle will lead to overaction of the yoke muscle, since greater innervation is required for contraction of the underacting muscle (Figure 12–4).

▶ Disjunctive Movements

A. Convergence (Figure 12–5)

As the eyes follow an approaching object, they must turn inward in order to maintain alignment of the visual axes with the object of regard. The medial rectus muscles are contracting and the lateral rectus muscles are relaxing under the influence of neural stimulation and inhibition. (Neural pathways of supranuclear control are discussed in Chapter 14.)

Convergence is an active process with a strong voluntary as well as involuntary component. An important consideration in evaluating the extraocular muscles in strabismus is convergence.

To test convergence, a small object is slowly brought toward the bridge of the nose. The patient's attention is directed to the object by saying, "Keep the image from going double as long as possible." Convergence can normally be maintained until the object is nearly to the bridge of the

nose. An actual numerical value is placed on convergence by measuring the distance from the bridge of the nose (in centimeters) at which the eyes "break" (ie, when the nonpreferred eye swings laterally so that convergence is no longer maintained). This point is termed the **near point of convergence,** and a value of up to 5 cm is considered within normal limits.

The ratio of accommodative convergence to accommodation (AC/A ratio) is a way of quantifying the relationship of convergence to accommodation. Accommodative convergence is elicited by viewing an accommodative target, that is, one that has resolvable contours or letters that stimulate accommodation. The result is commonly expressed as prism diopters of convergence per diopter of accommodation. The AC/A ratio is useful as a clinical and research tool to further investigate and clarify this relationship and has contributed significantly to our understanding, and therefore to the treatment, of accommodative esotropia—particularly in using bifocals and miotics, as described later in this chapter.

B. Divergence

Electromyography has established that divergence is an active process, not merely a relaxation of convergence. Clinically, this function is seldom tested except in considering the amplitudes of fusion.

▶ Sensory Examination

While many tests of the status of binocular vision have been devised, only a few need be mentioned here. The tests are for stereopsis, suppression, and fusion potential. All require the simultaneous presentation of two targets separately, one to each eye.

A. Binocular Vision and Stereopsis Testing

Binocular vision can be sub-divided into **simultaneous perception,** which requires sensory fusion, **fusion,** which requires sensory and motor fusion, and **stereopsis.** Tests for simultaneous perception and fusion depend upon presentation of different stimuli to each eye, such as with red/green or polarized glasses, and analysis of how well the stimuli can be fused. There are various tests of stereopsis. An example is **random dot stereograms.** A field of random dots is seen by each eye without any monocular depth clues,

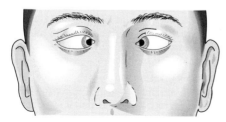

▲ **Figure 12–5.** Convergence. The position of the eyes at the normal near point of convergence (NPC) is shown above. The break point is within 5 cm of the bridge of the nose.

but dot-to-corresponding-dot correlation provides the necessary disparity that a form is seen in three dimensions if stereopsis is present.

B. Suppression Testing

The presence of suppression is readily demonstrated with the **Worth four-dot test.** Glasses containing a red lens over one eye and a green lens over the other are worn by the patient. A flashlight containing red, green, and white spots is viewed. The color spots are markers for perception through each eye, and the white dot, potentially visible to each eye, can indicate the presence of diplopia. The separation of the spots and the distance at which the light is held determine the size of the retinal area tested. Foveal and peripheral areas may be tested at distance and near, respectively.

C. Fusion Potential

In individuals with a manifest deviation, the status of binocular fusion potential can be determined by the red filter test. A red filter is placed over one eye. The patient is directed to look at a distance or near fixation light target. A red light and a white light are seen. Prisms are placed over one or both eyes in an attempt to bring the two images together. If fusion potential exists, the two images come together and are seen as a single pink light. If no fusion potential exists, the patient will continue to see one red and one white light.

OBJECTIVES & PRINCIPLES OF THERAPY OF STRABISMUS

The main objectives of strabismus treatment in children are (1) reversal of the deleterious sensory effects of strabismus (amblyopia, suppression, and loss of stereopsis) and (2) best possible alignment of the eyes by medical or surgical treatment. Even when normal stereopsis is not possible, the psychologic and sociologic benefit of straight eyes cannot be overestimated.

▶ Timing of Treatment in Children

A child can be examined at any age, and treatment for amblyopia or strabismus should be instituted as soon as the diagnosis is made. Neurophysiologic studies in animals have shown that the infant brain is quite responsive to sensory experience, and the quality of function possible later in life is greatly influenced by early life experiences. It has been shown that overall results are favorably influenced by early realignment of the eyes, preferably by age 2. Good eye alignment can be achieved later, but normal sensory adaptation becomes more difficult as the child grows older. By age 8, the sensory status is generally so fixed that deficient stereopsis cannot be effectively treated and amblyopia treatment is less likely to be successful.

▶ Medical Treatment

Nonsurgical treatment of strabismus includes treatment of amblyopia, the use of optical devices (prisms and glasses), pharmacologic agents, and orthoptics.

A. Treatment of Amblyopia

The elimination of amblyopia is crucial in the treatment of strabismus and is always one of the first goals. The strabismic deviation may lessen—rarely enlarge—following the treatment of amblyopia. Although some strabismologists feel that surgical results are more predictable and stable if there is good visual acuity in each eye preoperatively, others have reported equivalent results with earlier surgery and continued amblyopia treatment postoperatively.

1. **Occlusion therapy.** The mainstay of amblyopia treatment is occlusion. The sound eye is covered with a patch to stimulate the amblyopic eye. Glasses are also used if there is a significant refractive error or anisometropia. The two stages of successful amblyopia treatment are (1) initial improvement and (2) maintenance of the improved visual acuity.

   a. **Initial stage.** Full-time occlusion is the traditional initial treatment, although results from the Amblyopia Treatment Study have shown that it may not be needed. In some cases only part-time occlusion is used if the amblyopia is not too severe or the child is very young. As a guideline, full-time occlusion may be done for as many weeks as the child's age in years without risk of reduced vision in the sound eye. Occlusion treatment is continued in some form as long as visual acuity improves (occasionally up to a year). It is not worthwhile continuing to patch for more than 4 months if there is no improvement. In most cases, if treatment is started soon enough, substantial improvement or complete normalization of visual acuity can be achieved. Occasionally, there is no improvement even under ideal conditions. Poor compliance with treatment (peeking around a patch or inadequate enforcement of patching by the parents) may be a factor.

   b. **Maintenance stage.** Maintenance treatment consists of part-time patching to maintain the best possible vision beyond an age when amblyopia is likely to recur. The age at which a child is visually mature varies; for some it is as early as five or six years, while other children may respond to treatment in their early teens.

2. **Atropine penalization.** Some children are intolerant of occlusion therapy, or compliance with patching treatment may be poor. Atropine penalization is an effective alternative for patients when the nonamblyopic eye is emmetropic or hyperopic. Atropine causes cycloplegia, and therefore decreased accommodative ability. The exact mechanism of action of atropine in the treatment of amblyopia is unclear, as switching of fixation to the

amblyopic eye at near is not necessary for atropine penalization to be successful. The sound eye is atropinized, and the spectacle correction may be adjusted to optically penalize the sound eye, thus further encouraging use of the amblyopic eye. Atropine 1%, used daily or on weekends, is a useful and well-accepted treatment for many forms of amblyopia.

B. Optical Devices

1. **Spectacles.** The most important optical device in the treatment of strabismus is accurately prescribed spectacles. The clarification of the retinal image produced by glasses allows the natural fusion mechanisms to operate to the fullest extent. Small refractive errors need not be corrected. If there is significant hyperopia and esotropia, the esotropia is usually at least partially due to the uncorrected hyperopia (also known as refractive or accommodative esotropia). The full hyperopic correction should be prescribed when esotropia is present. If bifocals permit sufficient relaxation of accommodation to allow for near fusion, they should be used as well.

2. **Prisms.** Prisms produce optical redirection of the line of sight. Corresponding retinal elements are brought into line to eliminate diplopia. Correct sensory alignment of the eyes is also a form of antisuppression treatment. Used preoperatively, prisms can simulate the sensory effect that will follow successful surgery. In patients with horizontal deviation, prisms will show the patient's ability to fuse a simultaneous small vertical deviation, thus indicating whether surgery also needs to be done for the vertical component. In children with esotropia, prisms can be used preoperatively to predict a postoperative shift in position that might affect the surgical result, and the planned surgery can be modified accordingly (prism adaptation test).

   Prisms can be implemented in several ways. A particularly convenient form is the plastic Fresnel Press-On® prism. These plastic membranes can be stuck on the glasses and are very useful for diagnostic and temporary therapeutic purposes. Fresnel Press-On® prisms are available in powers up to 40 prism diopters. For permanent wear, prisms are best ground into the spectacle prescription, but the amount is usually limited to about 8 to 10 PD per lens as prismatic distortion, lens thickness, and chromatic aberration become prominent at higher strengths.

C. Botulinum Toxin

The injection of botulinum toxin type A (Botox) into an extraocular muscle produces a dose-dependent duration of paralysis of that muscle. The injection is given under electromyographic positional control using a monopolar electrode needle. The toxin is tightly bound to the muscle tissue. The doses used are so small that systemic toxicity does not occur.

Several days after botulinum injection, the chemical paralysis of the muscle allows the eye to be moved into the field of action of the antagonist muscle. During the time the eye is deviated, the chemically paralyzed muscle is stretched, whereas the antagonist muscle is contracted. As the paralysis resolves, the eye will gradually return toward its original position but with a new balance of forces that may reduce or eliminate the deviation. Two or more injections are often necessary to obtain a lasting effect.

D. Orthoptics

An orthoptist is trained in methods of testing and treating patients with strabismus. Orthoptists offer significant help to the ophthalmologist, particularly in the evaluation and diagnosis of the sensory and motor adaptations seen in strabismus. Evaluation of the sensory status is important in determining the fusional potential. An orthoptist may be able to aid in preoperative treatment, especially with patients who have amblyopia. At times, orthoptic training and instructions for "exercises" to be used at home can supplement and solidify surgical treatment.

▶ Surgical Treatment (Figure 12–6)
A. Surgical Procedures

A variety of changes in the rotational effect of an extraocular muscle can be achieved with surgery.

1. **Resection and recession.** Conceptually, the simplest procedures are strengthening and weakening. A muscle is strengthened by a procedure called **resection.** The muscle is detached from the eye, shortened by a measured amount, and then resewn to the eye, usually at the original insertion site. **Recession** is the standard weakening procedure. The muscle is detached from the eye and freed from fascial attachments. It is resewn to the eye a measured distance behind its original insertion. Recessions and resections are the usual surgeries performed on rectus muscles.

   The superior oblique is strengthened by tucking or advancing its tendon. This can be done by a graded amount. Superior oblique weakening is accomplished by a tenectomy (complete or partial division of the tendon) or one of several lengthening procedures. The inferior oblique can be weakened by disinsertion, myectomy, or recession. Anterior transposition of the inferior oblique is used in the treatment of dissociated vertical deviations.

2. **Shifting of the point of muscle attachment.** In addition to simple strengthening or weakening, the point of attachment of the muscle can be shifted; this may give the muscle a rotational action it did not previously have. For example, a temporal shift of both vertical rectus muscles on the same eye affects the horizontal position of the eye and improves abduction in cases of abducens palsy. Vertical shifts of the horizontal rectus muscles in opposite directions affect the horizontal eye position in upgaze and

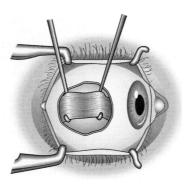

Exposure of lateral rectus

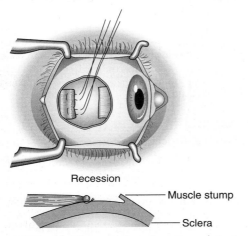

Recession

——— Muscle stump

——— Sclera

▲ **Figure 12–6.** Surgical correction of strabismus (right eye).

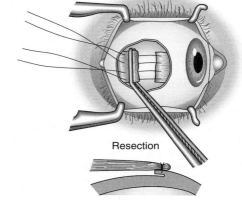

Resection

downgaze. This is done for A or V patterns, in which the horizontal deviation is more of an esodeviation in upgaze or downgaze, respectively.

The torsional effect of a muscle can also be changed. Tightening of the anterior fibers of the superior oblique tendon, known as the Harada-Ito procedure, gives that muscle enhanced torsional action.

3. **Faden procedure.** A special operation for muscle weakening is called the posterior fixation (Faden) procedure (Figure 12–7). In this operation, a new insertion of the muscle is created well behind the original insertion. This causes mechanical weakening of the muscle as the eye rotates into its field of action. When combined with recession of the same muscle, the Faden operation has a profound weakening effect on the muscle without significant alteration of the primary position of the eye. The procedure can be effective on vertical rectus muscles (dissociated vertical deviation) or horizontal muscles (high AC/A ratio, nystagmus, and other less common incomitant muscle imbalances).

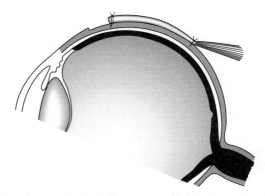

▲ **Figure 12–7.** Posterior fixation (Faden) procedure. The rectus muscle is tacked to the sclera far posterior to its insertion. This prevents unwrapping of the muscle as the eye turns into the muscle's field of action. The muscle is progressively weakened in its field of action. If this procedure is combined with recession, the alignment in primary position is also affected.

B. Choice of Muscles for Surgery

The decision concerning which muscles to operate on is based on several factors. The first is the amount of misalignment measured in the primary position. Modifications are made for significant differences in distance and near measurements. The medial rectus muscles have more effect on the angle of deviation for near and the lateral rectus muscles more effect for distance. For esotropia greater at near, both medial rectus muscles should be weakened. For exotropia greater at distance, both lateral rectus muscles should be weakened. For deviations approximately the same at distance and near, bilateral weakening procedures or unilateral recession/resection procedures are equally effective.

Surgical realignment affects only the muscular or mechanical part of a neuromuscular imbalance. Although most individuals respond in a predictable manner, variable responses may be due to differing mechanical properties of the muscles and surrounding tissues as well as variable innervational input. For these reasons, more than one operation may be required to obtain a satisfactory result.

C. Adjustable Sutures (Figure 12–8)

The development of adjustable sutures offers a great advantage in muscle surgery, particularly for reoperations and incomitant deviations. During the operation, the muscle is reattached to the sclera with a slip knot placed so that it is later accessible to the surgeon. After the patient has recovered sufficiently from the anesthesia to cooperate in the adjustment process, a topical anesthetic drop is placed in the eye and the suture can be tightened or loosened to change the eye position as indicated by cover testing. Adjustable sutures can be used on any rectus muscle for either recession or resection and on the superior oblique muscle for correction of torsion. Although any patient willing to cooperate is suitable, the method is usually not applicable for children under age 12.

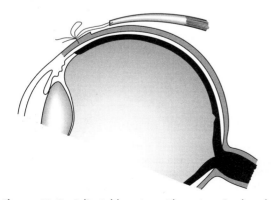

▲ **Figure 12–8.** Adjustable suture. The suture is placed on the sclera at any point that will be accessible to the surgeon. The bow is untied and the position of the muscle changed as desired.

ESOTROPIA (CONVERGENT STRABISMUS, "CROSSED EYES")

Esotropia is by far the most common type of strabismus. It is divided into two types: **paretic** (due to paresis or paralysis of one or both lateral rectus muscles) and **nonparetic** (comitant). Nonparetic esotropia is the most common type in infants and children; it may be accommodative, nonaccommodative, or partially accommodative. Most cases of childhood nonaccommodative esotropia are classified as **infantile esotropia,** with onset by age 6 months. The remainder occurs after age 6 months and are classified as **acquired nonaccommodative** esotropia. Paretic strabismus is uncommon in childhood but accounts for most new cases of strabismus in adults.

NONPARETIC ESOTROPIA

1. NONACCOMMODATIVE ESOTROPIA

A. Infantile Esotropia

Infantile esotropia is usually manifest by age 6 months, but may present later in the first year. The deviation is comitant, that is , the angle of deviation is approximately the same in all directions of gaze, and is usually not affected by accommodation. The cause, therefore, is not related to refractive error or paresis of an extraocular muscle. It is likely that the majority of cases are due to faulty innervational control, involving the supranuclear pathways for convergence and divergence and their neural connections to the medial longitudinal fasciculus. A smaller number of cases are due to anatomic variations such as anomalous insertions of horizontally acting muscles, abnormal check ligaments, or various other fascial abnormalities.

There is also good evidence that strabismus may have a multifactorial, genetically determined basis. Esophoria and esotropia are frequently passed on as an autosomal dominant trait. Siblings may have similar ocular deviations. An accommodative element is sometimes superimposed upon comitant esotropia, that is, correction of the hyperopic refractive error reduces but does not eliminate all of the deviation (partially accommodative esotropia—see later in the chapter). At least half of children with infantile esotropia will develop an accommodative esotropia as preschoolers, despite successful surgical alignment as infants.

The deviation is often large (= 40 PD) in infantile esotropia. Abduction may be limited but can be demonstrated with oculocephalic maneuvers. Vertical deviations may be observed after 18 months of age as a result of overaction of the oblique muscles or dissociated vertical deviation. Nystagmus, latent (LN) or manifest latent (MLN), is frequently present (see Chapter 14). The most common refractive error is low to moderate hyperopia.

The eye that appears to be straight is the eye used for fixation. Almost without exception, it is the eye with better vision or lower refractive error (or both). If there is anisometropia, there will probably be some amblyopia as well. If at various times either eye is used for fixation, the patient is said to show spontaneous alternation of fixation; in this case, vision will be equal or nearly equal in both eyes. In some cases, the eye preference is determined by the direction of gaze. For example, with large-angle esotropia, there is a tendency for the right eye to be used in left gaze and the left eye in right gaze (cross fixation).

Infantile esotropia is treated surgically. Preliminary nonsurgical treatment may be indicated to ensure the best possible result. Amblyopia should be treated aggressively. Glasses should be tried if there is more than 3 D of hyperopia to determine if reducing accommodation has a favorable effect on the deviation.

Surgery is performed after treatment of amblyopia has been completed. Once reproducible measurements are obtained, surgery should be scheduled as early as reasonably possible since there is ample evidence that sensory results are better the sooner the eyes are aligned. Many procedures have been recommended, but the two most popular are (1) weakening of both medial rectus muscles and (2) recession of the medial rectus and resection of the lateral rectus on the same eye.

B. Acquired Nonaccommodative Esotropia

This type of esotropia develops in childhood, usually after the age of 2 years. There is little or no hyperopia, and thus no accommodative component to the deviation. The angle of strabismus is often smaller than in infantile esotropia but may increase with time. Otherwise, clinical findings are the same as for infantile esotropia. Treatment is surgical and follows the same guidelines as for infantile esotropia.

2. ACCOMMODATIVE ESOTROPIA

Accommodative esotropia occurs when there is a normal physiologic mechanism of accommodation with an associated overactive convergence response but insufficient relative fusional divergence to hold the eyes straight. There are two pathophysiologic mechanisms at work, singly or together: (1) sufficiently high hyperopia, requiring so much accommodation to clarify the image that esotropia results because of the associated of convergence and (2) a high AC/A ratio, accompanied by mild to moderate hyperopia (1.5 D or more).

A. Accommodative Esotropia Due to Hyperopia (Figure 12–9)

Accommodative esotropia due to hyperopia typically begins at age 2–3 years but may occur earlier or later. Deviation is variable prior to treatment. Glasses with full cycloplegic refraction allow the eyes to become aligned.

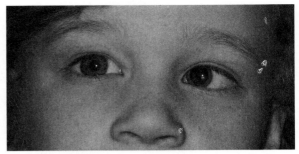

A

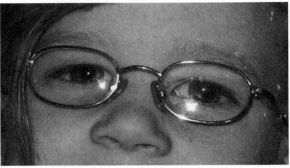

B

▲ **Figure 12–9.** Accommodative esotropia due to hyperopia. **(A)** Hyperopic individual requiring so much accommodation for clear vision that accommodative convergence causes esotropia. **(B)** Normal ocular alignment is achieved with full correction of hyperopia with corrective lenses.

B. Accommodative Esotropia due to High AC/A Ratio

In accommodative esotropia due to a high ratio of accommodative convergence to accommodation (AC/A ratio), the deviation is greater at near than at distance. The refractive error is hyperopic. Treatment is with glasses with full cycloplegic refraction plus bifocals or miotics to relieve excess deviation at near.

3. PARTIALLY ACCOMMODATIVE ESOTROPIA

A mixed mechanism—part muscular imbalance and part accommodative/convergence imbalance—may exist. Although glasses, bifocals, and miotics decrease the angle of deviation, the esotropia is not eliminated. Surgery is performed for the nonaccommodative component of the deviation with the choice of surgical procedure as described for infantile esotropia.

PARETIC (INCOMITANT) ESOTROPIA (ABDUCENS NERVE PALSY) (FIGURES 12–2 AND 12–10)

Incomitant strabismus results from paresis or restriction of action of one or more extraocular muscles. Incomitant esotropia is usually due to paresis of one or both lateral rectus muscles as a result of unilateral or bilateral abducens nerve palsy. Other causes are fracture of the medial orbital wall with entrapment of the medial rectus muscle, Graves' ophthalmopathy causing fibrosis of the medial rectus muscles, and Duane's retraction syndrome (see later in the chapter). Abducens nerve palsy is most frequently seen in adults with systemic hypertension or diabetes, in which case spontaneous resolution usually begins within 3 months (see Chapters 14 and 15). It may also be the first sign of intracranial tumor, increased intracranial pressure, or inflammatory disease. Associated neurologic signs are then important clues. Head trauma is another frequent cause of abducens palsy.

Incomitant esotropia is also seen in infants and children, but much less commonly than comitant esotropia. These cases may result from birth injuries affecting the lateral rectus muscle directly, from injury to the nerve, or, less commonly, from a congenital anomaly of the muscle or its fascial attachments.

In abducens palsy, the esotropia is characteristically greater with the affected eye fixing, at distance than at near, and on gaze to the affected side. Paresis of the right lateral rectus causes esotropia that is more marked with the right eye fixing, becomes greater on right gaze and, if paresis is mild, little or no deviation on left gaze. If the lateral rectus muscle is totally paralyzed, the eye will not abduct past the midline. Bilateral abducens palsy will cause an esotropia that increases on gaze to either side.

Acquired abducens palsy is initially managed by occlusion of the paretic eye or with prisms. Botulinum toxin type A injection into the antagonist medial rectus muscle may provide symptomatic relief but does not appear to influence the final outcome. If lateral rectus function in incomplete palsies has not recovered after 6 months, medial rectus botulinum toxin type A injections may be used on a long-term basis to allow fusion—and hence abolition of diplopia in straight-ahead gaze or to facilitate prism therapy. However, horizontal rectus muscle surgery, involving resection of the lateral recti and recession of the medial rectus is usually performed. Adjustable sutures are useful in achieving the largest possible area of binocular single vision. In complete palsies that have failed to improve after 6 months, surgical transposition of the insertions of the superior and inferior rectus muscles to the insertion of the lateral rectus muscle, sometimes combined with posterior fixation sutures of the temporal borders of the vertical recti is indicated. Botulinum toxin may be used as an adjunct to surgery when medial rectus restriction is severe. Full abduction cannot be restored, but fusion in primary position, with or without the aid of prisms, and a

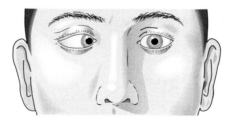

Primary position: right esotropia

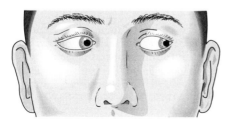

Left gaze: no deviation

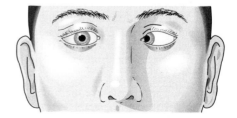

Right gaze: left esotropia

▲ **Figure 12–10.** Incomitant strabismus (paretic). Paresis of right lateral rectus muscle, with left eye fixing.

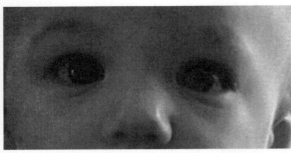

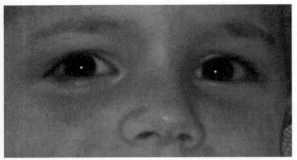

A

B

▲ **Figure 12–11. (A)** Toddler with pseudoesotropia. **(B)** Same child 3 years later without any intervention.

reasonable field of binocular single vision can usually be achieved. Abducens palsy in infants and children may cause amblyopia, so these patients must be followed carefully and the amblyopia treated appropriately.

► Pseudoesotropia

Pseudoesotropia is the illusion of crossed eyes in an infant or toddler when no strabismus is present (Figure 12–11). This appearance is usually caused by a flat, broad nasal bridge and prominent epicanthal folds that cover a portion of the nasal sclera, giving the impression that the eyes are crossed. This very common condition may be differentiated from true misalignment by the corneal light reflection appearing in the center of the pupil of each eye when the child fixes a light. With normal facial growth and increasing prominence of the nasal bridge, this pseudoesotropic appearance gradually disappears. Of course, true esotropia may be present in association with this common infantile facial configuration.

▼ EXOTROPIA (DIVERGENT STRABISMUS)

Exotropia is less common than esotropia, particularly in infancy and childhood. Its incidence increases gradually with age. Not infrequently, a tendency to divergent strabismus

beginning as exophoria progresses to **intermittent exotropia** and finally to **constant exotropia** if no treatment is given. Other cases begin as constant or intermittent exotropia and remain stationary. As in esotropia, there may be a hereditary element in some cases, but neurologic impairment and developmental delay are more common than in esotropia. Exophoria and exotropia (considered as a single entity of divergent deviation) are frequently passed on as autosomal dominant traits, so that one or both parents of an exotropic child may demonstrate exotropia or a high degree of exophoria.

► Descriptive Classification of Exotropia

Exotropia can also be classified on a descriptive basis as being an excess of divergence or an insufficiency of convergence, but this should not be assumed to imply that the cause of the deviation is understood.

A. Basic Exotropia

Distance and near deviations are approximately equal.

B. Divergence Excess

Distance deviation is significantly larger than near deviation.

C. Pseudodivergence Excess

Distance deviation is significantly larger than near deviation: however, use of a +3 diopter lens for near measurement will cause the near deviation to become approximately equal to the distance deviation.

D. Convergence Insufficiency

Near deviation is significantly larger than distance deviation.

1. INTERMITTENT EXOTROPIA

► Clinical Findings

Intermittent exotropia accounts for well over half of all cases of exotropia. The onset of the deviation may be in the first year, and practically all have presented by age 5. The history often reveals that the condition has become progressively worse. A characteristic sign is closing one eye in bright light (Figure 12–12). The manifest exotropia first becomes noticeable with distance fixation. The patient usually fuses at near, overcoming moderate to large angle exophoria. Convergence is frequently excellent. There is no correlation with a specific refractive error.

Since a child fuses at least part of the time, amblyopia is uncommon, and, when present, it is mild. For distance, with one eye deviated, there is suppression of that eye and normal retinal correspondence with little or no amblyopia.

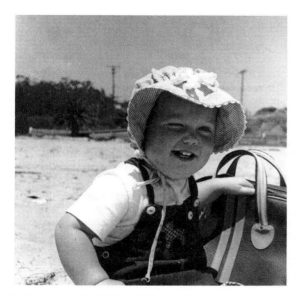

▲ **Figure 12–12.** Child with intermittent exotropia squinting in sunlight.

▶ Treatment

A. Medical Treatment

Nonsurgical treatment is largely confined to refractive correction and amblyopia therapy. If the AC/A ratio is high, the use of minus lenses may delay surgery for a while. Occasionally, antisuppression or convergence exercises may be of temporary benefit.

B. Surgical Treatment

Most patients with intermittent exotropia require surgery when their fusional control deteriorates. Deterioration of control is documented over time by an increasing percentage of time the manifest exotropia is observed, an enlarging angle of deviation, decreasing control for near fixation, and worsening in the patient's measured distance and near stereoscopic abilities. Surgery may also alleviate diplopia or other asthenopic symptoms, but recurrence of exotropia is frequent.

The choice of procedure depends on the measurements of the deviation. Bilateral lateral rectus muscle recession is preferred when the deviation is greater at distance. If there is more deviation at near, it is best to undertake resection of a medial rectus muscle and recession of the ipsilateral lateral rectus muscle. Surgery on one or even two additional horizontal muscles may be necessary for very large deviations (>50 PD). It is desirable to obtain slight overcorrection in the immediate postoperative period for best long-term results.

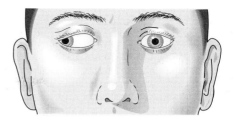

▲ **Figure 12–13.** Right exotropia.

2. CONSTANT EXOTROPIA (FIGURE 12–13)

Constant exotropia is less common than intermittent exotropia. It may be present at birth or may occur when intermittent exotropia progresses to constant exotropia. Because children with infantile exotropia are at risk for neurologic impairment and developmental delays, pediatric neurologic consultation is indicated in all such cases. Exotropia may also have its onset later in life, particularly following loss of vision in one eye. Except for cases due to loss of vision ("sensory exotropia"), the underlying cause is usually not known.

▶ Clinical Findings

Constant exotropia may be of any degree. With chronicity or poor vision in one eye, the deviation can become quite large. Adduction may be limited, and hypertropia also may be present. There is suppression if the deviation was acquired by age 6–8; otherwise, diplopia may be present. If exotropia is due to very poor vision in one eye, there may be no diplopia. Amblyopia is uncommon in the absence of anisometropia, and spontaneous alternation of fixation is frequently observed.

▶ Treatment

Surgery is nearly always indicated. The choice and amount are as described for intermittent exotropia. Slight overcorrection in an adult may result in diplopia. Most patients adjust to this, especially if they have been forewarned of the possibility. If one eye has reduced vision, the prognosis for maintenance of a stable position is less favorable, with the strong possibility that the exotropia will recur following surgery. Botulinum toxin type A injections can be useful as primary treatment in small deviations or as supplementary treatment in significant surgical overcorrections or undercorrections.

▼ A & V PATTERNS

A horizontal deviation may be vertically incomitant, that is, the deviation is different in upgaze versus downgaze (A or V pattern). An A pattern shows more esodeviation or less exodeviation in upgaze compared to downgaze. A V pattern shows less esodeviation or more exodeviation in upgaze compared to downgaze. An A pattern is diagnostically significant when greater than 10 PD and a V pattern when greater than 15 PD. These patterns are frequently associated with overaction of the oblique muscles, inferior obliques for V patterns and superior obliques for A patterns.

When surgically treating an A or V pattern, oblique muscle overaction must be treated if present. If little or no oblique overaction exists, vertical offsets of one tendon width of the horizontal muscles are utilized. The insertions of the medial rectus muscles are displaced toward the narrow end of the pattern (in V esotropia, recessed medial rectus muscles are moved down), and lateral rectus muscles are displaced toward the open end (in V exotropia, the insertions of the recessed lateral rectus muscles are moved up).

HYPERTROPIA (MANIFEST VERTICAL STRABISMUS) (FIGURE 12–14)

Vertical deviations are customarily named according to the higher eye, regardless of which eye has the better vision and is used for fixation. They are less common than horizontal deviations, commonly present after childhood, and have many causes.

Congenital palsy of the superior oblique muscle is a common cause of pediatric hypertropia, but may not present until adulthood. Congenital anatomic anomalies, such as in craniosynostoses, may result in muscle attachments in abnormal locations. Occasionally, there are anomalous fibrous bands that attach to the eye. The superior oblique is the most commonly paretic vertical muscle because of its susceptibility to closed head trauma. The vertical rectus muscles are commonly involved in orbital trauma, typically entrapment of the inferior rectus in an orbital floor fracture, and in Graves' ophthalmopathy causing fibrosis of the inferior rectus, thus limiting the upward movement of the eye and possibly pulling it downward. Orbital tumors, brain stem and other intracranial lesions, including strokes and inflammatory disease such as multiple sclerosis, and even myasthenia gravis can all produce hypertropias. Many of these specific entities are discussed in Chapters 13 and 14.

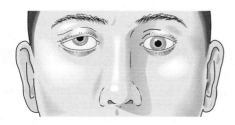

▲ **Figure 12–14.** Right hypertropia.

► Clinical Findings

The clinical findings vary, depending on the cause. The history is particularly important in diagnosis of hypertropias. Diplopia is almost invariably present if strabismus develops past age 6–8. As in other forms of strabismus, sensory adaptation occurs if the onset is before this age range. Suppression and anomalous retinal correspondence may be present in gaze directions where there is manifest strabismus, whereas in gaze directions without manifest strabismus, there may be no suppression and normal stereopsis. Abnormal head position (AHP) may comprise head tilt, head turn, or chin depression or elevation, or a combination.

The ocular misalignment may be of any magnitude and usually changes with the direction of gaze because most hypertropias are incomitant. The deviation tends to be greatest in the field of action of one of the four vertically acting muscles, and should be assessed without and with correction of any AHP. Prism and cover measurements in primary and cardinal positions and assessment of any AHP are the mainstays of the clinical evaluation and may often be diagnostic. The **three-step test** comprising (1) determination of which eye is higher in primary position, (2) determination of whether the vertical deviation increases on left or right gaze, and (3) the Bielchowsky head tilt test (see later in the chapter), will usually indicate which extraocular muscle is primarily responsible for the hypertropia. A fourth step of identification of cyclotorsion in each eye, such as with the double Maddox rod test (see later in the chapter), can be helpful in diagnosis of skew deviation due to intracranial disease. Observation of ocular rotations for limitations and overactions can also be of great value but the abnormalities may be subtle.

Paresis of the superior oblique usually presents with hypertropia on the involved side, increasing on gaze to the opposite side, with a head tilt to the opposite side. Other motility patterns can be seen when the deviation is of long standing, due to contractures of other vertically acting muscles. The **Bielschowsky head tilt test** (Figure 12–15) is particularly useful to confirm the diagnosis of superior oblique paresis. The test exploits the differing effects of each vertical muscle on torsion and elevation. Thus, with a paretic right superior oblique when the head is tilted to the right, the superior rectus and superior oblique contract to intort the eye and maintain the position of the retinal vertical meridian as much as possible. The superior rectus elevates the eye, and the superior oblique depresses the eye. Because of weakness of the superior oblique muscle, the vertical forces do not cancel out as they normally would, and right hypertropia increases. In head tilt to the left, the intorting muscles for the right eye relax and the right inferior oblique and right inferior rectus both contract to extort the eye. Both the paretic right superior oblique and the right superior rectus relax, and hypertropia is minimized. Hypertropia should be measured by prism and alternate cover testing with the head tilted to either side, as well as in the nine cardinal positions.

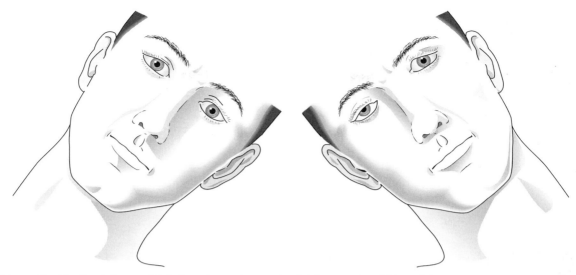

▲ **Figure 12–15.** Head tilt test (Bielschowsky test). Paresis of right superior oblique. **(A)** Hypertropia is minimized on tilting the head to the sound side. The right eye may then extort and the intorting superior oblique and superior rectus relax. **(B)** When the head is tilted to the paretic side, the intorting muscles contract together, but their vertical actions do not cancel out as usual, because of superior oblique paresis. Hypertropia is worse with head tilt to the paretic side.

There may be an associated **cyclotropia,** especially with superior oblique dysfunction. To measure a cyclotropia, the **double Maddox rod test** is used. In a trial frame, a red and white Maddox rod are aligned vertically, one over each eye. With the patient's head held straight and fixing a light, one rod is gradually turned until the observed lines are parallel to each other and to normal horizontal orientation. The angle of tilt is then read from the angular scale on the trial frame. Superior oblique paresis results in excyclotorsion of the affected eye. Skew deviation, which is hypertropia due to a supranuclear lesion, usually caused by brainstem or cerebellar disease, causes conjugate ocular torsion of both eyes, for example, excyclotorsion of the left eye and incyclotorsion of the right eye.

▶ **Treatment**

A. Medical Treatment

For smaller and more comitant deviations, a prism may be all that is required. For constant diplopia, one eye may need to be occluded, particularly if there is torisonal diplopia because this cannot be corrected with a prism. Any underlying cause may require specific treatment.

B. Surgical Treatment

Surgery is often indicated if the deviation, head tilt and/or diplopia persist (Figure 12–16). The choice of procedure depends on quantitative measurements and the pattern of misalignment. The use of adjustable sutures (Figure 12–8) may be helpful in fine-tuning the effect of vertical muscle surgery.

▼ SPECIAL FORMS OF STRABISMUS

DUANE RETRACTION SYNDROME

Duane retraction syndrome is typically characterized by marked limitation of abduction, mild limitation of adduction, retraction of the globe and narrowing of the palpebral fissure on attempted adduction, and, frequently, upshoot or downshoot of the eye in adduction. It is one type of Congenital Cranial Dysinnervation Disorder (CCDD), in which a cranial nerve fails to develop properly, and the target muscles are instead abnormally innervated by another cranial nerve. Marcus Gunn Jaw winking is another form of CCDD.

Duane retraction syndrome is usually monocular, with the left eye more often affected. Most cases are sporadic, although some families with dominant inheritance have been described. A variety of other anomalies may be associated, such as dysplasia of the iris stroma, heterochromia, cataract, choroidal coloboma, microphthalmos, Goldenhar's syndrome, Klippel–Feil syndrome, cleft palate, and anomalies of the face, ear, or extremities, and Duane retraction syndrome is a feature of thalidomide embryopathy. The causes of the motility defects are varied, and some anomalies of muscle structure have been found. Most cases can be explained by inappropriate innervation to the lateral rectus and sometimes to other muscles as well. Sherrington's law of reciprocal innervation is not obeyed, because nerve fibers of the oculomotor nerve to the medial rectus may also go to the lateral rectus. This accounts for

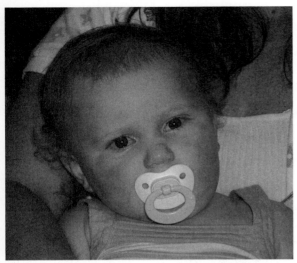

A

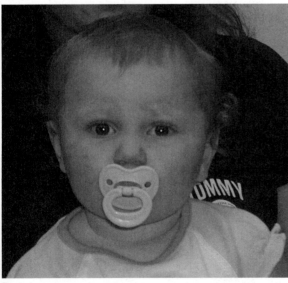

B

▲ **Figure 12–16. (A)** Head tilt due to congenital left superior oblique palsy. **(B)** Resolution of head tilt following extraocular muscle surgery.

simultaneous contraction of the medial and lateral rectus muscles (co-contraction), causing retraction of the globe in adduction. Cases with proved absence of the abducens nucleus and nerve have been documented.

▶ Treatment

Only when a primary position misalignment or a significant compensatory head turn exists is surgical treatment indicated.

The goal is to obtain straight eyes in the primary position and to horizontally expand the field of single vision. Recession of the medial rectus on the affected side is performed if any esotropia is present in the primary position. For more severe cases, temporal transposition of the vertical rectus muscles accompanied by weakening of the medial rectus muscle, either by adjustable recession or botulinum toxin A, is often indicated.

DISSOCIATED VERTICAL DEVIATION

Dissociated vertical deviation is frequently associated with infantile esotropia and rarely with an otherwise normal muscle balance. The exact cause is not known, though it is logical to assume it from faulty supranuclear innervation of extraocular muscles.

▶ Clinical Findings

Each eye drifts upward under cover, frequently with extorsion and a small exotropic shift, and then returns to its resting binocular position when the cover is removed. Occasionally, the upward drifting will occur spontaneously, causing a noticeable vertical misalignment. Most cases are bilateral, though asymmetry of involvement is common. There are usually no other symptoms, although a head tilt to one side is sometimes observed.

▶ Treatment

Treatment is indicated if the frequency or magnitude of the intermittent manifest vertical deviation is unacceptable. Nonsurgical treatment is limited to refractive correction to maximize the potential of motor fusion and therapy for amblyopia. Surgical results have been variable and can be disappointing. A popular and successful procedure is graded recession of the superior rectus, occasionally combined with posterior fixation (Faden) sutures. Anterior transposition of the inferior oblique insertion immediately adjacent to the lateral border of the inferior rectus muscle can be used to treat this disorder, especially when the inferior oblique muscle is overacting. Inferior rectus resection is an occasional surgical option.

BROWN'S SYNDROME (SUPERIOR OBLIQUE TENDON SHEATH SYNDROME)

Brown's syndrome is due to fibrous adhesions or inflammation in the superior nasal quadrant of the orbit involving the superior oblique tendon and trochlea, which mechanically limit elevation of the eye. Limitation of elevation is most marked in the adducted position, and improvement in elevation occurs gradually as the eye is abducted. The main differential diagnosis is paresis of the inferior oblique muscle. Forced duction testing is diagnostic, since there is an upward restriction to elevation in adduction when Brown's syndrome is present. The condition is usually unilateral and idiopathic, though rarely it may be due to trauma, inflammation, or tumor.

Surgical treatment is limited to those cases where there is an AHP to compensate for hypotropia or cyclotropia of the involved eye. The objective is to free the mechanical adhesions and weaken the superior oblique muscle via a superior oblique tenotomy (with or without a tendon spacer). Although controversial as to its timing, weakening of the ipsilateral inferior oblique may be needed to compensate for the iatrogenic fourth nerve palsy. Normalization of the head position may occur, but restoration of full motility is seldom achieved.

HETEROPHORIA

Heterophoria is deviation of the eyes that is held in check by binocular vision. Almost all individuals have some degree of heterophoria, and small amounts are considered normal. Larger amounts may cause symptoms depending on the level of effort required by the individual to control latent muscle imbalance.

▶ Clinical Findings

The symptoms of heterophoria may be clear-cut (intermittent diplopia) or vague ("eyestrain" or asthenopia). Diplopia may come on only with fatigue or with poor lighting conditions, as in night driving. Usage requirements for the eyes and personality type are additional factors. Thus, there is no degree of heterophoria that is clearly abnormal, though larger amounts are more likely to be symptomatic. Except for hyperopia, high AC/A ratios, and mild cases of muscle paresis not resulting in frank heterotropia, the fundamental causes of heterophorias are unknown.

Asthenopia is sometimes caused by uncorrected refractive errors as well as by muscle imbalance. One possible mechanism is **aniseikonia,** in which an image seen by one eye is a different size and shape from that seen by the other eye, preventing sensory fusion. Spectacles with unequal lens powers in the two eyes can cause asthenopia by creating prismatic displacement of the image in one eye for gaze away from the optic axis that is too large to control (induced prism). Another mechanism that may produce symptoms is a change in spatial perception due to the curvature of the lenses or astigmatic corrections (see Chapter 21). Anisometropia is more likely to cause symptoms when its onset is sudden, that is, after a scleral buckle procedure with relative myopia of the affected eye.

The symptoms encountered in asthenopia take a wide variety of forms. There may be a feeling of heaviness, tiredness, or discomfort of the eyes, varying from a dull ache to deep pain located in or behind the eyes. Headaches of all types occur. Easy fatigability, blurring of vision, and diplopia, especially after prolonged use of the eyes, also occur. Symptoms are more common for near visual work than for distance. Frequently, an aversion to reading develops. Symptoms can be brought on by fatigue or illness or following the ingestion of medications or alcohol.

▶ Diagnosis

The diagnosis of heterophoria is based on prism and cover measurements. Relative fusional vergence amplitudes are measured. While the patient views an accommodative target at distance or near, prisms of increasing strength are placed in front of one eye. The fusional vergence amplitude is the amount of prism the patient is able to overcome and still maintain single vision. Measurements are done with base-out, base-in, base-up, and base-down prisms. The important feature is the size of the amplitudes in comparison to the angle of heterophoria. While one cannot give exact norms for normal relative fusion vergence, guidelines for typical normal findings are as follows: at distance, convergence is 14 PD, divergence is 6 PD, and vertical is 2.5 PD; at near, convergence is 35 PD, divergence is 15 PD, and vertical is 2.5 PD.

▶ Treatment

Heterophoria requires treatment only if symptomatic. Untreated heterophoria or asthenopia does not cause any permanent damage to the eyes. Treatment methods are all aimed at reducing the effort required to achieve fusion or at changing muscle mechanics so that the muscle imbalance itself is reduced.

A. Medical Treatment

1. **Accurate refractive correction.** Occasionally, poor visual acuity is found in the presence of symptomatic heterophoria. Spectacles providing clear vision are sometimes all that is needed to alleviate symptoms. The clearer image allows the patient's fusional capacity to function to its fullest.

2. **Manipulation of accommodation.** In general, esophorias are treated with antiaccommodative therapy and exophorias by stimulating accommodation. Plus lenses often work well for esophoria, especially if hyperopia is present, by reducing accommodative convergence. A high AC/A ratio may be effectively treated with plus lenses, sometimes combined with bifocals or miotics.

3. **Prisms.** The use of prisms requires the wearing of glasses; for some patients, this is unacceptable. A trial of plastic Fresnel press-on prisms should be made before ground-in prisms are ordered. For optical reasons, larger amounts of prismatic correction produce visual distortions limiting the use of prisms in higher strengths. Furthermore, very thick lenses can result. The usual practice is to prescribe about one-third to one-half of the measured deviation, which often allows more comfortable fusion to occur. Prisms can be useful for esophoria, exophoria, and vertical phorias as well.

4. **Botulinum toxin type A (Botox) injection.** This treatment is well suited to producing small to moderate shifts in ocular alignment and has been used as a substitute for surgical weakening of one muscle. The main disadvantage is that the resulting effect may be variable or wear off completely months later.

B. Surgical Treatment

Surgery should be done only after medical methods have failed. Muscles are chosen for correction according to the measured deviation at distance and near in various directions of gaze. Sometimes only one muscle needs adjustment. Adjustable sutures can be very helpful (Figure 12–8).

REFERENCES

Baker JD: Twenty-year follow-up of surgery for intermittent exotropia. J AAPOS 2008;12;227. [PMID 18455937]

Buck D et al: Presenting features and early management of childhood intermittent exotropia in the UK: inception cohort study. Br J Ophthalmol 2009;93:1620. [PMID: 19605936]

Choi MY, Hyung SM, Hwang JM: Unilateral recession-resection in children with exotropia of the convergence insufficiency type. Eye 2007;21;344. [PMID 16327792]

Cotter SA et al: Fixation preference and visual acuity testing in a population-based cohort of preschool children with amblyopia risk factors. Ophthalmology 2009;116;145. [PMID 18962921]

Dobson V et al: Optical treatment reduces amblyopia in astigmatic children who receive spectacles before kindergarten. Ophthalmology 2009;116:1002. [PMID: 19232733]

Ekdawi NS et al: Postoperative outcomes in children with intermittent exotropia from a population-based cohort. J AAPOS 2009;13;4. [PMID 18848478]

Guyton DL: Ocular torsion reveals the mechanisms of cyclovertical strabismus. Invest Ophthalmol Vis Sci 2008;49;847. [PMID 18326702]

Hatt SR et al: The effects of strabismus on quality of life in adults. Am J Ophthalmol 2007;144;643. [PMID 17707329]

Hatt SR et al: Variability of control in intermittent exotropia. Ophthalmology 2008;115;371. [PMID 17629562]

Hatt SR et al: Variability of stereoacuity in intermittent exotropia. Am J Ophthalmol 2008;145;556. [PMID 18201680]

Li T, Shotton K: Conventional occlusion versus pharmacologic penalization for amblyopia. Cochrane Database Syst Rev 2009;4:CD006460. [PMID: 19821369]

MacEwen CJ et al: Is the maximum hypermetropic correction necessary in children with fully accommodative esotropia? Br J Ophthalmol 2008; 92:1329. [PMID 18408081]

Mohney BG: Common forms of childhood strabismus in an incidence cohort. Am J Ophthalmol 2007;144;465. [PMID 17765436]

Mohney BG et al: Age at strabismus diagnosis in an incidence cohort of children. Am J Ophthalmol 2007;144;467. [PMID 17765437]

Pediatric Eye Disease Investigator Group: A randomized trial of atropine versus patching for treatment of moderate amblyopia: follow-up at age 10 years. Arch Ophthalmol 2008;126;1039. [PMID 18695096]

Pediatric Eye Disease Investigator Group: Instability of ocular alignment in childhood esotropia. Ophthalmology 2008;115;2266. [PMID 18973948]

Pediatric Eye Disease Investigator Group: Interobserver reliability of the prism and alternate cover test in children with esotropia. Arch Ophthalmol 2009; 127:59. [PMID 19139339]

Repka MX et al: Treatment of severe amblyopia with weekend atropine: results from 2 randomized clinical trials. J AAPOS 2009;13:258. [PMID: 19541265]

Rowe et al: Botulinum toxin for the treatment of strabismus. Cochrane Database Syst Rev 2009;15:CD006499. [PMID 19370637]

Shotton K et al: Interventions for unilateral refractive amblyopia. Cochrane Database Syst Rev 2008;4:CD005137. [PMID: 18843683]

Strominger MB et al: Dissociated vertical deviation and inferior oblique overaction. J Pediatr Ophthalmol Strabismus 2009;46:132. [PMID 19496491]

Orbit

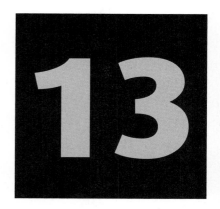

John H. Sullivan, MD

Orbital disease usually arises within the orbit or by spread from adjacent structures, particularly the paranasal sinuses. The etiology may be inflammatory, due to infection; neoplastic, either benign or malignant and arising from bone, muscle, nerve, blood vessels, or connective tissue; or due to vascular anomalies, including arteriovenous malformations and arterial fistulas. Orbital lesions may also be due to metastatic tumors. Thus, orbital disease may be due to serious and sometimes life-threatening entities.

PHYSIOLOGY OF SYMPTOMS

An increase in orbital contents results in displacement of the globe. Since the orbit has rigid bony walls except anteriorly (see Chapter 1), such displacement usually manifests predominantly as forward protrusion of the globe (**proptosis**), which is the hallmark of orbital disease. Swelling within the muscle cone displaces the globe directly anteriorly (**axial proptosis**), whereas swelling outside the muscle cone will also cause sideways or vertical displacement (**non-axial proptosis**).

Bilateral involvement generally indicates systemic disease, such as Graves' disease. The term "exophthalmos" is often used when describing proptosis associated with Graves' disease.

Pulsating proptosis may be due to carotid-cavernous fistula, arterial orbital vascular malformation, or transmission of cerebral pulsations due to a defect of the superior orbital roof, as in the sphenoid dysplasia of type 1 neurofibromatosis. Proptosis that increases on bending the head forward or with Valsalva's maneuver is a sign of venous orbital vascular malformation (orbital varices) or meningocele. **Intermittent proptosis** may be the result of a sinus mucocele. The Hertel exophthalmometer (see Chapter 2) is the standard method of quantifying the magnitude of proptosis. Serial measurements are most accurate if performed by the same individual with the same instrument. **Pseudoproptosis** is apparent proptosis in the absence of orbital disease. It may be due to high myopia, buphthalmos, or lid retraction.

Proptosis does not impair vision unless there are corneal changes due to exposure, but the orbital process itself, particularly if it arises from, involves, or compresses the optic nerve, or if it causes compression of the globe, resulting in distortion of the retina and possibly elevation of intraocular pressure, may impair vision. A relative afferent pupillary defect (RAPD) or impairment of color vision may identify optic nerve dysfunction before there is significant reduction of visual acuity.

Limitation of ocular movements resulting in diplopia (double vision) may be due to direct involvement of the extraocular muscles, interference with their mechanisms of action, or dysfunction of the oculomotor, trochlear, or abducens nerves. Pain may occur as a result of rapid expansion, inflammation, or infiltration of sensory nerves.

Disease involving the superior orbital fissure produces a characteristic combination of diplopia, resulting from disturbance of function of the oculomotor, trochlear, and abducens nerves, corneal and facial anesthesia (ophthalmic division of trigeminal nerve), and possibly proptosis, known as the **superior orbital fissure syndrome**. Lesions at the orbital apex also result in optic nerve dysfunction (**orbital apex syndrome**). (In the **cavernous sinus syndrome**, there is diplopia and trigeminal dysfunction, potentially involving all three divisions. There may be proptosis due to venous congestion but not optic nerve dysfunction.)

DIAGNOSTIC STUDIES

▶ Computed Tomography and Magnetic Resonance Imaging

Imaging by **computed tomography** (CT) (Figures 13–1 and 13–2) was a major advance in orbital diagnosis. Due to continued improvement in resolution quality, rapidity of scanning, and multi-planar imaging with manipulation of images to produce three-dimensional reconstructions, it retains an

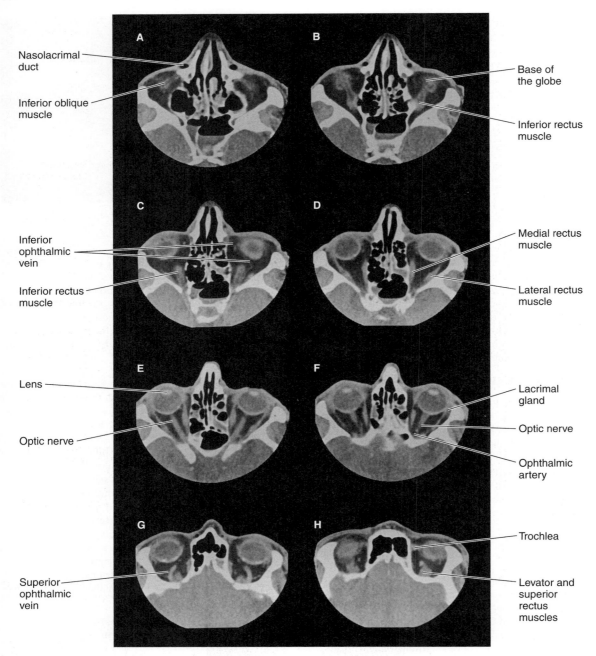

Nasolacrimal duct

Inferior oblique muscle

Base of the globe

Inferior rectus muscle

Inferior ophthalmic vein

Inferior rectus muscle

Medial rectus muscle

Lateral rectus muscle

Lens

Optic nerve

Lacrimal gland

Optic nerve

Ophthalmic artery

Superior ophthalmic vein

Trochlea

Levator and superior rectus muscles

▲ **Figure 13–1.** Normal CT scan showing the anatomy of the orbit. Axial CT sections, thickness 1.5 mm. A: Lowest section. H: Highest section. Note clear delineation of individual muscles, optic nerve, and major veins within the orbital fat.

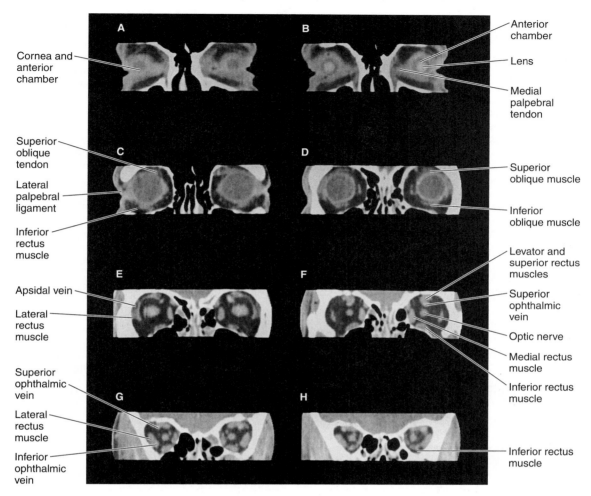

A:
Cornea and anterior chamber

B:
Anterior chamber
Lens
Medial palpebral tendon

C:
Superior oblique tendon
Lateral palpebral ligament
Inferior rectus muscle

D:
Superior oblique muscle
Inferior oblique muscle

E:
Apsidal vein
Lateral rectus muscle

F:
Levator and superior rectus muscles
Superior ophthalmic vein
Optic nerve
Medial rectus muscle
Inferior rectus muscle

G:
Superior ophthalmic vein
Lateral rectus muscle
Inferior ophthalmic vein

H:
Inferior rectus muscle

▲ **Figure 13–2.** Coronal computer reconstructions from axial CT sections. A: Most anterior section. H: Most posterior section. Note detailed demonstration of ocular and orbital structures.

important role. **Magnetic resonance imaging** (MRI) provides additional information on changes within soft tissues and the optic nerve but is less useful for bony changes. It is contraindicated in the presence of a ferrous intraorbital or intracranial foreign body.

Ultrasonography

The use of ultrasonography in the diagnosis of orbital disease has largely been supplanted by CT and MRI. Although it is a noninvasive and inexpensive form of imaging, its usefulness in both A and B mode is limited to the anterior portion of the orbit. It is of greatest value in the hands of the clinician-ultrasonographer capable of interpreting "real-time" images.

It provides a noninvasive method of diagnosing carotid artery–cavernous sinus fistula (see later in the chapter).

Venography

Venography is rarely useful in defining the extent of orbital venous disease. Although the diagnosis can be made by MRI, contrast injection into the orbital veins via a scalp vein can sometimes reveal the presence of varices that have escaped detection by CT.

Angiography

Selective carotid (catheter) angiography with bone subtraction is sometimes necessary to diagnose orbital vascular disorders. In carotid artery–cavernous sinus fistula, CT angiography may provide sufficient detail for diagnosis but catheter angiography is required to delineate the extent of involvement and for treatment by embolization.

► Radiography

Plain x-rays may be sufficient for initial diagnosis of orbital fractures. However, the thin walls of the orbit are difficult to visualize even with tomography, and CT with three-dimensional reconstructions is usually needed to determine the extent of injury, as well as for preoperative and possibly intraoperative planning of surgical reconstruction. CT will also show orbital soft tissue injury and hemorrhage, and may identify ocular damage, including globe rupture, intraocular hemorrhage, and lens dislocation. Dacryocystography and radionuclide scanning can be helpful in localizing the site of lacrimal obstructions.

► Fine-Needle Aspiration Biopsy

Fine-needle aspiration biopsy is an invasive procedure that has proved very useful in orbital diagnosis. Cytology specimens can be aspirated from a lesion, the exact location of which is determined by CT. Cytopathology can be inconclusive but is often invaluable.

▼ DISEASES & DISORDERS OF THE ORBIT

INFLAMMATORY DISORDERS

1. GRAVES' OPHTHALMOPATHY (SEE ALSO CHAPTER 15)

Graves' ophthalmopathy is a syndrome of clinical and imaging abnormalities caused by deposition of mucopolysaccharides and infiltration with chronic inflammatory cells of the orbital tissues, particularly the extraocular muscles. It usually occurs in association with autoimmune hyperthyroidism (Graves' disease), but exactly the same disease process can occur in association with autoimmune hypothyroidism (Hashimoto's thyroiditis); thyroid dysfunction due to amiodarone; thyroid antibodies (antimicrosomal (thyroperoxidase) or antithyroglobulin antibodies, or thyroid-simulating immunoglobulins) without thyroid dysfunction; and occasionally no clinical or laboratory evidence of thyroid dysfunction and no thyroid antibodies, even on long-term follow-up. It is thought to be an autoimmune disease but which antigens and antibodies are important in its pathogenesis remains uncertain. It is associated with other autoimmune diseases, including myasthenia gravis. It is exacerbated by cigarette smoking and radioiodine therapy. (Graves' ophthalmopathy or orbitopathy, dysthyroid ophthalmopathy or orbitopathy, and (dys)thyroid eye disease or orbital disease are interchangeable terms.)

► Clinical Findings

Some degree of ophthalmopathy, usually mild and typically including upper eyelid retraction, occurs in a high percentage of hyperthyroid patients. Severe ophthalmopathy with marked proptosis and restricted motility occurs in about 5% of cases of Graves' disease (Figure 13–3).

Graves' ophthalmopathy is the most common cause of unilateral or bilateral proptosis in adults or children. The accompanying upper eyelid retraction, manifesting as disproportionately greater exposure of sclera superiorly than inferiorly, and lid lag, manifesting as impaired descent of the upper eyelid on downward gaze, distinguishes it from other causes of proptosis.

Ocular surface discomfort is very common in all stages of the disease, in some cases due to superior limbic keratoconjunctivitis (see Chapter 5). Incomplete eyelid closure (lagophthalmos) results from proptosis and lid retraction, and corneal exposure may be present even in mild cases. Ptosis in association with thyroid ophthalmopathy is usually due to coexistent myasthenia gravis, which may also contribute to ocular motility disturbance.

The extraocular muscle involvement of thyroid ophthalmopathy begins with lymphocytic infiltration and edema of the rectus muscles, typically the inferior and medial recti. The inflamed muscles may become fibrotic and permanently restricted. Diplopia usually begins in the upper field of gaze. All extraocular muscles may eventually be involved, and there may be no position of gaze free of diplopia. Tethering of the inferior recti results in elevation of intraocular pressure on upgaze, or in severe cases even on looking straight ahead.

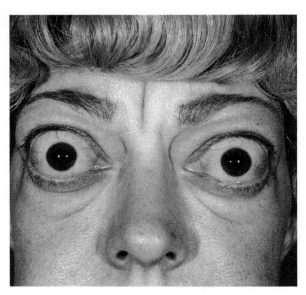

▲ **Figure 13–3.** Graves' ophthalmopathy.

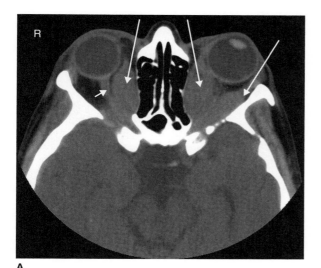

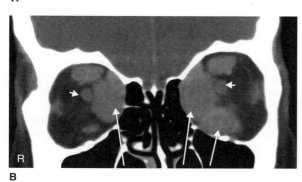

▲ **Figure 13–4.** CT scan of Graves' ophthalmopathy.
A: Axial section showing markedly enlarged medial recti
and left lateral rectus **(arrows)** and distortion of right
optic nerve **(arrowhead). B:** Coronal section showing
optic nerves **(arrowheads)** and markedly enlarged
medial recti and left inferior rectus **(arrows).**

If the extraocular muscles become markedly enlarged
(Figure 13–4), there may be compression of the optic nerve at
the orbital apex, not necessarily accompanied by significant
proptosis. Early signs include an afferent pupillary defect
and impairment of color vision, followed by reduction of visual
acuity. Blindness is liable to occur if compression is unrelieved.

▶ **Treatment**

Management should be multidisciplinary. An endocrinolo-
gist should manage the thyroid status, optimal control being
crucial to ameliorating the orbital disease. If hyperthyroidism cannot be controlled by drug therapy, thyroid surgery is

preferable to radioiodine therapy. Whether thyroid surgery
improves ophthalmopathy is uncertain. Radioidone therapy
is relatively contraindicated and prophylactic steroid therapy
needs to be considered if it needs to be administered.
Cigarette smoking should be discouraged.

Ocular surface problems, including exposure keratitis, can
usually be controlled with topical lubricants. Compressive
optic neuropathy, or proptosis with severe exposure keratitis
uncontrolled by lubricants, requires emergency treatment, initially with high-dose systemic steroids (oral prednisolone
80–100 mg/day or intravenous methylprednisolone therapy
1 g/day for 3 days repeated weekly for 3 weeks). If this is unsuccessful, either acutely or in the long term, including due to steroid complications, surgical decompression of the orbit is usually
performed. Several techniques have been devised using external
or transnasal endoscopic approaches. All aim to expand the
orbital volume by removal of the bony walls, usually the orbital
floor, medial wall, and possibly lateral wall, with incision of the
orbital periosteum. There is a risk of causing or exacerbating
diplopia and a lesser risk of orbital infection. Orbital radiotherapy may be an effective alternative in patients unsuitable for
surgery but should be avoided in diabetics with retinopathy.
Exposure keratitis due to severe proptosis may respond to lateral
tarsorrhaphy.

Whether oral corticosteroids (prednisone up to 60 mg/day),
with or without additional immunosuppressants, or orbital
radiotherapy should be used in active disease not complicated
by optic neuropathy or severe corneal exposure is controversial. Systemic steroids commonly result in improvement in
symptoms, but the potential for complications limits their
long-term use. Pulsed high-dose intravenous steroids appear
to be more effective with fewer adverse effects than long-term
oral therapy.

Eyelid retraction is often more disturbing than proptosis—
both functionally, because of exposure keratitis, and cosmetically. Surgical orbital decompression may improve lid
retraction, but correction of the retraction by lid surgery is safer
and camouflages proptosis to some extent. The upper and
lower lid retractors (aponeurosis and sympathetic muscles) can
be lengthened by inserting a spacer such as eye bank sclera. Small
amounts (2 mm) of lid retraction can be corrected by disin-
serting the retractors from the upper tarsal border. Once the
ophthalmopathy is inactive, surgical orbital decompression can
be performed for cosmetically unacceptable proptosis, but the
risks of surgery need to be borne in mind.

Double vision may not be sufficiently bothersome to require
treatment. While the ophthalmopathy is active, prisms
or occlusion may be helpful. Strabismus surgery should not
be undertaken until the ophthalmopathy is inactive and the
ocular motility disturbance has been stable for at least 6 months.
Tight muscles, usually inferior and medial recti, are recessed
using adjustable sutures. Most patients can achieve at least a
small area of binocular single vision in a useful position of
gaze. Torsional diplopia, the result of oblique muscle involvement, complicates management. Botulinum toxin is rarely

helpful in the acute or chronic stages of the disease. Some patients have intractable diplopia despite all attempts at correction.

2. PSEUDOTUMOR

A frequent cause of proptosis in adults and children is inflammatory pseudotumor. (The term "pseudotumor" was adopted to indicate a non-neoplastic process that produces the sentinel sign of an orbital neoplasm, ie, proptosis.) In some cases it is due to vasculitis, most commonly Wegener's granulomatosis, possibly in its limited form that may not be associated with positive serum antineutrophil cytoplasmic antibodies (ANCA). The inflammatory process can be diffuse or localized, specifically involving any orbital structure (eg, myositis, dacryoadenitis, superior orbital fissure syndrome, or optic perineuritis) or cell type (eg, lymphocytes, fibroblasts, histiocytes, and/or plasma cells). There may be extension to involve the cavernous sinuses and intracranial meninges. Onset is usually rapid, and pain is often present.

Pseudotumor is usually unilateral; when both orbits are involved, it is more often a manifestation of vasculitis. The differential diagnosis includes Graves' ophthalmopathy and orbital lymphoma.

Treatment with systemic NSAIDs, systemic corticosteroids, if necessary with other immunosuppressants (eg, cyclophosphamide) if there is underlying vasculitis, and rarely radiation, is usually effective, but there is a sclerosing variant that is very resistant to treatment. Surgery tends to exacerbate the inflammatory reaction, but biopsy may be required to confirm the diagnosis in recurrent or recalcitrant cases.

ORBITAL INFECTIONS

1. ORBITAL CELLULITIS (FIGURE 13–5) AND PRESEPTAL CELLULITIS

Orbital (postseptal) cellulitis, which is bacterial infection deep to the orbital septum, is the most common cause of proptosis in children. Immediate treatment is essential because delay can lead to blindness, due to optic nerve compression or infarction, or death, due to septic cavernous sinus thrombosis or intracranial sepsis. Although most cases occur in children, aged and immunocompromised individuals may also be affected.

The orbit is surrounded by the paranasal sinuses, and part of their venous drainage is through the orbit. Most cases of childhood orbital cellulitis arise from extension of acute sinusitis through the thin ethmoid bones, and thus the organisms usually responsible are *Streptococcus pneumoniae*, other streptococci, *Haemophilus influenza* (in countries where *H influenza* type b (Hib) immunization is not carried out in early infancy), and less commonly *Staphylococcus aureus*, including methicillin-resistant *S aureus* (MRSA), or

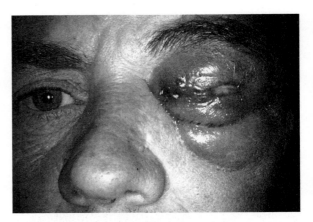

▲ **Figure 13–5.** Orbital cellulitis. Abscess draining through upper eyelid.

Moraxella catarrhalis. In adolescents and adults, when there is often chronic sinus infection, anaerobic organisms may also be involved. If there is a history of trauma, usually penetrating orbital injury but possibly from animal bites, *S aureus*, including methicillin-resistant *S aureus* (MRSA), or Group A β-hemolytic streptococci are commonly responsible.

In comparison **preseptal cellulitis**, which is bacterial infection superficial to the orbital septum, is usually caused by spread of infection arising within the eyelid, such as from a horedolum (see Chapter 4), surgical or traumatic wound, or an insect or animal bite.

▶ Clinical Findings

Orbital cellulitis is characterized by fever, pain, eyelid swelling and erythema, proptosis, chemosis, limitation of extraocular movements, and leukocytosis. Non-axial proptosis suggests sub-periosteal or intraorbital abscess. Extension to the cavernous sinus produces contralateral orbital involvement, trigeminal dysfunction, and more marked systemic illness. Intracranial extension causes meningitis and possibly brain abscess.

Few orbital diseases, except for mucormycosis (see later in the chapter), progress as rapidly as bacterial infection. Preseptal cellulitis, in which there is systemic illness with eyelid swelling and erythema but no proptosis, chemosis, or limitation of extraocular movements, is the main differential diagnosis but may also mimic the initial stages of orbital cellulitis. Other entities to be considered are rhabdomyosarcoma in children, pseudotumor, and Graves' ophthalmopathy.

A CT scan or MRI may be helpful to distinguish between preseptal and postseptal cellulitis, and is particularly important when there is concern about development of an abscess (Figure 13–6) or to identify a foreign body. MRI is better than

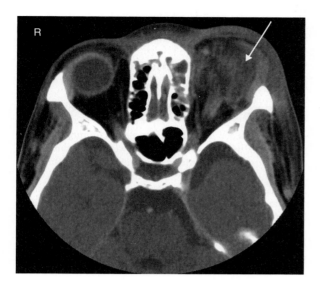

▲ **Figure 13–6.** Axial CT scan of left orbital abscess (arrow).

CT to detect cavernous sinus thrombosis. Plain x-rays alone can only identify the presence of sinusitis.

▶ Treatment

Treatment of orbital cellulitis should be initiated before the causative organism is identified. As soon as nasal, conjunctival, and blood cultures are obtained, antibiotics should be administered. Intravenous therapy is generally used, initially with a cephalosporin, such as the third-generation agents cefotaxime and ceftriaxone, or a β-lactamase-resistant drug, such as nafcillin, imipinen, or piperacillin/tazobactam. Possible anaerobic infection requires addition of metronidazole or clindamycin. Cepahalosporins are appropriate if there is a history of trauma, unless MRSA infection is likely, in which case vancomycin or clindamycin is required. For patients with penicillin hypersensitivity, vancomycin, levofloxacin, and metronidazole are recommended. Success with oral ciprofloxacin and clindamycin has been reported in uncomplicated cases.

Early consultation with an otolaryngologist is important. Nasal decongestants and vasoconstrictors help drain the paranasal sinuses. Most cases respond promptly to antibiotics. Those cases that do not respond may require surgical drainage of the paranasal sinuses. Orbital abscesses usually require surgical drainage, the route being determined by the results of CT or MRI.

Preseptal cellulitis can usually be treated with oral antibiotics, such as amoxicillin/clavulanate, but the patient should be monitored closely for development of postseptal cellulitis. Therapy should be adjusted if there is high likelihood of MRSA infection or if there is a dirty wound, in which case gram-negative organisms may need to be covered.

2. MUCORMYCOSIS

Diabetics and immunocompromised patients are at risk of developing severe and often fatal fungal infections of the orbit. The organisms are of the zygomycetes group, which have a tendency to invade vessels and create ischemic necrosis. Infection usually begins in the sinuses and erodes into the orbital cavity. A necrotizing reaction destroys muscle, bone, and soft tissue, not necessarily causing florid signs of orbital inflammation but severe pain, visual loss, ophthalmoplegia, and systemic upset. Examination of the nose and palate characteristically reveals black, necrotic mucosa, a smear of which shows broad branching hyphae.

Without treatment, the infection gradually erodes into the cranial cavity, resulting in meningitis, brain abscess, and death usually within days to weeks. Treatment is difficult and often inadequate. It consists of correction of the underlying disease combined with surgical debridement and administration of amphotericin B intravenously and, if possible, locally. Posaconazole is another potentially useful antifungal.

CYSTIC LESIONS INVOLVING THE ORBIT

1. DERMOID

Dermoids are not true neoplasms but benign choristomas arising from embryonic tissue not usually found in the orbit. Orbital dermoids arise from surface ectoderm and often contain epithelial structures such as keratin, hair, and even teeth. Most are cystic and filled with an oily fluid that can incite a severe inflammatory reaction if liberated into the orbit. Most dermoids occur in the superior temporal quadrant of the orbit, but they can occur at any bony suture line.

CT shows a sharp, round bony defect from the pressure of a slowly growing mass affixed to the periosteum.

Epidermoid cyst is a superficial keratin-filled mass, usually near the superior orbital rim. It may be congenital or posttraumatic. Excision is usually not difficult.

A **dermolipoma** is a solid mass of fatty material that occurs below the conjunctival surface, usually in the region of the lateral canthus (Figure 13–7). Hair growth on the overlying conjunctiva is not uncommon. Dermolipomas are often much larger than they appear to be, and excision may cause considerable damage to vital structures, particularly the lacrimal gland ductules leading to tear deficiency. If treatment is necessary, limited excision is usually advised.

2. SINUS MUCOCELE

Obstruction of drainage from a paranasal sinus may lead to its expansion to form a mucocele. Frontal or ethmoid sinus mucoceles typically present with progressive non-axial proptosis, whereas sphenoid sinus mucocele present with optic

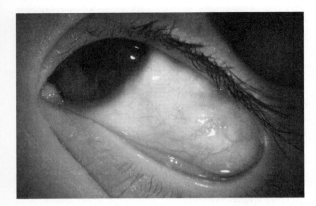

▲ **Figure 13-7.** Dermolipoma.

neuropathy. In either case the presentation may be rapid if there is infection. CT will usually make the diagnosis (Figure 13–8). MRI may be required to differentiate from dermoid cyst and to define the extent of the lesion. Treatment is surgical, sometimes by an endoscopic approach. Otolaryngologic and/or neurosurgical assistance is likely to be required.

3. MENINGOCELE

Erosion of the meninges into the orbital cavity through a congenital dehiscence in the bony sutures creates a cystic mass filled with cerebrospinal fluid known as a meningocele. If there is also brain tissue it is known as a meningoencephalocele. The resultant fluctuant mass in the superior medial orbit typically enlarges with Valsalva's maneuver. Most cases

are present at birth, but those arising from the sphenoid bone may not become apparent until adolescence.

VASCULAR ABNORMALITIES INVOLVING THE ORBIT

1. ARTERIOVENOUS MALFORMATION

Arteriovenous malformations are an uncommon cause of proptosis. Orbital venous anomalies (varices) produce intermittent proptosis, sometimes associated with pain and transient reduction of vision. Some degree of proptosis can be induced with Valsalva's maneuver or by placing the head in a dependent position. There may be acute exacerbations due to hemorrhage. MRI scan is usually diagnostic. Endovascular embolization is the preferred method of treatment. Surgery is very difficult, with risk of permanent impairment of vision.

2. CAROTID ARTERY–CAVERNOUS SINUS FISTULA

The diagnosis of high flow (direct) carotid artery–cavernous sinus fistulas is usually straightforward. Although sometimes occurring spontaneously due to rupture of an intracavernous internal carotid artery aneurysm, they usually follow severe head trauma causing damage to the intracavernous internal carotid. Physical signs include marked orbital congestion with chemosis, pulsating proptosis, raised intraocular pressure, retinal hemorrhages, and ophthalmoplegia, as well as a loud bruit.

Low-flow (indirect) shunts (dural carotid cavernous sinus fistula) are usually spontaneous, most commonly being associated with diabetes and systemic hypertension,

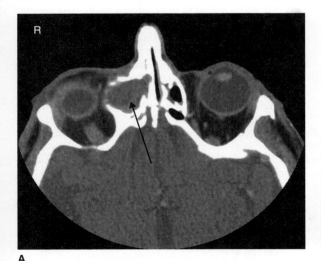

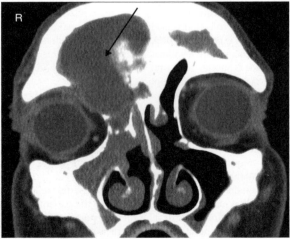

▲ **Figure 13–8.** CT scan of right fronto-ethmoidal mucocele **(arrows). A:** Axial section. **B:** Coronal section.

and diagnosis may be delayed by misdiagnosis such as chronic conjunctivitis. Orbital congestion, arterializations of episcleral vessels, elevated intraocular pressure, mild proptosis, and possibly a faint bruit are the typical features.

Orbital ultrasound blood flow studies with color Doppler imaging provide a noninvasive method of diagnosing carotid artery–cavernous sinus fistula, by demonstrating reversal of flow ("arterialization") in the superior ophthalmic vein. Definitive diagnosis requires angiography, often initially by CT or MR angiography, but proceeding to catheter angiography for identification of the sites of fistulization and determining whether they are amenable to treatment. High-flow fistulas generally need to be treated by transvenous or intra-arterial balloon or coil embolization, or parent vessel occlusion. Many low-flow fistulas resolve spontaneously but intra-arterial or transvenous embolization may be required.

▼ PRIMARY ORBITAL TUMORS

CAPILLARY HEMANGIOMA

Capillary hemangiomas are common benign tumors that sometimes involve the eyelids and orbit (Figure 13–9). Superficial lesions are reddish (strawberry nevus), and deeper lesions are more bluish. Over 90% become apparent before the age of 6 months. They tend to enlarge rapidly in the first year of life and regress slowly over 6–7 years. Lesions within the orbit may cause strabismus or proptosis. Involvement of the eyelids may induce astigmatism or occlude vision, resulting in amblyopia.

Small superficial lesions require no treatment and are best allowed to spontaneously regress. Deep orbital lesions are often associated with significant morbidity with or without treatment. The most common dilemma, however, is the rapidly growing lid lesion in a preverbal infant.

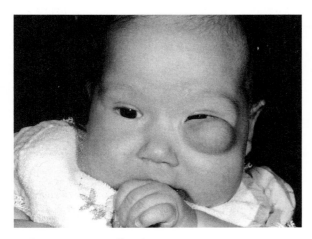

▲ **Figure 13–9.** Capillary hemangioma.

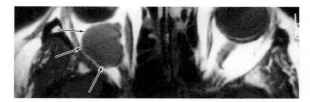

▲ **Figure 13–10.** MRI of cavernous hemangioma **(arrows)** of the right orbit. (Courtesy of D Char.)

Parents are often unwilling to wait for spontaneous regression and plead for treatment even if amblyopia is not a threat. The use of intralesional depot corticosteroids has been found to be effective in many instances and has evolved as the preferred method of treatment in most cases. Corticosteroids are thought to have an antiangiogenic effect that inhibits capillary proliferation and induces vascular constriction. Other forms of treatment are sometimes necessary, including prolonged compression, systemic corticosteroids, sclerosing agents, cryotherapy, laser surgery, radiation, and surgical resection.

CAVERNOUS HEMANGIOMA (FIGURE 13–10)

Cavernous hemangiomas are benign, grow slowly, and usually become symptomatic in middle life. Most occur in women. They most often lie within the muscle cone, producing axial proptosis, hyperopia, and, in many cases, choroidal folds. Unlike capillary hemangiomas, they do not tend to regress spontaneously. Surgical excision is usually successful and is indicated if the patient is symptomatic.

LYMPHANGIOMA

In its early stages, lymphangioma may be very similar to hemangioma—even histologically such that some authors have suggested a primarily venous origin. Both usually begin in infancy, although lymphangioma may present later in life. Lymphangioma does not regress and is characterized by intermittent hemorrhage and gradual worsening. Large blood cysts may cause proptosis and diplopia and require evacuation.

The tumor is often multifocal and frequently occurs in the soft palate and other areas of the face as well as the orbit. On histologic examination, it consists of large serum-filled channels and lymphoid follicles. Treatment can be for the purpose of either acute decompression of a hemorrhagic blood cyst or eradication of the tumor. Needle aspiration of blood or extirpation of a specific cyst may be temporarily effective. Sclerosing agents are sometimes useful. Excision of tumor by any method is seldom satisfactory. The risk of amblyopia is similar to that associated with capillary hemangioma.

RHABDOMYOSARCOMA (FIGURE 13–11)

Rhabdomyosarcoma is the most common primary malignant tumor of the orbit in childhood. Presentation is before

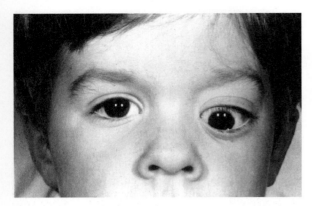

▲ **Figure 13–11.** Rhabdomyosarcoma.

age 10, and rapid growth is characteristic. The tumor may destroy adjacent orbital bone and spread into the brain. The combination of external megavoltage radiation and chemotherapy has improved the survival rate of these patients from less than 50%, when orbital exenteration was used, to over 90% today.

NEUROFIBROMA

Neurofibromatosis 1 (von Recklinghausen's disease) is inherited as an autosomal dominant trait. The responsible gene is on chromosome 17. Plexiform neurofibromas are characteristic and can distort the eyelids (Figure 13–12) and orbit. The presence of iris Lisch nodules and cutaneous cafe au lait spots helps confirm the diagnosis. The sphenoid bone is often defective; the associated orbital defect may lead to pulsating exophthalmos or enophthalmos. Optic nerve gliomas produce signs (proptosis) and symptoms (visual loss) in 5% of affected individuals; imaging has shown that many more patients harbor asymptomatic optic nerve gliomas. Some of

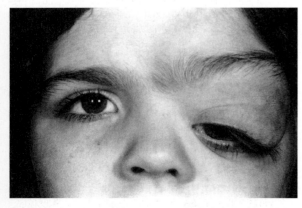

▲ **Figure 13–12.** Pexiform neurofibroma of upper eyelid in neurofibromatosis 1.

these patients also develop meningiomas and, rarely, malignant peripheral nerve sheath tumors.

OPTIC NERVE GLIOMA

Approximately 75% of symptomatic optic nerve gliomas become apparent before age 10. Twenty-five to fifty percent are associated with neurofibromatosis 1. They are low-grade astrocytomas. Those anterior to the chiasm tend to behave in a benign fashion and may regress spontaneously; those in and posterior to the chiasm may be more aggressive. Visual loss and optic atrophy are the most common signs. Proptosis occurs if the tumor is in the orbit.

Treatment is controversial. There are no compelling statistics to indicate that any form of treatment is applicable to all cases. Some believe that these tumors do not require treatment, others that they require surgical excision, radiotherapy, or chemotherapy. If progressive tumor growth and visual loss can be clearly documented, radiotherapy is often effective in stabilizing or even improving vision. There is a risk of secondary damage to the central nervous system such that chemotherapy is advocated as a better option, but there is little long-term follow-up data. In blind eyes with marked proptosis, the patient's cosmetic appearance can often be improved by excising the tumor through a lateral orbitotomy.

LACRIMAL GLAND TUMORS

Fifty percent of masses presenting in the lacrimal gland are epithelial tumors; one-half of these are malignant. Inflammatory masses and lymphoproliferative tumors comprise the other 50%. The most common epithelial tumor is the pleomorphic adenoma (benign mixed tumor). These tumors should be excised—not biopsied—because of their propensity for recurrence and malignant transformation.

A malignant tumor of the lacrimal gland is suspected when the patient presents with pain and destructive bony changes are evident on CT. Biopsy should be performed through the eyelid to avoid tumor seeding in the orbit. Orbital exenteration with ostectomy is required if there is to be any chance of survival. Even with radical treatment, the prognosis is poor.

LYMPHOMA

Lymphomatous tumors of the orbit are divided into lymphomas, of which the most common type is extranodal marginal zone (MALT) lymphoma, and reactive lymphoid hyperplasia, which is classified as atypical or benign. Immunologic and DNA hybridization techniques can help the pathologist determine whether a given lesion is a monoclonal proliferation (and presumably malignant) or a benign polyclonal proliferation. However, lymphomas can have associated benign reactive lesions; benign polyclonal lesions can have small clones of B lymphocytes; and monoclonal tumors often remain localized and behave in a benign fashion.

The differential diagnosis includes orbital infection and pseudotumor, with or without systemic vasculitis. Pain is more common with benign inflammatory processes than with malignant lymphomas.

The prognosis for both polyclonal lymphoid proliferations and well-differentiated B-cell monoclonal lesions is excellent. If disease is confined to the orbit, treatment for both monoclonal and polyclonal lesions is with radiation. Amongst patients with lymphoma or atypical reactive lymphoid hyperplasia confined to the orbit at presentation, the overall risk of systemic lymphoma at 10 years is 33%, being much more likely if there was initially bilateral orbital disease.

HISTIOCYTOSIS

Proliferation of Langerhans cells with characteristic cytoplasmic granules comprises a spectrum of disease that includes what were formerly classified as unifocal and multifocal eosinophilic granuloma, Hand–Schuller–Christian disease (multifocal lytic skull lesion, proptosis, and diabetes insipidus), and Letterer–Siwe disease (cutaneous, visceral, and lymph node involvement). The younger the child at the time of diagnosis, the greater the chance of multifocal disease.

The orbital lesions can be treated with surgical curettement, corticosteroid injections, or low-dose radiation.

▼ METASTATIC TUMORS

Metastatic tumors reach the orbit by hematogenous spread, since the orbit is devoid of lymphatics. In adults, breast, lung or prostate cancer, or melanoma are the usual primaries. In children, the most common metastatic tumor is neuroblastoma, which is often associated with spontaneous periocular hemorrhage as the rapidly growing tumor becomes necrotic. Metastatic tumors are much more common in the choroid than in the orbit, probably because of the nature of the blood supply.

Many metastatic orbital tumors respond to radiation, some to chemotherapy. Small localized tumors that are symptomatic can sometimes be completely or partially excised. Neuroblastomas in children under 11 months have a relatively good prognosis. Adults with metastatic tumors in the orbit have a very limited life expectancy.

▼ SECONDARY TUMORS

Basal cell, squamous cell, and sebaceous gland carcinomas may spread locally into the anterior orbit. Nasopharyngeal carcinomas—most commonly from the maxillary sinus—and intracranial meningiomas may invade the orbit, the latter by spreading along the optic nerve sheath.

REFERENCES

Acharya SH et al: Radioidoine therapy (RAI) for Graves' disease (GD) and the effect on ophthalmopathy: a systematic review. Clin Endocrinol 2008;69:943. [PMID: 18429949]

Arat YO, Mawad ME, Boniuk M: Orbital venous malformations: current multidisciplinary treatment approach. Arch Ophthalmol 2004;122:1151. [PMID: 15302655]

Arneja JS, Mulliken JB: Resection of amblyogenic periocular hemangiomas: indications and outcomes. Plast Reconstr Surg 2010;125:274. [PMID: 20048618]

Bartalena L, Tanda ML: Clinical practice. Graves' ophthalmopathy. N Engl J Med 2009;360:994. [PMID: 19264688]

Bell RB, Markiewicz MR: Computer-assisted planning, stereolithographic modeling, and intraoperative navigation for complex orbital reconstruction: a descriptive study in a preliminary cohort. J Oral Maxillofac Surg 2009;67:2559. [PMID: 19925972]

Bradley EA et al: Orbital radiation for Graves' ophthalmopathy: a report by the American Academy of Ophthalmology. Ophthalmology 2008;115:398. [PMID: 18082885]

Cannon PS et al: Our experience using primary oral antibiotics in the management of orbital cellulitis in a tertiary referral centre. Eye 2009;23:612. [PMID: 18309335]

Chen LZ et al: Retrospective study on the endovascular embolization for traumatic carotid cavernous fistula. Chin J Traumatol 2010;13:30. [PMID: 20109363]

Demirci H et al: Orbital lymphoproliferative tumors: analysis of clinical features and systemic involvement in 160 cases. Ophthalmology 2008;115:1626. [PMID: 18440641]

Dickinson J, Perros P: Thyroid-associated orbitopathy: who and how to treat. Endocrinol Metab Clin North Am. 2009;38:373. [PMID: 1932847]

European Group on Graves' Orbitopathy (EUGOGO): Outcome of orbital decompression for disfiguring proptosis in patients with Graves' orbitopathy using various surgical procedures. Br J Ophthalmol 2009;93:1518. [PMID: 19028743]

Gawley SD, Bingham EA, McGinnity G: Visual outcomes of treated periocular capillary haemangiomas in childhood: a 10-year review. Acta Ophthalmol 2010 Feb 12. [Epub ahead of print] [PMID: 20156200]

Jung WS et al: The radiological spectrum of orbital pathologies that involve the lacrimal gland and the lacrimal fossa. Korean J Radiol 2007;8:336. [PMID: 17673845]

Karcioglu ZA et al: Orbital rhabdomyosarcoma. Cancer Control 2004;11:328. [PMID: 15377992]

Kubal WS: Imaging of orbital trauma. Radiographics 2008;28:1729. [PMID: 18936032]

Lee TJ et al: Extensive paranasal sinus mucoceles: a 15-year review of 82 cases. Am J Otolaryngol 2009;30:234–238. [PMID: 19563933]

Liu GT: Optic gliomas of the anterior visual pathway. Curr Opin Ophthalmol 2006;17:427. [PMID: 16932058]

Loo JL, Looi AL, Seah LL: Visual outcome in patients with paranasal mucoceles. Ophthal Plast Reconstr Surg 2009;25:126. [PMID: 19300156]

Lowery AJ, Kerin MJ: Graves' ophthalmopathy: the case for thyroid surgery. Surgeon 2009;7:290. [PMID: 19848063]

McKinsley SH et al: Microbiology of pediatric orbital cellulitis. Am J Ophthalmol 2007;144:497. [PMID: 17698020]

Mendenhall WM, Lessner AM: Orbital pseudotumor. Am J Clin Oncol 2009 Sep 4. [Epub ahead of print] [PMID: 19738455]

Rootman J: Vascular malformations of the orbit: hemodynamic concepts. Orbit 2003:22:103. [PMID: 12789590]

Rudloe TF et al: Acute periorbital infections: who needs emergent imaging? Pediatrics 2010 Mar 1. [Epub ahead of print] [PMID: 20194288]

Sautter NB et al: Paranasal sinus mucoceles with skull-base and/or orbital erosion: is the endoscopic approach sufficient? Ototlaryngol Head Neck Surg 2008;139:570. [PMID: 18922346]

Schekenbach K et al: Emerging therapeutic options in fulminant invasive rhinocerebral mucormycosis. Auris Nasus Larynx 2009 Oct 24. [Epub ahead of print] [PMID: 19857939]

Shields JA et al: Orbital cysts of childhood: classification, clinical features, and management. Surv Ophthalmol 2004;49:281. [PMID: 15110666]

Shields JA et al: Review: primary epithelial malignancies of the lacrimal gland. The 2003 Ramon L. Font lecture. Ophthal Plast Reconstr Surg 2004;20:10. [PMID: 14752304]

Sikdera S. Weinberg RS: Thyroid Eye Disease: pathogenesis and treatment. Ophthalmologica 2010;224:199. [PMID: 19940525]

Smoker WR et al: Vascular lesions of the orbit: more than meets the eye. Radiographics 2008;28:185. [PMID: 18203938]

Stålberg P et al: Surgical treatment of Graves' disease: evidence-based approach. World J Surg 2008;32:1269. [PMID: 18327526]

Stiebel-Kalish H et al: Treatment modalities for Graves' ophthalmopathy: systematic review and metaanalysis. J Clin Endocrinol Metab 2009;94:2708. [PMID: 19491222]

Tjoumakaris SI, Jabbour PM, Rosenwasser RH: Neuroendovascular management of carotid cavernous fistulae. Neurosurg Clin N Am 2009;20:447. [PMID: 19853804]

Vaidhyanath R et al: Lacrimal fossa lesions: pictorial review of CT and MRI features. Orbit 2008;27:410. [PMID: 19085295]

Valenzuela AA et al: Orbital metastasis: clinical features, management and outcome. Orbit 2009;28:153. [PMID: 19839900]

Vannucchi G et al: Graves' orbitopathy activation after radioactive iodine therapy with and without steroid prophylaxis. J Clin Endocrinol Metab 2009;94:3381. [PMID: 19567525]

Warrier S et al: Orbital arteriovenous malformations. Arch Ophthalmol 2008;126:1669. [PMID: 19064847]

Wiess AH, Kelly JP: Reappraisal of astigmatism induced by periocular capillary hemangioma and treatment with intralesional corticosteroid injection. Ophthalmology 2008;115:390. [PMID: 17588666]

Neuro-Ophthalmology

Paul Riordan-Eva, FRCOphth, and
William F. Hoyt, MD

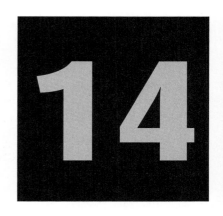

As demonstrated by their common embryological origin, the retinas and anterior visual pathways (optic nerves, optic chiasm, and optic tracts) are an integral part of the brain, providing a substantial proportion of total sensory input. They frequently give important diagnostic clues to central nervous system disorders. Intracranial disease frequently causes visual disturbances because of destruction of or pressure upon some portion of the optic pathways. Cranial nerves III, IV, and VI, which control ocular movements, may be involved, and nerves V and VII are also intimately associated with ocular function.

THE SENSORY VISUAL PATHWAY

▶ Topographic Overview (Figures 14–1 and 14–2)

Cranial nerve II subserves the special sense of vision. Light is detected by the rods and cones of the retina, which may be considered the special sensory end organ for vision. The cell bodies of these receptors extend processes that synapse with the bipolar cell, the second neuron in the visual pathway. The bipolar cells synapse, in turn, with the retinal ganglion cells. Ganglion cell axons comprise the nerve fiber layer of the retina and converge to form the optic nerve. The nerve emerges from the back of the globe and travels posteriorly within the muscle cone to enter the cranial cavity via the optic canal.

Intracranially, the two optic nerves join to form the optic chiasm (Figure 14–1). At the chiasm, more than half of the fibers (those from the nasal half of the retina) decussate and join the uncrossed temporal fibers of the opposite nerve to form the optic tracts. Each optic tract sweeps around the cerebral peduncle toward the lateral geniculate nucleus, where it will synapse. All of the fibers receiving impulses from the right hemifields of each eye thus make up the left optic tract and project to the left cerebral hemisphere. Similarly, the left hemifields project to the right cerebral hemisphere. Twenty percent of the fibers in the tract subserve pupillary function. These fibers leave the tract just anterior to the nucleus and pass via the brachium of the superior colliculus to the midbrain pretectal nucleus. The remaining fibers synapse in the lateral geniculate nucleus. The cell bodies of this structure give rise to the geniculocalcarine tract. This tract passes through the posterior limb of the internal capsule and then fans into the optic radiations that traverse parts of the temporal and parietal lobes en route to the occipital (calcarine, striate, or primary visual) cortex.

▶ Analysis of Visual Fields in Localizing Lesions in the Visual Pathways

In clinical practice, lesions in the visual pathways may be localized by examination of the central and peripheral visual fields. The technique (perimetry) is discussed in Chapter 2.

Figure 14–3 shows the types of field defects caused by lesions in various locations of the pathway. Lesions anterior to the chiasm (of the retina or optic nerve) cause unilateral field defects; lesions anywhere in the visual pathway posterior to the chiasm cause contralateral homonymous defects (affecting the same side of the visual field in each eye). Chiasmal lesions usually cause bitemporal defects.

Test objects of different intensities, sizes, and possibly colors are used to evaluate field defects thoroughly. A sloping border (ie, larger field defect to a dimmer, smaller or colored rather than white test object) suggests edema or compression. Ischemic or vascular lesions tend to produce steep borders (ie, the field defect is the same size no matter what the intensity, size, or color of the test object).

The more congruous the homonymous field defects (ie, the more similar the defect in size, shape, and location in the two eyes), the farther posterior the lesion is likely to be in the visual pathway. A lesion in the occipital region tends to cause identical defects in each field, whereas optic tract lesions tend to cause incongruous (dissimilar) homonymous field defects.

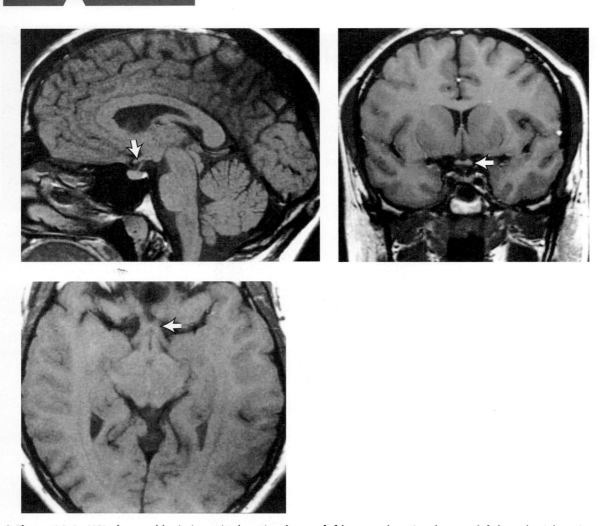

▲ **Figure 14–1.** MRI of normal brain in sagittal section **(upper left),** coronal section **(upper right),** and axial section **(lower left).** The white arrows indicate the chiasm.

Particularly in lesions of the occipital cortex, where the central field is represented posteriorly and the upper field inferiorly (Figure 14–4), there is a correlation between the visual field defect and the location of the lesion. Owing to the dual vascular supply to the occipital lobe—from the middle and posterior cerebral circulation—occipital infarcts may spare or damage the occipital pole. This leads to sparing or loss of the central field on the side of the hemianopia, respectively referred to as macular sparing (Figure 14–5) and macular splitting. Occipital lesions may also produce the phenomenon of residual sight, in which responses to movement, for example, may be demonstrable in the hemianopic field in the absence of form vision.

A complete homonymous hemianopia, wherever the site of the lesion, should still have intact visual acuity in each eye since macular function is still present in the retained visual field.

▼ THE OPTIC NERVE

A wide variety of diseases affect the optic nerve (Table 14–1). Clinical features particularly suggestive of optic nerve disease are an afferent pupillary defect, poor color vision, and optic disk changes. It is important to remember that the optic disk may be normal in the early stages of disease affecting the retrobulbar optic nerve, particularly compression by an intracranial lesion, even when there has been severe loss of visual acuity and field. Axons can be dysfunctional long before they become atrophic.

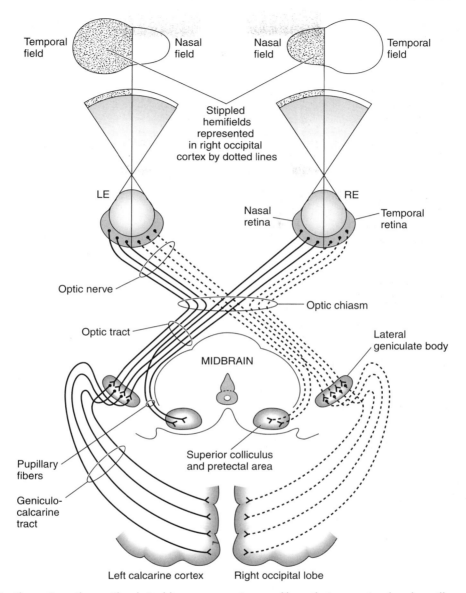

▲ **Figure 14–2.** The optic pathway. The dotted lines represent nerve fibers that carry visual and pupillary afferent impulses from the left half of the visual field.

Optic disk swelling occurs predominantly in diseases directly affecting the anterior portion of the optic nerve but also occurs with raised intracranial pressure and compression of the intraorbital optic nerve. Optic disk swelling can be a crucial clinical sign, such as in the diagnosis of anterior ischemic optic neuropathy, in which optic disk swelling must be present in the acute stage for the diagnosis to be made on clinical grounds. Central retinal vein occlusion, ocular hypotony, and intraocular inflammation can produce optic disk swelling, and hence the misleading impression of optic nerve disease.

Optic atrophy (Figure 14–6) is a nonspecific response to optic nerve damage from any cause. Since the optic nerve consists of retinal ganglion cell axons, optic atrophy may be the consequence of primary retinal disease, such as central retinal artery occlusion or retinitis pigmentosa. Excavation of the optic nerve head (optic disk cupping) is generally a sign of glaucomatous optic neuropathy, but it

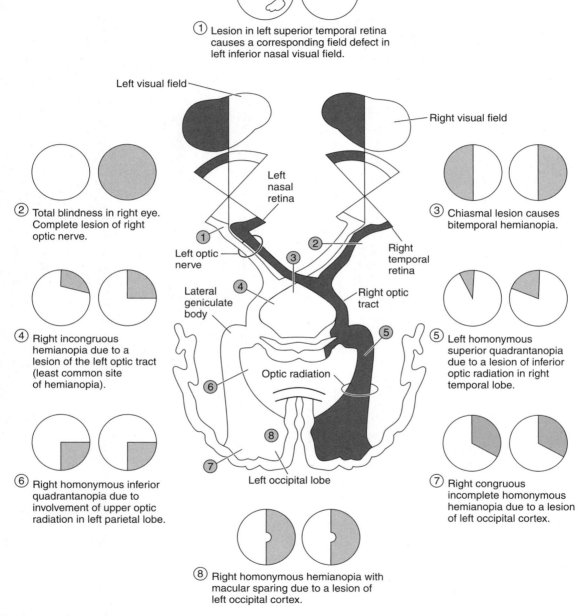

Normal blind spots

① Lesion in left superior temporal retina causes a corresponding field defect in left inferior nasal visual field.

Left visual field

Right visual field

② Total blindness in right eye. Complete lesion of right optic nerve.

③ Chiasmal lesion causes bitemporal hemianopia.

Left nasal retina

Right temporal retina

① Left optic nerve

Lateral geniculate body

Right optic tract

④ Right incongruous hemianopia due to a lesion of the left optic tract (least common site of hemianopia).

⑤ Left homonymous superior quadrantanopia due to a lesion of inferior optic radiation in right temporal lobe.

Optic radiation

⑥ Right homonymous inferior quadrantanopia due to involvement of upper optic radiation in left parietal lobe.

Left occipital lobe

⑦ Right congruous incomplete homonymous hemianopia due to a lesion of left occipital cortex.

⑧ Right homonymous hemianopia with macular sparing due to a lesion of left occipital cortex.

▲ **Figure 14–3.** Visual field defects due to various lesions of the optic pathways.

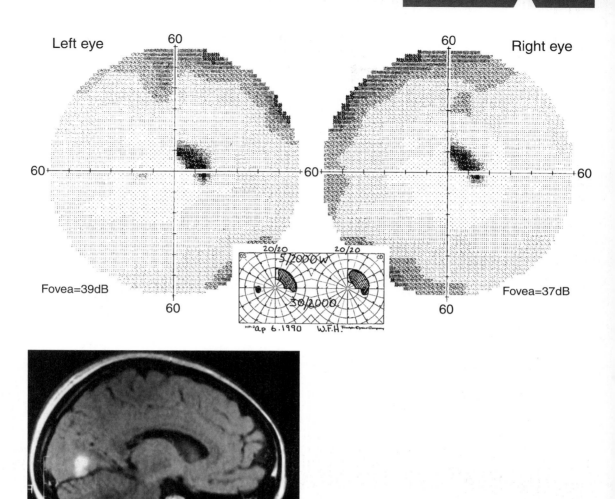

▲ Figure 14–4. Occipital lobe abscess. **Top:** Automated perimetry and tangent screen examination showing homonymous, congruous, paracentral scotoma in right upper visual fields. **Bottom:** Parasagittal MRI showing lesion involving left inferior calcarine cortex. (Reproduced, with permission, from Horton JC et al: The representation of the visual field in human striate cortex. A revision of the classic Holmes map. Arch Ophthalmol 1991;109:816.)

may occur with any cause of optic atrophy. Segmental pallor and attenuated retinal blood vessels are often the consequence of anterior ischemic optic neuropathy. Hereditary optic neuropathies usually produce bilateral temporal segmental disk pallor with preferential loss of papillomacular axons. Peripapillary exudates occur with optic

disk swelling, due to inflammation (papillitis), ischemic optic neuropathy, raised intracranial pressure (papilloedema), or severe systemic hypertension. (The term "neuroretinitis" for retinal exudates, including a macular star, due to optic disk swelling, of whatever cause, is a misnomer in that there is no inflammation of the retina, the

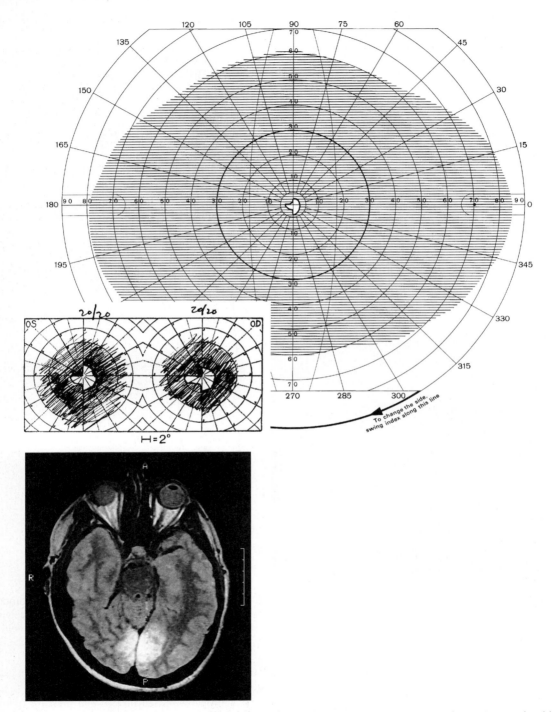

▲ **Figure 14–5.** Bilateral occipital infarcts with bilateral macular sparing. **Top:** Tangent screen and superimposed Goldmann visual fields of both eyes showing bilateral homonymous hemianopia with macular sparing, greater in the right hemi-field. **Bottom:** Axial MRI showing sparing of occipital poles. (Reproduced, with permission, from Horton JC et al: The representation of the visual field in human striate cortex. A revision of the classic Holmes map. Arch Ophthalmol 1991;109:816.)

Table 14–1. Etiologic Classification of Diseases of the Optic Nerve

Inflammatory (optic neuritis)
Demyelinative
  Multiple sclerosis
  Neuromyelitis optica (Devic's disease)
  Postviral (measles, mumps, chickenpox, influenza, infectious
    mononucleosis)
  Postimmunization
  Acute disseminated encephalomyelitis
Immune-mediated
  Systemic lupus erythematosus
Granulomatous
  Sarcoidosis
Direct infection
  Herpes zoster, syphillis, tuberculosis, cryptococcosis,
    cytomegalovirus, Lyme disease, cat-scratch disease
Contiguous inflammatory disease
  Intraocular inflammation
  Orbital disease
  Sinus disease, including mucormycosis
  Intracranial disease: meningitis, encephalitis

Vascular (ischemic optic neuropathy)
Nonarteritic anterior ischemic optic
  neuropathy
Systemic vasculitis
  Giant cell arteritis (arteritic anterior ischemic optic neuropathy),
    systemic lupus erythematosus, polyarteritis nodosa
Diabetic papillopathy
Posterior ischemic optic neuropathy
  Sudden massive blood loss (eg, trauma, gastrointestinal
    hemorrhage)
  Radiation optic neuropathy

Raised intracranial pressure (papilledema)
Intracranial mass: cerebral tumor, abscess,
  subdural hematoma
Arteriovenous malformation
Subarachnoid hemorrhage
Meningitis or encephalitis
Hydrocephalus
Pseudotumor cerebri
  Cerebral or jugular venous sinus occlusion
  Secondary pseudotumor cerebri: oral contraceptives, tetracyclines,
    steroid therapy, steroid withdrawal, hypervitaminosis A, uremia,
    hypoparathyroidism, obstructive sleep apnea, respiratory failure
  Idiopathic intracranial hypertension
Spinal tumor
Acute idiopathic polyneuropathy (Guillain–Barré syndrome)
Mucopolysaccharidosis
Craniosynostosis

Optic nerve compression
Intracranial disease: meningioma, pituitary adenoma,
  craniopharyngioma, supraclinoid internal carotid aneurysm,
  meningeal carcinomatosis, basal meningitis
Orbital disease: dysthyroid eye disease, idiopathic orbital
  inflammatory disease, orbital neoplasm, orbital abscess
Optic nerve sheath meningioma

Nutritional and toxic
Vitamin deficiencies: vitamin B_{12}, vitamin B_1 (thiamin), folate
Tobacco-alcohol amblyopia
Heavy metals: lead, thallium, arsenic
Drugs: ethambutol, isoniazid, linezolid, disulfiram, tamoxifen,
  quinine, chloramphenicol, amiodarone, chemotherapeutic agents
Chemicals: methanol, ethylene glycol

Trauma
Direct optic nerve injury
Indirect optic nerve injury
Optic nerve avulsion

Hereditary optic atrophy
Leber's hereditary optic neuropathy (mitochondrial inheritance)
Autosomal hereditary optic atrophy
  Dominant (juvenile) optic atrophy
  Recessive (infantile) optic atrophy
  Wolfram's syndrome (DIDMOAD: diabetes insipidus, diabetes
    mellitus, optic atrophy, deafness)
Inherited neurodegenerative diseases
  Hereditary spinocerebellar ataxia (Friedreich's ataxia)
  Hereditary motor and sensory neuropathy (Charcot–Marie–Tooth
    disease)
  Lysosomal storage disorders

Neoplastic infiltration
Glioma, leukemia, lymphoma, meningeal carcinomatosis,
  astrocytic hamartoma, melanocytoma, hemangioma

Optic nerve anomalies
Hypoplasia
Dysplasia (including "morning glory syndrome," coloboma, and
  optic nerve pit)
Tilted disks, including situs inversus, and scleral crescents
Megalopapilla
Myelinated nerve fibers
Persistent hyaloid system
Prepapillary vascular loops
Optic nerve head drusen
Hyperopic pseudopapilledema

Glaucomatous optic neuropathy (see Chapter 11: Glaucoma)
Optic atrophy secondary to retinal disease

exudates being a response to the anterior optic nerve disease (Figure 14–7 A). The term is more reasonably applied if there is inflammation of the retina and optic nerve (Figure 14–7 B). Signs of prior disk edema are peripapillary gliosis and atrophy, chorioretinal folds, and internal limiting membrane wrinkling.

In general, there is a correlation between degree of optic disk pallor and loss of acuity, visual field, color vision, and pupillary responses, but the relationship varies according to the underlying etiology. The major exception to this rule is compressive optic neuropathy, in which optic disk pallor is generally a late manifestation.

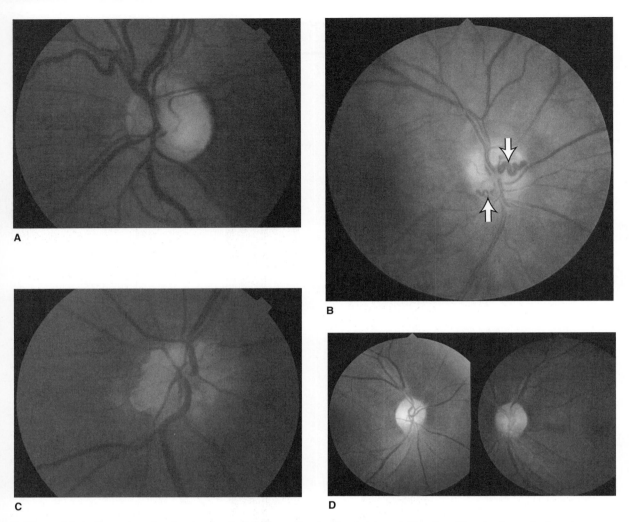

▲ **Figure 14–6.** Examples of optic atrophy. **A:** Primary optic atrophy due to nutritional amblyopia. See color insert. **B:** Secondary optic atrophy with retinochoroidal collaterals **(arrows)** due to optic nerve sheath meningioma. **C:** Optic atrophy with optic disk drusen. See color insert. **D:** Pallor (atrophy) of right optic disk due to nerve compression by sphenoid meningioma. The left disk is normal.

OPTIC NEURITIS

Inflammatory optic neuropathy (optic neuritis) may be due to a variety of causes (Table 14–1), but the most common is demyelinative disease, including multiple sclerosis. Retrobulbar neuritis is an optic neuritis that occurs far enough behind the optic disk that the disk remains normal during the acute episode. Papillitis is disk swelling caused by inflammation at the nerve head (intraocular optic nerve) (Figure 14–8). Loss of vision is the cardinal symptom of optic neuritis and is particularly useful in differentiating papillitis from papilledema, with which it may be confused on ophthalmoscopic examination.

1. DEMYELINATIVE OPTIC NEURITIS

In adults demyelinative optic neuritis is usually unilateral and occurs chiefly in women (about 3:1), with onset mostly in the third or fourth decade of life. It is associated with multiple sclerosis in up to 85% of cases, depending on several factors, including gender, racial origin, and duration of follow-up. In children there is much lower risk of progression

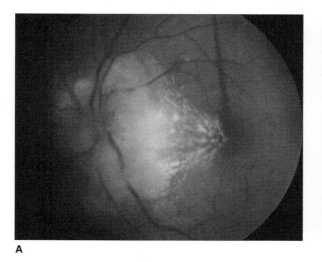

A

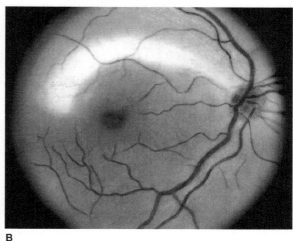

B

▲ **Figure 14–7. A:** Retinal exudates due to optic disk swelling. **B:** Arcuate neuroretinitis due to acute retinal necrosis syndrome. (B: Reproduced, with permission, from Margolis T et al: Acute retinal necrosis syndrome presenting with papillitis and arcuate neuroretinitis. Ophthalmology 1988;95:937.)

to multiple sclerosis, optic neuritis commonly following a viral infection or immunization and affecting both eyes simultaneously.

▶ Clinical Features

Visual loss is generally subacute, developing over 2–7 days. In adults, approximately one-third of patients have vision better than 20/40 during their first attack, and slightly more than one-third have vision worse than 20/200. Color vision and contrast sensitivity are correspondingly impaired. In over 90% of cases, there is pain in the region of the eye, and about 50% of patients report that the pain is exacerbated by eye movement.

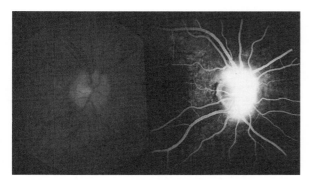

▲ **Figure 14–8.** (A, B) Mild disk swelling in demyelinative papillitis, with disk leakage on fluorescein angiography.

Almost any field defect is possible. With manual perimetry a central scotoma is most commonly found. Central visual field testing by automated perimetry most commonly shows diffuse loss. The pupillary light response is sluggish, and if the optic nerves are asymmetrically involved, a relative afferent pupillary defect will be present.

Optic disk swelling (papillitis) occurs in one third of adult cases and two thirds of childhood cases. Marked edema is unusual. Peripapillary flame-shaped hemorrhages occur in less than 10% of adult cases and vitreous cells in less than 5%. Retinal exudates and cotton-wool spots don't occur and are indicative of an infectious inflammatory or non-inflammatory optic neuropathy.

Without treatment vision usually improves, visual acuity being better than 20/30 within 2 weeks in the majority of adult cases.

▶ Investigation & Differential Diagnosis

In typical cases, clinical diagnosis is adequate and no other investigation is required. If there are atypical features—particularly failure of vision to begin to recover by 6 weeks after onset—other diagnoses must be considered, especially compressive optic neuropathy, for which magnetic resonance imaging (MRI) or computed tomography (CT) should be performed. Other entities to be considered are optic neuritis due to sarcoidosis or systemic lupus erythematosus, anterior ischemic optic neuropathy, Leber's hereditary optic neuropathy, toxic amblyopia, and vitamin B_{12} deficiency, of which the last two usually present with symmetrical bilateral visual loss.

Papillitis needs to be differentiated from papilledema (optic disk swelling due to raised intracranial pressure)

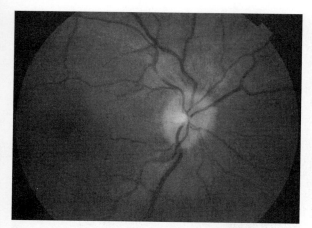

▲ **Figure 14–9.** Mild papilledema. The disk margins are blurred superiorly and inferiorly by the thickened layer of nerve fibers entering the disk.

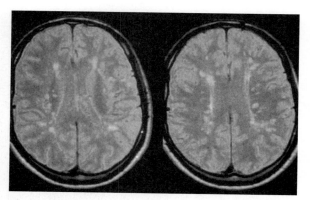

▲ **Figure 14–10.** Cerebral hemisphere white matter lesions on MRI associated with acute demyelinative optic neuritis.

(Figure 14–9). In papilledema, which usually causes bilateral optic disk changes, there is often greater elevation of the optic nerve head, normal corrected visual acuity, normal pupillary response to light, and an intact visual field except for an enlarged blind spot. If there has been acute papilledema with vascular decompensation (ie, hemorrhages and cotton-wool spots) or chronic papilledema with secondary ischemia of the optic nerve, visual field defects can include nerve fiber bundle defects and nasal quadrantanopias. Differentiation between papilledema and papillitis is particularly difficult when papilledema is asymmetric and/or associated with visual loss or papillitis is bilateral and/or associated with minimal visual impairment. Diagnosis may depend on associated symptoms particularly headache and results of MRI and lumbar puncture, as well as subsequent clinical course.

During an acute episode of optic neuritis, MRI shows gadolinium enhancement, increased signal, and sometimes swelling of the affected nerve. The gadolinium enhancement and optic nerve swelling resolve, but the increased signal persists. Brain MRI at presentation shows white matter lesions in about 50% of patients with isolated optic neuritis (Figure 14–10). This does not establish a diagnosis of multiple sclerosis, although it does indicate an increased risk of subsequent development of clinically definite multiple sclerosis (see later in the chapter).

The visual evoked response (VER) from the affected eye may show reduced amplitude or increased latency during the acute episode of optic neuritis. This in itself is not particularly helpful in diagnosis except in distinguishing retrobulbar optic neuritis from subclinical maculopathy, in which there will be abnormalities of the electroretinogram (ERG). Following recovery of vision after an episode of optic neuritis, the VER will continue to show an increased latency in about one-third of cases, and this finding can be useful in the identification of past episodes of demyelinative optic neuritis in patients undergoing investigation for possible multiple sclerosis.

▶ **Treatment**

Steroid therapy by whatever route—either intravenously (methylprednisolone, 1 g/d for 3 days with or without a subsequent tapering course of oral prednisolone), orally (methylprednisolone, 500 mg/d to 2 g/d for 3–5 days with or without subsequent oral prednisolone, or prednisolone, 1 mg/kg/d tapered over 10–21 days), or by retrobulbar injection—accelerates recovery of vision but does not influence the ultimate visual outcome. In the large multicenter Optic Neuritis Treatment Trial from the United States, oral prednisolone alone increased the risk of recurrent optic neuritis in either eye, but this result has not been replicated.

▶ **Prognosis**

Vision continues to improve slowly over many months, with recovery of acuity to 20/40 or better occurring in over 90% of cases at both 1 year and 15 years from onset. Poorer vision during the acute episode is correlated with poorer visual outcome, but even loss of all perception of light can be followed by recovery of acuity to 20/20. Poor visual outcome is also associated with longer lesions in the optic nerve, especially if there is involvement of the nerve within the optic canal. In general, there is close correlation between recovery of visual acuity, contrast sensitivity, and color vision. If the disease process is sufficiently destructive, retrograde optic atrophy results, nerve fiber bundle defects appear in the retinal nerve fiber layer (Figure 14–11), and the disk becomes pale. Factors that correlate with subsequent development of multiple sclerosis include female sex, lack of optic disk swelling during the acute phase, brain MRI abnormalities, and cerebrospinal fluid oligoclonal bands. In the Optic Neuritis

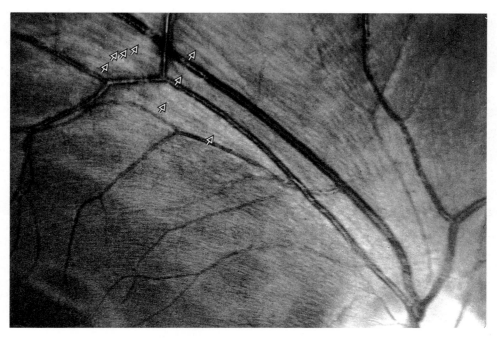

▲ **Figure 14–11.** Retinal nerve fiber layer in demyelinating optic neuropathy of multiple sclerosis. The upper temporal nerve fiber bundles show multiple slit-like areas of thinning **(arrows)** representing retrograde axonal atrophy from subclinical disease in the optic nerve. Vision in the eye was 20/20.

Treatment Trial, the overall 15-year risk of developing clinically definite multiple sclerosis following a first episode of demyelinative optic neuritis was 50%. It ranged from 25% in those with normal brain MRI at presentation to 72% in those with any white matter lesions. In men with optic disk swelling in the acute phase and no brain MRI abnormality, the 15-year risk was only 4%. Neurologic impairment in patients who develop clinically definite multiple sclerosis is generally mild and MRI abnormalities may be predictive.

In patients with a first episode of optic neuritis, which is designated a clinically isolated syndrome, and abnormal brain MRI at presentation, interferon β and glatiramer acetate have been shown to reduce the risk of clinically definite multiple sclerosis. Whether patients should be treated with such disease modifying therapy after a first episode of optic neuritis needs to be determined on an individual basis, according to their likely risk of subsequent episodes of demyelination and bearing in mind the relatively mild likely disability after further episodes and the potential side effects of treatment. The benefit is likely to increase if the patient develops frequent relapses.

2. MULTIPLE SCLEROSIS

Multiple sclerosis is typically a chronic relapsing and remitting demyelinating disorder of the central nervous system.

The cause is unknown. Some patients develop a chronically progressive form of the disease, either following a period of relapses and remissions (secondary progressive) or, less commonly, from the outset (primary progressive). Characteristically, the lesions occur at different times and in noncontiguous locations in the nervous system—that is, "lesions are disseminated in time and space." Onset is usually in young adult life; the disease rarely beginning before 15 years or after 55 years of age. There is a tendency to involve the optic nerves and chiasm, brainstem, cerebellar peduncles, and spinal cord, although no part of the central nervous system is protected. The peripheral nervous system is seldom involved.

▶ Clinical Features

Optic neuritis may be the first manifestation. There may be recurrent episodes, and the other eye usually becomes involved. The overall incidence of optic neuritis in multiple sclerosis is 90%, and the identification of symptomatic or subclinical optic nerve involvement is an important diagnostic clue.

Diplopia is a common early symptom, due most frequently to internuclear ophthalmoplegia that is frequently bilateral (Figure 14–12). Less common causes are lesions of the sixth or third cranial nerve within the brainstem.

Nystagmus is a common early sign, and unlike most manifestations of the disease (which tend toward remission), it is often permanent (70%).

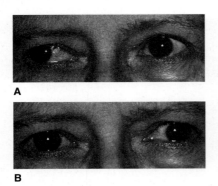

A

B

▲ **Figure 14–12. (A, B)** Bilateral internuclear ophthalmoplegia due to multiple sclerosis.

Intraocular inflammation may occur, particularly subclinical peripheral retinal venous sheathing, which can be highlighted by fluorescein angiography.

In addition to ocular disturbances, there may be motor weakness with pyramidal signs, ataxia, limb incoordination with intention tremor, dysarthria, urinary and/or bowel disturbance, and sensory disturbance, particularly paresthesias.

▶ Investigation

Diagnosis of multiple sclerosis traditionally relied upon clinical evidence of white matter disease of the central nervous system disseminated in time and space (Schumacher criteria), subsequently supported by MRI and cerebrospinal fluid abnormalities (Poser criteria). Increasingly, emphasis is being placed on MRI abnormalities, in the brain and spinal cord, supported by clinical features and cerebrospinal fluid abnormalities, to establish dissemination in time and space (McDonald criteria), thus facilitating earlier diagnosis.

Cerebrospinal fluid oligoclonal bands that are not present in the serum—representing intrathecal production of immunoglobulins—are characteristic but not diagnostic. There may be cerebrospinal fluid lymphocytosis or a mildly raised cerebrospinal fluid protein concentration during an acute relapse.

Retinal nerve fiber layer defects consistent with a subclinical optic neuritis can be detected in 68% of multiple sclerosis patients. The VER may help confirm involvement of the visual pathway. It has been reported to be abnormal in 80% of definite, 43% of probable, and 22% of suspected cases of multiple sclerosis.

▶ Course, Treatment, & Prognosis

The course of disease is unpredictable. Optic neuritis rather than brainstem or spinal cord disease as the initial manifestation is associated with a better prognosis. Relapses and remissions are characteristic, permanent disability tending to increase with each relapse. Pregnancy or the number of pregnancies has no effect on disability, but there is an increased risk of relapse just after delivery. Onset during pregnancy has a more favorable outcome than onset unrelated to pregnancy. Elevation of body temperature may exacerbate disability (Uhthoff's phenomenon), particularly visual impairment.

Steroid treatment, usually oral or intravenous methylprednisolone, is useful in hastening recovery from acute relapses but does not influence the final disability or the frequency of subsequent relapses. Interferon β glatiramer acetate, mitoxantrone, and natalizumab reduce the rate and severity of relapses and slow the progression of brain MRI abnormalities but the effect on long-term disability is still being determined. Many immunosuppressant treatments have been tested for progressive disease with no significant benefit.

3. OTHER TYPES OF OPTIC NEURITIS

Neuromyelitis optica (Devic's disease) is characterized by recurrent optic neuritis and transverse myelitis that may resemble severe multiple sclerosis, but lesions on brain MRI are atypical for multiple sclerosis; spinal cord lesions are long and necrotic; there may be a cellular cerebrospinal fluid response; severe disability is common; and there is a specific probably pathogenic serum auto-antibody, NMO-IgG. The clinical outcome is variable. Approximately 50% of patients progress to death within the first decade due to the paraplegia, but the remainder may have a prolonged remission and, ultimately, a better prognosis than patients with multiple sclerosis. Treatment is with systemic steroids or if necessary plasmapheresis for the acute episodes, followed by long-term immunosuppression, primarily targeted at humoral immunity, according to disease activity.

Particularly in children, 1–2 weeks following a viral infection or immunization there may be an episode of optic neuritis, often with simultaneous bilateral involvement. There is no association with subsequent development of multiple sclerosis. In some cases, the acute disease causes more extensive neurologic involvement manifesting as an encephalomyelitis, which overlaps with acute disseminated encephalomyelitis, in which optic neuritis is also often bilateral.

Optic neuropathy in systemic lupus erythematosus may be immune-mediated, with features of inflammatory disease, or due to small blood vessel occlusion, with features of ischemic disease (see later in the chapter). Inflammatory optic neuropathy may occur in sarcoidosis, sometimes as the first manifestation. Generally there is rapid response to steroid therapy, but long-term treatment with steroids and/or other immunosuppressants is often required. Such disease occurring in individuals in whom no evidence of sarcoidosis or other systemic disease can be identified has been termed idiopathic granulomatous optic neuropathy or chronic relapsing inflammatory optic neuropathy (CRION).

Herpes zoster—particularly herpes zoster ophthalmicus—may be complicated by optic neuropathy. This is probably due to vasculitis as well as direct neural invasion, and the prognosis is poor even with antiviral and steroid therapy. Other types of primary infection of the optic nerve, such as by syphilis, tuberculosis, cryptococcosis, and cytomegalovirus, are becoming more common with the increasing numbers of severely immunocompromised individuals such as those with AIDS. Lyme disease and cat-scratch disease are important causes of optic neuritis associated with macular star formation.

Intraocular inflammation may lead to direct involvement of the anterior optic nerve with visual loss or to optic disk swelling without apparent reduction in optic nerve function. Optic nerve involvement is an important cause of permanent visual loss in cellulitis or vasculitis of the orbit. The association between sinusitis and optic neuritis is less strong than once thought, but the occurrence of visual loss in the presence of sphenoid or posterior ethmoid sinus disease may indicate a causal relationship, particularly if there is a sinus mucocele. In diabetic or immunocompromised patients, mucormycosis is an important cause of rapidly progressive sinus disease with optic and other cranial nerve involvement (see Chapter 13).

ANTERIOR ISCHEMIC OPTIC NEUROPATHY

Anterior ischemic optic neuropathy is characterized by pallid disk swelling associated with acute loss of vision; often there are one or two peripapillary splinter hemorrhages (Figure 14–13). The disorder is due to infarction of the retrolaminar optic nerve (the region just posterior to the lamina cribrosa) from occlusion or decreased perfusion of the short posterior ciliary arteries. Fluorescein angiography in the acute stage shows decreased perfusion of the optic disk, often segmental in the nonarteritic form but usually diffuse in the arteritic form and disk leakage in the late phase. There may be associated perfusion defects in the peripapillary choroid.

Nonarteritic anterior ischemic optic neuropathy occurs generally in the sixth or seventh decade and is associated with arteriosclerosis, diabetes, hypertension, and hyperlipidemia. Low optic cup to disk ratio is almost always present. Optic nerve head drusen and increased intraocular pressure are predisposing factors. Systemic hypotension during the

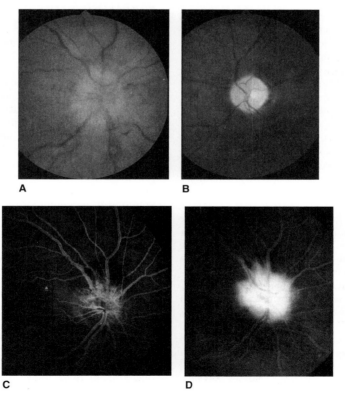

A

B

C

D

▲ **Figure 14–13.** Pseudo-Foster Kennedy syndrome due to sequential anterior ischemic optic neuropathy. **A:** Swollen right optic disk with hemorrhages due to current ischemic episode. See color insert. **B:** Atrophy of left optic disk due to previous ischemia. **C:** Early phase of fluorescein angiogram of right eye showing poor perfusion of optic disk and dilated superficial disk capillaries. **D:** Late phase of fluorescein angiogram showing disk leakage.

early morning may be an important etiologic factor. The precise relationship between phosphodiesterase inhibitors for erectile dysfunction and ischemic optic neuropathy is uncertain. In younger patients, vasculitis (eg, systemic lupus erythematosus, antiphospholipid antibody syndrome, and polyarteritis nodosa), migraine, and inherited prothrombotic states (deficiencies of protein C, protein S, or antithrombin III and activated protein C resistance) should be considered and appropriately treated. The visual loss is generally abrupt, but it may be progressive over 1–2 weeks. Impairment of visual acuity varies from slight to no light perception; visual field defects are usually nasal (characteristically inferior with a relative altitudinal pattern). In over 40% of cases, there is spontaneous improvement in visual acuity. No treatment has been shown to provide long-term benefit. Low-dose aspirin therapy may reduce the risk of involvement of the fellow eye, which occurs in up to 40% of individuals. Recurrences in the same eye are rare. As the acute process resolves, a pale disk usually without "glaucomatous" cupping results.

It is particularly important to identify **arteritic anterior ischemic optic neuropathy** due to giant cell arteritis. This causes severe visual loss with the risk of complete blindness if treatment is delayed. It occurs in elderly people and is associated with painful and tender temporal arteries, pain on mastication (jaw claudication), general malaise, and muscular aches and pains (polymyalgia rheumatica). The diagnosis is usually based on an anterior ischemic optic neuropathy and high erythrocyte sedimentation rate (ESR) and C-reactive protein (CRP) in an elderly patient, with or without associated local or systemic features, but the ESR and CRP may be normal. Other ocular manifestations of giant cell arteritis are central retinal artery occlusion, cilioretinal artery occlusion, retinal cotton-wool spots, ophthalmic artery occlusion, and diffuse ocular ischemia. Diagnosis is established by temporal artery biopsy, looking particularly for inflammatory cell infiltration, often but not always including giant cells, and prominent disruption of the internal elastic lamina.

Treatment with high-dose systemic steroids should be started as soon as a clinical diagnosis of arteritic anterior ischemic optic neuropathy has been made without waiting for the result of temporal artery biopsy, which should be performed within 1 week after starting treatment. Oral prednisolone, 80–100 mg/d, is usually adequate as a starting dose. Intravenous hydrocortisone, 250–500 mg, can be given if there is likely to be a delay in instituting oral therapy. Intravenous methylprednisolone may improve final visual outcome and certainly should be considered in patients with bilateral disease—including those with transient episodes of visual loss in the second eye—and in patients whose visual loss progresses or whose systemic manifestations and high ESR do not respond despite oral therapy. Steroid dosage can usually be reduced to about 40 mg prednisolone per day over 4 weeks but then should be more gradually tapered and discontinued after 9–12 months overall as long as there has been no recurrence of disease activity. Thirty percent of patients require long-term steroid therapy.

Diabetics occasionally develop mild, chronic, usually bilateral disk swelling with little change in visual function, so-called **diabetic papillopathy.** This is thought to represent microvascular disease affecting the optic disk circulation. It is sometimes confused with optic disk neovascularization because of the leakage of dye from the disk on fluorescein angiography. **Posterior ischemic optic neuropathy,** in which there is no optic disk swelling during the acute stage of the disease, may occur from massive blood loss, such as from trauma or bleeding peptic ulcer, nonocular surgery, particularly lumbar spine surgery in the prone position, radiotherapy, usually treatment for skull base or sinus tumors 12–18 months previously, giant cell arteritis, or mucormycosis. In general, the diagnosis of posterior ischemic optic neuropathy should not be considered until other causes, particularly a compressive lesion, have been excluded. Radiation optic neuropathy produces a characteristic pattern of gadolinium enhancement on MRI and may be helped by early hyperbaric oxygen therapy.

PAPILLEDEMA (FIGURES 14–9 AND 14–14 TO 14–16)

Papilledema is by definition optic disk swelling due to raised intracranial pressure, of which the most common causes are cerebral tumors, abscesses, subdural hematoma, arteriovenous malformations, subarachnoid hemorrhage, hydrocephalus, meningitis, and encephalitis.

In ophthalmology practice, a frequent cause is **idiopathic intracranial hypertension.** This is characterized by raised intracranial pressure, no neurologic or neuroimaging abnormality except for anything attributable to the raised intracranial pressure, such as sixth cranial nerve palsy, and normal cerebrospinal fluid constituents. It is a diagnosis of exclusion, and a number of other causes of the syndrome of pseudotumor cerebri must be excluded, such as cerebral venous sinus occlusion, tetracycline or vitamin A (retinoid) therapy, and particularly in men, obstructive sleep apnea.

Less common causes of papilledema are spinal tumors, acute idiopathic polyneuropathy (Guillain–Barré syndrome), mucopolysaccharidosis, and craniosynostoses, in which various factors, including decreased cerebrospinal fluid absorption, abnormalities of spinal fluid flow, and reduced cranial volume, contribute to the raised intracranial pressure.

For papilledema to occur, the subarachnoid space around the optic nerve must be patent and connect the retrolaminar optic nerve through the bony optic canal to the intracranial subarachnoid space, thus allowing increased intracranial pressure to be transmitted to the retrolaminar optic nerve. There, slow and fast axonal transport is blocked, and axonal distention, particularly noticeable at the superior and inferior poles of the optic disk, occurs as the first sign of papilledema.

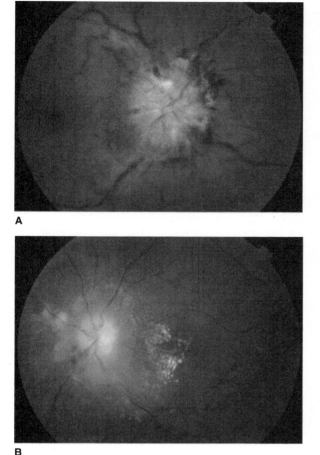

A

B

▲ **Figure 14–14.** Acute papilledema. **(A)** Optic disk swelling with cotton-wool spots and hemorrhages. **(B)** Retinal exudates. See color insert.

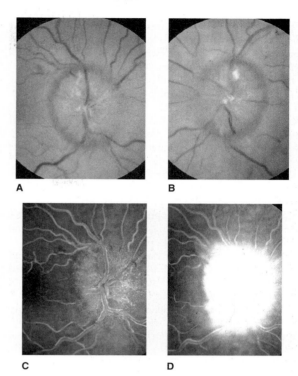

A   **B**

C   **D**

▲ **Figure 14–15.** Chronic papilledema with prominent disk swelling, capillary dilation, and retinal folds but few hemorrhages or cotton-wool spots **(A)** and **(B).** Fluorescein angiography demonstrates the capillary dilation in its early phase **(C)** and marked disk leakage in its late phase **(D).**

Hyperemia of the disk with dilated surface capillaries, blurring of the peripapillary disk margin, and loss of spontaneous venous pulsations are the signs of mild papilledema. Circumferential peripapillary retinal folds (Paton's lines) also develop. In acute papilledema, probably as a consequence either of markedly elevated or rapidly increasing intracranial pressure, there are hemorrhages and cotton-wool spots on and around the optic disk, indicating vascular and axonal decompensation with the attendant risk of acute optic nerve damage and visual field defects (Figure 14–14). There may also be peripapillary edema (which can extend to the macula), retinal exudates (Figure 14–14), and choroidal folds. In chronic papilledema (Figure 14–15), which is likely to be the consequence of prolonged, moderately raised intracranial pressure, a process of compensation appears to limit the

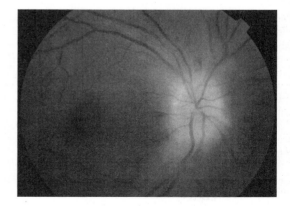

▲ **Figure 14–16.** Atrophic papilledema in idiopathic intracranial hypertension. The disk is pale and mildly elevated with blurred margins. The white areas surrounding the macula are reflected light from the vitreo-retinal interface. See color insert.

optic disk changes such that there are few if any hemorrhages or cotton-wool spots. With persistent raised intracranial pressure, the hyperemic elevated disk gradually becomes gray-white as a result of astrocytic gliosis and neural atrophy with secondary constriction of retinal blood vessels, thus leading to the stage of atrophic papilledema (Figure 14–16). There may also be retinochoroidal collaterals (previously known as opticociliary shunts) linking the central retinal vein and the peripapillary choroidal veins, which develop when the retinal venous circulation is obstructed in the prelaminar region of the optic nerve. (Other causes of retinochoroidal collaterals are central retinal vein occlusion, optic nerve sheath meningioma (Figure 14–6), optic nerve glioma, and optic nerve head drusen.) The presence of drusen-like deposits within the swollen optic nerve head, which indicates that the swelling is likely to have been present for several months, characterizes vintage papilledema.

It takes 24–48 hours for early papilledema to occur and 1 week to develop fully. It takes 6–8 weeks for fully developed papilledema to resolve following adequate treatment. Transient visual obscurations are a characteristic symptom of papilledema. Acute papilledema may reduce visual acuity by causing hyperopia and occasionally is associated with optic nerve infarction, but in most cases vision is normal apart from blind spot enlargement. Chronic, particularly atrophic or vintage, papilledema is associated with gradual constriction of the peripheral visual field, particularly inferonasal loss. Sudden reduction of intracranial pressure or systolic perfusion pressure may precipitate severe visual loss in any stage of papilledema.

Papilledema is often asymmetric. It may even appear to be unilateral, although fluorescein angiography in such cases usually shows leakage from both disks. Papilledema occurs late in glaucoma and will not occur at all if there is optic atrophy or if the optic nerve sheath on that side is not patent. The Foster Kennedy syndrome is papilledema on one side with optic atrophy due to optic nerve compression on the other, commonly due to skull-base meningiomas. However, it can be mimicked (pseudo-Foster Kennedy syndrome) by ischemic optic neuropathy when optic disk swelling due to a new episode of ischemic optic neuropathy is associated with optic atrophy in the fellow eye due to a previous episode (Figure 14–13).

Papilledema can be mimicked by buried optic nerve head drusen, small hyperopic disks, and myelinated nerve fibers (Figure 14–17).

The treatment of papilledema must be directed to the underlying cause. **Idiopathic intracranial hypertension** generally affects obese young women, and maintained weight loss is then an important treatment objective. The major morbidity is visual loss due to papilledema, but headaches may also be troublesome. Oral acetazolamide—usually 250 mg one to four times daily but up to 500 mg four times daily in severe cases—or diuretics such as furosemide are usually effective in reducing optic disk swelling. Cerebrospinal fluid shunting or optic nerve sheath fenestration may be

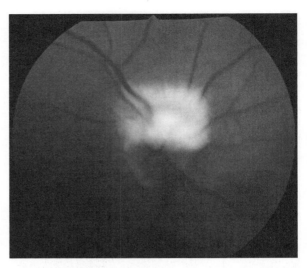

▲ **Figure 14–17.** Large patch of myelinated nerve fibers originating from superior edge of the disk. (Right eye).

undertaken if there is severe or progressive loss of vision or if medical therapy is not tolerated. Repeated lumbar punctures are rarely indicated except as a temporary measure prior to surgical therapy. Headaches usually respond to control of intracranial pressure, but other treatments may be required. It is essential that patients with idiopathic intracranial hypertension undergo regular visual field assessments by perimetry.

OPTIC NERVE COMPRESSION

Optic nerve compression is often amenable to treatment, and early recognition is vital to optimal outcome. The possibility of optic nerve compression should be considered in any patient with signs of optic neuropathy or visual loss not explained by an intraocular lesion. Optic disk swelling may occur with intraorbital optic nerve compression, but in many cases, particularly when the optic nerve compression is intracranial, the optic disk shows no abnormality until optic atrophy develops or there is papilledema from associated raised intracranial pressure. (Examination for signs of optic nerve disease, particularly a relative afferent pupillary defect, is thus crucial in assessment of the patient with unexplained visual loss.) Investigation of possible optic nerve compression requires early imaging by MRI or CT. If no structural lesion is identified and meningeal disease is suspected, it may be necessary to proceed to cerebrospinal fluid examination.

Intracranial meningiomas that may compress the optic nerve include those arising from the sphenoid wing, the tuberculum sellae (suprasellar meningioma), and the olfactory groove. Sphenoid wing meningiomas also produce proptosis, ocular motility disturbance, and trigeminal sensory loss (Figure 14–18). Surgical excision is generally effective in debulking intracranial meningiomas, but complete excision is often very difficult to achieve and recurrence rates

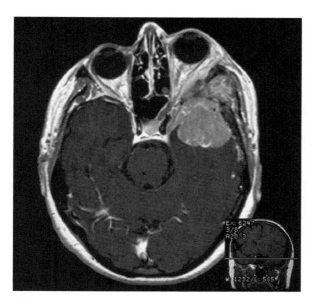

▲ **Figure 14–18.** Axial MRI of sphenoid wing meningioma causing proptosis.

are relatively high. Radiotherapy may be indicated as adjuvant or primary treatment. Pituitary adenoma and craniopharyngioma are discussed in the section on chiasmal disease (see later in the chapter). The management of orbital causes of optic nerve compression is discussed in Chapter 13.

Primary optic nerve sheath meningioma is a rare tumor most commonly presenting, like other types of meningioma, in middle-aged women (Figure 14–19). Five percent of cases

are bilateral. Visual loss is slowly progressive. The classic clinical features are a pale, slightly swollen optic disk with retinochoroidal collaterals, but in most cases the collateral vessels are not present (Figure 14–6). Stereotactic radiotherapy is the preferred treatment.

NUTRITIONAL & TOXIC OPTIC NEUROPATHIES

The usual clinical features of nutritional or toxic optic neuropathy are subacute, progressive, symmetrical visual loss, with central field defects (Figure 14–20), poor color vision, and the development of temporal disk pallor (Figure 14–6).

1. VITAMIN DEFICIENCY

Optic nerve involvement is relatively uncommon in vitamin B_{12} deficiency, but it may be the first manifestation of pernicious anemia. Thiamin (vitamin B_1) deficiency is generally a feature of severe malnutrition, and, as discussed below, there is an overlap with tobacco-alcohol amblyopia. Folate deficiency alone is a rare cause of optic neuropathy.

2. TOBACCO-ALCOHOL AMBLYOPIA

Nutritional amblyopia is probably a more accurate term for this entity. Usually it occurs in individuals with poor dietary habits, with heavy alcohol consumption and heavy smoking often being associated. Strict vegetarianism without vitamin supplementation may contribute. Much consideration has been given to other toxic causes, such as cyanide from tobacco producing low vitamin stores and low levels of sulfur-containing amino acids, but experimental studies with cyanide in primates have not confirmed this theory.

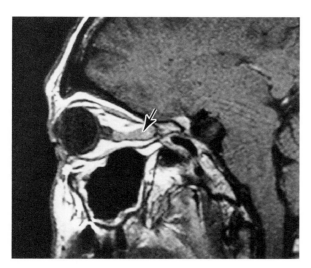

▲ **Figure 14–19.** MRI of tubular optic nerve sheath meningioma.

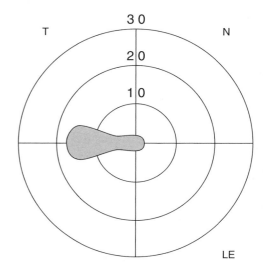

▲ **Figure 14–20.** Nutritional amblyopia showing centrocecal scotoma. VA = 20/200.

Drug-induced optic neuropathy must be excluded. Leber's hereditary optic neuropathy, pernicious anemia, methanol poisoning, the rare chronic optic neuropathy of primary progressive multiple sclerosis, or macular disease may cause diagnostic confusion.

There is bilateral loss of central vision, generally reducing visual acuity to less than 20/200, but it can be asymmetric. Central visual fields reveal scotomas that nearly always include both fixation and the blind spot (centrocecal scotoma) (Figure 14–20).

Adequate diet plus thiamine, folic acid, and vitamin B_{12} supplements may be effective if presentation is not delayed. Withdrawal of tobacco and alcohol is advisable and may hasten the cure, but adequate nutrition or vitamin B_{12} supplements can be effective despite continued excessive intake of alcohol or tobacco. Improvement usually begins within 1–2 months, although in occasional cases significant improvement may not occur for 1 year. Visual function can but may not return to normal. Permanent optic atrophy or at least temporal disk pallor can occur depending on the stage of disease at the time treatment was started (Figure 14–6). Loss of the ganglion cells of the macula and destruction of myelinated fibers of the optic nerve—and sometimes of the chiasm as well—are the main histologic changes.

3. HEAVY METAL POISONING

Chronic lead exposure, or thallium (present in depilatory cream) or arsenic poisoning can produce a toxic effect on the optic nerve.

4. DRUG-INDUCED OPTIC NEUROPATHY

Ethambutol, isoniazid, linezolid, disulfiram, and tamoxifen can all cause optic neuropathy, which usually improves with prompt cessation of the drug with or without nutritional supplements. Quinine overdose produces optic neuropathy, narrowed retinal arterioles and irregular, poorly reactive pupils. Chloramphenicol in high doses causes optic neuropathy. Amiodarone has been associated with bilateral optic neuropathy with chronic disk swelling, but the relationship is not necessarily causal. It characteristically also induces a verticillate keratopathy. Various chemotherapeutic agents may cause optic neuropathy, especially with high-dose or intra-arterial therapy.

5. CHEMICAL-INDUCED OPTIC NEUROPATHY: METHANOL POISONING

Absorption, usually oral, of methanol, which is used widely in the chemical industry as antifreeze, solvent varnish, or paint remover, causes visual impairment, sometimes progressing to complete blindness. Whitish, striated edema of the peripapillary retina is a characteristic sign.

Treatment consists of correction of the acidosis with intravenous sodium bicarbonate and oral or intravenous administration of ethanol to compete with, and thus prevent the slower metabolism of methanol into its byproducts. Hemodialysis is indicated for blood methanol levels over 50 mg/dL.

OPTIC NERVE TRAUMA

Direct optic nerve injury occurs in penetrating orbital trauma, including local anesthetic injections for ocular surgery, and in mid-facial fractures involving the optic canal. Visual loss due to indirect optic nerve trauma, which refers to optic nerve damage secondary to distant skull injury, occurs in approximately 1% of all head injuries. The site of injury is usually the forehead, often without skull fracture, and the probable mechanism of optic nerve injury is transmission of shock waves through the orbital walls to the orbital apex. Optic nerve avulsion usually results from an abrupt rotational injury to the globe, such as from being poked in the eye with a finger.

Surgery may be indicated to relieve orbital, subperiosteal, or optic nerve sheath hemorrhage or to treat orbital fractures. High-dose systemic steroids for direct or indirect optic nerve injury and decompression of the bony optic canal for indirect injury have been advocated, but their value is uncertain. There is no effective treatment for optic nerve avulsion.

HEREDITARY OPTIC ATROPHY

1. LEBER'S HEREDITARY OPTIC NEUROPATHY

Leber's hereditary optic neuropathy is a rare disease characterized by sequential subacute optic neuropathy usually in males aged 11–30 years. The underlying genetic abnormality is a point mutation in mitochondrial DNA (mtDNA), with over 90% of affected families harboring a mutation at position 11778, 14484, or 3460. mtDNA is exclusively derived from the mother, and thus, in accordance with the general pattern of mitochondrial (maternal) inheritance (see Chapter 18), the mutation is transmitted through the female line—but for unexplained reasons the disease rarely manifests in carrier females. Once an individual is known to have the disorder, it is possible without further genetic testing to predict which other family members are at risk, with matrilineal nephews, that is, sons of the affected individual's sisters, being particularly at risk.

Blurred vision and a central scotoma usually appear first in one eye and later—within days, weeks, or months—in the other eye. During the acute episode, there may be swelling of the optic disk and peripapillary retina with dilated telangiectatic small blood vessels on their surface, but characteristically there is no leak from the optic disk during fluorescein angiography. Both optic nerves eventually become atrophic, and vision is usually between 20/200 and counting fingers. The 14484 mutation is associated with recovery of vision but not until many months after the initial onset of visual loss. Total loss of vision or recurrences of visual loss usually do not occur. Leber's neuropathy may be associated with a multiple sclerosis-like illness (particularly in affected females), cardiac conduction defects, and dystonia.

Diagnosis is by identification of one of the three mtDNA point mutations. No treatment is known to be effective. Because high tobacco and alcohol consumption may precipitate visual loss in susceptible individuals, carriers of a pathogenic point mutation, particularly males, should be advised not to smoke and to avoid high alcohol consumption.

Optic atrophy also occurs in other mitochondrial disorders, either as a manifestation of primary optic neuropathy—for example, myoclonic epilepsy and ragged red fibers (MERRF) and mitochondrial myopathy, lactic acidosis, and stroke-like episodes (MELAS)—or secondary to retinal degeneration, for example, Kearns–Sayre syndrome. Wolfram's syndrome (see later in the chapter) is also probably the result of a mitochondrial disorder.

2. AUTOSOMAL HEREDITARY OPTIC ATROPHY

Autosomal dominant (juvenile) optic atrophy generally has an insidious onset in childhood, with slow progression of visual loss throughout life. It is often detected as mild reduction in visual acuity by childhood vision screening programs. There is characteristically a centrocecal scotoma with impaired color vision. Temporal optic disk pallor is usually present, although often mild, and mild disk cupping is occasionally seen. Diagnosis is by identification of other affected family members. The genetic defect has been mapped to the long arm of chromosome 3, but a diagnostic genetic test is not yet available. Rarely, the disease is associated with congenital or progressive deafness or ataxia.

Autosomal recessive (infantile) optic atrophy manifests as severe visual loss, present at birth or within 2 years and accompanied by nystagmus. It can be associated with progressive hearing loss, spastic quadriplegia, and dementia, although an inborn error of metabolism must first be considered. Wolfram's syndrome consists of juvenile diabetes insipidus, diabetes mellitus, optic atrophy, and deafness (DIDMOAD). Although there is a recessive pattern of inheritance, with the gene defect localized to chromosome 4, the underlying metabolic abnormality is probably a defect in cellular energy production, as in the mitochondrial diseases.

3. OPTIC ATROPHY WITH INHERITED NEURODEGENERATIVE DISEASES

Various neurodegenerative diseases with onset in the years from childhood to early adult life are manifested by steadily progressive neurologic and optic atrophy to a variable extent. Examples are hereditary spinocerebellar ataxias (Friedreich's ataxia), hereditary motor and sensory neuropathy (Charcot–Marie–Tooth disease), and the lysosomal storage disorders. Most of the sphingolipidoses late in their course are associated with optic atrophy. The leukodystrophies (Krabbe's, metachromatic leukodystrophy, adrenoleukodystrophy, globoid dystrophy, Pelizaeus–Merzbacher disease, Schilder's disease) are associated with optic atrophy earlier. Canavan's spongy degeneration and glioneuronal dystrophy (Alper's

disease) are associated with optic atrophy as well. In Refsum's disease, optic atrophy is secondary to the pigmentary retinopathy. Optic atrophy can occur in the mucopolysaccharidoses due to hydrocephalus from meningeal involvement or due to mucopolysaccharides in glial cells of the optic nerve.

NEOPLASTIC OPTIC NERVE INFILTRATION

In leukemia (usually acute leukemia), non-Hodgkin's lymphoma, and disseminated carcinoma, optic nerve infiltration with marked visual loss and optic disk swelling may develop. Optic nerve glioma is discussed below, together with chiasmal glioma. Other primary neoplasms of the optic nerve include the astrocytic hamartoma of tuberous sclerosis, melanocytoma, and hemangioma, all rarely causing any visual disturbance.

OPTIC NERVE ANOMALIES

There are a large number of congenital optic nerve anomalies. They may be associated with other anomalies of the head since closure of the fetal fissure, ocular melanogenesis, and development of the optic disks occur at the same time as development of the skull and face.

Optic nerve hypoplasia, dysplasia, and coloboma have all been associated with basal encephaloceles and with varying intracranial anomalies, including agenesis of the corpus callosum (de Morsier's syndrome) and pituitary-hypothalamic dysfunction (especially growth hormone deficiency). Hypoplastic optic nerves are small, with normal-sized retinal blood vessels (Figure 14–21). They are associated with a wide range of visual acuities, astigmatism, a peripapillary halo that

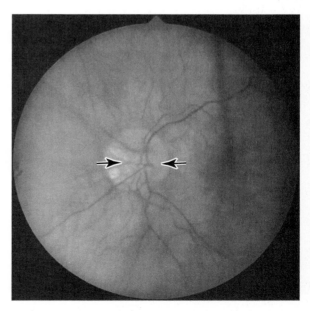

▲ **Figure 14–21.** Optic nerve hypoplasia. (Arrows indicate optic disk margins.) See color insert.

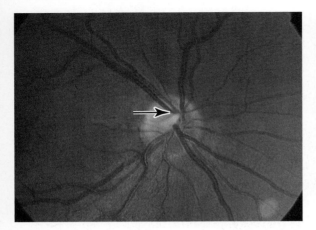

▲ **Figure 14–22.** Superior segmental optic nerve hypoplasia with superior entrance of central retinal artery **(arrow).**

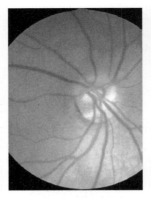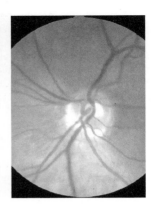

▲ **Figure 14–24.** Bilateral tilted optic disks.

may have a pigmented rim (double-ring sign), and various visual field defects. Superior segmental optic nerve hypoplasia (topless optic disk) usually occurs in children born to mothers with type 1 diabetes. It is characterized by superior disk entrance of the central retinal artery, superior disk pallor (Figure 14–22), and inferior visual field loss. Dysplastic optic disks usually are associated with poor vision and show abnormal vasculature, retinal pigment epithelium, and glial tissue. They are often surrounded by a chorioretinal pigmentary disturbance. Dysplastic disks have been reported with trisomy 4q. The papillorenal syndrome has been reported with dysplastic disks and colobomas. Colobomas of the optic nerve have been called "pseudoglaucoma" because of their resemblance to glaucomatous cupping (Figure 14–23). Disk

colobomas or hypoplasia when associated with chorioretinal lacunae, absence of the corpus callosum, and focal seizures constitute Aicardi's syndrome. This can also include retrobulbar cysts. Optic disk pits are usually not associated with any visual symptoms, but they can be mistaken for glaucomatous cupping, particularly if there is an associated field defect. Optic disk pits may present later in life as a consequence of serous detachment of the macula.

Tilted disks, which occur in 3% of normal subjects, may also be seen with hypertelorism or the craniofacial dysostoses (Crouzon's disease, Apert's disease). They are oval disks with usually an inferior scleral crescent and an associated area of fundus hypopigmentation (Figure 14–24). They may be mistaken for papilledema. They may also produce predominantly upper temporal field defects, which may be mistaken for bitemporal loss due to chiasmal dysfunction. Scleral crescents are particularly common in myopic eyes.

Megalopapilla may be mistaken for optic atrophy due to the prominence of the lamina cribrosa. Myelinated nerve fibers usually extend into the retina from the disk but occasionally are just seen in the retinal periphery (Figure 14–17). They always follow the course of the retinal nerve fiber layer. Remnants of the embryonic hyaloid system range from tissue fragments on the optic disk (Bergmeister's papilla) to strands extending to the posterior lens capsule. Prepapillary vascular loops are distinct from the hyaloid system and occasionally become obstructed, leading to branch retinal artery occlusion.

Optic nerve head drusen are clinically apparent in about 0.3% of the population but are found on ultrasound or histopathologic studies in up to 2%. They are exclusively found in white individuals. In children, they are usually buried within the disk substance, and thus are not visible on clinical examination but cause elevation of the disk surface and mimic papilledema. The optic disk is characteristically small, with no physiologic cup and an anomalous pattern of the retinal vessels. With increasing age and loss of overlying axons, optic nerve head drusen become exposed, being apparent as "lumpy-bumpy" yellow crystalline excrescences,

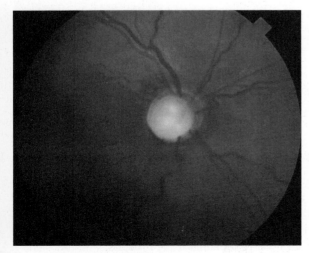

▲ **Figure 14–23.** Optic disk coloboma.

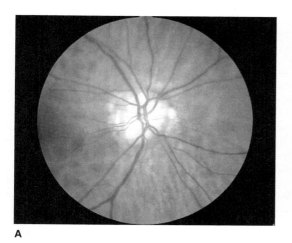
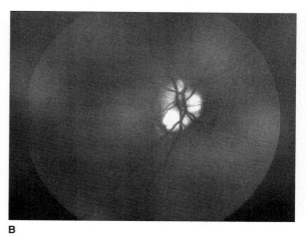

▲ **Figure 14–25.** Optic nerve head drusen **(A)** exhibiting autofluorescence **(B).**

highlighted by retroillumination of the disk substance (Figure 14–6). On fluorescein angiography, exposed drusen are autofluorescent and result in accumulation of dye within the disk substance (Figure 14–25). Buried drusen are best diagnosed by orbital ultrasound or thin-slice CT scanning, which detects their associated calcification. Optic nerve head drusen are usually bilateral. They can rarely cause visual loss, either by optic neuropathy or choroidal neovascularization. Hyperopic eyes may also have small elevated disks, resembling buried optic nerve head drusen and similarly mimicking papilledema (pseudo-papilledema).

▼ THE OPTIC CHIASM

In general, lesions of the chiasm cause bitemporal hemianopic visual field defects. Initially these defects are typically incomplete and are often asymmetric. As the disease progresses, the temporal hemianopia becomes complete but central visual acuity is preserved until there is also loss of the nasal visual fields or associated optic nerve dysfunction. Most diseases that affect the chiasm are neoplastic, vascular, and inflammatory processes being uncommon.

PITUITARY TUMORS

The anterior lobe of the pituitary gland is the site of origin of pituitary tumors (Figure 14–26), which manifest as pituitary dysfunction, loss of vision, cranial nerve palsies including extraocular muscle palsies, and a mass lesion on CT scan or MRI, arising from the pituitary sella and extending into the suprasellar and/or parasellar regions.

Visual assessment, especially documentation of visual fields, as well as endocrine assessment, is vital to decisions about management. Prolactinomas are generally treated medically in the first instance with dopamine agonists such as cabergoline, bromocriptine, or pergolide. Other pituitary macroadenomas generally undergo transsphenoidal hypophysectomy. Radiotherapy may be used as an adjuvant to surgery or for recurrent disease. Visual acuity and visual fields may improve dramatically after the chiasm is decompressed. The initial appearance of the optic nerve head does not predict the ultimate visual outcome, but optic atrophy is a poor prognostic sign.

CRANIOPHARYNGIOMA

Craniopharyngiomas are an uncommon group of tumors arising from epithelial remnants of Rathke's pouch (80% of the population normally have such remnants) and

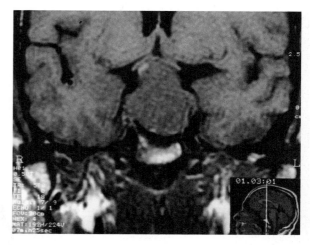

▲ **Figure 14–26.** Coronal MRI showing large pituitary adenoma elevating and distorting the optic chiasm.

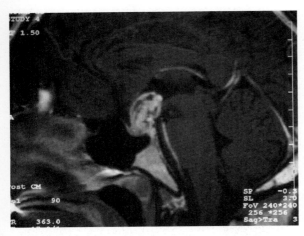

▲ Figure 14–27. Sagittal MRI showing contrast-enhanced suprasellar craniopharyngioma.

characteristically become symptomatic between the ages of 10 and 25 years but occasionally not until the 60s and 70s. They are usually suprasellar (Figure 14–27) but occasionally intrasellar. The signs and symptoms vary tremendously with the age of the patient and the exact location of the tumor as well as its rate of growth. When a suprasellar tumor occurs, asymmetric chiasmatic or tract field defects are prominent. Papilledema is more common than in pituitary tumors. Optic nerve hypoplasia can be seen with tumors presenting in infancy. Pituitary deficiency may result, and involvement of the hypothalamus may cause stunted growth. Calcification of parts of the tumor contributes to a characteristic radiologic appearance, especially in children.

Treatment consists of surgical removal—as complete as possible but limiting damage to the hypothalamus. Adjunctive radiotherapy is often used, particularly if there has been incomplete surgical removal.

SUPRASELLAR MENINGIOMAS

Suprasellar meningiomas arise from the meninges covering the tuberculum sellae and the planum sphenoidale, with a high proportion of patients being female. Visual loss, due to involvement of the optic chiasm and nerves, is often the presenting feature. Diagnosis is usually possible on the neuroimaging appearance. Treatment consists of surgical removal, possibly combined with adjuvant radiotherapy if there has been incomplete excision or the histopathology shows an aggressive tumor.

CHIASMATIC & OPTIC NERVE GLIOMAS

Gliomas of the anterior visual pathway, more commonly arising in the optic nerve but sometimes arising in the optic chiasm, are rare, usually indolent disorders of children,

particularly associated with neurofibromatosis 1 (see later in the chapter). About 70% of cases present before the age of 7 years, with visual loss, proptosis, strabismus, or nystagmus. Occasionally onset is sudden, with rapid loss of vision. There may be optic disk swelling, but optic atrophy is more common. Visual field defects reveal an optic nerve or chiasmal syndrome. Neuroimaging may reveal optic nerve expansion or a mass in the region of the chiasm and hypothalamus. Treatment depends on the location of the tumor and its clinical course. Chemotherapy can be given during a tumor growth spurt, irradiation being avoided because of adverse effects on the developing brain, and optic nerve resection is sometimes done when an optic nerve tumor aggressively starts to extend intracranially toward the chiasm, but generally management is conservative.

Malignant glioma of the anterior visual pathways is a rare disease of elderly men. There is a rapid clinical course to bilateral blindness and death due to invasion of the base of the brain. There is no effective treatment.

▼ THE RETROCHIASMATIC VISUAL PATHWAYS

Cerebrovascular disease and tumors are responsible for most lesions of the retrochiasmatic visual pathways, although almost any intracranial disease process can involve these structures.

Retrochiasmatic lesions produce contralateral homonymous visual field defects. Anterior partial lesions, in the optic tract, lateral geniculate nucleus, or geniculocalcarine tract (optic radiation), tend to produce incongruous (or dissimilar) visual field defects with more involvement in the eye with the nasal defect. Posterior partial lesions, in the geniculocalcarine tract or occipital cortex, tend to produce more congruous visual field defects. Once any retrochiasmatic lesion becomes complete, incongruity cannot be assessed, and this sign loses its localizing ability. Any unilateral retrochiasmatic lesion should spare visual acuity since the visual pathway in the other hemibrain is intact.

Lesions of the optic tract or lateral geniculate nucleus are uncommon. After several weeks to months, the disks may become pale, more marked in the contralateral eye, with corresponding retinal nerve fiber layer defects. In optic tract lesions, there may be a contralateral relative afferent pupillary defect. The optic tract and lateral geniculate nucleus have at least a dual blood supply, so that primary vascular lesions are uncommon. Most cases are due to trauma, tumors, and arteriovenous malformations.

Lesions involving the geniculocalcarine tract do not result in optic atrophy (due to the synapse at the geniculate nucleus) unless the lesion is longstanding, usually congenital. The inferior portion of the geniculocalcarine tract passes through the temporal lobe and the superior portion through the parietal lobe, with macular function between them. Lesions of the inferior portion result in predominantly superior visual field defects. Processes affecting the anterior and midtemporal lobes are commonly neoplastic; posterior temporal lobe and parietal processes can be either vascular or neoplastic. An insidious onset with mild and multiple neurologic deficits would be more typically neoplastic, whereas an acute event would be more typically vascular.

Vascular lesions of the occipital lobe are common and account for over 80% of cases of isolated homonymous visual field loss in patients over age 50 years. Macular function is represented at the most posterior tip of each occipital lobe, the representation of increasingly peripheral visual field lying increasingly anterior. Due to the frequent presence of a dual blood supply, vascular occlusions may selectively spare the posterior cortex to produce homonymous defects with macular sparing, or conversely involve the posterior occipital cortex to produce homonymous congruous macular scotomas. The cortical centers involved in the generation of optokinetic nystagmus lie in the area between the occipital and temporal lobes and in the posterior parietal area, which are within the vascular territory of the middle cerebral artery. Optokinetic nystagmus asymmetry characteristically occurs in parietal lesions but not in occipital lesions. An asymmetric optokinetic nystagmus combined with an occipital visual field defect indicates a process not respecting vascular territories, and thus suggests a tumor (Cogan's sign). Posterior reversible encephalopathy syndrome, which can be due to severe systemic hypertension, such as in eclampsia, diabetic hyperglycemia, or drugs, including cyclosporin and tacrolimus, characteristically involves the posterior cerebral hemispheres causing homonymous hemianopia, or even cortical blindness, and visual perceptual abnormalities. CT and MRI demonstrate structural cerebral lesions with remarkable clarity (Figures 14–4, 14–5, 14–28, and 14–29). Visual disturbance with dementia is suggestive of the predominantly visual variants of Alzheimer's disease and sporadic Creutzfeldt–Jakob disease, both characterized by a paucity of imaging changes initially.

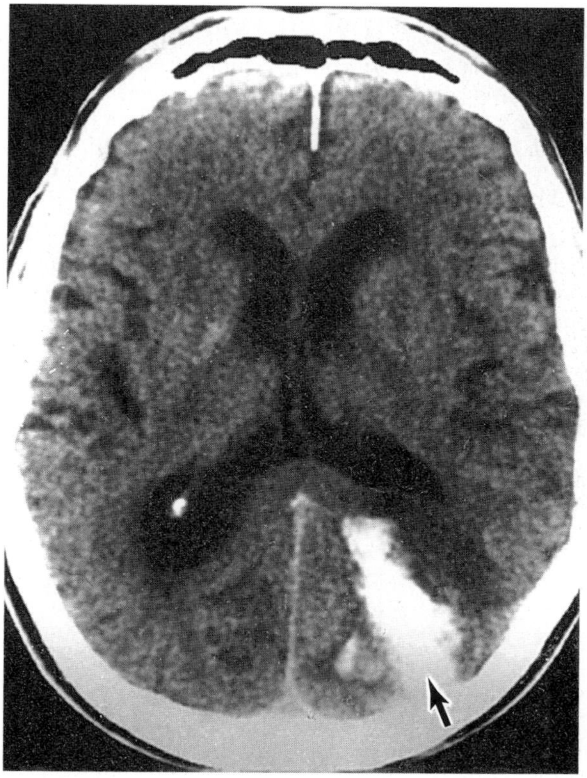

▲ **Figure 14–28.** Axial CT showing occipital hematoma **(arrow)** resulting from a bleeding arteriovenous malformation. This lesion produced homonymous hemianopia and headache.

▼ THE PUPIL

The size of the normal pupil varies at different ages, from person to person, and with different emotional states, levels of alertness, degrees of accommodation, and ambient room light. The normal pupillary diameter is about 3–4 mm, smaller in infancy, and tending to be larger in childhood and again progressively smaller with advancing age. Pupillary size relates to varying interactions between the sympathetically innervated iris dilator, with supranuclear control from the frontal (alertness) and occipital lobes (accommodation). The pupil also normally responds to respirations (ie, hippus). Twenty to forty percent of normal patients have a slight difference in pupil size (physiologic anisocoria), usually less than 1 mm. Mydriatic agents work more effectively on blue eyes than on brown eyes.

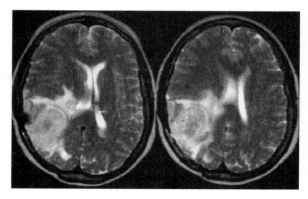

▲ **Figure 14–29.** Axial MRI of parietal meningioma with secondary cerebral edema.

► Neuroanatomy of the Pupillary Pathways

Evaluation of pupillary responses is important in localizing lesions involving the optic pathways. The examiner should be familiar with the neuroanatomy of the pathways for the pupillary responses to light and near (Figure 14–30).

A. Light Reflex

The pupillary response to light is a pure reflex with an entirely subcortical pathway. Whereas previously retinal photoreceptors were thought to be the sole receptors for the pupillary light reflex, melanopsin-expressing retinal ganglion cells in the inner retina are now known to be involved. The afferent pupillary fibers are included within the optic nerve and visual pathways until they exit the optic tract just prior to the lateral geniculate nucleus. Having decussated in the chiasm—in the same way as the visual sensory fibers—they enter the midbrain through the brachium of the superior colliculus and synapse in the pretectal nucleus. Each pretectal nucleus decussates neurons dorsal to the cerebral aqueduct to the ipsilateral and contralateral Edinger–Westphal nucleus via the posterior commissure and the periaqueductal gray matter. A synapse then occurs in the Edinger–Westphal nucleus of the oculomotor nerve. The efferent pathway is via the third nerve to the ciliary ganglion in the lateral orbit. The postganglionic fibers go via the short ciliary nerves to innervate the sphincter muscle of the iris.

Light shone into the right eye produces an immediate direct response in the right eye and an immediate indirect consensual response in the left eye (Figure 14–31). The intensity of this response in each eye is proportionate to the light-carrying ability of the directly stimulated optic nerve.

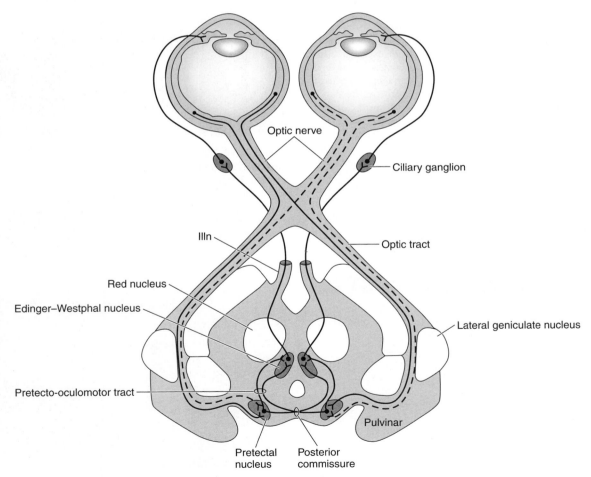

▲ **Figure 14–30.** Diagram of the path of the pupillary light reflex. (Reproduced, with permission, from Walsh FB, Hoyt WF: Clinical Neuro-Ophthalmology, 3rd ed. Vol 1. Williams & Wilkins, 1969.)

Light stimulus

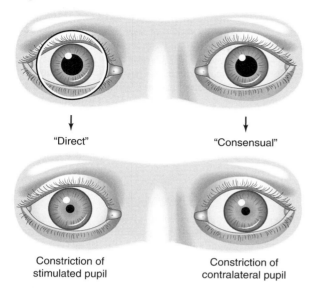

"Direct" "Consensual"

Constriction of stimulated pupil   Constriction of contralateral pupil

▲ **Figure 14–31.** Normal pupillary light reflex.

B. The Near Response

When the eyes look at a near object, three responses occur—accommodation, convergence, and constriction of the pupil—bringing a sharp image into focus on corresponding retinal points. The final common pathway is mediated through the oculomotor nerve with a synapse in the ciliary ganglion. The afferent pathway enters the midbrain ventral to the Edinger–Westphal nucleus and sends fibers to both sides of the cortex. Although the three components are closely associated, the near response cannot be considered a pure reflex, since each component can be neutralized while leaving the other two intact—that is, by prisms (neutralizing convergence), by lenses (neutralizing accommodation), and by weak mydriatic drugs (neutralizing miosis). It can occur even in a blind person who is instructed to look at his nose.

AFFERENT PUPILLARY DEFECT

One of the most important assessments to make in a patient complaining of decreased vision is whether it is due to an ocular problem (eg, cataract) or to a potentially more serious optic nerve problem. If an optic nerve lesion is present, the pupillary light response (both the direct response in the stimulated eye and the consensual response in the fellow eye) is less intense when the involved eye is stimulated than when the normal eye is stimulated. This phenomenon is called a relative afferent pupillary defect (RAPD) (Figure 14–32). It will be present also if there is a large retinal or severe macular lesion. Even dense cataract does not impair the pupillary light response. Other causes of unilateral decreased vision

without an afferent pupillary defect include refractive error, media opacity other than cataract such as corneal opacity or vitreous hemorrhage, amblyopia, and functional visual loss. In a lesion of the brachium of the superior colliculus, it is possible for a relative afferent pupillary defect to be present when visual function is normal.

Absolute afferent pupillary defect is the term applied when there is no pupillary response to light stimulation of a completely blind (amaurotic) eye. Light shone into the normal eye would still induce a consensual response in the blind eye (Figure 14–33).

An afferent pupillary defect can still be identified if one pupil is either not visible, due to corneal disease, or is unable to respond due to structural damage or damage to its innervation, for example, third nerve palsy, by examination of the normal pupil.

Diffuse illumination

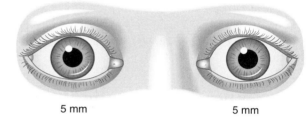

5 mm   5 mm

Light on normal eye

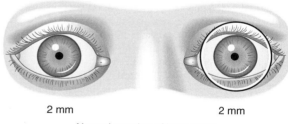

2 mm   2 mm

Normal reaction of both pupils

Light on eye with afferent defect

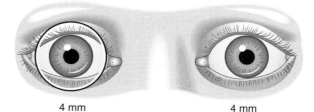

4 mm   4 mm

Decreased reaction of both pupils

▲ **Figure 14–32.** Relative afferent pupillary defect.

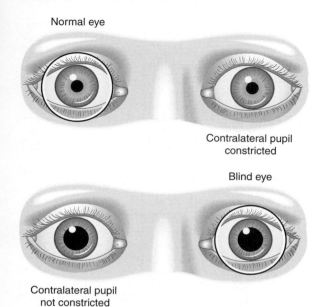

Normal eye

Contralateral pupil
constricted

Blind eye

Contralateral pupil
not constricted

▲ **Figure 14–33.** Absolute afferent (amaurotic) pupillary defect.

PUPILLARY LIGHT-NEAR DISSOCIATION

The light reflex normally produces more miosis than the near response. The reverse is known as pupillary light-near dissociation. This is most commonly due to an afferent pupillary defect (such as in optic nerve disease) because the pupillary light reflex to stimulation of the affected eye is reduced but the near response is normal. It occurs also in lesions of the ciliary ganglion or of the midbrain, in which the light reflex pathway is relatively dorsal and the near response pathway relatively ventral. Causes include tonic pupil (see later in the chapter), midbrain tumors and infarcts, diabetes, chronic alcoholism, encephalitis, and central nervous system degenerative disease.

Argyll Robertson pupils, which are usually bilateral, are typically small (less than 3 mm in diameter), commonly irregular and eccentric, do not respond to light stimulation but do respond to a near stimulus, and dilate poorly with mydriatics as a consequence of concomitant iris atrophy. They are strongly suggestive of central nervous system syphilis.

TONIC PUPIL

Tonic pupil is characterized by light-near dissociation, delayed dilation after a near stimulus (tonic near response), segmental iris constriction, and constriction in response to a weak (0.1%) solution of pilocarpine (denervation hypersensitivity). It results from damage to the ciliary ganglion or the short ciliary nerves. In the acute stage, the pupil is dilated

and accommodation is impaired. The pattern of recovery is influenced by fibers in the short ciliary nerves subserving the near response outnumbering those subserving the light reflex by 30:1. Accommodation usually recovers fully, but incomplete reinnervation of the iris results in segmental iris constriction and pupillary light-near dissociation. The pupil usually becomes smaller than the pupil in the fellow eye.

Tonic pupil is usually an isolated benign entity, presenting in young women. It may be associated with loss of deep tendon reflexes (Adie's syndrome). Subsequent involvement of the other eye over a period of 10 years occurs in 50% of individuals, but bilateral tonic pupils may be due to autonomic neuropathy. Tonic pupil may occur after retinal laser photocoagulation.

HORNER'S SYNDROME

Horner's syndrome is caused by a lesion of the sympathetic pathway either (1) in its **central portion,** which extends from the posterior hypothalamus through the brainstem to the upper spinal cord (C8–T2); or (2) in its **preganglionic portion,** which exits the spinal cord and synapses in the superior cervical (stellate) ganglion; or (3) in its **postganglionic portion,** from the superior cervical ganglion via the carotid plexus and the ophthalmic division of the trigeminal nerve, by which it enters the orbit. The sympathetic fibers then follow the nasociliary branch of the ophthalmic division of the trigeminal nerve and the long ciliary nerves to the iris and innervate Müller's muscle and the iris dilator. Iris dilator muscle paresis causes miosis, which is more evident in dim light. Melanocyte maturation in the iris depends on sympathetic innervation; thus, a less pigmented (bluer) iris occurs in congenital or longstanding acquired Horner's syndrome. Paresis of Müller's muscle produces ptosis. Unilateral miosis, ptosis, and absence of sweating on the ipsilateral face and neck make up the complete syndrome. Sweating on the face is normal in postganglionic lesions because postganglionic fibers to the face for sweating follow the external rather than the internal carotid artery.

Central Horner's syndrome may be due to brainstem infarction, particularly lateral medullary infarction (Wallenberg's syndrome), syringomyelia, or cervical cord tumor. Preganglionic Horner's syndrome may be due to cervical rib, cervical vertebral fractures, apical pulmonary lesions—particularly bronchogenic carcinoma (Pancoast's syndrome)—or brachial plexus injuries. Postganglionic Horner's syndrome may be due to carotid artery dissection, skull base tumors, or cluster headache. The localization of central and preganglionic Horner's syndrome is often apparent from the associated clinical features. Sudden-onset isolated painful Horner's syndrome, particularly with a recent history of neck trauma or associated with pain in the neck or jaw, necessitates urgent investigation for carotid dissection, which may lead to thrombotic or embolic stroke. Horner's syndrome associated with chronic facial pain, particularly if associated with fifth, sixth, third, fourth, or second cranial nerve palsy, requires investigation for skull-base tumor. In most cases of isolated congenital Horner's syndrome no etiology is identified. Birth trauma is a commonly identified cause and neuroblastoma is occasionally responsible. Unexplained acquired Horner's syndrome in infants requires imaging for neuroblastoma.

Pharmacologic testing with topical cocaine in the conjunctival sac differentiates Horner's syndrome, in which the pupil does not dilate, from physiologic anisocoria. Topical apraclonidine, which causes dilation of the affected but not the normal pupil, can also be used. Testing with hydroxyamphetamine drops differentiates central and preganglionic from postganglionic lesions, but they are difficult to obtain.

▼ EXTRAOCULAR MOVEMENTS

This section deals with the neural apparatus that controls eye movements and causes them to move simultaneously, up or down and side to side, as well as in convergence or divergence.

The neural control of eye movements is ultimately controlled by alterations in activity in the nuclei and nerve fibers of the oculomotor, trochlear, and abducens nerves. These are referred to as the nuclear and infranuclear pathways. Coordination of eye movements requires connections between these ocular motor nuclei, the internuclear pathways. The supranuclear pathways are responsible for generation of the commands necessary for the execution of the appropriate movement, whether it be voluntary or involuntary.

▶ Classification & Examination of Eye Movements

Eye movements are either fast or slow. Fast eye movements include voluntary or involuntary refixation movements (saccades) and the fast phases of vestibular and optokinetic nystagmus (see later in the chapter). The fast eye movement system is tested by command refixation movements and by the fast phase of vestibular and optokinetic nystagmus.

Slow eye movements include pursuit movements, which track a slowly moving target once the saccadic system has placed the target on the fovea and which are tested by asking a patient to follow a slow, smoothly moving target, the slow phase movements generated by vestibular stimuli, the slow phase of optokinetic nystagmus, and vergence movements, which, unlike all the other forms of eye movements, involve dysconjugate movements of the two eyes.

Under physiologic conditions, vestibular stimulation occurs from head movements. The resulting slow eye movements, known as the **vestibulo-ocular responses (VOR),** compensate for the head motion such that the position of the eyes in space remains static and steady visual fixation can be maintained. The **doll's head maneuver** is a clinical method of testing the VOR. The patient is asked to fixate on a target while the examiner moves the head in a horizontal or vertical plane. If the VOR is deficient, the compensatory eye movements are insufficient and must be supplemented by saccadic movements to maintain fixation. The head motion must be rapid; otherwise, pursuit mechanisms dominate the ocular motor response. In the unconscious patient, the doll's head maneuver is used to assess brainstem function. Since the pursuit and saccadic systems are not operative, the head movements can be slow. Absence of the VOR leads to failure of the eyes to move within the orbit. Other methods of vestibular stimulation are whole body rotation and caloric testing (see later in the chapter).

▶ Generation of Eye Movements
A. Physiology

1. **Fast eye movements**—Understanding of the control of eye movements is most complete in the case of saccadic movements. Similar mechanisms are thought to apply to the fast phases of nystagmus. The generation of a saccade involves a **pulse** of increased innervation to move the eye in the required direction and a **step** increase in tonic innervation to maintain the new position in the orbit by counteracting the visco-elastic forces working to return the eye to the primary position. The pulse is produced by the **burst cells of the saccadic generator.** The step change in tonic innervation is produced by the **tonic cells of the neural integrator,** so called because it effectively integrates the pulse to produce the step. There is a close relationship between the amplitude of movement and its peak velocity, larger movements having greater peak velocities. Loss of the saccadic generator function leads to slowing of saccades. Loss of the neural integrator function leads to a failure of maintenance of the desired final position, ie, a failure of gaze holding. Clinically, this usually manifests as a gaze-evoked nystagmus, with a drift of the eyes toward the primary position followed by a corrective saccade back to the desired position of gaze.

2. **Slow eye movements**—The slow phase movements generated by vestibular stimuli are a direct response to the detection of movement by the semicircular canals. The canals are acceleration detectors, but their output is integrated to produce a velocity signal that is then conveyed to the ocular motor nuclei. The generation of pursuit movements is less well understood. The slow phase of optokinetic nystagmus is in part a pursuit movement, but there is also an additional specific optokinetic movement generated by the perception of movement of the background of the visual scene. This optokinetic movement appears to be generated by the pathways involved in generating slow-phase vestibular movements but with an input from the retina, either via cortical centers or directly via a subcortical pathway. Vergence eye movements are generated in response to retinal disparity, that is, stimulation of noncorresponding retinal loci by the object of regard. Electromyography has established divergence as an active process, not a relaxation of convergence.

B. Anatomy

1. **Brainstem centers for fast eye movements**—The saccadic generator for horizontal eye movements lies in the paramedian pontine reticular formation. The output from this structure is channeled through the abducens nucleus, which contains both the motor neurons for the abducens nerve and the cell bodies of inter-neurons, which pass via the medial longitudinal fasciculus to innervate the motor neurons in the contralateral medial rectus subnucleus of the oculomotor nerve. The neural integrator for horizontal eye movements appears to be located close to the paramedian pontine reticular formation in the nucleus prepositus hypoglossi.

   The saccadic generator for vertical movements is in the rostral interstitial nucleus of the medial longitudinal fasciculus in the rostral midbrain. The pathway to the ocular motor nuclei for upward movements involves the posterior commissure, dorsal to the cerebral aqueduct, and its nucleus. The corresponding pathway for downward eye movements is less well defined. Neural integration for vertical eye movements seems to take place in both the interstitial nucleus of Cajal, close to the rostral interstitial nucleus of the medial longitudinal fasciculus in the midbrain and in the vestibular nuclei in the medulla.

2. **Cortical centers for fast eye movements**—Voluntary saccades are initiated in the frontal lobe (frontal eye field area 8). The pathway descends through the basal ganglia and the anterior limb of the internal capsule into the brainstem, terminating in the midbrain pretectal area for vertical movements and crossing to the paramedian pontine reticular formation in the opposite side of the pons for horizontal movements. The generation of involuntary (reflexive) saccades, in response to a target appearing in the peripheral field of vision, depends on activity within the superior colliculus, which receives information from the occipital cortex and also directly from the retina in a purely subcortical pathway.

3. **Brainstem centers for slow eye movements**—The processing of information from the semicircular canals occurs in the vestibular nuclei, which then connect directly to the ocular motor nuclei. These pathways from the vestibular nuclei in the medulla to the pons and midbrain pass in a number of fiber tracts, including the medial longitudinal fasciculus.

4. **Cortical centers for slow eye movements**—Pursuit movements originate in the occipital cortex. The pathway descends through the posterior limb of the internal capsule to the midbrain and ipsilateral paramedian pontine reticular formation. The slow phase of optokinetic nystagmus is likely to be generated at least in part in area V5 (or MT) at the junction of the occipital and temporal lobes, which is involved in motion detection. The descending pathway probably accompanies the pathway for pursuit movements. Vergence eye movements are generated in the occipital cortex, and the pathway also probably descends via the posterior limb of the internal capsule, together with the pathway for pursuit movements, to terminate in the rostral midbrain near or in the oculomotor nucleus. Impulses then pass directly to each medial rectus subnucleus and via the medial longitudinal fasciculus to the abducens nuclei. It is not clear whether convergence and divergence are controlled by the same or separate brainstem centers.

ABNORMALITIES OF EYE MOVEMENTS

Owing to the multiplicity of pathways involved in the supranuclear control of eye movements, with origins in different areas of the brain and an anatomic separation in the brainstem of the horizontal and vertical eye movement systems, disorders of the supranuclear pathways characteristically produce a dissociation of effect upon the various types of eye movements. Thus, the clinical clues to a supranuclear lesion are a differential effect on horizontal and vertical eye movements or upon saccadic, pursuit, and vestibular eye movements. In diffuse brainstem disease, such features may not be apparent, and differentiation from disease at the neuromuscular junction or within the extraocular muscles on clinical grounds can be difficult.

Disease of the internuclear pathways results in a disruption of the conjugacy of eye movements. In infranuclear disease, the pattern of eye movement disturbance usually complies with that expected of a lesion involving one or more cranial nerves or their nuclei.

1. LESIONS OF THE SUPRANUCLEAR PATHWAYS

▶ Cerebral Hemispheres

A seizure focus in the frontal lobe may cause involuntary turning of the eyes to the opposite side. Destructive lesions cause transient deviation to the same side, and the eyes cannot be turned quickly and voluntarily (saccadic movement) to the opposite side. This is called frontal gaze palsy, and recovery occurs when the opposite frontal eye field substitutes. Ocular pursuit to the opposite side is retained. There is no diplopia.

Smooth ocular pursuit may be lost with posterior lesions of the hemispheres. The patient is unable to follow a slowly moving object in the direction of the gaze palsy. The command (fast) eye movement is not lost, so pursuit is "saccadic."

Phenytoin can significantly affect saccades. Sedative agents and carbamazepine can alter smooth pursuit eye movements.

▶ Brainstem

Lesions of the posterior commissure of the midbrain cause impairment of conjugate upgaze. Lesions dorsal and medial to the red nuclei produce a downgaze paresis.

Dorsal midbrain syndrome (Parinaud's syndrome) is characterized by loss of voluntary upward gaze, convergence-retraction nystagmus, pupillary light-near dissociation, and eyelid retraction (Collier's sign). There may also be insufficiency or spasm of convergence and/or accommodation, and loss of voluntary downward gaze. Conjugate horizontal ocular movements are usually not affected. The syndrome results from tectal or pretectal lesions affecting the periaqueductal area. Pineal tumors, hydrocephalus, midbrain infarcts or arteriovenous malformations, and trauma may be responsible.

Lesions of the paramedian pontine reticular formation produce an ipsilateral horizontal gaze palsy affecting saccadic and pursuit movements. Vestibular slow-phase movements are preserved owing to the direct pathway from the vestibular nuclei to the abducens and oculomotor nuclei.

Lesions of the brainstem that cause gaze palsies include vascular accidents, arteriovenous malformations, multiple sclerosis, tumors (pontine gliomas, cerebellopontine angle tumors), and encephalitis.

▶ Spasm of the Near Response

Spasm of the near response, also known as convergence or accommodative spasm, is usually caused by functional disease, but it may be caused by a midbrain lesion. It is characterized by convergent strabismus with diplopia, miotic pupils, and spasm of accommodation (induced myopia).

In functional disease, the features are usually intermittent and provoked by eye movement examination. Cyclopentolate 1%, one drop in each eye twice daily, with reading glasses to compensate for loss of accommodation may be helpful. Psychiatric consultation may be indicated.

▶ Convergence Insufficiency

Convergence insufficiency is characterized by diplopia for near vision in the absence of any impairment of adduction on monocular testing, refractive error, particularly presbyopia, having been excluded. It is caused by functional disease or dysfunction of the supranuclear pathway for convergence in the midbrain. In organic lesions, pupillary miosis still occurs when convergence is attempted, whereas in functional disease, it does not.

2. INTERNUCLEAR OPHTHALMOPLEGIA

The medial longitudinal fasciculus is an important fiber tract extending from the rostral midbrain to the spinal cord. It contains many pathways connecting nuclei within the brainstem, particularly those concerned with extraocular movements. The most common manifestation of damage to the medial longitudinal fasciculus is an internuclear ophthalmoplegia, in which conjugate horizontal eye movements are disrupted owing to failure of coordination between the abducens nerve nucleus in the pons and the oculomotor nerve nucleus in the midbrain. The lesion in the brainstem is ipsilateral to the eye with the adduction failure and contralateral to the direction of horizontal gaze that is abnormal. In the mildest form of internuclear ophthalmoplegia, the clinical abnormality is restricted to a slowing of saccades in the adducting eye, producing transient diplopia on lateral gaze. In the most severe form, there is complete loss of adduction on horizontal gaze, producing constant diplopia on lateral gaze (Figure 14–12). Convergence is characteristically preserved in internuclear ophthalmoplegia except when the lesion is in the midbrain, when the convergence mechanisms may also be affected. Another feature of internuclear ophthalmoplegia is nystagmus in the abducting eye on attempted horizontal gaze, which is at least in part a result of compensation for the failure of adduction in the other eye. In bilateral internuclear ophthalmoplegia, there may also be an upbeating nystagmus on upgaze due to failure of control of gaze holding in the upward direction, and the eyes may be divergent; this is known as the wall-eyed bilateral internuclear ophthalmoplegia (WEBINO) syndrome.

Internuclear ophthalmoplegia may be due to multiple sclerosis (particularly in young adults), brainstem infarction (particularly in older patients), tumors, arteriovenous malformations, Wernicke's encephalopathy, and encephalitis. Bilateral internuclear ophthalmoplegia is most commonly due to multiple sclerosis.

A horizontal gaze palsy combined with an internuclear ophthalmoplegia, due to a lesion of the abducens nucleus or paramedian pontine reticular formation extending into the ipsilateral medial longitudinal fasciculus, affects all horizontal eye movements in the ipsilateral eye and adduction in the contralateral eye. This is known as a "one-and-a-half syndrome," or paralytic pontine exotropia.

3. NUCLEAR & INFRANUCLEAR CONNECTIONS

▶ Ocular Motor Nerve Palsies

Ocular motor nerve palsies result in impairment of eye movements, the pattern being determined by which extraocular muscles are involved, ocular misalignment, which at least in the acute stage also varies in severity with different gaze positions according to which muscles are paretic, and ptosis if there is palsy of the levator palpebrae superioris muscle. Misalignment of the visual axes results in diplopia, unless there is suppression, which more commonly develops in children than adults. Dizziness or disequilibrium may be associated but disappears with monocular patching. Abnormal head posture may develop. In sixth nerve palsy, there is head turn to the side of the palsy, and in fourth nerve palsy, there is head tilt to the opposite side. Paresis of an extraocular muscle can be simulated by restriction of action of the yoke muscle, for example limitation of abduction may be due to medial rectus restriction rather than lateral rectus paresis. Assessment of saccadic velocity may be helpful, but forced duction tests may need to be performed. Saccadic velocity may also help identify which muscle is paretic, for instance in differentiating superior oblique from inferior rectus palsy.

There is wide variation in the site of damage and etiology in ocular motor nerve palsies. Nuclear lesions have specific localizing features. Fascicular lesions within the brainstem resemble peripheral nerve lesions but usually can be differentiated on the basis of other brainstem signs. Any extraocular muscle palsy that occurs with minor head trauma (subconcussive injuries) should be investigated for an intracranial lesion. In ischemic (microvascular) palsies, recovery by 4 months is the rule. Palsies that have not started to recover by then—especially those involving the sixth nerve—should be evaluated for another cause, particularly a structural lesion. Urgent investigation should be undertaken when there is evidence of multiple cranial nerve dysfunction or for any extraocular muscle palsy in a young adult. Assessment of any ocular motor nerve palsy must include assessment of second, fifth, and seventh cranial nerve function.

▶ Oculomotor Nerve (III)

The motor fibers arise from a group of nuclei in the central gray matter ventral to the cerebral aqueduct at the level of the superior colliculus. The midline central caudal nucleus innervates both levator palpebrae superioris muscles. The paired superior rectus subnuclei innervate the contralateral superior rectus. The efferent fibers decussate immediately and pass through the opposite superior rectus subnucleus. The subnuclei for the medial rectus, inferior rectus, and inferior oblique muscles are also paired structures but innervate the ipsilateral muscles. The fascicle of the oculomotor nerve courses through the red nucleus and the inner side of the substantia nigra to emerge on the medial side of the cerebral peduncles. The nerve runs alongside the sella turcica, in the outer wall of the cavernous sinus, and through the superior orbital fissure to enter the orbit. The superior branch innervates the levator palpebrae and superior rectus muscles and the inferior branch of all other muscles and the sphincter.

The parasympathetics arise from the Edinger–Westphal nucleus just rostral to the motor nucleus of the third nerve and pass via the inferior division of the third nerve to the ciliary ganglion. From there the short ciliary nerves are distributed to the sphincter muscle of the iris and to the ciliary muscle.

A. Oculomotor Palsy

Lesions of the third nerve nucleus typically affect the ipsilateral medial and inferior rectus and inferior oblique muscles, both levator muscles, and both superior rectus muscles. There will be bilateral ptosis and bilateral limitation of elevation as well as limitation of adduction and depression ipsilaterally.

From the fascicle of the nerve in the midbrain to its eventual termination in the orbit, third nerve palsy produces purely ipsilateral dysfunction. The exact pattern depends on the extent of the palsy, but in general the ipsilateral eye is turned out by the intact lateral rectus muscle and slightly depressed by the intact superior oblique muscle. The eye may only be moved laterally. (Incyclotorsion from the action of the intact superior oblique muscle can be observed by watching a small blood vessel on the medial conjunctiva as depression of the eye is attempted.) There can be a dilated fixed pupil, absent accommodation, and ptosis of the upper lid, often severe enough to cover the pupil. The pattern of pupil abnormality may be influenced by concomitant Horner's syndrome (sympathetic paresis) resulting in a relatively small unreactive pupil or aberrant regeneration (see later in the chapter).

Ischemia, intracranial aneurysm, head trauma, and intracranial tumors are the most common causes of third nerve palsy in adults. Causes of ischemic (microvascular) palsy include diabetes mellitus, hypertension, hyperlipidemia, and systemic vasculitis. Aneurysm usually arises from the junction of the internal carotid and posterior communicating arteries. Intracranial tumor may cause oculomotor palsy by direct damage to the nerve or due to mass effect. Pupillary dilation, initially unilateral and then bilateral, is an important sign of herniation of the medial temporal lobe through the tentorial hiatus (tentorial herniation) due to a rapidly expanding supratentorial mass. Bilateral peripheral third nerve palsies can be caused by interpeduncular lesions, such as basilar artery aneurysm.

A useful guide clinically is that in ischemic lesions the pupillary responses are spared, whereas in compression, including aneurysmal, the pupil is involved, initially loss of reactivity and then also dilation. Less than 5% of vascular third nerve palsies are associated with complete pupillary palsy, and in only 15% there is partial pupillary palsy. Painful isolated third nerve palsy with pupillary involvement necessitates emergency investigation for ipsilateral posterior communicating artery aneurysm. Such investigation may also be indicated in painful isolated third nerve palsy without pupillary involvement and in young patients with painless isolated third nerve palsy with pupillary involvement.

Monocular elevator paralysis—inability to elevate one eye in both abduction (superior rectus) and adduction (inferior oblique)—can be due to paresis of the superior division of the third nerve (tumor, sinusitis, postviral) but also occurs as a congenital defect or in thyroid ophthalmopathy, orbital myositis, orbital floor fracture, myasthenia gravis, and midbrain stroke.

Third nerve palsies in children may be congenital or may be due to ophthalmoplegic migraine, meningitis, or postviral.

B. Oculomotor Synkinesis (Aberrant Regeneration of the Third Nerve)

This phenomenon is characterized by inappropriate activation of muscles innervated by the oculomotor nerve, including (1) lid dyskinesias due to inappropriate activation of levator palpebrae superioris either on horizontal gaze (eyelid elevates on attempted adduction) or on vertical gaze (eyelid elevates on attempted depression ("pseudo-Graefe's sign");

(2) adduction or retraction on attempted upgaze due to inappropriate activation of medial rectus or inferior rectus; (3) pupillary constriction on attempted adduction or depression; and (4) a monocular vertical optokinetic nystagmus response (due to coactivation of superior rectus, inferior oblique and inferior rectus muscles fixing the involved eye, allowing only the normal eye to respond to the moving target).

Oculomotor synkinesis most commonly occurs in congenital third nerve palsy or during recovery from acute third nerve palsy due to trauma or aneurysmal compression (secondary oculomotor synkinesis). It may also occur as a primary phenomenon in chronic compression, usually due to an internal carotid aneurysm or meningioma in the cavernous sinus. Oculomotor synkinesis is not a feature of ischemic oculomotor palsy.

C. Cyclic Oculomotor Palsy

Cyclic oculomotor palsy can complicate congenital third nerve palsy; it is a rare, predominantly unilateral event, with a typical third nerve palsy showing cyclic spasms every 10–30 seconds. During these intervals, ptosis improves and accommodation increases. This phenomenon continues unchanged throughout life but decreases with sleep and increases with greater arousal.

D. Marcus Gunn Phenomenon (Jaw-Winking Syndrome)

This rare usually congenital condition consists of elevation of a ptotic eyelid upon movement of the jaw. Acquired cases occur after damage to the oculomotor nerve with subsequent innervation of the lid (levator palpebrae superioris) by a branch of the fifth cranial nerve.

▶ Trochlear Nerve (IV)

Motor (entirely crossed) fibers arise from the trochlear nucleus just caudal to the third nerve at the level of the inferior colliculus; they then run posteriorly, decussate in the anterior medullary velum, and wind around the cerebral peduncles. The fourth nerve travels near the third nerve along the wall of the cavernous sinus to the orbit, where it supplies the superior oblique muscle. The fourth nerve is unique among the cranial nerves in arising from the dorsal brainstem.

A. Trochlear Palsy

Congenital trochlear palsy is probably not usually neurogenic in origin but due to developmental anomaly within the orbit. It may present in childhood with an abnormal head posture (see later in the chapter) or in childhood or adult life with eyestrain or diplopia due to reduced ability to overcome the vertical ocular deviation (decompensation). Acquired trochlear palsy is commonly traumatic. The nerve is vulnerable to injury at the site of exit from the dorsal aspect of the brainstem. Both nerves may be damaged by severe trauma as they decussate in the anterior medullary velum, resulting in bilateral superior oblique palsies. Acquired trochlear palsy may also be ischemic (microvascular) or secondary to posterior fossa surgery. Rarely, posterior fossa tumors may present with an isolated trochlear palsy.

Superior oblique palsy results in upward deviation (hypertropia) of the eye, which increases when the patient looks down and to the opposite side. In addition, in acquired palsy, there is excyclotropia; therefore, one of the diplopic images will be tilted with respect to the other. Thus, torsional diplopia indicates an acquired palsy and lack of torsional symptoms indicates a congenital palsy. Tilting the head toward the involved side increases the vertical ocular deviation (Bielschowsky head tilt test). Tilting the head away from the side of the involved eye may relieve the diplopia, and patients frequently adopt such a head tilt. History of an abnormal head posture during childhood, which may be confirmed by review of family photographs and a large vertical prism fusion range, are strong clues that a trochlear palsy is congenital. In bilateral traumatic palsy, there is usually a chin-down head posture. Strabismus surgery is effective in decompensated congenital palsy not controlled by prisms and for unresolved acquired palsy.

B. Superior Oblique Myokymia

Contrary to its name, this is an uncommon acquired tremor of the superior oblique muscle, affecting only one eye. The patient complains of episodes of torsional and/or vertical oscillopsia or double vision, which may be precipitated by looking down, such as when reading. Various anticonvulsants, typically carbamazepine, or β-blocker eye drops can be beneficial. Superior oblique muscle surgery may be undertaken. The cause may be compression of the trochlear nerve by an aberrant artery, for which intracranial surgery may be successful.

▶ Abducens Nerve (VI)

Motor (entirely uncrossed) fibers arise from the nucleus in the floor of the fourth ventricle in the lower portion of the pons near the internal genu of the facial nerve. Piercing the pons, the fibers emerge anteriorly, the nerve running a long course over the tip of the petrous portion of the temporal bone into the cavernous sinus. It enters the orbit with the third and fourth nerves to supply the lateral rectus muscle.

A. Abducens Nucleus Lesion

The abducens nucleus contains the motor neurons to the ipsilateral lateral rectus and the cell bodies of interneurons innervating the motor neurons to the contralateral medial rectus. It is the final common relay point for all horizontal conjugate eye movements, and a lesion within the nucleus will produce an ipsilateral horizontal gaze palsy affecting all types of eye movement, including vestibular movements. This contrasts with a lesion of the paramedian pontine reticular formation, in which vestibular movements are preserved.

B. Abducens Nerve Palsy (see Also Chapter 12)

This is the most common single extraocular muscle palsy. Abduction of the eye is reduced or absent; esotropia is present in the primary position and increases with distance fixation and upon gaze to the affected side. Ischemia (arteriosclerosis, diabetes, migraine, and hypertension) is a common cause. However, increased intracranial pressure, in which the abducens palsy is a false localizing sign, intracranial tumors, particularly at the base of the skull, trauma, meningitis, demyelination, dural arteriovenous fistula, and intracranial hypotension including after lumbar puncture are other causes. Infections can produce sixth nerve palsy from direct involvement, as in middle ear infection, ischemia, or meningitis. Arnold–Chiari malformation (congenital downward displacement of the cerebellar tonsils) can produce sixth nerve palsy due to traction but can also produce a distance esotropia without limitation of abduction due to cerebellar dysfunction. A child with a sixth nerve palsy should be evaluated for a brainstem tumor (glioma) or inflammation if trauma was not present or if trauma was minimal. Möbius' syndrome (congenital facial diplegia) can be associated with a sixth nerve or conjugate gaze palsy. Pseudo-sixth nerve palsies can occur in Duane's syndrome, spasm of the near response, thyroid eye disease, myasthenia, or long-standing strabismus and in medial rectus entrapment by an ethmoid fracture.

C. Duane's Syndrome

Duane's syndrome is uncommon (<1% of cases of strabismus) and in almost all cases congenital. It is a stationary, nearly always unilateral condition characterized by complete or partial deficiency of abduction, with retraction of the globe and narrowing of the lid fissure on adduction. Congenital absence of the sixth nerve with coinnervation of the lateral rectus by a branch of the third nerve is the likely cause in most cases and other congenital anomalies are common. The visual handicap is seldom severe. Visual acuity is usually normal. Unless there is a marked abnormal head posture, strabismus surgery is best avoided.

D. Gradenigo's Syndrome

Gradenigo's syndrome is characterized by pain in the face (from irritation of the trigeminal nerve) and abducens palsy. The syndrome is produced by disease of the tip of the petrous bone and most often occurs as a rare complication of otitis media with mastoiditis or petrous bone tumors.

▶ Syndromes Affecting Cranial Nerves III, IV, & VI

A. Superior Orbital Fissure Syndrome

All the ocular motor nerves pass through the superior orbital fissure and can be affected by tumor, inflammation, or trauma involving the fissure.

B. Orbital Apex Syndrome

This syndrome is similar to the superior orbital fissure syndrome with the addition of optic nerve signs and usually greater proptosis. It is also caused by tumor, inflammation, or trauma.

C. Sudden Complete Ophthalmoplegia

Complete ophthalmoplegia of sudden onset can be due to extensive brainstem vascular disease, Wernicke's encephalopathy, Fisher's syndrome, bulbar poliomyelitis, pituitary apoplexy, basilar aneurysm, meningitis, diphtheria, botulism, or myasthenic crisis.

4. THE CEREBELLUM

The cerebellum has an important modulating influence on the function of the neural integrators. Thus, it is involved in gaze holding and the control of saccades, particularly the relationship between the pulse and the step of saccade generation. Cerebellar dysfunction produces gaze-evoked nystagmus, by its influence on gaze holding, and abnormalities of saccades, including saccadic dysmetria in which the saccadic amplitude is inaccurate, and postsaccadic drift due to a mismatch between the pulse and step of the saccade.

The cerebellum is also important in the control of pursuit eye movements, and cerebellar dysfunction may thus result in broken (saccadic) pursuit. It may also result in ocular misalignment, vertical due to skew deviation or horizontal.

▼ MYASTHENIA GRAVIS

Myasthenia gravis is characterized by abnormal fatigability of striated muscles after repetitive contraction that improves after rest and often is first manifested by weakness of the extraocular muscles. Unilateral fatiguing ptosis is a frequent first sign, with subsequent bilateral involvement of extraocular muscles, so that diplopia is often an early symptom. Unusual ocular presentations may simulate gaze palsies, internuclear ophthalmoplegias, vertical nystagmus, and progressive external ophthalmoplegia. Generalized weakness of the arms and legs, difficulty in swallowing, weakness of jaw muscles, and difficulty in breathing may follow rapidly in untreated cases. The weakness often worsens as the day progresses but can be improved by a nap. There are no sensory changes.

The incidence of the disease is in the range of 1:30,000 to 1:20,000. Myasthenia gravis usually affects young adults aged 20–40 (70% are under 40 years of age), although it may occur at any age and can be misdiagnosed as functional, especially because the weakness can be greater in exciting or embarrassing situations. Older patients are more commonly male and are more likely to have a thymoma.

The onset may follow an upper respiratory infection, stress, pregnancy, or any injury, and the disease has been noted as a transitory condition in newborn infants of myasthenic mothers. Drugs, including β-blockers (eg, propranolol), penicillamine, statins, lithium, aminoglycoside antibiotics, chloroquine, and phenytoin, may induce, unmask, or exacerbate the disease. Myasthenia gravis has been associated with hyperthyroidism (5%), thyroid abnormalities (15%), autoimmune diseases (5%), and diffuse metastatic carcinoma (7%).

In about one-third of cases, the disease is confined to the extraocular muscles at onset. In about two-thirds of these cases, the disease will become generalized with time, usually within the first year.

The differential diagnosis includes chronic progressive external ophthalmoplegia, oculopharyngeal muscular dystrophy, myotonic dystrophy, ocular motor cranial nerve palsies, and brainstem lesions including encephalitis, botulism, and multiple sclerosis.

The disease has its origin at the neuromuscular junction, especially at the postsynaptic site, primarily due to antibodies against it and the presynaptic site. Anti-acetylcholine receptor antibodies are diagnostic. They are present in 80%–90% of patients with systemic myasthenia and 40%–60% of patients with pure ocular myasthenia, but the titers do not correlate with severity of disease. Antibody-positive patients should undergo chest CT or MRI to detect thymic enlargement. Thymomas occur in 15% of patients. A large proportion of patients with generalized myasthenia gravis without acetylcholine receptor antibodies have antibodies against muscle-specific receptor tyrosine kinase (MuSK). These patients tend to be female, with predominant cranial and bulbar muscle involvement, frequent respiratory crises, and poorer response to treatment. MuSK antibody myasthenia gravis may also present with pure ocular disease.

Cholinesterase destroys acetylcholine at the neuromuscular junction, and cholinesterase-inhibiting drugs may improve the condition by increasing the amount of acetylcholine available to the damaged postsynaptic site. Intravenous edrophonium or intramuscular neostigmine can be used for diagnosis. In the edrophonium (Tensilon) test, pretreatment with intravenous atropine is recommended. Edrophonium, 2 mg (0.2 mL), is given intravenously over 15 seconds. If no response occurs in 30 seconds, an additional 5–7 mg (0.5–0.7 mL) is given. The test is most helpful when marked ptosis is present. Significant improvement in muscle function constitutes a positive response and confirms the diagnosis of myasthenia gravis. Slightly positive edrophonium tests can occur in neurogenic palsies, and there may be false-negative results when myasthenia is complicated by muscle wasting. Documented improvement of ptosis with rest or application of ice can be helpful for diagnosis.

Repetitive nerve stimulation, especially of the facial or proximal muscles, can demonstrate abnormal muscle fatigability (more than 10% decrease in the response is diagnostic of myasthenia). Variation in size and shape of motor unit potentials is noted on needle electromyography of affected muscles, and single-fiber studies show increased variability (jitter) in the temporal pattern of action potentials from muscle fibers of the same motor unit. Orbicularis oculi single-fiber electromyography is particularly useful in diagnosis of ocular myasthenia.

Myasthenia can be treated with pyridostigmine, systemic steroids, other immunosuppressants such as azathioprine, immunoglobulins, and plasmapheresis according to the severity of disease. During severe exacerbations, artificial ventilation may be necessary. Thymectomy may be indicated in patients with thymoma (although it may not influence the severity of the myasthenia) and in patients with early-onset generalized disease without evidence of thymoma—in one-third of whom it may produce complete remission without the need for immunosuppressants. Ocular myasthenia tends to respond less well to anticholinesterase agents than generalized disease, but the response to systemic steroids is usually good. Extraocular muscle surgery can be undertaken but should be delayed until the ocular motility deficit has been stable for a long time.

Myasthenia is generally a chronic disease with a tendency to pursue a relapsing and remitting course. The prognosis depends on the extent of the disease, the response to medication and thymectomy, and the careful management of severe exacerbations.

CHRONIC PROGRESSIVE EXTERNAL OPHTHALMOPLEGIA

This rather rare disease is characterized by slowly progressive inability to move the eyes and severe early ptosis yet normal pupillary responses. It may begin at any age and progresses over a period of 5–15 years to complete external ophthalmoplegia. It is a form of mitochondrial myopathy and may be associated with other manifestations of mitochondrial disease, such as pigmentary degeneration of the retina, deafness, cerebellar-vestibular abnormalities, seizures, cardiac conduction defects, and peripheral sensorimotor neuropathy, in which case the term "ophthalmoplegia-plus" may be applied. Onset before 15 years of age of chronic progressive external ophthalmoplegia, heart block, and pigmentary retinopathy constitutes the Kearns–Sayre syndrome. Chronic progressive external ophthalmoplegia is associated with deletions of mitochondrial DNA, which are more frequent and more extensive in the cases with nonocular manifestations.

NYSTAGMUS (TABLE 14–2)

Nystagmus is defined as repetitive, rhythmic oscillations of one or both eyes in any or all fields of gaze, initiated by a slow eye movement. The waveform may be pendular, in which the movements in each direction have equal speed, amplitude, and duration; or jerk, in which the slow movement in one direction is followed by a rapid corrective return to the

Table 14–2. Classification of Nystagmus

Physiologic nystagmus
   End-point nystagmus
   Optokinetic nystagmus
   Stimulation of semicircular canals (physiologic vestibular nystagmus)
      Rotatory
      Caloric

Pathologic nystagmus
   Congenital nystagmus
      With sensory abnormality
      Without sensory abnormality (congenital idiopathic motor nystagmus)
      Latent nystagmus (LN)
      Manifest latent nystagmus (MLN)
   Acquired pendular nystagmus
      Infantile visual deprivation
      Spasmus nutans
      Oculopalatal myoclonus
   Vestibular nystagmus
      Peripheral vestibular nystagmus
      Central vestibular nystagmus
         Downbeat nystagmus
         Upbeat nystagmus
   Gaze-evoked nystagmus
   Gaze-paretic nystagmus
   Convergence-retraction nystagmus
   Seesaw nystagmus
   Periodic alternating nystagmus

Mimics of nystagmus
   Saccadic intrusions
   Spontaneous eye movements in coma
   Voluntary nystagmus

original position (fast component). By convention, the direction of jerk nystagmus is given as the direction of the corrective fast phase and not the direction of the primary slow phase.

Jerk nystagmus is classified as grade I, present only with the eyes directed toward the fast component; grade II, present also with the eyes in primary position; or grade III, present even with the eyes directed toward the slow component. The movements of pendular or jerk nystagmus may be horizontal, vertical, torsional, oblique, circular, or a combination of these. The direction may change depending on the direction of gaze.

The **amplitude** of nystagmus is the extent of the movement; the **rate** of nystagmus is the frequency of oscillation. Generally speaking, the faster the rate, the smaller the amplitude and vice versa. Nystagmus is usually conjugate but is occasionally dysconjugate, as in convergence-retraction nystagmus and seesaw nystagmus.

Nystagmus is also occasionally dissociated (more marked in one eye than the other), as in internuclear ophthalmoplegia, spasmus nutans, monocular visual loss, and acquired

pendular nystagmus and with asymmetric muscle weakness in myasthenia gravis.

Physiology of Symptoms

Reduced visual acuity is caused by inability to maintain steady fixation. The patient may complain of illusory movement of objects (oscillopsia), which is usually indicative of acquired rather than congenital nystagmus and is particularly severe in vestibular disease. Head tilting is usually involuntary, to decrease the nystagmus. The head is turned toward the fast components in jerk nystagmus or set so that the eyes are in a position that minimizes ocular movement in pendular nystagmus. Head nodding may occur in congenital nystagmus and is a characteristic feature of spasmus nutans. Nystagmus is noticeable and cosmetically disturbing except when excursions of the eye are very small.

PHYSIOLOGIC NYSTAGMUS

Three types of nystagmus can be elicited in the normal person.

End-Point (End-Gaze) Nystagmus

Normal individuals may have nystagmus on extreme horizontal gaze, which disappears when the eyes are moved centrally by a few degrees. It is primarily horizontal but may have a slight torsional component and greater amplitude in the abducting eye.

Optokinetic Nystagmus

This type of nystagmus may be elicited in all normal individuals, most easily by means of a rotating drum with alternating black and white lines but in fact by any repetitive targets in the visual field, such as repetitive telephone poles as seen from a window of a fast-moving vehicle. The slow component follows the object, and the fast component moves rapidly in the opposite direction to fixate on the succeeding object. A unilateral or asymmetric horizontal response usually indicates a deep parietal lobe lesion, especially a tumor. It occurs as a result of a deficit in the slow (pursuit) phase. Anterior cerebral (ie, frontal lobe) lesions may inhibit this response only temporarily when an acute saccadic gaze palsy is present, which suggests the presence of a compensatory mechanism that is much greater than for lesions situated farther posteriorly. Asymmetry of response in the vertical plane suggests a brainstem lesion. Since it is an involuntary response, this test is especially useful in detecting functional visual loss. A large mirror filling the patient's central field at near can be rotated from side to side and will induce an optokinetic nystagmus if vision is present.

Stimulation of Semicircular Canals

The three semicircular canals of each inner ear sense movements of the head in space, being primarily sensitive to acceleration. The neural output of the vestibular system, after processing within the vestibular and related brainstem nuclei, is a velocity signal. This is transmitted, principally via the medial longitudinal fasciculus on each side of the brainstem, to the ocular motor nuclei to produce the necessary compensatory eye movements (**VOR**) for maintaining a stable position of the eyes in space, and hence optimal vision. Vestibular signals also pass to the cerebellum and cerebral cortex.

Stimulation of the semicircular canals results in a compensatory eye movement. In the unconscious subject with an intact brainstem, this leads to a tonic deviation of the eyes, whereas in the conscious subject, a superimposed corrective fast-phase movement, returning the eyes back toward the straight-ahead position, results in a jerk nystagmus. These tests are useful methods of investigating vestibular function in conscious subjects and, in the case of caloric stimulation, brainstem function in comatose patients.

A. Rotatory Physiologic Nystagmus (Bárány Rotating Chair)

When the head is tilted 30° forward, the horizontal semicircular canals lie horizontally in space. Rotation, such as in a Bárány chair, then leads to a horizontal jerk nystagmus with the compensatory slow-phase eye movement opposite to the direction of turning and the corrective fast phase in the direction of turning. Owing to impersistence of the vestibular signal during continued rotation, the nystagmus abates. Once the rotation stops, there is a vestibular tone in the opposite direction, which results in a jerk nystagmus with the fast phase away from the original direction of turning (postrotatory nystagmus). Since the subject is stationary, postrotatory nystagmus is often easier to analyze than the nystagmus during rotation.

B. Caloric Stimulation

With the head tilted 60° backward, the horizontal semicircular canals lie vertically in space. Water irrigation of the auditory canal then generates convection currents predominantly within the horizontal rather than the vertical semicircular canals. Cold water irrigation induces a predominantly horizontal jerk nystagmus with a fast phase opposite to the side of irrigation, and warm water irrigation induces a similar jerk nystagmus with a fast phase toward the side of irrigation. (The mnemonic device is "COWS": cold-opposite, warm-same.) Caloric nystagmus is made more obvious by the patient wearing Frenzel's spectacles, which eliminate patient fixation and provide a magnified view for the examiner. It is important to verify that the tympanic membrane is intact before performing irrigation of the external auditory canal.

PATHOLOGIC NYSTAGMUS

▶ Congenital Nystagmus

Congenital nystagmus is nystagmus present within 6 months after birth. Ocular instability is usual at birth, due to poor visual fixation, but this abates during the first few weeks of life. The presence of spontaneous nystagmus is always pathologic.

Congenital impairment of vision or visual deprivation due to lesions in any part of the eye or optic nerve can result in nystagmus at birth or soon thereafter. Causes include corneal opacity, cataract, albinism, achromatopsia, bilateral macular disease, aniridia, and optic atrophy. By definition, congenital idiopathic motor nystagmus has no associated underlying sensory abnormality, although visual performance is limited by the ocular instability. Typically it is not present at birth but becomes apparent between 3 and 6 months of age.

At one time it was thought that congenital pendular nystagmus was indicative of an underlying sensory abnormality whereas congenital jerk nystagmus was not. Eye movement recordings have shown this not to be true, both pendular and jerk waveforms being seen whether there is a sensory abnormality or not. Indeed, in many cases, a mixed pattern of alternating pendular and jerk waveforms is seen. Congenital nystagmus, particularly the idiopathic motor type with its potential for better visual fixation, generally undergoes a progressive change in its waveform during early childhood. There is development of periods of relative ocular stability, that is, relatively slow eye velocity, known as foveation periods since they are thought to be an adaptive response to maximize the potential for fixation, and hence to improve visual acuity. In addition, congenital nystagmus with a jerk nystagmus has a characteristic waveform in which the slow phases have an exponentially increasing velocity. This is known as CN-type waveform, and with very few exceptions its presence signifies that the nystagmus has been present since early childhood. This can be a particularly useful feature in determining that nystagmus noted in adulthood is not of recent onset.

Congenital nystagmus is usually horizontal and conjugate. Vertical and torsional components are only occasionally present. The direction of any jerk component often varies with the direction of gaze, but an important feature in comparison to many forms of acquired nystagmus is that there is no additional vertical component on vertical gaze. In most patients with congenital nystagmus, there is a direction of gaze (null zone) in which the nystagmus is relatively quiet. If this null zone is away from primary position, a head turn may be adopted to place the eccentric position straight ahead. In a few cases, the position of the null zone varies to produce one type of periodic alternating nystagmus. Congenital nystagmus is usually decreased in intensity by convergence, and some patients will adopt an esotropia (nystagmus blockage). Anxiety and increased "effort to see" will often increase the intensity of congenital nystagmus, and thus reduce visual acuity.

Once congenital nystagmus has been noted, it is important to identify any underlying sensory abnormality, if only to determine the visual potential. This may require electrodiagnostic studies. Extraocular muscle surgery is predominantly indicated for patients with a marked head turn. Supramaximal recessions of the horizontal rectus muscles reduce the intensity of congenital nystagmus, but the effect is only temporary. Gabapentin and/or memantine may be beneficial.

In general, **latent nystagmus** means nystagmus that increases in intensity when one eye is covered, which is a characteristic feature of congenital nystagmus. There is also a specific type of latent nystagmus, known as **LN,** which is predominantly seen in infantile esotropia. LN is a horizontal jerk nystagmus with the fast phase toward the side of the fixing eye—with the left eye covered, there is a rightward nystagmus, and with the right eye covered, a leftward nystagmus. LN also becomes more marked when one eye is covered, only then being apparent on clinical examination, but eye movement recordings show that the nystagmus is always present. **Manifest latent nystagmus (MLN)** is a particular type of LN in which the nystagmus is always apparent on clinical examination. It occurs in patients with LN when binocular function is lost, that is, the equivalent of one eye being covered. This may be because of loss of sight in one eye or even from the development of a divergent squint. If binocular function is restored, MLN will revert to LN.

Acquired Pendular Nystagmus

Any child who develops bilateral visual loss before 6 years of age may also develop a pendular nystagmus, and indeed the acquisition of a pendular nystagmus during infancy necessitates further investigation. A specific syndrome of acquired pendular nystagmus in childhood is **spasmus nutans.** This is a bilateral, generally horizontal (occasionally vertical), fine, dissociated pendular nystagmus, associated with head nodding and an abnormal head posture. There is a benign form, which may be familial, with onset before age 2 and spontaneous improvement during the third or fourth year. Spasmus nutans may also rarely be the first manifestation of an anterior visual pathway glioma.

In adults, acquired pendular nystagmus is a feature of brainstem disease, usually multiple sclerosis or brainstem stroke. There may be horizontal, vertical, or torsional components or even a combination of components to produce oblique or elliptical trajectories. The syndrome of **oculopalatal myoclonus** characteristically develops several months after a brainstem stroke. There is a pendular nystagmus with synchronous movements variably involving the soft palate, larynx, and diaphragm as well as producing head titubation. (The term "myoclonus" is a misnomer since the abnormal movements are a form of tremor.) The associated hypertrophy of the inferior olivary nucleus in the medulla and other evidence suggest a disruption of the dentato-rubro-olivary pathway between the brainstem and the cerebellum as the underlying pathogenesis. Various drug treatments have been tried for adult acquired pendular nystagmus, of which gabapentin, memantine, and baclofen have produced the best

although still limited results. Base-out prisms may also be tried.

Vestibular Nystagmus

Abnormalities of vestibular tone result in abnormal activation of the vestibulo-ocular pathways and abnormal neural drive to the extraocular muscles. Loss of function in the left horizontal semicircular canal is equivalent to activation of the right horizontal semicircular canal, as would normally be produced by a rightward head turn. The oculomotor response is conjugate leftward slow-phase movement of the eyes. The corrective fast-phase response is rightward in direction, and a right-beating horizontal nystagmus is thus generated. The pattern of response to dysfunction of one or more semicircular canals can be similarly derived to give the full possible range of **peripheral vestibular nystagmus,** although in clinical practice it is the effect of dysfunction of the horizontal canals that usually predominates. As a general rule, peripheral vestibular lesions are destructive and the fast phase of the resulting nystagmus is away from the side of the lesion. Since the neural signal of the vestibulo-ocular pathways is a velocity signal, the slow phase of peripheral vestibular nystagmus has a constant velocity. This gives rise to the characteristic saw-tooth waveform on eye movement recordings.

Peripheral vestibular nystagmus is not dependent on visual stimuli and thus is still present in the dark, or with the eyes closed, as well as in blind individuals. It is, however, inhibited by visual fixation or, conversely, accentuated by wearing Frenzel's spectacles, and this is an important factor in the normal dampening over 2–3 weeks of peripheral vestibular nystagmus. Head position does not usually influence peripheral vestibular nystagmus except in benign paroxysmal positional vertigo, in which elicitation of the characteristic pattern of nystagmus with the Hallpike maneuver is a specific diagnostic feature. Other clinical features associated with peripheral vestibular disease are vertigo, tinnitus, and deafness, the latter two reflecting the close association between the vestibular and auditory systems. Causes of peripheral vestibular disease are labyrinthitis, Meniere's disease, trauma (including surgical destruction of one labyrinth), and vascular, inflammatory, or neoplastic lesions of the vestibular nerves.

Central vestibular nystagmus is an acquired jerk nystagmus due to disease in the central vestibular pathways of the brainstem and cerebellum. It has a variety of forms, but characteristic types are a purely torsional or vertical jerk nystagmus and the syndromes of downbeat and upbeat nystagmus, which are probably the result of imbalance in vestibular tone from the vertical semicircular canals. Central vestibular nystagmus is frequently elicited or enhanced by specific head positions, presumably as a result of modulation by input from the peripheral vestibular apparatus. It is not dampened by visual fixation and does not spontaneously abate in intensity with time. Other clinical features reflect the associated brainstem and cerebellar dysfunction and include abnormalities of smooth pursuit eye movements other than those due to the nystagmus itself. Causes of central vestibular nystagmus include lesions of the vestibular nuclei (brainstem demyelination, including multiple sclerosis, inflammation, and stroke, particularly thrombosis of the posteroinferior cerebellar artery leading to lateral medullary infarction—Wallenberg's syndrome).

Downbeat nystagmus is a downward-beating nystagmus, usually present in primary position. It is often most obvious on gaze down and to the side, when the nystagmus becomes oblique, with the horizontal component in the direction of lateral gaze. Downbeat nystagmus is characteristically associated with lesions at the cervicomedullary junction, notably Chiari malformation and basilar invagination, and all patients should undergo MRI to exclude such lesions. Other causes are cerebellar degeneration, demyelinating disease, hydrocephalus, anticonvulsants, and lithium. Clonazepam or aminopyridines may be beneficial.

Upbeat nystagmus is characterized by an upward-beating nystagmus in primary position, which usually increases, although it may reduce in intensity on upgaze. It is virtually always the result of brainstem disease but occasionally reflects cerebellar disease. It is seen in brainstem encephalitis, demyelination, and tumors and also as a toxic side effect of barbiturates, alcohol, and anticonvulsants. Baclofen or aminopyridines may be beneficial.

Gaze-Evoked & Gaze-Paretic Nystagmus

Maintenance of steady eccentric gaze is dependent on the neural integrator system, which produces the tonic extraocular muscle activity necessary to overcome the viscous and elastic orbital forces acting to return the globe to primary position. Reduction in activity of the neural integrator results in eccentric gaze being negated by a slow drift of the globe toward primary position. Since the force acting to produce this central drift reduces with decreasing eccentricity, this slow drift has an exponentially decreasing velocity. Additional corrective fast eye movements, returning the eye to the desired eccentric position, result in nystagmus beating in the direction of gaze, whether it is horizontal, vertical, or oblique.

End-point nystagmus (see earlier in the chapter) is the physiologic manifestation of the inability of the neural integrator to maintain steady eye position in extreme eccentric gaze. Gaze-evoked nystagmus is the result of pathologic failure of the neural integrator system. In its mildest form it manifests only on moderate horizontal gaze, whereas in its most severe form nystagmus is present with any movement away from primary position. In many cases of gaze-evoked nystagmus, there is also **rebound nystagmus**—following return of the eyes to primary position from a position of eccentric gaze, a jerk nystagmus beating away from the direction of the eccentric gaze develops after a latent period and lasts for a short period.

The neural integrator is situated in the brainstem but is highly dependent on cerebellar inputs. Thus, gaze-evoked nystagmus may be a manifestation of either brainstem or, especially, cerebellar disease. Often there are other cerebellar eye movement abnormalities, such as saccadic dysmetria and disruption of smooth pursuit. The most common causes of gaze-evoked nystagmus are cerebellar diseases, sedatives, and anticonvulsants. Cerebellopontine angle neoplasms, such as vestibular schwannomas (acoustic neuromas), may produce a combination of gaze-evoked nystagmus and a peripheral vestibular nystagmus beating toward the opposite side (Brun's nystagmus).

Reduction in the supranuclear input into the neural integrator or in the ability of the peripheral oculomotor system to facilitate its function will lead to nystagmus with the same basic characteristics as gaze-evoked nystagmus. Thus, conditions ranging from gaze palsy through oculomotor cranial nerve palsies and myasthenia gravis to extraocular muscle disease can manifest with nystagmus on eccentric gaze in the direction of the affected eye movements. This is termed gaze-paretic nystagmus and should be excluded whenever the possibility of a gaze-evoked nystagmus is being considered so as to avoid misdirected investigation.

Convergence-Retraction Nystagmus

Convergence-retraction nystagmus is a feature of the dorsal midbrain (Parinaud's) syndrome either from intrinsic lesions (tumor, hemorrhage, infarction, or inflammation) or extrinsic lesions, particularly pineal tumors and hydrocephalus. On attempted upgaze, which is usually defective, the eyes undergo rapid convergent movements with retraction of the globes. This is best elicited as the patient watches downward-moving stripes on an optokinetic tape or drum. Electromyographic studies have shown cocontraction of extraocular muscles and loss of normal agonist–antagonist reciprocal innervation. Convergence-retraction nystagmus may represent asynchronous, opposed, adducting saccades due to inappropriate activation of the medial rectus muscles.

Seesaw Nystagmus

Seesaw nystagmus is characterized by rising intorsion of one eye and falling extorsion of the other—and then the reverse. It may have a pendular or jerk waveform. Although it is uncommon, it occurs with acquired and congenital chiasmal lesions in association with a bitemporal hemianopia, and midbrain lesions. There does not appear to be a single underlying pathogenesis, but it is likely that dysfunction of the interstitial nucleus of Cajal or the rostral interstitial nucleus of the medial longitudinal fasciculus is important in the cases with midbrain disease.

Periodic Alternating Nystagmus

This is a horizontal jerk nystagmus regularly alternating between leftward and rightward directions, each phase lasting approximately 2 minutes. The acquired form usually results from cerebellar disease, such as cerebellar degenerations, congenital hindbrain anomalies, such as Chiari malformation, multiple sclerosis, or anticonvulsant therapy. It characteristically responds to baclofen. It may also occur with bilateral blindness and be suppressed if vision is restored. Periodic alternation may also be a feature of congenital nystagmus (see earlier in the chapter).

MIMICS OF NYSTAGMUS

Abnormal spontaneous eye movements may be the result of unwanted saccadic eye movements (saccadic intrusions), which include square-wave jerks, macrosaccadic oscillations, ocular flutter, and opsoclonus. These are generally due to cerebellar disease. There is also a variety of abnormal eye movements that occur in coma, including ocular bobbing, ocular dipping, and ping-pong gaze. Superior oblique myokymia (see earlier in the chapter) is a tremor of the superior oblique muscle leading to episodic monocular vertical or torsional oscillopsia.

▶ Voluntary Nystagmus

About 5% of normal individuals can generate short bursts of ocular oscillations that resemble small-amplitude, fast, horizontal pendular nystagmus. Eye movement recordings show the movements to be rapidly alternating saccades. Recognition of the entity is important to avoid unnecessary investigation.

▼ CEREBROVASCULAR DISORDERS OF OPHTHALMOLOGIC IMPORTANCE

▶ Vascular Insufficiency & Occlusion of the Internal Carotid Artery

Transient episodes of visual loss most often result from retinal emboli (amaurosis fugax), usually from carotid disease but possibly from cardiac valvular disease or cardiac arrhythmia (see Chapter 15). They also occur in thrombotic disorders such as hyperviscosity states or antiphospholipid syndrome and from other causes of impaired ocular or cerebral perfusion such as giant cell arteritis, migraine, vertebrobasilar ischemia (see later in the chapter), severe hypotension, or shock. The visual loss from retinal emboli is characteristically described as a curtain descending across the vision of one eye, with complete loss of vision for 5–10 minutes, and then complete recovery. There may be associated transient ischemic attacks (TIAs) or completed strokes of the ipsilateral cerebral hemisphere. In other causes of transient visual loss, there may be constriction of the visual field from the periphery to the center, "graying" rather than complete loss of vision, and involvement of both eyes simultaneously. Fleeting episodes of visual loss that last a few seconds (transient visual obscurations) may occur in papilledema, affecting one or both eyes together, or monocularly with orbital tumors.

Cholesterol, platelet-fibrin, and calcific are the three main types of retinal emboli. Cholesterol emboli (Hollenhorst plaques) may be visible with the ophthalmoscope as small, glistening, yellow-red crystals situated at bifurcations of the retinal arteries. The nonreflective gummy white plugs filling retinal vessels, which characterize platelet-fibrin emboli, are less commonly seen because they quickly disperse and traverse the retinal circulation. Calcific emboli, which usually originate from damaged cardiac valves, have a duller, white-gray appearance compared with cholesterol emboli. Retinal emboli may also produce branch or, particularly in the case of calcific emboli, central retinal arterial occlusions.

In patients with amaurosis fugax, high-grade (70%–99%) stenosis of the internal carotid artery, as determined by ultrasound or angiographic studies, is an indication for carotid endarterectomy to reduce the risk of cerebral hemisphere stroke. Low-grade (0%–29%) and probably medium-grade (30%–69%) stenoses are best treated medically, usually with low-dose (81 mg/d) aspirin. Incidentally, noted cholesterol retinal emboli in asymptomatic individuals are associated with a tenfold increased risk of cerebral infarction, but the role of carotid endarterectomy in such individuals is uncertain.

In the acute stages of embolic retinal arterial occlusion, treatment with ocular massage, anterior chamber paracentesis, rebreathing into a paper bag to increase inhaled CO_2 level, and intravenous acetazolamide may lead to displacement of the embolus and recovery of vision. After 12 hours, the clinical picture is usually irreversible, although many exceptions to this rule have been reported. Visual acuity better than counting fingers on presentation has a better prognosis with vigorous treatment. Embolic retinal arterial occlusion has a poorer 5-year survival rate due to attendant cardiac disease or stroke than occlusion due to thrombotic disease.

Slow flow (venous stasis) retinopathy is a sign of generalized ocular ischemia and indicative of severe carotid disease, usually with complete occlusion of the ipsilateral internal carotid artery. It is characterized by venous dilation and tortuosity, retinal hemorrhages, macular edema, and eventual neovascular proliferation. It resembles diabetic retinopathy, but the changes occur more in the retinal midperiphery than the posterior pole. In more severe cases, there may be vasodilation of the conjunctiva, iris neovascularization, neovascular glaucoma, and frank anterior segment ischemia with corneal edema, anterior uveitis, and cataract. Diagnosis is most easily confirmed by demonstration of reversal of blood flow in the ipsilateral ophthalmic artery using orbital ultrasound, but further investigation by angiography is usually required to determine the full extent of arterial disease. Carotid endarterectomy may be indicated but carries a risk of precipitating or exacerbating intraocular neovascularization. The role of panretinal laser photocoagulation in treating intraocular neovascularization is uncertain.

▶ Occlusion of the Middle Cerebral Artery

This disorder may produce severe contralateral hemiplegia, hemianesthesia, and homonymous hemianopia. The lower quadrants of the visual fields (upper radiations) are most apt to be involved. Aphasia may be present if the dominant hemisphere is involved.

Vascular Insufficiency of the Vertebrobasilar Arterial System

Brief episodes of transient bilateral blurring of vision commonly precede a basilar artery stroke. An attack seldom leaves any residual visual impairment, and the episode may be so minimal that the patient or doctor does not heed the warning. The blurring is described as a graying of vision just as if the house lights were being dimmed at a theater. Episodes seldom last more than 5 minutes (often only a few seconds) and may be associated with other transient symptoms of vertebrobasilar insufficiency. Antiplatelet drugs can decrease the frequency and severity of vertebrobasilar symptoms.

Occlusion of the Basilar Artery

Complete or extensive thrombosis of the basilar artery nearly always causes death. With partial occlusion or basilar "insufficiency" due to arteriosclerosis, a wide variety of brainstem and cerebellar signs may be present. These include nystagmus, supranuclear oculomotor signs, and involvement of cranial nerves III, IV, VI, and VII.

Prolonged anticoagulant therapy has become the accepted treatment of partial basilar artery thrombotic occlusion.

Occlusion of the Posterior Cerebral Artery

Occlusion of the posterior cerebral artery seldom causes death. Occlusion of the cortical branches (most common) causes homonymous hemianopia, usually superior quadrantic (the artery supplies primarily the inferior visual cortex). Lesions on the left in right-handed persons can cause aphasia, agraphia, and alexia if extensive with parietal and occipital involvement. Involvement of the occipital lobe and splenium of the corpus callosum can cause alexia (inability to read) without agraphia (inability to write); such a patient would not be able to read his or her own writing. Occlusion of the proximal branches may produce the thalamic syndrome (thalamic pain, hemiparesis, hemianesthesia, choreoathetoid movements) and cerebellar ataxia.

Subdural Hemorrhage

Subdural hemorrhage results from tearing or shearing of the veins bridging the subdural space from the pia mater to the dural sinus. It leads to an encapsulated accumulation of blood in the subdural space, usually over one cerebral hemisphere. It is nearly always caused by head trauma. The trauma may be minimal and may precede the onset of neurologic signs by weeks or even months.

In infants, subdural hemorrhage produces progressive enlargement of the head with bulging fontanelles. Ocular signs include strabismus, pupillary changes, papilledema, and retinal hemorrhages.

In adults, the symptoms of chronic subdural hematoma are severe headache, drowsiness, and mental confusion, usually appearing hours to weeks (even months) after trauma. Symptomatology is similar to that of cerebral tumors. Papilledema is present in 30%–50% of cases. Retinal hemorrhages occur in association with papilledema. Ipsilateral dilation of the pupil is the most common and most serious sign and is an urgent indication for immediate surgical evacuation of blood. Unequal, miotic, or mydriatic pupils can occur, or there may be no pupillary signs. Other signs, including vestibular nystagmus and cranial nerve palsies, also occur. Many of these signs result from herniation and compression of the brainstem, and therefore often appear late with stupor and coma.

CT scan or MRI confirms the diagnosis.

Treatment of acute large subdural hematoma consists of surgical evacuation of the blood; small hematomas may be simply followed with careful observation. Without treatment, the course of large hematomas is progressively downhill to coma and death. With early and adequate treatment, the prognosis is good.

Subarachnoid Hemorrhage

Subarachnoid hemorrhage most commonly results from ruptured congenital berry aneurysms of the circle of Willis in the subarachnoid space. It may also result from trauma, birth injuries, intracranial hemorrhage, hemorrhage associated with tumors, arteriovenous malformations, or systemic bleeding disorders.

The most prominent symptom of subarachnoid hemorrhage is sudden, severe headache, usually occipital and often associated with signs of meningeal irritation (eg, stiff neck). Drowsiness, loss of consciousness, coma, and death may occur rapidly.

Treatment of intracranial aneurysm prior to rupture greatly improves prognosis. An expanding posterior communicating artery aneurysm may present with painful isolated third nerve palsy with pupillary involvement, which thus necessitates emergency investigation. Oculomotor palsy with associated numbness and pain in the distribution of the ipsilateral trigeminal nerve may be caused by supraclinoid, internal carotid, or posterior communicating artery aneurysm. Subarachnoid hemorrhage with optic nerve dysfunction suggests an ophthalmic artery aneurysm. If it occurs, papilledema develops after subarachnoid hemorrhage has occurred. Various types of intraocular hemorrhage occur infrequently (pre-retinal hemorrhages are the most common—Terson's syndrome) and carry a poor prognosis for life when they are both early and extensive, since they reflect rapid severe elevation of intracranial pressure.

Subarachnoid hemorrhage may be diagnosed by CT scan or cerebrospinal fluid examination. CT angiography (CTA) or magnetic resonance angiography (MRA) may identify intracranial aneurysm and will exclude other causes of subarachnoid hemorrhage, but cerebral angiography is usually necessary to determine appropriate treatment, of which endovascular therapy or surgical ligation of the aneurysm neck or of the parent arterial trunk are the main options. Supportive treatment, including control of blood pressure and vasodilator therapy, are important during the acute phase of subarachnoid hemorrhage.

Migraine

Migraine is a common episodic illness of unknown cause and varied symptomatology characterized by unilateral headache (which usually alternates sides), visual disturbances, nausea, and vomiting. There is usually a family history. The disease usually manifests between ages 15 and 30 years. It is more common and more severe in women. Many factors, including emotional ones, may predispose or contribute to the attacks.

Photophobia is common during a migraine attack. Visual auras characteristically consist of a repeating triangular colored pattern ("fortification spectrum"), beginning in the center of vision and moving with increasing speed across the same side of the visual field of each eye. The whole episode usually lasts 15–30 minutes. It may be followed by a homonymous hemianopia on the same side that lasts for several hours. Permanent visual field loss rarely develops. It may be due to cerebral infarction but should also arouse suspicion of an underlying arteriovenous malformation. Migrainous visual auras frequently have a less typical pattern. Migraine sufferers may also suffer episodes of transient monocular visual loss (see earlier in the chapter) thought to be due to either retinal or choroidal vasospasm.

PHAKOMATOSES

The phakomatoses are a group of diseases characterized by multiple hamartomas occurring in various organ systems and at variable times.

NEUROFIBROMATOSIS

Neurofibromatosis is a generalized hereditary disease characterized by multiple tumors of the skin, central nervous system, peripheral nerves, and nerve sheaths. Other developmental anomalies, particularly of the bones, may be associated. There are two distinct dominant conditions, both due to inactivating mutations of tumor suppressor genes. Neurofibromatosis 1 is associated with tumors primarily of astrocytes and neurons, whereas neurofibromatosis 2 is associated with tumors of the meninges and Schwann cells. There is no racial predominance. The manifestations may be present at birth but often become apparent during pregnancy, during puberty, and at menopause.

Neurofibromatosis 1 (Recklinghausen's disease) is characterized by multiple café au lait spots (six or more greater than 1.5 cm in diameter) (99%), peripheral neurofibromas, which are usually nodular but may be diffuse (plexiform) and usually cutaneous but may involve deep structures,

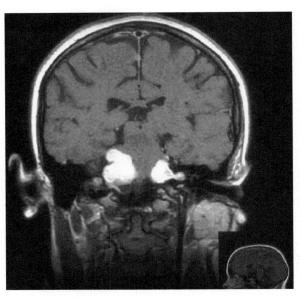

▲ **Figure 14–34.** Coronal MRI of bilateral acoustic neuromas in neurofibromatosis 2.

axillary freckling, and Lisch nodules (iris hamartomas) (93%). Its gene lies on chromosome 17. The frequency is 1:3000 live births, with 100% penetrance but variable expressivity. When lesions are confined to the skin, the prognosis is good. The disease tends to be fairly stationary, with only slow progression over long periods of time. Neurofibromas may need to be removed, for instance to relieve spinal nerve root compression. They may undergo sarcomatous degeneration.

A defining feature of **neurofibromatosis 2** is bilateral vestibular schwannomas (Figure 14–34), but unilateral vestibular schwannoma, other intracranial or spinal schwannoma, multiple intracranial or intraspinal meningiomas, or gliomas may occur. Café au lait spots and peripheral neurofibromas may be present. Its gene lies on chromosome 22. The frequency is 1:35,000.

Ophthalmic Features

In neurofibromatosis 1, as well as Lisch nodules, there may be neurofibromas of the lids, either cutaneous nodular or subcutaneous plexiform (rubbery "bag of worms"). Corneal nerves are often prominent. There may be congenital glaucoma. Anterior visual pathway glioma (see earlier in the chapter) is particularly associated with neurofibromatosis 1, bilateral optic nerve disease being pathognomonic, and many are asymptomatic (30%–80%). A subgroup with nerves having a thickened nerve core and a low-density perineural proliferation are more likely to be symptomatic. Treatment depends on disease location and progression, which is probably less severe than in patients without neurofibromatosis 1.

About 75% of patients with neurofibromatosis 2 have early posterior subcapsular lens opacities. Epiretinal membranes, combined pigment epithelial and retinal hamartomas, optic disk gliomas, and optic nerve sheath meningiomas occur with increased frequency in neurofibromatosis 2.

VON HIPPEL–LINDAU DISEASE

Usually presenting in the second decade and rarely after age 45, von Hippel–Lindau disease is due to a mutation on chromosome 3. Inheritance is autosomal dominant with high penetrance. The incidence is approximately 1:40,000. The most common manifestation is retinal capillary hemangioma. Other manifestations are cerebellar hemangioblastoma; cysts of the kidneys, pancreas, and epididymis; pheochromocytoma; and renal cell carcinoma.

Retinal capillary hemangioma usually develops in the peripheral retina (Figure 10–36). Occasionally, it develops adjacent to the optic disk (juxtapapillary). In the peripheral retina, it initially manifests as dilation and tortuosity of retinal vessels, followed by development of an angiomatous lesion with hemorrhages and exudates. A stage of massive exudation, retinal detachment, and secondary glaucoma occurs later and will cause blindness if left untreated. Among all patients with retinal capillary hemangioma, about 80% have von Hippel–Lindau disease, and they usually have multiple lesions. Among patients with solitary retinal capillary hemangioma, the prevalence of von Hippel–Lindau disease is about 45%. The diagnosis is usually obvious by personal or family history but may become apparent after screening for associated lesions or after genetic testing. Sporadic retinal capillary hemangioma not associated with von Hippel–Lindau disease usually presents in the fourth decade. Any patient with bilateral retinal capillary hemangiomas or multiple lesions in eye—either at presentation or developing during follow-up—must be assumed to have von Hippel–Lindau disease.

▶ Treatment & Prognosis

Retinal capillary hemangiomas may be treated with laser photocoagulation, cryotherapy, or plaque radiotherapy. All patients, particularly those with von Hippel–Lindau disease, need regular screening for detection of new lesions. Patients with von Hippel–Lindau disease also need regular screening for development of central nervous system and abdominal disease. Presymptomatic detection of the lesions of von Hippel–Lindau disease greatly improves the prognosis. First-degree relatives of patients with von Hippel–Lindau disease also need to undergo regular screening. Genetic testing increasingly allows identification of individuals specifically at risk.

STURGE–WEBER SYNDROME

This uncommon nonfamilial disease with unknown inheritance is recognizable at birth by a characteristic nevus flammeus (port wine stain, or venous angioma) on one side of the face. There is corresponding angiomatous involvement (leptomeningeal angiodysplasia) of the meninges and brain, which causes seizures (85%), mental retardation (60%), and cerebral atrophy. Since the cortical lesions calcify, they can be seen on plain skull x-rays after infancy. Unilateral infantile glaucoma on the affected side frequently develops if there is extensive involvement of the conjunctiva with hemangioma of the episclera and anterior chamber anomalies. Lid or conjunctival involvement nearly always implies ultimate intraocular involvement and glaucoma. Forty percent of patients with a port wine stain on the face develop choroidal hemangioma, usually diffuse rather than circumscribed, on the same side.

▶ Treatment & Prognosis

There is no effective treatment for Sturge–Weber syndrome. The glaucoma is difficult to control. Choroidal hemangioma may require treatment with laser photocoagulation or radiotherapy.

WYBURN–MASON SYNDROME

Wyburn–Mason syndrome is a rare disorder of multiple arteriovenous malformations, variably involving the retina, other portions of the anterior visual pathway, the midbrain, the maxilla, and the mandible, all on the same side of the head.

Headaches and seizures are the common presenting symptoms. Large, tortuous, dilated vessels covering extensive areas of the retina are an important diagnostic clue and can cause cystic retinal degeneration with decreased vision. Optic atrophy without retinal lesions can also occur.

ATAXIA–TELANGIECTASIA

Ataxia–telangiectasia is an autosomal recessive disorder characterized by skin and conjunctival telangiectases, cerebellar ataxia, and recurrent sinopulmonary infections. All signs and symptoms are progressive with time, but the ataxia appears first as the child begins to walk, and the telangiectases appear between 4 and 7 years of age. Mental retardation also occurs. The recurrent infections relate to thymic deficiencies and corresponding T-cell abnormalities as well as to deficiency of immunoglobulins. Saccadic and eventually pursuit abnormalities produce a supranuclear ophthalmoplegia.

TUBEROUS SCLEROSIS (BOURNEVILLE'S DISEASE)

Tuberous sclerosis is characterized by the triad of adenoma sebaceum, epilepsy, and mental retardation, although 40%–50% of affected individuals have normal intelligence. Adenoma sebaceum (angiofibromas) occur in 90% of patients over the age of 4 years, and the number of lesions increases with puberty. These flesh-colored papules are

1–2 mm in diameter and have a butterfly distribution on the nose and malar area; they can also occur in the subungual and periungual areas. Ashleaf-shaped hypopigmented ovals can be present on the skin even of neonates and are best seen under Wood's (ultraviolet) light.

Retinal astrocytomas appear as oval or circular white areas in the peripheral fundus and, like optic nerve astrocytomas, characteristically have a mulberry-like appearance (Figure 10–35). Renal hamartomas occur in 70%–80% of patients. Subependymal nodules in the periventricular areas of the brain can calcify and appear as candle-wax gutterings or drippings on radiologic studies. MRI can show actively growing subependymal nodules. These can become astrocytomas. Seizures occur in 70% of patients, often starting within the first year of life.

The disease is inherited sporadically (80%) or as an autosomal dominant disorder with low penetrance. The prevalence may be 1:7000 if patients with the incomplete form of the disease are included. Vision is generally normal, and progression of retinal hamartomas is rare. The prognosis for life relates to the degree of central nervous system involvement. In severe cases, death can occur in the second or third decade; if there is minimal central nervous system involvement, life expectancy should be normal.

CEREBROMACULAR DEGENERATION

The genetically determined (autosomal recessive) lysosomal storage disorders may affect the neural elements of the retina. The clinical forms are classified by the age at onset and the enzyme deficiency. The pathologic changes are present prenatally. Clinical manifestations occur as a critical level of intraneuronal lipid deposition is reached, resulting in a progressive disease, including dementia, visual disturbance, and neuromotor deterioration.

The striking ocular finding of a cherry-red spot in the macula is seen in a number of lysosomal storage disorders, for example, gangliosidosis (Tay–Sachs disease, Sandhoff disease, and generalized GM_1), Niemann–Pick type A (sphingomyelin lipidosis), neuraminidase deficiency (sialidosis and Goldberg syndrome), and Farber disease. A halo occurs from loss of transparency of the ganglion cell ring of the macula, which accentuates the central red of the normal choroidal vasculature. Optic atrophy is also prominent in Tay–Sachs disease and Niemann–Pick type A. Retinal degeneration without a macular cherry-red spot occurs in mucopolysaccharidoses and in the lipopigment storage disorder, neuronal ceroid lipofuscinosis.

Eye movement disorders occur in the lysosomal storage disorders, Niemann–Pick type C (vertical supranuclear gaze palsy) and juvenile (type 3) Gaucher's disease (horizontal supranuclear gaze palsy), and occasionally in Refsum's disease, a disorder of lipid metabolism, and abetalipoproteinemia, the latter two disorders more typically being associated with pigmentary retinopathy.

REFERENCES

Abou Zeid N, Bhatti MT: Acute inflammatory demyelinating optic neuritis: evidence-based visual and neurological considerations. Neurologist 2008;14:207. [PMID: 18617847]

Agarwal S, Kushner BJ: Results of extraocular muscle surgery for superior oblique myokymia. J AAPOS 2009;13:472. [PMID: 19716737]

Antonio-Santos AA, Eggenberger ER: Medical treatment options for ocular myasthenia gravis. Curr Opin Ophthalmol 2008;19:468. [PMID: 18854691]

Bartynski WS: Posterior reversible encephalopathy syndrome, part 1: fundamental imaging and clinical features. AJNR Am J Neuroradiol 2008;29:1036. [PMID: 18356474]

Bartynski WS: Posterior reversible encephalopathy syndrome, part 2: controversies surrounding pathophysiology of vasogenic edema. AJNR Am J Neuroradiol 2008;29:1043. [PMID: 18403560]

Beck RW, Gal RL: Treatment of acute optic neuritis. A summary of findings from the Optic Neuritis Treatment Trial. Arch Ophthalmol 2008;126:994. [PMID: 18625951]

Biswas J et al: Ocular manifestation of storage diseases. Curr Opin Ophthalmol 2008;19:507. [PMID: 18854696]

Bonhomme GR et al: Pediatric optic neuritis: brain MRI abnormalities and risk of multiple sclerosis. Neurology 2009;72:881. [PMID: 19273821]

Borchert M, Garcia-Filion P: The syndrome of optic nerve hypoplasia. Curr Neurol Neurosci Rep 2008;8:395. [PMID: 18713575]

Brazis PW: Clinical review: the surgical treatment of idiopathic pseudotumour cerebri (idiopathic intracranial hypertension). Cephalalgia 2008;28:1361. [PMID: 19037972]

Brazis PW. Isolated palsies of cranial nerves III, IV, and VI. Semin Neurol 2009;29:14. [PMID: 19214929]

Bruce BB et al: Traumatic homonymous hemianopia. J Neurol Neurosurg Psychiatry 2006;77:986. [PMID: 16574725]

Bruce BB et al: Idiopathic intracranial hypertension in men. Neurology 2009;72:304. [PMID: 18923135]

Bruce BB, Biousse V, Newman NJ: Third nerve palsies. Semin Neurol 2007;27:257. [PMID: 17577867]

Chen CS, Miller NR: Ocular ischemic syndrome: review of clinical presentations, etiology, investigation, and management. Compr Ophthalmol Update 2007;8:17. [PMID: 17394756]

Comi G et al: Effect of glatiramer acetate on conversion to clinically definite multiple sclerosis in patients with clinically isolated syndrome (PreCISe study): a randomised, double-blind, placebo-controlled trial. Lancet 2009;374:1503. [PMID: 19815268]

Dale RC, Brilot, Banwell B: Pediatric central nervous system inflammatory demyelination: acute disseminated encephalomyelitis, clinically isolated syndromes, neuromyelitis optica, and multiple sclerosis. Curr Opin Neurol 2009;22:233. [PMID: 19434783]

Fraser JA et al: The treatment of giant cell arteritis. Rev Neurol Dis 2008;5:140. [PMID: 18838954]

Galal A et al: Determinants of postoperative visual recovery in suprasellar meningiomas. Acta Neurochir (Wien) 2010;152:69. [PMID: 19707716]

Golnik KC: Cavitary anomalies of the optic disc: neurologic significance. Curr Neurol Neurosci Rep 2008;8:409. [PMID: 18713577]

Hayreh SS: Management of non-arteritic anterior ischemic optic neuropathy. Graefes Arch Clin Exp Ophthalmol 2009;247:1595. [PMID: 19916247]

Hornyak M, Digre K, Couldwell WT: Neuro-ophthalmologic manifestations of benign anterior skull base lesions. Postgrad Med 2009;121:103. [PMID: 19641276]

Johnson FR et al: Multiple sclerosis patients' benefit-risk preferences: serious adverse event risks versus treatment efficacy. J Neurol 2009;256:554.

Kappos L et al: Long-term effect of early treatment with interferon beta-1b after a first clinical event suggestive of multiple sclerosis: 5-year active treatment extension of the phase 3 BENEFIT trial. Lancet Neurol 2009;8:987. [PMID: 19748319]

Kawasaki A, Kardon RH: Intrinsically photosensitive retinal ganglion cells. J Neuro-Ophthalmol 2007;27:195. [PMID: 17895821]

Kawasaki A, Purvin V: Giant cell arteritis: an updated review. Acta Ophthalmol 2009;87:13. [PMID: 18937808]

Kedar S et al: Pediatric homonymous hemianopia. J AAPOS 2006;10:249. [PMID: 16814179]

Kedar S et al: Congruency in homonymous hemianopia. Am J Ophthalmol 2007;143:772. [PMID: 17362865]

Kerr NM, Chew SSSL, Danesh-Meyer HV: Non-arteritic anterior ischaemic optic neuropathy: a review and update. J Clin Neurosci 2009;16:994. [PMID: 19596112]

Komotar RJ, Roguski M, Bruce JN: Surgical management of craniopharyngiomas. J Neurooncol 2009;92:283. [PMID: 19357956]

Lee AG: Neuroophthalmological management of optic pathway gliomas. Neurosurg Focus 2007;23:E1. [PMID: 18004957]

Luneau K, Newman NJ, Biousse V: Ischemic optic neuropathies. Neurologist 2008;14:341. [PMID: 19008740]

McLean RJ, Gottlob I. The pharmacological treatment of nystagmus: a review. Expert Opin Pharmacother 2009;10:1805. [PMID: 19601699]

Merle H et al: Natural history of the visual impairment of relapsing neuromyelitis optica. Ophthalmology 2007;114:810. [PMID: 17141316]

Miller DH et al: Differential diagnosis of suspected multiple sclerosis:

a consensus approach. Multiple Sclerosis 2008;14:1157. [PMID: 18805839]

Miller DH, Leary SM: Treatment of clinically isolated syndrome: to be PreCISe. Lancet 2009;374:1475. [PMID: 19815269]

Mughal M, Longmuir R: Current pharmacologic testing for Horner syndrome. Curr Neurol Neurosci Rep 2009;9:384. [PMID: 19664368]

Muppidi S, Wolfe GI: Muscle-specific receptor tyrosine kinase antibody-positive and seronegative myasthenia gravis. Front Neurol Neurosci 2009;26:109. [PMID: 19349708]

Newman NJ: Perioperative visual loss after nonocular surgeries. Am J Ophthalmol 2008;145:604. [PMID: 18358851]

Optic Neuritis Study Group: Visual function 15 years after optic neuritis: a final follow-up report from the Optic Neuritis Treatment Trial. Ophthalmology 2008;115:1079. [PMDI: 17976727]

Optic Neuritis Study Group: Multiple sclerosis risk after optic neuritis. Final Optic Neuritis: Treatment Trial follow-up. Arch Neurol 2008;65:727. [PMID: 18541792]

Proulx AA, Strong MJ, Nicolle DA: Creutzfeldt-Jakob disease presenting with visual manifestations. Can J Ophthalmol 2008;43:591. [PMID: 18982039]

Pula JH, Eggenberger E: Posterior reversible encephalopathy syndrome. Curr Opin Ophthalmol 2008;19:479. [PMID: 18854692]

Rucker JC: Oculomotor disorders. Semin Neurol 2007;27:244. [PMID: 17577866]

Swanton JK et al: Early MRI in optic neuritis: the risk for disability. Neurology 2009;72:542. [PMID: 19204264]

Taylor D: Developmental abnormalities of the optic nerve and chiasm. Eye 2007;21:1271. [PMID: 17914430]

Volpe NJ: The Optic Neuritis Treatment Trial. A definitive answer and profound impact with unexpected results. Arch Ophthalmol 2008;126:996. [PMID: 18625952]

Wall M: Idiopathic intracranial hypertension (pseudotumor cerebri). Curr Neurol Neurosci Rep 2008;8:87. [PMID: 18460275]

Walsh MT, Couldwell WT: Management options for cavernous sinus meningiomas. J Neurooncol 2009;92:307. [PMID: 19357958]

Wang X et al: Giant cell arteritis. Rheumatol Int 2008;29:1. [PMID: 18716781]

Wingerchuk DM et al: The spectrum of neuromyelitis optica. Lancet Neurol 2007;6:805. [PMID: 17706564]

Yonghong J et al: Detailed magnetic resonance imaging findings of the ocular motor nerves in Duane's retraction syndrome. J Pediatr Ophthalmol Strabismus 2009;46:278. [PMID: 19791724]

Young NP, Weinshenker BG, Lucchinetti CF: Acute disseminated excephalomyelitis: current understanding and controversies. Semin Neurol 2008;28:84. [PMID: 18256989]

Yu-Wai-Man P et al: Inherited mitochondrial optic neuropathies. J Med Genet 2009;46:145. [PMID: 19001017]

Zhang X et al: Homonymous hemianopias: clinical-anatomic correlations in 904 cases. Neurology 2006;66:906. [PMID: 16567710]

Zhang X et al: Natural history of homonymous hemianopia. Neurology 2006;66:901. [PMID: 16567709]

Zhang X et al: Homonymous hemianopia in stroke. J Neuroophthalmol 2006;26:180. [PMID: 16966935]

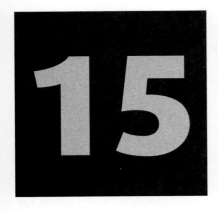

Ocular Disorders Associated with Systemic Diseases

Edward Pringle, MRCP, MRCOphth, and
Elizabeth M. Graham, FRCP, FRCOphth

Examination of the eye provides invaluable information for the diagnosis and monitoring of systemic disease. Nowhere else in the body can a microcirculatory system be directly visualized, investigated with such precision or neural tissue so easily examined, and nowhere else are the results of minute focal lesions so devastating. Many systemic diseases involve the eyes, and therapy demands some knowledge of the vascular, rheologic, and immunologic nature of these diseases.

▼ VASCULAR DISEASE

NORMAL ANATOMY & PHYSIOLOGY

The blood supply to the eye is from the ophthalmic artery, which is the first branch of the internal carotid artery (see Chapter 1). The first branches of the ophthalmic artery are the central retinal artery and the long posterior ciliary arteries. The retina is perfused by retinal and choroidal vessels that provide contrasting anatomic and physiologic circulations. The retinal arteries correspond to arterioles in the systemic circulation. They function as end arteries and feed a capillary bed consisting of small capillaries (7 μm) with tight endothelial junctions. Dependent on this anatomic arrangement is the maintenance of the blood-retina barrier, and this system is autoregulated, there being no autonomic nerve fibers. Most of the blood within the eye, however, is in the choroidal circulation, which is characterized by a high flow rate, autonomic regulation, and an anatomic arrangement with collateral branching and large capillaries (30 μm), all of which have fenestrations in juxtaposition to Bruch's membrane. Examination of the retinal vessels is facilitated by the use of red-free light and fluorescein angiography, whereas indocyanine green angiography gives further information about the choroidal vessels.

CLINICAL MANIFESTATIONS

▶ Hemorrhages

The sources of fundal hemorrhages may be arteries, capillaries, or veins, and their configurations depend on the site and severity of the disruption of vascular integrity (Figure 15–1). They usually indicate some abnormality of the retinal or choroidal vascular system but they may be caused by any condition that alters the efficacy of the endothelial barrier. The contribution of systemic factors should be considered in relation to (1) vessel wall disease (eg, hypertension, diabetes), (2) blood disorders (eg, thrombocytopenia, anemia, leukemia), and (3) reduced perfusion (eg, carotid artery–cavernous sinus fistula, acute blood loss).

A. Preretinal Hemorrhages

These result from damage to superficial disk or retinal vessels, which commonly are the consequence of retinal neovascularization, and are usually large with a crescentic shape, a gravity-dependent fluid level forming the superior border, and the extent of posterior vitreous detachment determining the lower border.

B. Linear Hemorrhages

These lie in the superficial nerve fiber layer and their shape, often so-called flame-shaped, reflects the orientation of the retinal ganglion cell axons in the affected area of the fundus.

C. Punctate Hemorrhages

These are situated deeper in the substance of the retina, their source being capillaries and smaller venules. Their circular appearance reflects the compact arrangement of the deeper retinal tissues.

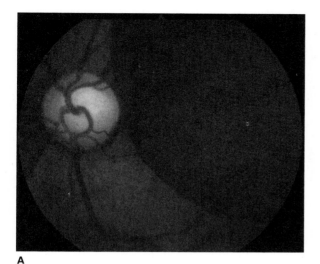

A

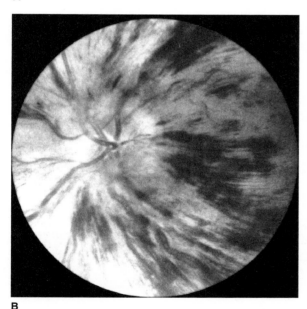

B

▲ **Figure 15–1.** See color insert. **A:** Large preretinal hemorrhage due to severe straining. **B:** Flame-shaped retinal hemorrhages in the nerve fiber layer radiating out from the optic disk. Three days before the photograph was taken, the patient experienced sudden loss of vision, which left him with light perception only.

D. Subretinal Hemorrhages

Normally there are no blood vessels between the retina and the choroid, but these may arise due to optic disk abnormalities or whenever there is subretinal neovascularization. They are large and red, with a well-defined margin and no fluid level.

E. Hemorrhages under the Retinal Pigment Epithelium

Hemorrhages situated under the retinal pigment epithelium are usually dark and large, their source being choroidal vessels. They need to be differentiated from choroidal melanomas and hemangiomas.

F. White Centered Hemorrhages (Roth's Spots)

Although commonly thought to be peculiar to subacute bacterial endocarditis, superficial retinal hemorrhages with pale or white centers are not pathognomonic of any disease process. They may be due to (1) a cotton-wool spot (see later in the chapter) with surrounding hemorrhage; (2) retinal hemorrhage in combination with extravasation of white blood cells (eg, leukemia); or (3) retinal hemorrhage with central resolution.

▶ Acute Ocular Ischemia

A. Optic Disk Infarction (Anterior Ischemic Optic Neuropathy)

Impairment of the blood supply to the optic disk produces sudden visual loss, usually with an altitudinal field defect, and sectoral pallid swelling of the optic disk. The primary abnormality is complete or partial interruption of the choroidal blood supply to the disk, while the retinal capillaries on the surface of the disk appear dilated. Fluorescein angiography confirms the circulatory alterations (Figure 15–2). Pathologic studies show infarction of the retrolaminar region of the optic nerve. The explanation for the vulnerability of the short posterior ciliary vessels supplying this region is unclear.

The most common cause is non-arteritic anterior ischemic optic neuropathy (NAION), in which the optic disk is small, the so-called "disk at risk," and hypertension and arteriosclerotic disease are the commonly identified additional factors in middle age, although it is uncertain whether vascular occlusion or a perfusion deficit is the precipitating event. With increasing likelihood with increasing age over 50 years, optic disk infarction may be caused by giant cell arteritis. Other systemic vasculitides (such as ANCA-associated vasculitis) may also present with anterior ischemic optic neuropathy. The visual loss is usually less severe than in GCA and the disc may not be small as in NAION. Bilateral optic disk infarction can be seen after sudden hypotension following acute blood loss, but posterior (retrobulbar) optic nerve infarction without optic disc changes in the acute stage is more typical.

B. Choroidal Infarction

This is extremely rare, although certain clinical appearances have been attributed to ciliary vessel occlusion. These include small pale areas in the equatorial region that resolve to leave

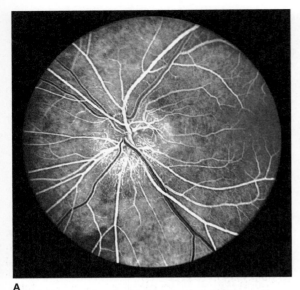

A

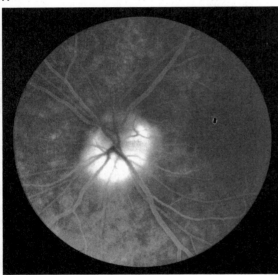

B

▲ **Figure 15–2.** Ischemic optic neuropathy. Sudden visual loss in a 48-year-old man produced a complete inferior altitudinal field loss. **A:** Fluorescein angiogram shows impaired filling of the upper part of the disk with dilation of retinal capillaries at the lower part of the disk. **B:** Photograph taken 10 minutes after injection shows leakage of dye mainly at the lower part of the disk.

mottled pigmentary areas (Elschnig's spots) due to necrosis of the pigment epithelium. Larger infarcts may occur and may be triangular (Amalric's sign) or linear (Siegrist streaks) (Figure 15–3).

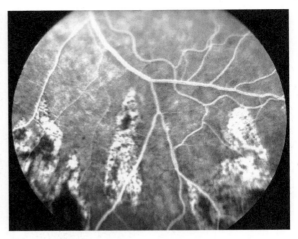

▲ **Figure 15–3.** Anti-phospholipid antibody syndrome. Fluorescein angiogram demonstrates choroidal infarcts in a patient who presented with multiple strokes.

C. Retinal Infarction or Ischemia

The funduscopic appearance of arteriolar occlusion depends on the size of the vessel occluded, the duration of occlusion, and the time course. Occlusion of major arterioles (retinal arteries) produces total, hemispheric, or segmental pallid swelling of the retina, with corresponding visual loss (Figure 15–4) (see Chapter 10). Central retinal artery occlusion is usually due to atherosclerosis but can result from embolic disease. It can also be a manifestation of giant cell arteritis in the elderly. Branch retinal artery occlusion is more commonly due to emboli (see later in the chapter).

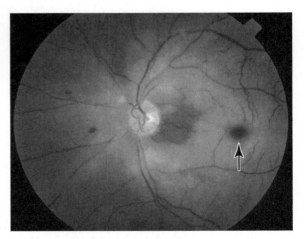

▲ **Figure 15–4.** Central retinal artery occlusion, with pallid retinal swelling and a "cherry red spot" at the fovea **(arrow)** in a patient with hypertension.

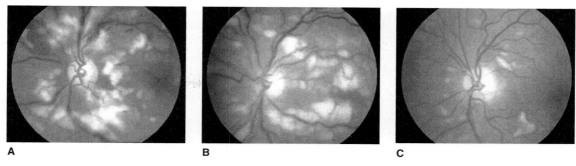

A   **B**   **C**

▲ **Figure 15–5.** Cotton-wool spots. Numerous cotton-wool spots are seen in the posterior poles in three patients. **(A)** A young woman with acute systemic lupus erythematosus and neurologic disease. **(B)** A young man with pancreatitis (Purtscher's retinopathy). **(C)** A patient with HIV infection. Cotton-wool spots resolve over 6 weeks regardless of their cause.

A cotton-wool spot (Figure 15–5), representing interruption of axoplasmic transport in the axons of the retinal nerve fiber layer due to superficial retinal ischemia, is usually due to occlusion of a precapillary retinal arteriole but occasionally may result from more proximal impairment of retinal blood flow. It consists of pale, slightly elevated swelling usually one-fourth to one-half the size of the optic disk. Pathologic examination shows distention of neurons, with cytoid bodies (Figure 15–6); electron microscopy shows accumulation of axoplasm and organelles.

D. Transient Retinal Ischemia due to Emboli (Amaurosis Fugax)

Episodes of complete monocular visual loss with full recovery after 5–10 minutes, the beginning and end often being described as a curtain passing vertically across the vision, are characteristic of transient retinal ischemia due to transit of platelet-fibrin emboli through the retinal circulation (amaurosis fugax). Paresthesias or weakness in the contralateral limbs confirm involvement of the vascular territory of the internal carotid artery, with embolization into the ophthalmic and middle cerebral arteries.

Retinal emboli most commonly arise from carotid artery disease (see Chapter 14). A cardiac cause such as atrial fibrillation, mitral or aortic valve disease, or subacute infective endocarditis needs to be considered, particularly in patients under 40 years of age or those with a history of cardiac disease. It is important for the ophthalmologist to search the fundus for emboli, although frequently they are not seen; auscultate for carotid bruits and cardiac murmurs; check the pulse for atrial fibrillation; and arrange investigations for disease of the carotids, including for underlying risk factors, and cardiac disease as appropriate. Retinal emboli, whether or not associated with retinal dysfunction, indicate a risk of stroke and the incidental discovery of usually cholesterol emboli should prompt similar assessment.

The three main types of retinal emboli are:

1. **Cholesterol emboli**—These so-called Hollenhorst plaques usually arise from an atheromatous plaque in the carotid artery. They initially lodge at the bifurcation of retinal arterioles, are refractile, and may appear larger than the vessel that contains them but may not obstruct the blood flow (Figure 15–7). Passage of a cholesterol embolus may result in permanent focal arteriolar whitening.

2. **Platelet-fibrin emboli**—These are usually broken up as they traverse the retinal circulation, and hence are rarely seen, although occasionally they produce retinal infarction. Usually arising from abnormalities of the great vessels or heart, they may be reduced by drugs that reduce platelet aggregation (eg, aspirin).

3. **Calcific emboli**—Originating from damaged cardiac valves, these solid emboli usually lodge permanently within a retinal arteriole, producing complete occlusion and infarction of the distal retina.

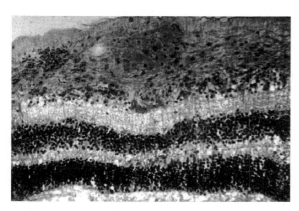

▲ **Figure 15–6.** Cotton-wool spot. Histologic examination shows cytoid bodies and distended neurons in the superficial retinal layers. Deeper retinal layers are normal. (Courtesy of N Ashton.)

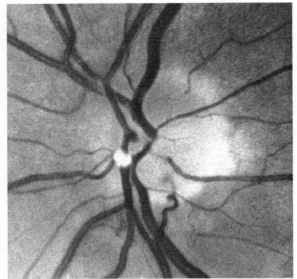

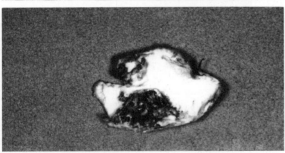

▲ **Figure 15–7.** Cholesterol embolus (Hollenhorst plaque). **Top:** A cholesterol embolus at the optic disk, which is refractile and appears larger than the vessel that contains it. A collateral vessel is seen at the lower border of the disk. **Bottom:** Surgical specimen from a patient with a similar embolus shows an atheromatous ulcer at the bifurcation of the common carotid artery.

Table 15–1. Causes of Transient Visual Loss

Retinal emboli (amaurosis fugax) or cerebral emboli
Carotid artery stenosis, ulceration, or dissection
Basilar or vertebral artery disease (cerebral not retinal emboli)
Cardiac dysrhythmia (eg, atrial fibrillation)
Cardiac valvular disease (eg, mitral leaflet prolapse)
Left ventricular aneurysm with mural thrombus secondary to myocardial infarction

Arterial occlusive disease
Internal carotid artery occlusion
Basilar or vertebral artery occlusion
Arteritis (eg, giant cell arteritis)

Hematologic disease
Anemia
Polycythemia
Macroglobulinemia
Sickle cell disease

Other
Systemic hypertension
Systemic hypotension
   Drugs
   Cardiac dysrhythmia
   Impaired left ventricular function
   Autonomic dysfunction (eg, diabetes mellitus)
   Endocrine dysfunction (eg, Addison's disease)
   Blood loss
   Shock
Migraine, including retinal (choroidal) migraine
Raised intraocular pressure
Raised intracranial pressure

► Central Retinal Vein Occlusion (Figure 15–8)

Central retinal vein occlusion is an important cause of visual morbidity in elderly people, particularly those with hypertension or glaucoma.

Fundus examination shows dilated tortuous veins with retinal and macular edema, hemorrhages all over the posterior pole, and cotton-wool spots. The arterioles are usually attenuated, indicating generalized microvascular disease.

Fluorescein angiography demonstrates two types of response: a nonischemic type, with dilation of retinal vessels and edema; and an ischemic type, with large areas of capillary nonperfusion or evidence of retinal or anterior segment neovascularization. In less than 10% of ischemic but over 80% of nonischemic central retinal vein occlusions, the ultimate visual acuity is better than 20/200.

Central retinal vein occlusion has an increased incidence in certain systemic conditions such as hypertension, hyperlipidemia, diabetes mellitus, collagen-vascular diseases, chronic renal failure, and hyperviscosity syndromes (eg, myeloma, Waldenström's macroglobulinemia). Smoking is also a risk

There are several other causes of transient visual loss, including cerebral emboli, arterial occlusive disease, including giant cell arteritis, hematologic disease, systemic hypertension, systemic hypotension that may be due to various entities, migraine, raised intraocular pressure, and raised intracranial pressure (Table 15–1).

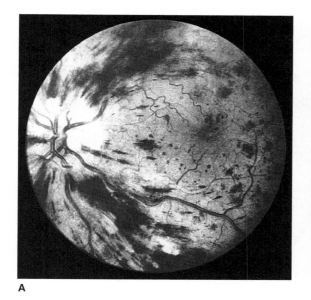 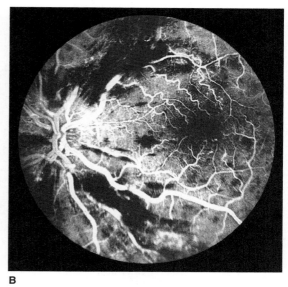

A **B**

▲ **Figure 15–8.** Central retinal vein occlusion. **A:** Photograph shows linear hemorrhages in the nerve fiber layer and punctate hemorrhages in the deeper retinal layers. **B:** Fluorescein angiogram shows dilation of the veins.

factor. Central retinal vein occlusion is associated with increased mortality from ischemic heart disease, including myocardial infarction. Investigations include measurement of serum lipids, plasma proteins, plasma glucose, and assessment of blood viscosity by hemoglobin, hematocrit, and fibrinogen estimations. In young patients, the antiphospholipid antibody syndrome should be excluded, and protein C, protein S, factor V Leiden, homocysteine, and antithrombin III levels should be measured to exclude abnormalities of the thrombolytic system. If hypertension is present, simple renal function tests, including urea and electrolytes, estimation of creatinine clearance, microscopic examination of the urine, and renal ultrasound are indicated.

Treatment of retinal vein occlusion is unsatisfactory. Randomized controlled trials treating patients with hemodilution have reported variable results. Trials with anticoagulants and fibrinolytic agents have not been successful. Intravitreal vascular endothelial growth factor (VEGF) inhibitors or steroid may be indicated, and surgical procedures are being investigated (see Chapter 10). In ischemic central retinal vein occlusion, pan-retinal laser photocoagulation is effective in preventing and treating secondary neovascular glaucoma.

Occasionally, central retinal vein occlusion occurs in young people and may be associated with cells in the vitreous. Rheologic investigations are usually negative, and the prognosis for vision is good.

Retinal Branch Vein Occlusion (Figure 15–9)

Occlusion of a branch vein should be viewed as part of the spectrum of central retinal vein occlusion. Investigations are similar in the two conditions, but arterial disease—particularly

hypertension—is common. Branch retinal vein occlusion occurs more frequently in the superotemporal and inferotemporal regions and particularly at sites where arteries cross over veins, and only rarely where veins cross over arteries.

The roles of laser treatment, intravitreal anti-VEGF agents or steroid, and surgery in the management of branch retinal vein occlusion are discussed in Chapters 10 and 24.

ATHEROSCLEROSIS & ARTERIOSCLEROSIS

The process of atherosclerosis occurs in larger arteries and is due to fatty infiltration of a patchy nature occurring in the intima and associated with fibrosis. Involvement of smaller vessels (ie, < 300 μm) by diffuse fibrosis and hyalinization is termed arteriosclerosis. The retinal vessels beyond the disk are less than 300 μm; therefore, involvement of the retinal arterioles should be termed arteriosclerosis, whereas involvement of the central retinal artery is properly termed atherosclerosis.

Atherosclerosis is a progressive change developing in the second decade, with lipid streaks in larger vessels, progressing to a fibrous plaque in the third decade. In the fourth and fifth decades, ulceration, hemorrhages, and thrombosis occur, and the lesion may be calcified. Destruction of the elastic and muscular elements of the media produces ectasia and rupture of the large vessels, although in smaller vessels obstruction is usually seen. The clinical results of atherosclerosis are seen several decades after the onset of the process. Factors contributing to atheroma include hyperlipidemia, hypertension, and obesity.

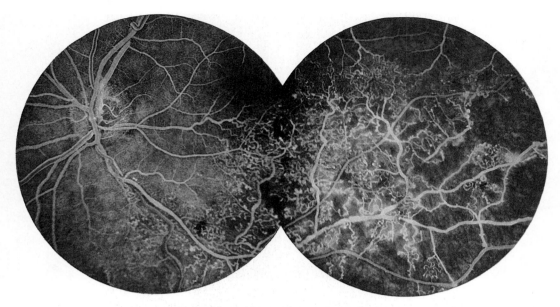

▲ **Figure 15–9.** Retinal branch vein occlusion. The affected segment of retina shows changes of reduced perfusion. This results in irregularity of the arterioles and veins, areas of capillary closure, and dilated capillaries with microaneurysms.

Arteriosclerosis is characterized by an enhanced light reflection, focal attenuation, and irregularity of caliber. These signs may also be seen in the arterioles of normotensive individuals in middle age. In elderly individuals with arteriosclerosis and associated mild hypertension, it is difficult to differentiate the changes of arteriosclerosis from those due to hypertension.

▶ Appearance of Retinal Vessels

A normal arteriolar wall is transparent, so that what is actually seen is the column of blood within the vessel. A thin, central light reflection in the center of the blood column appears as a yellow refractile line about one-fifth the width of the column. As the walls of the arterioles become infiltrated with lipids and cholesterol, the vessels become sclerotic. As this process continues, the vessel wall gradually loses its transparency and becomes visible; the blood column appears wider than normal, and the thin light reflection becomes broader. The grayish yellow fat products in the vessel wall blend with the red of the blood column to produce a typical "copper wire" appearance. This indicates moderate arteriosclerosis. As sclerosis proceeds, the blood column-vessel wall light reflection resembles "silver wire," which indicates severe arteriosclerosis; at times, even occlusion of an arteriolar branch may occur.

Red-free light (a white light with a green filter) allows details of hemorrhages, focal irregularity of blood vessels, and nerve fibers to be seen more clearly (Figure 15–10).

HYPERTENSIVE RETINOCHOROIDOPATHY

The appearance of the fundus in hypertensive retinochoroidopathy is determined by the degree of elevation of the blood pressure and the state of the retinal arterioles. In mild to moderate systemic hypertension, the retinal signs may be subtle. Focal attenuation of a major retinal arteriole is one of the earliest signs. Diffuse arteriolar attenuation, broadening of the arteriolar light reflex, and arteriovenous crossing changes also occur. However, in young patients with accelerated malignant hypertension, an extensive retinopathy is seen, with hemorrhages, retinal infarcts (cotton-wool spots), choroidal infarcts, and occasionally serous detachment of the retina. Severe disk edema is a prominent feature and may be accompanied by a macular star of hard exudates (Figure 15–11). Vision may be impaired and may deteriorate further if blood pressure is reduced too quickly.

In contrast, elderly patients with arteriosclerotic vessels are unable to respond in this manner, and their vessels are thus protected by the arteriosclerosis. It is for this reason that elderly patients seldom exhibit florid hypertensive retinochoroidopathy (Figure 15–12).

In young patients with hypertension, fluorescein angiography demonstrates arteriolar attenuation and occlusion and capillary nonperfusion in relation to a cotton-wool spot, which is surrounded by abnormal dilated capillaries and microaneurysms with increased permeability. Resolution of the cotton-wool spots and the arteriolar changes occurs with successful hypotensive therapy. In elderly patients, the underlying arterio-sclerotic changes are irreversible.

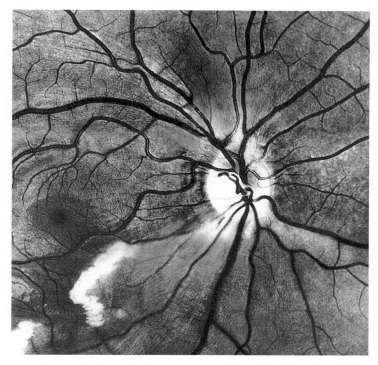

▲ **Figure 15–10.** Acute retinal infarction. Red-free photograph shows acute arterial occlusion in a congenitally anomalous vessel at the disk. The inferior retina is infarcted, but axoplasm has accumulated beneath the fovea in an irregular pattern owing to preserved neuronal function of the distal ganglion cells.

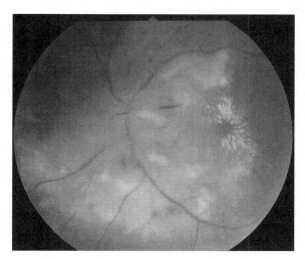

▲ **Figure 15–11.** Accelerated hypertension in a young woman manifesting as marked optic disk edema, macular star of hard exudates, serous retinal detachment, and retinal hemorrhages and cotton-wool spots. See color insert.

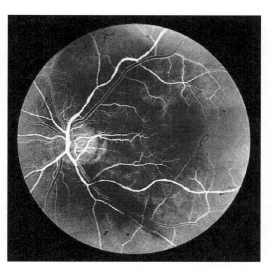

▲ **Figure 15–12.** Accelerated hypertension. Fluorescein angiogram in an elderly woman showing marked arteriolar constriction and irregularity but few signs of florid retinopathy.

▶ Other Forms of Hypertensive Retinochoroidopathy

A severe retinochoroidopathy may be seen in advanced renal disease, in patients with pheochromocytoma, and in preeclampsia–eclampsia. All such patients should receive a complete medical workup to establish the nature of the hypertension.

CHRONIC OCULAR ISCHEMIA

Reduction in the retinal arteriovenous pressure gradient may produce acute signs of ocular ischemia (see preceding pages) or the less frequently recognized chronic changes.

▶ Carotid Occlusive Disease

Carotid occlusive disease usually presents in middle-aged and elderly patients and is due to involvement of both the carotid artery and its smaller branches. Contributory factors include hypertension, smoking, and hyperlipidemia.

In anterior segment ischemia, patients develop iritis, intraocular pressure changes, and pupillary abnormalities. In retinal ischemia (Figure 15–13A), patients show evidence of capillary dilation and hemorrhages, capillary occlusion, new vessels at the optic disk, and cotton-wool spots.

▶ Carotid Artery–Cavernous Sinus Fistula

Carotid artery–cavernous sinus fistula results from a communication between the carotid artery or its branches and the cavernous sinus. Direct fistulas occur as a consequence of rupture of the intracavernous internal carotid artery, due to aneurysm, weakened vessel wall (eg, collagen vascular disease and Ehler's Danlos syndrome), or trauma. They usually have an acute, florid presentation and commonly require closure. Indirect (dural) fistulas are chronic and mild. They are associated with diabetes and systemic hypertension and may be a consequence of thrombosis of dural veins. Frequently they resolve spontaneously. Clinical features of carotid artery–cavernous sinus fistulas include dilated conjunctival and episcleral vessels, elevated intraocular pressure, dilated retinal vessels with hemorrhages and fluorescein leakage (Figure 15–13B), ophthalmoplegia (usually lateral rectus), and bruit. Computed tomography (CT) and magnetic resonance imaging (MRI) show thickened ocular muscles and a dilated superior ophthalmic vein, the latter being a differentiating feature from thyroid eye disease. Reversal of flow ("arterializations") in the superior ophthalmic vein is a characteristic finding on orbital ultrasound blood flow studies. When required, closure of carotid artery–cavernous sinus fistulas is usually achieved by interventional radiological techniques.

IDIOPATHIC (BENIGN) INTRACRANIAL HYPERTENSION (PSEUDOTUMOR CEREBRI)

Idiopathic intracranial hypertension is characterized by raised intracranial pressure with normal cerebrospinal fluid

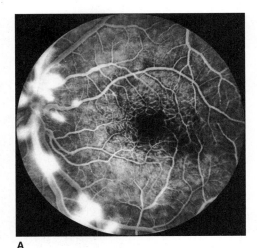

A

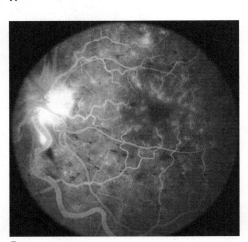

B

▲ **Figure 15–13. A:** Fluorescein angiogram of left fundus in a patient with chronic ocular ischemia secondary to Takayasu's disease. Note capillary dilation, leakage of dye, retinal hemorrhages, cotton-wool spots, and neovascularization of the optic nerve head. **B:** Fluorescein angiogram, showing leakage at optic disk and macula in a patient with chronic ocular ischemia secondary to dural arteriovenous fistula.

constituents and normal radiologic studies, particularly no evidence of cerebral venous sinus occlusion. The cause of the increased intracranial pressure is unknown, although diminished absorption of cerebrospinal fluid due to impaired venous sinus drainage is suspected. Usually patients are young overweight women and present with headache; transient visual obscurations, blurred vision, and diplopia are the ophthalmologic features. Etiologic factors that need to be excluded include (1) drug therapy, particularly tetracyclines, retinoids including

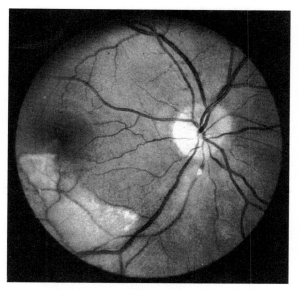

▲ **Figure 15–14.** Subacute bacterial endocarditis. Calcific embolus impacted in arteriole below the disk, producing a distal area of retinal infarction.

vitamin A, prolonged steroid therapy or in children steroid withdrawal, and possibly hormonal contraceptives; (2) endocrine abnormalities; and (3) sleep apnea syndrome. Idiopathic intracranial hypertension is very rare in adult men.

Initially visual fields are normal apart from enlarged blind spots due to papilledema. Generalized field constriction and inferonasal and arcuate defects may occur. CT or MRI usually shows distended optic nerve sheaths, flattened globes, and an empty pituitary sella. The aims of treatment are to minimize permanent visual loss, which occurs in up to 50% of patients, and relieve symptoms. Treatment options include weight loss, oral acetazolamide or other diuretics, cerebrospinal fluid shunt, and optic nerve sheath fenestration (see also Chapter 14).

SUBACUTE INFECTIVE ENDOCARDITIS

Inflammatory changes on the cardiac valves may produce multiple embolization with frequent ocular manifestations that range from retinal and choroidal infarction to a mild infective vitritis. The emboli may be composed of platelet-fibrin aggregates or calcified endocardial vegetations (Figure 15–14).

▼ HEMATOLOGIC & LYMPHATIC DISORDERS

LEUKEMIA

The ocular changes of leukemia occur primarily in those structures with a good blood supply, including the retina, the

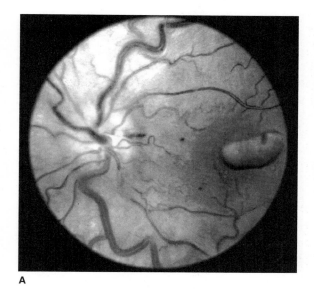

A

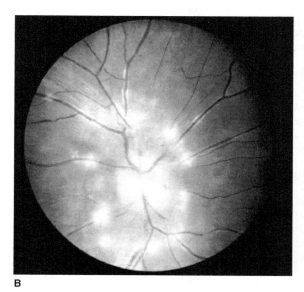

B

▲ **Figure 15–15.** **A:** Retinal changes in chronic myeloid leukemia, where dilated veins and hemorrhages may be seen. **B:** In acute lymphoblastic leukemia, infiltration of the disk may be seen.

choroid, and the optic disk (Figure 15–15). Changes are most common in the acute leukemias, where hemorrhages are seen in the nerve fiber and pre-retinal layers.

HYPERVISCOSITY SYNDROMES

Increased viscosity results in reduced flow ocular perfusion, producing dilation of the retinal arteries and veins, hemorrhages,

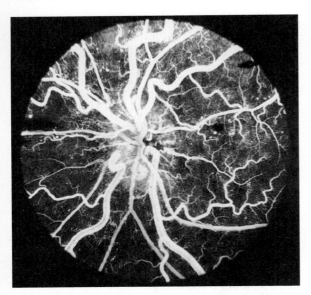

▲ **Figure 15–16.** Hyperviscosity syndrome. Dilated arteries and veins, with hemorrhages and microaneurysms in a patient with hyperviscosity due to elevated IgM levels.

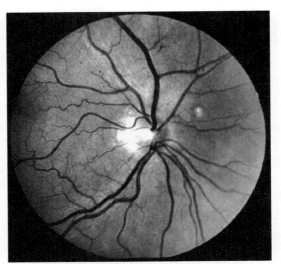

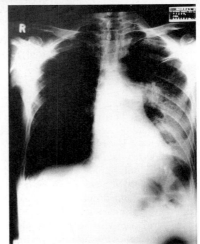

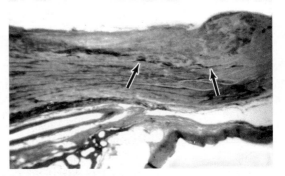

microaneurysms, and areas of capillary closure (Figure 15–16). The main causes are polycythemia, either primary or secondary, macroglobulinemia, and multiple myeloma. Treatment of the hyperviscosity can reverse the retinal changes.

SICKLE CELL DISEASE

Sickle cell hemoglobinopathies are heritable disorders in which the normal adult hemoglobin is replaced by sickle hemoglobin in the red cell. This causes "sickle-shaped" deformity of the red cell on deoxygenation.

Ocular abnormalities include conjunctival changes, with "comma-shaped capillaries," and retinal changes, including arterial occlusions and peripheral capillary closure, which leads to new vessel formation, particularly a sea-fan pattern. Retinal detachment may develop. Laser therapy is rarely needed, since the complexes fibrose and reperfusion can occur.

NEOPLASTIC DISEASE (FIGURE 15–17)

Neoplastic disease may involve the eye and optic pathways by direct spread, metastases, or immunologic mechanisms.

The consequences of metastatic spread depend on the size and site of the metastatic tumor and the site of the primary lesion. The most frequent primary tumor metastasizing to the eye is carcinoma of the breast in women and bronchial carcinoma in men (see Chapters 7 and 10). Most patients have a known history of cancer, but in a third of

▲ **Figure 15–17.** Neoplastic disease. **A:** Normal fundus of a patient with rapid visual loss in his only eye. **B:** Chest x-ray showed left lower lobe consolidation and a hilar mass. **C:** Carcinoma of the bronchus was confirmed at autopsy, and metastasis was found in the optic nerve in the region of the canal **(arrows).**

patients presenting with ocular metastasis the primary tumor has yet to be diagnosed. Visual loss may occur from nonmetastatic disease, due to so-called cancer-associated retinopathy (CAR), melanoma-associated retinopathy (MAR), each associated with specific retinal autoantibodies and characteristic electrophysiological abnormalities, or diffuse uveal melanocytic proliferation.

▼ METABOLIC DISORDERS

DIABETES MELLITUS

Diabetes mellitus is a complex metabolic disorder that involves the small blood vessels, often causing widespread damage to tissues, including the eyes.

The risk of ocular complications is increased by poor diabetic control but they still occur approximately 20 years after onset despite apparently adequate control. The lengthened life span of diabetics has resulted in a marked increase in the incidence of retinopathy and other ocular complications. The visual outlook is generally better for type 2 than for type 1 diabetics.

The possibility of diabetes should be considered in all patients with unexplained retinopathy, cataract, extraocular muscle palsy, optic neuropathy, or sudden changes in refractive error. Absence of glycosuria or a normal fasting blood glucose level does not exclude a diagnosis of diabetes.

▶ Diabetic Retinopathy (Figures 15–18 to 15–21)

Diabetic retinopathy is a common cause of blindness. In the Western world, it accounts for almost one-fourth of blind registrations and is the commonest cause of new blindness in the population of working age.

Good control of diabetes and hypertension retards the development of retinopathy and other diabetic complications.

Type 1 diabetics develop a severe form of retinopathy within 20 years in 60%–75% of cases even if under good

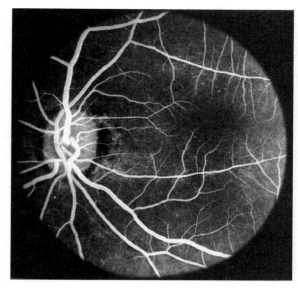

▲ **Figure 15–19.** Diabetic retinopathy. Fluorescein angiogram shows earliest stage with microaneurysm in the macular region.

control. The retinopathy is usually proliferative. In the usually older type 2 diabetic patients, retinopathy is more often nonproliferative, with the risk of severe central visual loss from maculopathy.

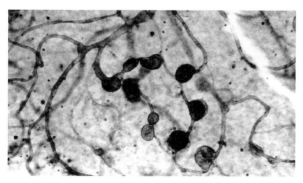

▲ **Figure 15–18.** Diabetic retinopathy stage I. Trypsin-digested whole mount showing microaneurysms of the retinal capillaries.

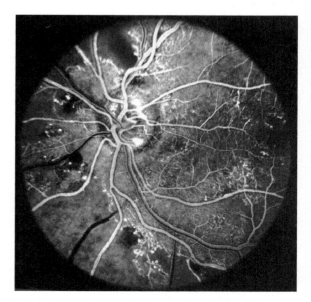

▲ **Figure 15–20.** Diabetic retinopathy. Fluorescein angiogram shows florid retinopathy of diabetes with extensive areas of capillary closure, dilated capillaries with microaneurysms, and early new vessel formation at the optic disk.

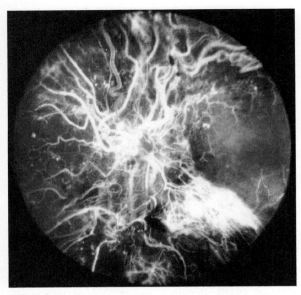

▲ **Figure 15–21.** Proliferative diabetic retinopathy. Fluorescein angiogram shows extensive growth of vessels into the vitreous with marked fluorescein leakage.

The clinical features and treatment of diabetic retinopathy are detailed in Chapter 10.

▶ Lens Changes

A. True Diabetic Cataract (Rare)

Bilateral cataracts occasionally occur with a rapid onset in severe juvenile diabetes. The lens may become completely opaque in several weeks.

B. Senile Cataract in the Diabetic (Common)

Typical senile nuclear sclerosis, posterior subcapsular changes, and cortical opacities occur earlier and more frequently in diabetics.

C. Sudden Changes in the Refraction of the Lens

Especially when diabetes is not well controlled, changes in blood glucose levels may cause changes in refractive power by as much as 3 or 4 diopters of hyperopia or myopia.

▶ Iris Changes

Glycogen infiltration of the pigment epithelium and sphincter and dilator muscles of the iris may cause diminished pupillary responses. The reflexes may also be altered by the autonomic neuropathy of diabetes.

Rubeosis iridis is a serious complication of the retinal ischemia that is also the stimulus to retinal neovascularization in severe diabetic retinopathy. Numerous small intertwining

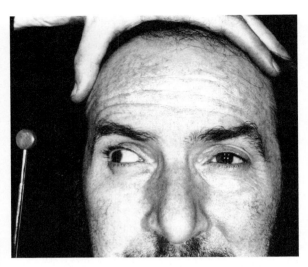

▲ **Figure 15–22.** Pupil-sparing third nerve palsy in diabetes mellitus. Sudden painful ophthalmoplegia, left ptosis, failure of adduction, and normal pupillary responses.

blood vessels develop on the anterior surface of the iris. Spontaneous hyphema may occur. Formation of peripheral anterior synechiae blocks aqueous outflow resulting in secondary (rubeotic) glaucoma.

▶ Extraocular Muscle Palsy (Figure 15–22)

This common occurrence in diabetes is manifested by a sudden onset of diplopia, caused by paresis of one or more extraocular muscles due to infarction of one of the ocular motor nerves. It may be the first manifestation of diabetes. When the third nerve is involved, pain may be a prominent symptom. Differentiation from a posterior communicating aneurysm is important; in diabetic third nerve palsy, the pupil is usually spared. Recovery of ocular motor function begins within 3 months after onset and usually is complete. The fourth and sixth nerves may be similarly involved.

▶ Optic Neuropathy

Visual loss is usually due to infarction of the optic disk (nonarteritic anterior ischemic optic neuropathy). Diabetic papillopathy manifests as chronic optic disk swelling, usually with mild visual impairment.

▼ ENDOCRINE DISEASES

Disturbances of the endocrine glands have a number of important ocular manifestations. By far the most important of these are due to disturbances of the thyroid gland, although parathyroid and pituitary abnormalities also produce significant ocular changes.

THYROID GLAND DISORDERS

1. GRAVES' DISEASE

The term Graves' disease denotes hyperthyroidism due to an autoimmune process. A small proportion of patients with Graves' disease develop characteristic eye signs known as Graves' ophthalmopathy or thyroid eye disease (see also Chapter 13). In addition to signs of thyrotoxicosis, patients may have pretibial myxedema and (rarely) clubbing of the fingers. The ophthalmopathy may appear before any manifestations of thyrotoxicosis. It also may occur in autoimmune hypothyroidism (Hashimoto's thyroiditis); thyroid dysfunction due to amiodarone (see later in the chapter); in association with thyroid antibodies without thyroid dysfunction; and occasionally in the absence of thyroid antibodies and clinical and laboratory evidence of thyroid dysfunction. It is exacerbated by radioiodine therapy, especially if the patient smokes cigarettes.

▶ Clinical Findings

Patients may present with nonspecific complaints such as dryness, discomfort, or prominence of the eyes. Mourits developed a clinical scoring system that uses the signs and symptoms which reflect the cardinal features of inflammation (Table 15–2). The Mourits score can be used to assess changes in disease activity with time and response to therapy.

A. Lid Retraction

Lid retraction is almost pathognomonic of thyroid disease, particularly when associated with exophthalmos. Lid retraction may be unilateral or bilateral and involve the upper and lower lids. It is often accompanied by restrictive myopathy, initially involving the inferior rectus and resulting in impaired

Table 15–2. The Mourits Classification System to Access Disease Activity in Graves' Ophthalmopathy

Pain
  Painful, oppressive feeling on or behind globe
  Pain on attempted up, side, or down gaze

Redness
  Redness of the eyelids
  Diffuse redness of the conjunctiva

Swelling
  Chemosis (conjunctival edema)
  Swollen caruncle
  Edema of the eyelids
  Increase in proptosis of 2 mm or more over a period of 1–3 months

Impaired function
  Decrease in visual acuity of one or more lines on the Snellen chart (using a pinhole) during a period of 1–3 months
  Decrease of eye movements in any direction equal to or more than 5° during a period of 1–3 months.

elevation of the eyes. The pathogenesis of lid retraction is diverse, including hyperstimulation of the sympathetic nervous system and direct inflammatory infiltration of the levator muscle. Restrictive myopathy of the inferior rectus muscle can cause lid retraction from the increased stimulation of the levator on attempted upgaze.

The system is based on the well-known signs of acute inflammation: pain (*dolor*), redness (*rubor*), swelling (*tumor*), and impaired function (*functio laesa*), defined by Celsus and Galen in antiquity. For each of the signs present, one point is given. The sum of these points defines the activity score.

B. Exophthalmos (Figure 15–23)

The degree of exophthalmos is extremely variable. Measurements using the Hertel or Krahn exophthalmome-

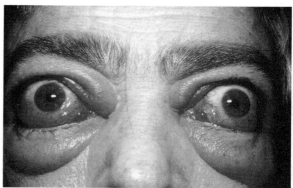

A

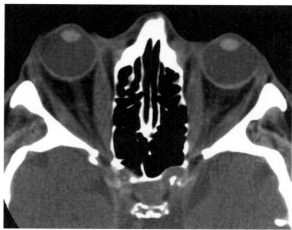

B

▲ **Figure 15–23.** Thyroid ophthalmopathy. **A:** Proptosis, lid edema, lid retraction, chemosis, ophthalmoplegia, and visual loss in thyroid eye disease. **B:** CT scan showing thickening of the extraocular muscles with optic nerve compression at the orbital apex.

ter range from mild (less than 24 mm) to severe (28 mm or more). The condition is usually asymmetric and may be unilateral. The increase in orbital contents that produces the exophthalmos is due to an increase in the bulk of the ocular muscles and the orbital fat, and thus it is clinically important to assess the resistance to manual retropulsion of the globe. MRI or CT scan (Figure 15–23) will differentiate exophthalmos due to an orbital tumor. MRI offers superior soft tissue resolution, and the intensity of signal in the extraocular muscles on short tau inversion recovery (STIR) sequences can be used to quantify disease activity. In some cases, thickening of the ocular muscles may be restricted to certain muscles only—commonly the inferior rectus or medial rectus.

C. Ophthalmoplegia

Limitation of elevation is the most frequent finding. This is mainly due to tethering of the inferior rectus muscle, which can be confirmed by substantial increase in intraocular pressure when the patient attempts to look up. Often there is mild limitation of ocular movements in all positions of gaze. Patients complain of diplopia, which may spontaneously return to normal or, if severe, may require corticosteroid treatment. If it remains static for 6–12 months, it can be relieved by operation on one or more extraocular muscles.

D. Retinal and Optic Nerve Changes

Compression of the globe by the orbital contents may produce elevation of the intraocular pressure and retinal or choroidal striae. Optic neuropathy associated with Graves' ophthalmopathy occasionally occurs either as a result of compression or due to ischemia of the optic nerve as it traverses the tense orbit, particularly at the orbital apex.

E. Corneal Changes

In some patients, superior limbic keratoconjunctivitis may be seen, although this is not specific for thyroid disease. In severe exophthalmos, corneal exposure and ulceration may occur.

▶ Pathogenesis of the Ocular Signs

The disease process affects the extraocular muscles, orbital fat, lacrimal glands, and orbital interstitial connective tissue. The extraocular muscles may become grossly distended. Histologically, they show intercellular edema secondary to increased concentrations of mucopolysaccharides, which are generated by orbital fibroblasts stimulated by activated lymphocytes. Eventually, fibrosis of the muscle ensues.

Graves' ophthalmopathy is an autoimmune disorder. The specific antigen involved is still not certainly known, although increasing evidence points to the TSH receptor expressed in retroocular preadipocyte fibroblasts. Patients usually have serum antibodies to thyroid microsomes (thyroperoxidase), thyroglobulin, and thyroid-stimulating immunoglobulins.

▶ Treatment

A. Medical Treatment

The primary medical treatment is maintaining euthyroidism, which may be best achieved by thyroidectomy. Severe cases with visual loss, disk edema, or corneal ulceration require urgent treatment, usually with high-dose oral corticosteroids (eg, prednisolone 100 mg daily), but alternatively with high-dose intravenous pulse therapy (eg, methylprednisolone 1 g daily for 3 days each week) and possibly with intra-orbital steroid injections. Immunosuppressive agents (eg, azathioprine) may play a supportive role by allowing a lower maintenance dose of corticosteroids in patients requiring long-term therapy. Plasmapheresis is occasionally used with good results in the treatment of refractory cases, but full immunosuppression must follow plasmapheresis to prevent rebound increase of immunoglobulins and recurrence of disease. Rituximab, an anti-CD20 monoclonal antibody, has also been shown to be effective in corticosteroid-resistant cases. Orbital radiotherapy may be useful to avoid or as a sequel to surgical decompression.

B. Surgical Treatment

Decompression of the orbit is achieved usually by removing the medial, inferior, and lateral walls via an external or endoscopic approach. Decompression of the orbital apex is essential for a successful outcome.

2. HYPOTHYROIDISM (MYXEDEMA)

Significant ocular signs are not common in myxedema, although the signs of thyroid ophthalmopathy may be seen. Hyperthyroid patients who subsequently become hypothyroid are at greater risk of ophthalmic involvement.

HYPOPARATHYROIDISM

Occasionally at thyroidectomy, the parathyroid glands are removed inadvertently, causing hypoparathyroidism. Spontaneous cases of hypoparathyroidism, although rare, should be suspected in young patients with cataracts. The blood calcium decreases, and serum phosphates are increased. Tetany may ensue and can be severe enough to cause generalized convulsions. The ocular manifestations consist of blepharospasm and twitching eyelids. Small, discrete, punctate opacities of the lens cortex develop that may eventually require lens extraction.

Treatment with calcium salts, calciferol, and dihydrotachysterol usually prevents further development of lens opacities, but anyone that has occurred prior to treatment remain.

VITAMINS & EYE DISEASE

VITAMIN A

Vitamin A is essential for the maintenance of epithelium throughout the body. Ocular changes resulting from vitamin A deficiency (Figure 15–24) are described in Chapter 6.

VITAMIN B

Acute thiamin (vitamin B_1) deficiency causes **Wernicke's encephalopathy,** typically characterized by confusion, ataxia, and nystagmus but also manifesting as ophthalmoplegia, and may result in **Korsakoff's psychosis.** It most commonly occurs in alcoholics. Urgent treatment with parenteral thiamin, initially intravenously, is essential.

Chronic thiamin deficiency produces **beriberi,** and 70% of patients with beriberi have ocular abnormalities. Epithelial changes in the conjunctiva and cornea produce dry eyes. Visual loss may occur as a result of optic atrophy.

Treatment is by oral, and if necessary intramuscular, thiamin, and correction of dietary deficiency.

Riboflavin (vitamin B_2) deficiency has been said to cause a number of ocular changes. Rosacea keratitis, peripheral corneal vascularization, seborrheic blepharitis, and secondary conjunctivitis have all been attributed to riboflavin deficiency. **Niacin (nicotinic acid) deficiency (pellagra)** is quite common in alcoholics and is characterized by dermatitis, diarrhea, and dementia. Ocular involvement is rare, but optic neuritis or retinitis may develop. Both riboflavin and niacin deficiency are treated with oral supplementation.

Vitamin B_{12} deficiency (pernicious anemia) is discussed in Chapter 14.

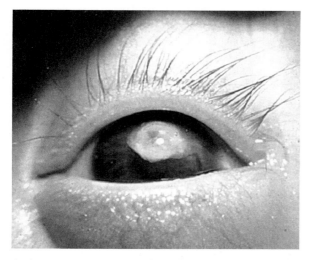

▲ **Figure 15–24.** Keratomalacia due to xerophthalmia in a 5-month-old child.

VITAMIN C

In vitamin C (ascorbic acid) deficiency (scurvy), hemorrhages may develop in a variety of sites, for example, skin, mucous membranes, body cavities, the orbits, and subperiosteally in the joints. Hemorrhages may also occur into the lids, subconjunctival space, anterior chamber, vitreous cavity, and retina.

Treatment is with oral ascorbic acid and correction of dietary deficiency.

GRANULOMATOUS DISEASES

Many of the so-called granulomatous infectious diseases, including tuberculosis, brucellosis, leprosy, and toxoplasmosis, undergo a chronic course with frequent exacerbations and remissions. The eye is often involved, particularly by anterior uveitis.

TUBERCULOSIS

Ocular tuberculosis results from endogenous spread from systemic foci. The incidence of eye involvement is less than 1% in known cases of pulmonary tuberculosis. A granulomatous panuveitis may occur; the iritis (anterior uveitis; see Chapter 7) is treated with topical mydriatics and corticosteroids. Systemic antituberculosis therapy is essential in the treatment of established cases of tuberculous uveitis. Retinal "cold" abscesses may occur (Figure 15–25). In miliary tuberculosis, many small, discrete yellowish nodules are visible ophthalmoscopically in the choroid at the posterior pole of the eye. Tuberculosis may also cause ocular motor cranial nerve palsies, papilloedema, or damage to the optic nerves or optic chiasm from basal meningitis, vasculitis, or direct infiltration, including mass lesion (tuberculoma). There has been a recent increase in the incidence of tuberculosis as a result of the spread of the human immunodeficiency virus (HIV) epidemic.

SARCOIDOSIS (FIGURES 15–26 AND 15–27)

Sarcoidosis is a multisystem disease characterized by noncaseating granulomatous infiltration of affected tissues. The prevalence in North America is 10–80 per 100,000 population, with wide racial and geographic variations: blacks are affected almost 10 times more commonly than whites. Patients may present with pulmonary, ocular, joint, cutaneous, and reticuloendothelial system manifestations. A granulomatous uveitis may be accompanied by cells in the vitreous, periphlebitis, disk swelling, retinal neovascularization, and choroidal disease. New vessels may require photocoagulation. Infiltrative optic neuropathy is a rare cause of severe and progressive loss of vision.

The ocular and systemic disease may require treatment with corticosteroids and occasionally immunosuppressant agents.

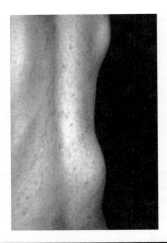

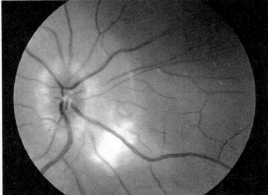

▲ **Figure 15–25.** Tuberculosis. Cold abscess. A young man presented with a swelling on his back **(A)** and a choroidal lesion **(B)**. Aspiration of the abscess revealed *Mycobacterium* tuberculosis.

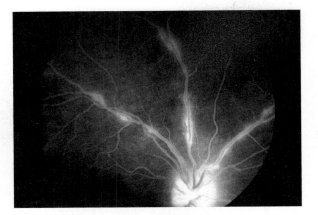

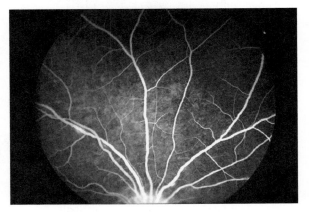

▲ **Figure 15–26.** Sarcoidosis. Focal periphlebitis and disk leakage may respond dramatically to systemic corticosteroids. **A:** Before treatment. **B:** After 6 weeks of treatment with prednisolone, 30 mg daily.

EALES' DISEASE

This disease was originally reported in young men in poor general health who experienced recurrent vitreous hemorrhages from areas of retinal neovascularization, but it is a diagnosis of exclusion. The same clinical features occur in tuberculosis, sarcoidosis, systemic lupus erythematosus, sickle cell disease, and diabetes, all needing to be excluded by appropriate investigations before the diagnosis of Eales's disease can be made. Photocoagulation of the new vessels can reduce the chance of further vitreous hemorrhage. Patients should stop smoking.

LEPROSY (HANSEN'S DISEASE)

Leprosy is a chronic granulomatous disorder caused by *Mycobacterium leprae,* an acid-fast bacillus. The World Health Organization lists leprosy as one of the major health problems of developing countries. Over 2 million people in the world have leprosy, and of this number, 20%–50% have ocular involvement. In tropical countries, the infection is endemic.

Three major types of leprosy are recognized: lepromatous, tuberculoid, and dimorphous. The eye may be affected in any type of leprosy, but ocular involvement is more common in the lepromatous type. Ocular lesions are due to direct invasion by *M leprae* of the ocular tissues or of the nerves supplying the eye and adnexa. Since the organism appears to grow better at lower temperatures, infection is more apt to involve the anterior segment of the eye than the posterior segment.

▶ Clinical Findings

The early clinical signs of ocular leprosy are lagophthalmos, loss of the lateral portions of the eyebrows and eyelashes (madarosis), conjunctival hyperemia, and superficial keratitis

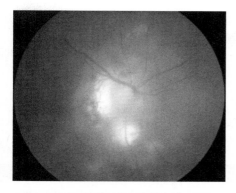

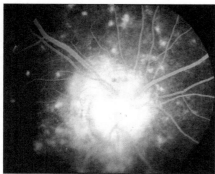

▲ **Figure 15–27.** Sarcoidosis. Retinal pigment epithelial and choroidal disease may be very distinctive **(A)** and highlighted by fluorescein angiography **(B)**.

(Figure 15–28), with interstitial keratitis—beginning typically in the superior temporal quadrant of the cornea—often supervening.

Scarring of the cornea from interstitial or exposure keratitis (or both) causes blurred vision and often blindness.

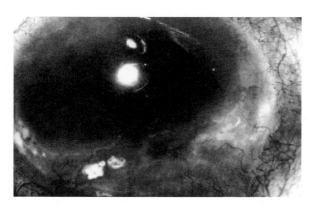

▲ **Figure 15–28.** Leprosy keratitis, left eye. (Courtesy of W Richards.)

Granulomatous iritis with lepromas (iris pearls) is common, and a low-grade iritis associated with iris atrophy and a pinpoint pupil may also occur. Hypertrophy of the eyebrows with deformities of the lids and trichiasis late in the course of the disease, and exposure keratitis, typically in the inferior and central cornea, can result from facial motor nerve palsy and absence of corneal sensation.

Ocular leprosy can be diagnosed on the basis of characteristic signs combined with a characteristic skin biopsy.

▶ Treatment

Leprosy is now treated with multidrug therapy, which includes dapsone, rifampin, and clofazimine, and the results in patients with early disease have been encouraging.

SYPHILIS

▶ Congenital Syphilis

The most common eye lesion in congenital syphilis is interstitial keratitis, but it is a late manifestation (discussed in Chapter 6). Chorioretinitis unassociated with interstitial keratitis may occur. Congenital syphilis is treated with large doses of penicillin, although usually it does not influence the interstitial keratitis.

▶ Acquired Syphilis

Ocular chancre (primary lesion) occurs rarely on the lid margins and follows the same course as a genital chancre.

Iritis and iridocyclitis occur in the secondary stage of syphilis along with the rash in about 5% of cases. The inflammation may involve the posterior segment producing a vitritis and punctate retinitis, as well as affecting the retinal pigment epithelium, retinal capillaries (Figure 15–29), and optic nerve.

TOXOPLASMOSIS

This disease is of great ocular importance. The etiologic organism is a protozoal parasite that infects a great number of animals and birds and has worldwide distribution. Felids are the definitive host.

▶ Congenital Toxoplasmosis (Figure 15–30)

Infection occurs in utero, and 40% of infants born to mothers who acquired toxoplasmosis during pregnancy—particularly during the third trimester—will be affected (see also Chapter 20).

A focal choroiditis is seen, usually in the posterior pole, and an active lesion is often related to an old healed lesion. Episodes of posterior uveitis and chorioretinitis usually represent reactivation of a congenital infection. Rarely, panuveitis may occur, or optic neuritis progressing to optic atrophy. Isolated anterior uveitis does not occur.

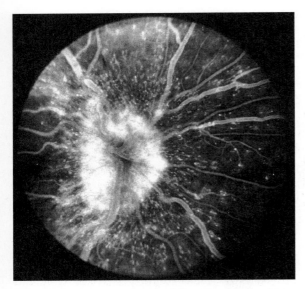

▲ **Figure 15-29.** Secondary syphilis. Bilateral visual loss occurred in a 24-year-old man. Late fluorescein photographs showed disk leakage with dilation and leakage of peripapillary capillaries.

Treatment with anti-protozoal agents, sometimes combined with systemic corticosteroids, reduces inflammation but does not prevent scar formation and is only given for disease that threatens vision (see Chapter 7). Subconjunctival or retrobulbar injection of corticosteroids is contraindicated because it may cause severe exacerbation of disease. Topical corticosteroids and cycloplegics may be useful.

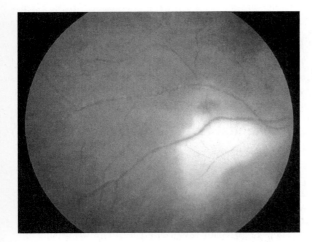

▲ **Figure 15-30.** Toxoplasmosis. Active area of chorioretinitis adjacent to scar with reaction in adjacent retinal arteriole.

▶ Acquired Toxoplasmosis

Acquired toxoplasmosis affects young adults and is characterized by general malaise, lymphadenopathy, sore throat, and hepatosplenomegaly similar to that seen in infectious mononucleosis. It is endemic in South America and in parts of sub-Saharan Africa. Toxoplasmic retinochoroiditis may rarely follow acquired systemic toxoplasmosis. The diagnosis is confirmed by the finding of both IgG and IgM antibodies.

▼ VIRAL DISEASES

HERPES SIMPLEX

There are two morphologic strains of the herpes simplex virus: type 1 and type 2. Ocular infections are usually produced by type 1, whereas genital infections are caused by type 2. The most common manifestation of herpes simplex is cold sores on the lips. The most common eye lesion is keratitis (see Chapter 6). Vesicular skin lesions can also appear on the skin of the lids and the lid margins. Herpes simplex may also cause iridocyclitis and, more rarely, retinitis (see later in the chapter) and severe encephalitis.

VARICELLA-ZOSTER (CHICKENPOX & HERPES ZOSTER)

First infection with varicella-zoster virus causes chickenpox (varicella). Swollen lids, conjunctivitis, vesicular conjunctival lesions, and (rarely) uveitis and optic neuritis may occur.

Herpes zoster is the response to the same virus in a partially immune person, that is, someone who has previously had chickenpox. It is usually confined to a single dermatome on one side and presents with malaise, headache, and fever followed by burning, itching, and pain in the affected area. The most common ophthalmic manifestation is herpes zoster ophthalmicus, and the ocular complications are caused by ischemia, viral spread, or a granulomatous reaction. The acute stage is characterized by a virulent rash, conjunctivitis, keratitis, episcleritis, and uveitis when the nasociliary nerve is involved.

Treatment is not usually required in varicella but should be considered in all cases of ophthalmic zoster. Oral acyclovir, 800 mg five times a day for 7–10 days, started within 72 hours after eruption of the rash, reduces ocular complications, including postherpetic neuralgia. Alternatives are famciclovir 500 mg three times daily or valacyclovir 1 g three times daily. In immunocompromised individuals, both herpes zoster, which may become disseminated, and varicella are likely to be severe and may be fatal. Intravenous acyclovir, 30 mg/kg/d in three divided doses, should be given for at least 7 days. Anterior uveitis requires topical steroids and cycloplegics.

Acute retinal necrosis has been described following chickenpox and herpes zoster (see later in the chapter).

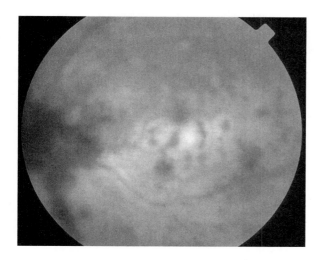

▲ **Figure 15–31.** Acute retinal necrosis due to varicella-zoster virus.

▶ Acute Retinal Necrosis

Acute retinal necrosis is a disease of healthy individuals. Patients present with anterior uveitis with fine keratic precipitates and severe occlusive retinal vasculitis. There is often more than one focus of retinitis, resulting in necrotic areas with discrete borders, which spread circumferentially and posteriorly from the midperipheral retina (Figure 15–31). In most cases, varicella-zoster virus or herpes simplex virus types 1 or 2 is implicated. Cytomegalovirus is less commonly responsible. Polymerase chain reaction (PCR) of vitreous samples is helpful to confirm the diagnosis and identify which virus is responsible. Initial treatment is with intravenous acyclovir. Intravenous foscarnet or cidofovir may be effective in infections resistant to acyclovir. Intravitreal ganciclovir or oral valganciclovir may also be used. A 3-month course of oral acyclovir reduces the chances of involvement of the second eye. The disease may result from reactivation of dormant virus, whose antigens have been found in all layers of the retina, pigment epithelium, and choroid. There may be an immunogenetic predisposition to the disease.

▶ Progressive Outer Retinal Necrosis

Progressive outer retinal necrosis is a form of necrotizing retinitis similar to acute retinal necrosis found in immunocompromised patients and attributed to herpes zoster. There is less inflammation, with multifocal onset in the posterior retina. It has faster progression and a worse outcome when compared with acute retinal necrosis. Retinal detachment may follow the retinal necrosis. Management is the same as for acute retinal necrosis.

CYTOMEGALIC INCLUSION DISEASE

Infection with cytomegalovirus (CMV), also a member of the herpesvirus group, may range from subclinical infection to classic manifestations of cytomegalic inclusion disease. The virus most frequently affects immunocompromised individuals (eg, those with HIV infection, organ transplant recipients). It manifests as a florid necrotizing retinitis with arteriolar occlusion, hemorrhage, and edema. The retinitis itself or secondary retinal detachment can be blinding. In HIV infection, CMV retinitis is more common when CD4 counts are very low.

First-line treatment of CMV retinitis is with intravenous ganciclovir or oral valganciclovir. A standard regimen is a 2-week induction course of intravenous therapy followed by maintenance oral therapy. Alternative treatment can be with a ganciclovir intraocular implant, cidofovir, or foscarnet. Neutropenia is the most important side effect of ganciclovir; renal damage, that of foscarnet. Ocular complications of cidofovir include uveitis, ocular hypotension, and ciliary body necrosis. Maintenance therapy is required unless the immunocompromise can be reversed, such as with highly active antiretroviral therapy (HAART) in HIV infection (see later in the chapter). Congenital CMV infection can cause microphthalmia, cataract, optic atrophy, and optic disk malformation. The differential diagnosis of congenital disease should include toxoplasmosis, rubella, herpes simplex infection, and syphilis. CMV rarely causes retinitis in the newborn.

POLIOMYELITIS

Bulbar poliomyelitis severe enough to cause lesions of the third, fourth, or sixth cranial nerve is usually fatal. In survivors, any type of internal or external ophthalmoplegia may result. Supranuclear abnormalities ("gaze" palsies, paralysis of convergence or divergence) are rare residual defects. Optic neuritis is uncommon. Treatment is purely symptomatic, although occasionally a residual extraocular muscle imbalance can be greatly improved by strabismus surgery.

RUBELLA (GERMAN MEASLES)

Maternal rubella during the first trimester of pregnancy causes serious congenital anomalies. The most common eye complication is cataract, which is bilateral in 75% of cases. Other congenital ocular anomalies are frequently associated with the cataracts, for example, uveal colobomas, nystagmus, microphthalmos, strabismus, retinopathy, and infantile glaucoma. Congenital cataract, especially if bilateral, may require surgical removal, but the prognosis is always guarded.

MEASLES (RUBEOLA)

Acute conjunctivitis is common early in the course of measles. Koplik's spots may be seen on the conjunctiva, and epithelial keratitis occurs frequently.

The treatment of the eye complications of measles is symptomatic unless there is secondary infection, in which case local antibiotic ointment is used.

MUMPS

The most common ocular complication of mumps is dacryoadenitis. A diffuse keratitis with corneal edema resembling the disciform keratitis of herpes simplex occurs rarely.

INFECTIOUS MONONUCLEOSIS

The disease process can affect the eye directly, causing keratitis, nongranulomatous uveitis, scleritis, conjunctivitis, retinitis, choroiditis, or optic neuritis. Complete recovery is usual, but residual visual loss can result.

VACCINATION

Optic neuritis can occur following any vaccination but is most often seen in children following administration of the combined measles-mumps-rubella (MMR) vaccine. Onset is usually within 2 weeks and is bilateral, with visual loss and sometimes pain on eye movements. Examination reveals bilateral disk edema, and MRI shows high signal in the optic nerves. Treatment is with oral corticosteroids, and complete recovery of vision is the anticipated outcome.

▼ FUNGAL DISEASE

CANDIDIASIS

Ocular involvement accompanies systemic candidal infection and candidemia in approximately two-thirds of cases. The initial lesion is a focal necrotizing granulomatous retinitis with or without choroiditis, characterized by fluffy white exudative lesions associated with cells in the vitreous overlying the lesion. Such lesions may spread to involve the optic nerve and macula. Endophthalmitis, Roth's spots, and exudative retinal detachment may occur. Spread into the vitreous cavity may result in formation of vitreous abscesses, sometimes described as "a string of pearls" (Figure 15–32). Anterior uveitis occurs, and a hypopyon may form.

Treatment consists of intravitreal amphotericin B combined with oral flucytosine and fluconazole, which are synergistic. Early vitrectomy may prevent macular damage.

MUCORMYCOSIS

Mucormycosis is a rare, often fatal infection occurring in debilitated patients, particularly poorly controlled diabetics. The fungi (rhizopus, mucor, and absidia) attack through the upper respiratory tract and invade the arterioles, producing necrotic tissue. Clinical features are the pathognomonic black hemipalate, proptosis, and an ischemic globe with blindness due to ophthalmic artery occlusion. Death occurs from cerebral abscess.

Treatment includes removal of the affected tissue, intravenous amphotericin B (preferably liposomal) or possibly posaconazole, and management of the underlying medical condition.

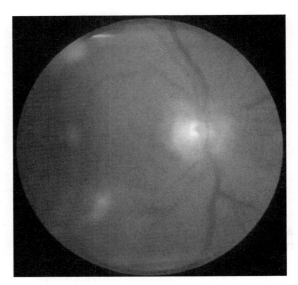

▲ **Figure 15–32.** Candidal endophthalmitis, with typical "string of pearls" appearance in the vitreous.

ACQUIRED IMMUNODEFICIENCY SYNDROME (AIDS)

AIDS is caused by HIV, a retrovirus. The virus infects mature T helper cells and leads to immunosuppression, the severity of which depends on the balance between the rates of destruction and replacement of T cells. The persistent immunodeficiency gives rise to opportunistic infections. The virus has been recovered from various body fluids, including blood, semen, saliva, tears, and cerebrospinal fluid.

▶ Transmission & Prevention of AIDS

Transmission of HIV is primarily by exchange of bodily fluids during sexual contact or through the use of contaminated needles by intravenous drug abuse. Transmission may also occur when contaminated blood products are transfused. The virus is not transmitted by casual contact, but because it is found in tears, conjunctival cells, and blood, health-care workers must take reasonable precautions when handling infectious waste or when at risk of contact with body fluids.

▶ Clinical Findings

The spectrum of clinical disease is wide, presumably due to the degree of immunologic damage and the frequency and nature of opportunistic infections. Typically, an acute flu-like illness occurs a few weeks after infection, followed months later by weight loss, fever, diarrhea, lymphadenopathy, and encephalopathy. The hallmark of AIDS is the high incidence of infections, which are frequently multiple, opportunistic, and severe. The incidence of opportunistic infections

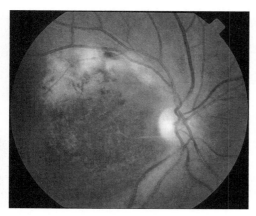

▲ **Figure 15–33.** Retinal changes in HIV infection— cytomegalovirus retinitis. See color insert.

increases with increasing immune deficiency. Herpes zoster, oral candida, and tuberculosis become more frequent as the CD4 count drops below 500 cells/mcL. When the CD4 cell count is below 200 cells/mcL infections with protozoa (such as *Pneumocystis* and *Toxoplasma*) and fungi (such as *Cryptococcus*) occur. *Cytomegalovirus* and *Mycobacterium avium-intracellulare* are seen when the CD4 count is below 100 cells/mcL.

The eye is involved in 30% of patients with AIDS. The most common abnormalities are retinal microvasculopathy with cotton-wool spots (Figure 15–33) and hemorrhages, and conjunctival vasculopathy characterized by comma vessels, sludging of the blood, and linear hemorrhages. The cause of these findings is unknown, but they are sometimes associated with increased plasma viscosity and may represent immune complex deposition. An intermediate uveitis may occur when there is a high viral load. Amongst the opportunistic infections, viral infections of the retina are most common, particularly cytomegalovirus (see earlier in the chapter). Involvement of the optic nerve results in gross optic disk edema and severe sudden and irreversible visual loss. Diagnosis is usually based on the clinical picture and confirmation of active viral replication as shown by PCR testing of blood, urine, cerebrospinal fluid, aqueous, or vitreous.

Treatment of HIV infection is complicated and individualized according to comorbidity and therapeutic response. Initially it involves "triple therapy"—a combination of 2 reverse transcriptase inhibitors and a protease inhibitor. These regimens may result in a dramatic drop in the HIV viral load, increase in CD4 count, and improved well-being. In this setting, patients with CMV retinitis may develop a "reconstitution uveitis" in which relative immune recovery is followed by panuveitis. It may be possible to stop anti-CMV therapy when the CD4 count has risen above 200/mcL for 3 months.

Acute retinal necrosis and progressive outer retinal necrosis (see earlier in the chapter) may occur. If the causative agent of the former is herpes simplex, concurrent encephalitis is common. Toxoplasma chorioretinitis is usually bilateral, acquired (congenital infections are rarely reactivated in AIDS), and associated with substantial vitreous reaction; candidal endophthalmitis is rarely seen except in drug addicts. Less common organisms that typically involve the choroid are *Pneumocystis jiroveci* (formerly *P carinii*), *Cryptococcus neoformans,* and *M avium-intracellulare.* Choroidal infection is blood-borne and portends imminent demise.

Herpes zoster ophthalmicus is a common presenting feature of HIV infection in sub-Saharan Africa and may be very severe, with anterior segment necrosis and ophthalmoplegia. Syphilis in association with HIV infection may produce severe blinding uveitis or optic neuropathy. Herpes simplex, molluscum contagiosum, and Kaposi's sarcoma frequently affect the eyelids and surrounding tissues. The combination of rifabutin and clarithromycin or cidofovir may precipitate symptomatic uveitis.

Neuroophthalmologic problems are divided into those related directly to HIV infection of the brain, such as optic neuropathy and supranuclear ophthalmoplegia, and those caused by cerebral abscesses or encephalitis, commonly due to cryptococcal infection, lymphoma, or toxoplasmosis.

▼ MULTISYSTEM AUTOIMMUNE DISEASES

SYSTEMIC LUPUS ERYTHEMATOSUS

Systemic or disseminated lupus erythematosus is a multisystem disease manifested by facial "butterfly skin lesions," pericarditis, Raynaud's phenomenon, renal involvement, arthritis, anemia, and central nervous system signs. Ocular findings include episcleritis and scleritis and keratoconjunctivitis sicca (in 25% of cases). Uveitis rarely occurs. Retinal involvement manifests as cotton-wool spots and arteriolar occlusions, as a result of immune complex deposition with associated choroidal vasculitis. This may herald life-threatening neurological and renal disease. The fundus picture may be complicated by a hypertensive retinochoroidopathy, which in severe cases can cause capillary occlusion or even proliferative retinopathy. An optic neuropathy may occur due to either an inflammatory or vaso-occlusive mechanism.

▶ Pathogenesis & Diagnosis

The disease is an immunologic disorder marked by the presence of circulating immune complexes. Antinuclear or antiphospholipid antibodies as well as antibodies to double-stranded DNA or ribonucleoprotein (anti-Sm) may be present. Active disease is associated with raised circulating immune complexes and reduced serum complement.

▶ Treatment

Systemic steroids and pulsed intravenous cyclophosphamide are most effective. Hydroxychloroquine, methotrexate, and azathioprine may be useful.

ANTI-PHOSPHOLIPID ANTIBODY SYNDROME

This diagnosis should be considered in patients with recurrent thromboembolism, recurrent fetal loss, livedo reticularis, thrombocytopenia, and neurologic disease without other features of systemic lupus erythematosus. Visual loss may be due to retinal vein or arterial occlusion or ischemic optic neuropathy. Choroidal infarcts may also occur (Figure 15–3). The diagnosis is confirmed by the presence of lupus anticoagulant and high-titer IgG and IgM anticardiolipin antibodies.

DERMATOMYOSITIS

In this rare disease, there is characteristically a degenerative subacute inflammation of the muscles, sometimes including the extraocular muscles. The lids are commonly a part of the generalized dermal involvement and may show marked swelling and erythema. Retinopathy with cotton-wool spots and hemorrhages may occur. High doses of systemic corticosteroids will frequently effect a remission that continues even after cessation of therapy. The ultimate prognosis is, however, poor.

SCLERODERMA

This rare chronic disease is characterized by widespread alterations in the collagenous tissues of the mucosa, bones, muscles, skin, and internal organs. Individuals of both sexes between 15 and 45 years of age are affected. The skin in local areas becomes tense and leathery, and the process may spread to involve large areas of the limbs, rendering them virtually immobile. The skin of the eyelids is often involved. Iritis and cataract occur less frequently. Retinopathy, similar to that which occurs in lupus erythematosus and dermatomyositis, may be present. Systemic corticosteroid treatment improves the prognosis.

POLYARTERITIS NODOSA

This collagen disease affects the medium-sized arteries, most commonly in men. There is intense inflammation of all the muscle layers of the arteries, with fibrinoid necrosis and a peripheral eosinophilia. The main clinical features include nephritis, hypertension, asthma, peripheral neuropathy, muscle pain with wasting, and peripheral eosinophilia. Cardiac involvement is common, although death is usually caused by renal dysfunction.

Ocular changes are seen in 20% of cases and consist of episcleritis and scleritis, which is often painless (see Chapter 7). When the limbal vessels are involved, guttering of the peripheral cornea may occur. A retinal microvasculopathy is common. Sudden dramatic visual loss may be due to an inflammatory steroid responsive optic neuropathy, ischemic

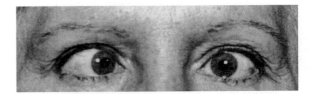

▲ **Figure 15–34.** Polyarteritis nodosa. Bilateral sixth nerve palsies.

optic neuropathy, or central retinal artery occlusion. Ophthalmoplegia may result from involvement of ocular motor cranial nerves (Figure 15–34). Systemic corticosteroids and cyclophosphamide are of some value. A few patients have a monophasic disease that resolves completely, but in the remainder, the long-term prognosis is uniformly bad.

WEGENER'S GRANULOMATOSIS

This granulomatous process shares certain clinical features with polyarteritis nodosa. The three diagnostic criteria are (1) necrotizing granulomatous lesions of the respiratory tract, (2) generalized necrotizing arteritis, and (3) renal involvement with necrotizing glomerulitis.

Ocular complications occur in 50% of cases, and proptosis resulting from orbital granulomatous formation occurs with associated ocular muscle or optic nerve involvement (Figure 15–35). If the vasculitis affects the eye, conjunctivitis, peripheral corneal ulceration, episcleritis, scleritis, uveitis, and retinal vasculitis may occur. Nasolacrimal duct obstruction is a rare complication.

Antineutrophil cytoplasmic antibodies, characteristically C-ANCA, are present in most cases with generalized disease and have both diagnostic and prognostic value, but they are found in only 30% of cases with disease limited to the head and neck. Combined corticosteroids and immu-

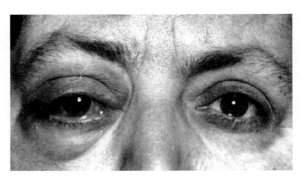

▲ **Figure 15–35.** Wegener's granulomatosis with proptosis, ptosis, and ophthalmoplegia. The condition has remained static for 10 years with use of corticosteroids and cyclophosphamide.

nosuppressives (particularly cyclophosphamide) often produce a satisfactory response. Rituximab has been advocated for refractory cases.

RHEUMATOID ARTHRITIS

Rheumatoid arthritis, a disease that is more common in women than in men, rarely presents with uveitis, but scleritis and episcleritis are comparatively common. The scleritis may herald exacerbation of the systemic disease, tends to occur with widespread vasculitis, and may lead to scleromalacia perforans (see Chapter 7).

Corticosteroid drops are helpful in episcleritis or anterior uveitis, but systemic treatment (nonsteroidal anti-inflammatory agents, corticosteroids, and other agents such as methotrexate or tumor necrosis factor inhibitors, although1> the last may exacerbate ocular inflammatory disease) is necessary for scleritis. Keratoconjunctivitis sicca is present in 15% of cases (see Chapter 4). Peripheral corneal melting may occur in more severe cases.

JUVENILE IDIOPATHIC ARTHRITIS (JUVENILE CHRONIC ARTHRITIS, JUVENILE RHEUMATOID ARTHRITIS, STILL'S DISEASE)

Ocular complications of juvenile idiopathic arthritis occur 3 times more frequently in girls with pauciarticular disease. The systemic disease appears to be disproportionately mild in children with severe visual loss, and diagnosis and treatment may therefore be delayed. Ocular involvement may occur before joint involvement. There is a chronic insidious uveitis with a high incidence of anterior segment complications (eg, posterior synechiae, cataract, secondary glaucoma, band-shaped keratopathy). Antinuclear antibodies are positive in 88% of patients with juvenile idiopathic arthritis who develop uveitis, whereas they are positive in only 30% of the group as a whole. Most cases are controlled with local corticosteroids and mydriatics, but severe cases require methotrexate and occasionally a short course of high-dose systemic corticosteroids.

SJÖGREN'S SYNDROME

Sjögren's syndrome is a systemic disorder with diverse features. The disease is characterized by keratoconjunctivitis sicca and xerostomia (dryness of the mouth). It may be secondary to a connective tissue disease, usually rheumatoid arthritis. It is more common in females. The onset of ocular symptoms occurs most frequently during the fourth, fifth, and sixth decades. Lymphoid proliferation is a prominent feature of Sjögren's syndrome and may involve the kidneys, the lungs, or the liver, causing renal tubular acidosis, pulmonary fibrosis, or cirrhosis. Lymphoreticular malignant disease such as reticulum cell sarcoma may complicate the benign course of Sjögren's syndrome many years after its onset.

The histopathologic changes in the lacrimal gland consist of infiltration of lymphocytes, histiocytes, and occasional plasma cells leading to atrophy and destruction of the glandular structures. These changes are part of the generalized polyglandular involvement in Sjögren's syndrome, which results in dryness of the eyes, mouth, skin, and mucous membranes.

Because of the relative inaccessibility of the lacrimal gland, the labial salivary gland biopsy serves as an important diagnostic procedure in patients with suspected Sjögren's syndrome in whom the diagnosis cannot be confirmed by the presence of serum antibodies to the extractable nuclear antigens Ro (SSA) and La (SSB).

GIANT CELL ARTERITIS (TEMPORAL OR CRANIAL ARTERITIS)

This is a disease of elderly patients (mostly women over age 60). Medium-sized arteries are involved, particularly the intima. Branches of the external carotid system are frequently involved, although pathologic studies have shown more diffuse arterial involvement. Polymyalgia rheumatica may precede or accompany the disease. Patients feel ill and have excruciating pain over the temporal or occipital arteries. Visual loss due to an ischemic optic neuropathy is frequent, and a few cases have a central retinal artery occlusion. Rarely visual loss is due to cortical blindness. Other central is nervous system signs include cranial nerve palsies and signs referable to brain stem lesions. Thoracic aortitis, possibly resulting in aneurysm, is frequently present. The diagnosis is confirmed by a high erythrocyte sedimentation rate (ESR) and a positive temporal artery biopsy. The ESR may be normal, but usually it is markedly elevated (80–100 mm in the first hour). It is important to make the diagnosis early because immediate systemic corticosteroid administration produces dramatic relief of pain and prevents further ischemic episodes. Disease activity is monitored by the clinical state and the erythrocyte sedimentation rate. The corticosteroid dose may have to be maintained for several years and should be kept below 5-mg prednisolone daily if possible, since toxic effects develop with higher doses.

IDIOPATHIC ARTERITIS OF TAKAYASU (PULSELESS DISEASE)

This disease, found most frequently in young women and occasionally in children, is a polyarteritis of unknown cause with increased predilection for the aorta and its branches. Manifestations may include evidence of cerebrovascular insufficiency, syncope, absence of pulsations in the upper extremities, and ophthalmologic changes compatible with chronic hypoxia of the ocular structures.

Thromboendarterectomy, prosthetic graft, and systemic corticosteroid therapy have been reported to be successful.

ANKYLOSING SPONDYLITIS

Ankylosing spondylitis occurs mainly in males 16–40 years of age. In most cases, an intermittent anterior uveitis is seen, but in a minority, anterior and posterior uveitis exists with glaucoma and cataracts developing in the long term (see

Chapter 7). In a few cases, aortic valve disease is also seen. There is a strong association with HLA-B27. Antigenic cross-reactivity is present between HLA-B27 and *Klebsiella pneumoniae,* but the etiology remains poorly understood.

REITER'S DISEASE

The diagnosis of Reiter's disease is based on a triad of signs that includes urethritis, conjunctivitis, and arthritis (see Chapter 16). Scleritis, keratitis, and uveitis may also occur.

BEHÇET'S DISEASE

Behçet's disease consists of the clinical triad of relapsing uveitis and aphthous and genital ulceration (Figure 15–36). Ocular signs occur in 75% of cases; the uveitis is severe, occasionally associated with hypopyon. Visual loss is due to inflammatory changes in the retinal vessels and retina, and there is a propensity to microvascular venous occlusions and retinal infiltrates. Treatment often involves multiple immunosuppression (eg, steroids, cyclosporine, azathioprine, and

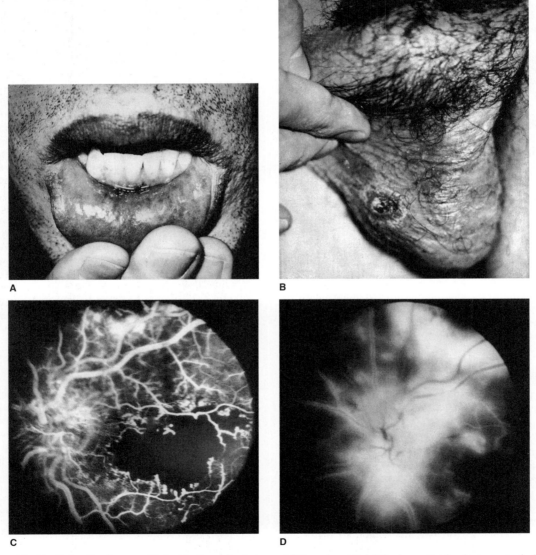

A

B

C

D

▲ **Figure 15–36.** Behçet's disease. Clinical features include oral **(A)** and genital **(B)** ulcers. Ocular features include increased capillary permeability and areas of retinal ischemia and infiltration **(C)**. Marked leakage of capillaries is seen in the late stages of fluorescein angiography **(D)**.

interferon), but despite manipulation with these drugs, the visual outcome is bad in 25% of cases. Ocular involvement is associated with the HLA-B51 haplotype, and tumor necrosis factor gene polymorphisms have been found more commonly in patients with severe ocular disease, as well as the prothrombotic Factor V Leiden mutation.

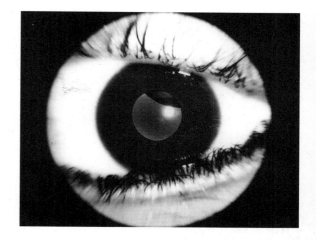

▼ HERITABLE CONNECTIVE TISSUE DISEASES

MARFAN'S SYNDROME (ARACHNODACTYLY) (FIGURE 15–37)

The most striking feature of this rare syndrome is increased length of the long bones, particularly of the fingers and toes. Other characteristics include scanty subcutaneous fat, relaxed ligaments, and, less commonly, other associated developmental anomalies, including congenital heart disease and deformities of the spine and joints. Ocular complications are often seen—in particular, dislocation of the lenses, usually superiorly and nasally. Less common ocular anomalies include severe refractive errors, megalocornea, cataract, uveal colobomas, and secondary glaucoma. There is a high infant mortality rate. Removal of a dislocated lens may be necessary. The disease is due to a mutation in the fibrillin-1 gene located on chromosome 15. Inheritance is autosomal dominant with variable expression, so that mild, incomplete forms of the syndrome are seen, but about 25% of affected individuals are due to new mutations.

OSTEOGENESIS IMPERFECTA (BRITTLE BONES & BLUE SCLERAS)

This rare autosomal dominant syndrome is characterized by multiple fractures, blue scleras, and, less commonly, deafness. The disease usually manifests soon after birth. The long bones are very fragile, fracturing easily and often healing with fibrous bony union. The bones become more fragile with age. The very thin sclera allows the blue color imparted by the underlying uveal tract to show through. There is usually no visual impairment. Occasionally, abnormalities such as keratoconus, megalo-cornea, and corneal or lenticular opacities are also present.

Ophthalmologic treatment is seldom necessary.

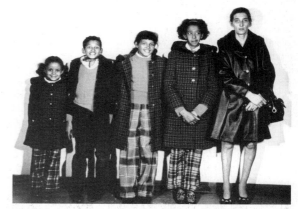

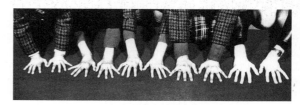

▲ **Figure 15–37.** Marfan's syndrome. Familial expression of upward dislocation of the lens **(A)** and arachnodactyly **(C)**.

▼ HEREDITARY METABOLIC DISORDERS

HEPATOLENTICULAR DEGENERATION (WILSON'S DISEASE)

This rare autosomal recessive disease of young adults—characterized by abnormal copper metabolism—causes changes in the basal nuclei, cirrhosis of the liver, and corneal pigmentation called the Kayser–Fleischer ring (see Chapter 6). The ring appears as a green or brown band peripherally at the level of Descemet's membrane and may only be visible with a slitlamp.

The disease is progressive and often results in death by age 40. Treatment of the abnormal copper metabolism can result in sustained clinical improvement in some cases.

CYSTINOSIS

This rare autosomal recessive derangement of amino acid metabolism causes widespread deposition of cystine crystals throughout the body. Dwarfism, nephropathy, and death in childhood from renal failure are the rule. Cystine crystals can be readily seen in the conjunctiva and cornea, where fine particles are seen predominantly in the outer third of the corneal stroma. Treatment with cysteamine may be beneficial.

ALBINISM

Oculocutaneous albinism consists of a heterogeneous group of conditions characterized by generalized reduction in or absence of melanin pigmentation and inherited as autosomal recessive traits. Mutations have been found on chromosomes 9, 11, and 15. At birth there is little or no cutaneous pigmentation, such that the skin and hair, including the eyebrows and eyelashes, are white or paler than expected. In severely affected cases, this situation persists throughout life, whereas in less affected individuals, some pigmentation and tanning with sun exposure can develop during childhood. The ocular manifestations are reduced visual acuity (generally 20/200), nystagmus, pale irides that transilluminate, hypopigmented fundi, and hypoplastic foveas. Photophobia is a prominent symptom. Ocular albinism, an X-linked recessive trait, has the same ocular features as oculocutaneous albinism but generally without cutaneous manifestations, although the skin may be paler than that of first-degree relatives. It is an important cause of congenital nystagmus. Female carriers may be identified by the presence of iris transillumination and retinal abnormalities. In all types of albinism there is a characteristic increase in the proportion of decussating axons in the optic chiasm, which can be identified by electrodiagnostic testing.

GALACTOSEMIA

Galactosemia is a rare autosomal recessive disorder of carbohydrate metabolism clinically manifested soon after birth by feeding problems, vomiting, diarrhea, abdominal distention, hepatomegaly, jaundice, ascites, cataracts, mental retardation, and elevated blood and urine galactose levels. Dietary exclusion of milk and all foods containing galactose and lactose for the first 3 years of life will prevent the clinical manifestations and will result in improvement of existing abnormalities. Even the cataract changes, which are characterized by vacuoles of the cortex, are reversible in the early stage.

Identification of the carrier state is possible by finding a 50% reduction of galactose 6-phosphatase.

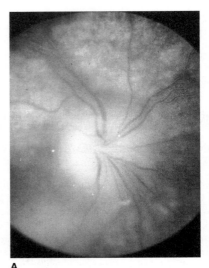

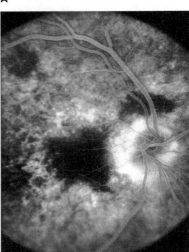

▲ **Figure 15–38.** Vogt–Koyanagi–Harada syndrome. Acute pigment epithelial disease with disk swelling and cells in the vitreous **(A)**. Three months later, disk swelling has subsided and pigment epithelial damage is seen **(B)**.

▼ MISCELLANEOUS SYSTEMIC DISEASES WITH OCULAR MANIFESTATIONS

VOGT–KOYANAGI–HARADA SYNDROME (FIGURE 15–38)

Bilateral uveitis associated with alopecia, poliosis, vitiligo, and hearing defects, usually in young adults, has been termed Vogt–Koyanagi disease. When the choroiditis is more exudative, serous retinal detachment occurs, and the complex is known as Harada's syndrome. There is a tendency toward recovery of visual function, but this is not always complete. Initial treatment is with local steroids and mydriatics, but systemic steroids in high doses are frequently required to prevent permanent visual loss.

ERYTHEMA MULTIFORME (STEVENS–JOHNSON SYNDROME)

Erythema multiforme is a serious mucocutaneous disease that occurs as a hypersensitivity reaction to drugs or food. Children are most susceptible. The manifestations consist of generalized maculopapular rash, severe stomatitis, and membranous conjunctivitis, sometimes leading to tear deficiency due to occlusion of the lacrimal gland ducts and symblepharon. In severe cases, corneal ulcers, perforations, and panophthalmitis can destroy all visual function. Systemic corticosteroid treatment often favorably influences the course of the disease and usually preserves useful visual function. Secondary infection with *Staphylococcus aureus* is common and must be vigorously treated with local antibiotics instilled into the conjunctival sac. Tear deficiency can be helped by instillation of artificial tears.

ROSACEA (ACNE ROSACEA)

This disease of unknown cause is primarily dermatologic, beginning as hyperemia of the face associated with acneiform lesions and eventually causing hypertrophy of tissues (such as rhinophyma). Chronic blepharitis due to staphylococcal infection or seborrhea is often present. Rosacea keratitis develops in about 5% of cases. Episcleritis, scleritis, and nongranulomatous iridocyclitis are rare ocular complications.

Careful attention to lid hygiene is essential. Topical corticosteroids help in controlling keratitis or iridocyclitis. Long-term systemic doxycycline or erythromycin therapy is often beneficial.

LYME DISEASE

Lyme disease is a vector-mediated multisystem illness caused by the spirochete *Borrelia burgdorferi*. The usual vectors are small ixodid ticks that have a complex three-host life cycle involving multiple mammalian and avian species.

The disease has three major stages. Initially, in the area of the tick bite, there develops the characteristic skin lesion of erythema chronicum migrans, often accompanied by regional lymphadenopathy, malaise, fever, headache, myalgia, and arthralgia. Several weeks to months later, there is a period of neurologic and cardiac abnormalities. After a few more weeks or even years, rheumatologic abnormalities develop—initially, migratory musculoskeletal discomfort, but later, a frank arthritis that may recur over several years.

Conjunctivitis is a frequent finding in the first stage. Cranial nerve palsies—particularly of the seventh but also of the third, fourth, or sixth cranial nerves—often occur in the neurologic phase. Other ophthalmologic abnormalities that have been reported include uveitis, ischemic optic neuropathy, optic disk edema and neuroretinitis with macular star, bilateral keratitis, and choroiditis with exudative retinal detachments.

Laboratory diagnosis is by demonstration of specific IgM and IgG antibodies in serum or cerebrospinal fluid. The spirochetes may also be isolated from these sources.

Doxycycline and ampicillin are effective in curing the initial infection but unfortunately may not prevent late complications.

IMMUNOSUPPRESSIVE AGENTS USED IN MANAGEMENT OF EYE DISEASE

Immunosuppressive agents are used to suppress inflammatory reactions within the eye, particularly those affecting the uveal tract but also the sclera, retina, and optic nerve. Frequently, the cause of inflammation is not known, and the use of these drugs is therefore empirical. All patients must have a full medical examination before treatment is started. Special consideration must be given to patients with infections and blood diseases, and regular blood counts must be performed during the course of treatment.

Corticosteroids (eg, prednisolone) are the mainstay of immunosuppressive treatment in ophthalmology. High doses (eg, 60 mg of prednisolone daily) may be required to control inflammation, and there is a high incidence of side effects. Weight gain, acne, and hirsutism are common; peptic ulceration, myopathy, osteoporosis, and avascular necrosis are less frequently encountered. Alternate-day regimens produce fewer side effects in some patients. Intravenous methylprednisolone (1 g per day given over 3 hours in dextrose saline for 3 days) is an effective method of controlling exacerbations in patients already taking high doses of corticosteroids.

Azathioprine may be used as a corticosteroid-sparing drug; 2.5 mg/kg daily is an effective dose, and the total course should not last longer than 18 months. Measurement of thiopurine methyltransferase (TPMT) allows modification of the azathioprine dose to reduce the risk of bone marrow toxicity.

Cyclosporine is an immunosuppressive agent isolated from the fermentation products of a fungus that was recovered from Norwegian soil. It has an effective immunomodulating action and causes suppression of T helper cells. It is a useful alternative drug for refractory sight-threatening noninfectious inflammatory eye disease in patients who have not responded to corticosteroids or in whom the optimal therapeutic dose of corticosteroids is associated with intolerable side effects. The recommended dose is 5 mg/kg orally daily. The most important side effect is renal toxicity, but liver toxicity may also occur. Close surveillance and monitoring of kidney and liver functions are mandatory. The drug should not be given to hypertensive patients. Reduction of the daily dose may be associated with troublesome rebound of the ocular inflammation.

Mycophenolate mofetil prevents lymphocyte proliferation, suppresses antibody synthesis, and decreases recruitment of leukocytes to sites of inflammation. It has been used successfully as a steroid-sparing agent in a variety of ocular inflammatory disorders, including uveitis and scleritis.

Cytotoxic agents are rarely indicated in the management of inflammatory eye disease except in severe cases of Behçet's syndrome and Wegener's granulomatosis. These drugs and their important side effects are listed in Table 15–3. Cytotoxic agents are sometimes used in the treatment of myasthenia gravis (Figure 15–39).

Table 15–3. Cytotoxic Agents Used in the Management of Inflammatory Eye Disease

Drug	Dose	Maximum Length of Treatment[1]	Side Effects
Azathioprine	2.5–3 mg/kg/d	1.5 y	Bone marrow depression, more likely if low thiopurine methyltransferase (TPMT) enzyme activity (usually leukopenia, but may be anemia, thrombocytopenia, and bleeding) (irreversible in elderly patients). Skin rashes, drug fever, nausea and vomiting, sometimes diarrhea. Hepatic dysfunction (raised liver enzymes, mild jaundice). Lymphoma.
Chlorambucil	0.05–0.2 mg/kg/d	2.5 y (4 g)	Moderate depression of peripheral blood count. Excessive doses produce severe bone marrow depression with leukopenia, thrombocytopenia, and bleeding. Lymphoma. Chlorambucil: Leukemia may occur. Large doses near puberty may cause infertility. Cyclophosphamide: Nausea and vomiting acutely. Alopecia and hemorrhagic cystitis (risk lessened by increased fluid intake after intravenous administration) occasionally. Infertility may occur.
Cyclophosphamide	1.5–2.5 mg/kg/d	3 y	
Colchicine	0.01–0.03mg/kg/d	5 y	Occasionally nausea, vomiting, abdominal pain, diarrhea. Rarely, hair loss, bone marrow depression, peripheral neuritis, myopathy.
Methotrexate	7.5–15 mg/wk	2.5 y (1.5 g)	Bone marrow depression. Skin rashes. Anorexia, nausea. Hepatic dysfunction with fibrosis, particularly in patients with excess alcohol consumption, obesity, and diabetes mellitus.
Mycophenolate mofetil	0.5–1.5 g twice daily	2 y	Gastrointestinal side effects are common. Myalgia, fatigue, headache. Leukopenia, lymphoma, nonmelanoma skin cancers all reported. Opportunistic infections: Mostly cytomegalovirus and herpes simplex.

[1]Numbers in parentheses are maximum cumulative doses.

Biologics are being used increasingly to modulate the immune response. Examples include monoclonal antibodies to proteins, such as cytokines (eg, tumor necrosis factor-α), cell adhesion molecules, cytokine receptors (anti-interleukin-2 receptor), or T cell subsets. Etanercept, a soluble tumor necrosis factor receptor, has been used with success in the treatment of rheumatoid arthritis and juvenile idiopathic arthritis. Rituximab, an anti-CD20 monoclonal antibody, has been shown to be effective in corticosteroid-resistant Graves' ophthalmopathy and Wegener's granulomatosis.

OCULAR COMPLICATIONS OF CERTAIN SYSTEMICALLY ADMINISTERED DRUGS (SEE ALSO CHAPTER 22)

AMIODARONE

Amiodarone is a benzofuran derivative used to treat cardiac dysrhythmias, such as atrial fibrillation, atrial flutter, ventricular fibrillation, and Wolff–Parkinson–White syndrome. Most patients develop small punctate deposits with a vortex pattern in the basal cell layer of the corneal epithelium (Figure 15–40). The severity of keratopathy is related to the total daily dose and is mild at a dose of less than 200 mg daily. The deposits rarely interfere with vision, and although they progress with continued treatment, even in low dosage, they always resolve

completely when treatment is stopped. A small percentage of patients develop thyroid ophthalmopathy, although the mechanism is not fully understood. Rarely, bilateral optic neuropathy may occur as a direct toxic effect and alternative anti-arhythmic agents may need to be considered.

ANTICHOLINERGICS (ATROPINE & RELATED SYNTHETIC DRUGS)

All of these drugs, when given preoperatively or for gastrointestinal disorders, may cause blurred vision because of a direct action on accommodation. They also tend to dilate the pupils, so that in patients with narrow anterior chamber angles, there is the added threat of angle-closure glaucoma.

ANTIDEPRESSANTS

Tricyclic antidepressants and monoamine oxidase inhibitors have an anticholinergic effect and theoretically may exacerbate open-angle glaucoma or provoke an attack of angle-closure glaucoma. However, these side effects are rare in clinical practice.

CHLORAMPHENICOL

Chloramphenicol, in addition to the possibility of causing severe blood dyscrasias, hepatic and renal disease, and gastrointestinal disturbances, can sometimes cause optic neuritis. This is especially true in children. Bilateral blurred vision

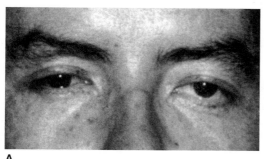

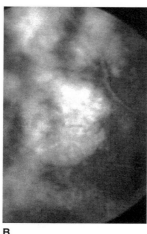

▲ **Figure 15–39.** Retinitis in an immunosuppressed patient. **A:** This patient with myasthenia gravis underwent thymectomy and received long-term immunosuppression with cytotoxic agents. **B:** He developed retinal necrosis and Ramsay Hunt syndrome following infection with herpes zoster.

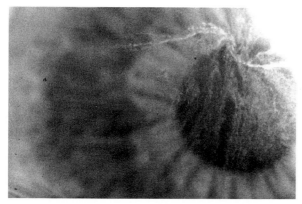

▲ **Figure 15–40.** Amiodarone keratopathy. (Courtesy of DJ Spalton.)

with central scotomas occurs. Stopping the drug does not always restore vision.

Isolated case reports of aplastic anemia occurring after topical chloramphenicol have not been substantiated.

CHLOROQUINE & HYDROXYCHLOROQUINE

Chloroquine is an effective antimalarial drug. With high dosage—often 250–750 mg daily administered for months or years—serious ocular toxicity has occurred. Corneal changes were described first and consisted of diffuse haziness of the epithelium and subepithelial area, occasionally sufficient to simulate an epithelial dystrophy. These changes cause only mild blurring of vision and are reversible upon drug withdrawal. Similar changes have been described in patients receiving quinacrine. Minimal corneal involvement is not necessarily an indication for discontinuance of chloroquine therapy.

A less common but more serious ocular complication of long-term chloroquine therapy is retinal damage, causing loss of central vision as well as constriction of peripheral visual fields. Pigmentary changes and edema of the macula, marked alteration of the retinal vessels, and in some cases peripheral pigmentary changes can be seen ophthalmoscopically. **Hydroxychloroquine** is a derivative of chloroquine that is regularly used in the treatment of collagen diseases (especially systemic lupus erythematosus), rheumatoid arthritis, and chronic skin disease, including discoid lupus and sarcoidosis. The range of ocular complications is the same as with chloroquine, but both their incidence and their severity are greatly reduced.

ORAL CONTRACEPTIVES

Although numerous reports suggest that in predisposed individuals, oral contraceptives can provoke or precipitate ophthalmic vascular occlusive disease or optic nerve damage, it is difficult to establish a definite cause and effect relationship. Optic neuritis, retinal arterial or venous thrombosis, and pseudotumor cerebri have been described in patients taking oral contraceptives. Since there is some uncertainty regarding the possibility of such ocular complications, oral contraceptives, particularly those containing estrogen, should be used only by healthy women with no history of vascular, neurologic, or ocular disease.

CORTICOSTEROIDS

Systemic corticosteroids can cause chronic open-angle glaucoma and usually posterior subcapsular cataracts with long-term therapy, and can provoke and worsen attacks of herpes simplex keratitis. Locally administered corticosteroids are much more potent in this respect and have the added disadvantage of causing fungal overgrowth if the corneal epithelium is not intact. Serous retinal detachments have been associated with systemic corticosteroids, particularly when these agents are used to treat the systemic vasculitides.

OXYGEN

Premature infants who are given supplemental oxygen are at increased risk of developing retinopathy of prematurity (see Chapters 10 and 17). In adults, administration of hyperbaric oxygen (3 atm) can cause constriction of the retinal arterioles.

PHENOBARBITAL & PHENYTOIN

Ocular complications relate to oculomotor involvement, producing nystagmus and weakness of convergence and accommodation. The nystagmus may persist for many months after cessation of the drug, and the degree of oculomotor abnormality is related to drug dosage. Early abnormalities include disturbance of smooth pursuit.

VIGABATRIN

Vigabatrin is an anticonvulsant that blocks gamma-aminobutyrate (GABA) transaminase. It causes irreversible visual field constriction in about 40% of patients and is no longer licensed for use in the United States. Patients receiving vigabatrin should undergo regular visual field testing. In young children, visual electrodiagnostic testing may be adequate.

PHENOTHIAZINES

The phenothiazines usually exert an atropine-like effect on the eye so that the pupils may be dilated, especially with large doses. Of greater clinical significance, however, are the pigmentary ocular changes, which include pigmentary retinopathy and pigment deposits on the corneal endothelium and anterior lens capsule. The corneal and lens pigmentation may cause blurring of vision, but the pigment deposits usually disappear several months after the drug is discontinued. In pigmentary retinopathy, there is a diminution of central vision, night blindness, diffuse narrowing of the retinal arteries, and occasionally severe blindness. The piperidine group (eg, thioridazine) has a higher risk of causing pigmentary retinopathy, and the maximum daily dose should not exceed 600 mg. The dimethylamine (eg, chlorpromazine) and the piperazine (eg, trifluoperazine) groups rarely produce retinal pigmentary changes.

All of these drugs can produce an extrapyramidal syndrome that may involve eye movements. Large doses can provoke profound hypotension, which may produce ischemic optic neuropathy.

Patients receiving large doses or prolonged treatment with phenothiazines should be questioned regarding visual disturbances and should have periodic ophthalmoscopic examinations.

QUININE

Quinine toxicity may cause bilateral blurred vision, as well as tinnitus and deafness. There is constriction of the visual field and, rarely, total blindness. The tendency is toward partial recovery, though usually there are permanent peripheral field defects. The ganglion cells of the retina are affected first, presumably as a result of vasoconstriction of the retinal arterioles. Varying degrees of retinal edema occur early. Optic atrophy is a late finding. Pupillary abnormalities are characteristic.

SEDATIVE TRANQUILIZERS

When taken regularly, the so-called minor tranquilizers can decrease tear production by the lacrimal gland, thus resulting in ocular irritation because of dry eyes. Tear production returns to normal when the tranquilizers are discontinued.

The principal drugs in this group are meprobamate, chlordiazepoxide, and diazepam.

TAMOXIFEN

A retinopathy consisting of intraretinal crystals in the macula, with visual loss, is seen in some patients receiving long-term tamoxifen therapy. It only occurs when the total lifetime dose has exceeded 90 g. Corneal crystals and optic neuropathy have also been reported.

RADIATION

Both optic neuropathy and retinopathy may occur months or years after radiation treatment to the head and neck, particularly to the sinuses or the parasellar region. The retinopathy manifests as cotton-wool spots, hemorrhages, and capillary closure, sometimes leading to retinal neovascularization. In the optic neuropathy, gadolinium-enhanced MRI reveals characteristic sharply demarcated lesions and hyperbaric oxygen therapy may be helpful if started soon after the onset of visual loss.

FETAL EFFECTS OF DRUGS

The visual pathways of the fetus are occasionally affected by drugs taken by the mother during pregnancy.

Phenytoin may cause optic nerve hypoplasia. Pigmentary retinopathy has been reported in a child of a mother taking **busulfan** for acute myeloid leukemia.

Warfarin is teratogenic and may produce a hypoplastic nose, stippled epiphyses, and skeletal abnormalities. Affected children may present with recurrent sticky eyes from obstruction of the nasolacrimal duct secondary to malformation of the nose. Other ocular abnormalities include optic atrophy, microphthalmia, and lens opacities.

REFERENCES

Acharya SH et al: Radioiodine therapy (RAI) for Graves' disease (GD) and the effect on ophthalmopathy: a systematic review. Clin Endocrinol 2008;69:943. [PMID: 18429949]

Ali A, Samson CM: Seronegative spondyloarthropathies and the eye. Curr Opin Ophthalmol 2007;18:476. [PMID: 18162999]

Anshu A, Cheng CL, Chee SP: Syphilitic uveitis: an Asian perspective. Br J Ophthalmol 2008;92:594. [PMID: 18441168]

Atkins EJ et al: Treatment of nonarteritic anterior ischemic optic neuropathy. Surv Ophthalmol 2010;55:47. [PMID: 20006051]

Bartalena L, Tanda ML: Clinical practice. Graves' ophthalmopathy. N Engl J Med 2009;360:994. [PMID: 19264688]

Bonfioli AA, Orefice F: Toxoplasmosis. Semin Ophthalmol. 2005;20:129. [PMID: 16282146]

Braakenburg AM et al: Human leukocyte antigen-B27-associated uveitis: long-term follow-up and gender differences. Am J Ophthalmol 2008;145:472. [PMID: 18282492]

Bradley EA et al: Orbital radiation for Graves' ophthalmopathy: a report by the American Academy of Ophthalmology. Ophthalmology 2008;115:398. [PMID: 18082885]

Brazis PW: Clinical review: the surgical treatment of idiopathic pseudotumour cerebri (idiopathic intracranial hypertension). Cephalalgia 2008;28:1361. [PMID: 19037972]

Calamia KT, Kaklamanis PG: Behçet's disease: recent advances in early diagnosis and treatment. Curr Rheumatol Rep 2008;10:349. [PMID: 18817637]

Chen CS, Miller NR: Ocular ischemic syndrome: review of clinical presentations, etiology, investigation, and management. Compr Ophthalmol Update 2007;8:17. [PMID: 17394756]

DelMonte DW, Bhatti MT: Ischemic optic neuropathy. Int Ophthalmol Clin 2009;49:35. [PMID: 19584621]

Dickinson J, Perros P: Thyroid-associated orbitopathy: who and how to treat. Endocrinol Metab Clin North Am 2009;38:373. [PMID: 1932847]

European Group on Graves' Orbitopathy (EUGOGO): Outcome of orbital decompression for disfiguring proptosis in patients with Graves' orbitopathy using various surgical procedures. Br J Ophthalmol 2009;93:1518. [PMID: 19028743]

Fonollosa A et al: Ocular syphilis–back again: understanding recent increases in the incidence of ocular syphilitic disease. Ocul Immunol Inflamm 2009;17:207. [PMID: 19585365]

Fraser JA et al: The treatment of giant cell arteritis. Rev Neurol Dis 2008;5:140. [PMID: 18838954]

Galor A et al: Comparison of antimetabolite drugs as corticosteroid-sparing therapy for noninfectious ocular inflammation. Ophthalmology 2008;115:1826. [PMID: 18579209]

Garrity JA, Bahn RS: Pathogenesis of Graves' ophthalmopathy: implications for prediction, prevention, and treatment. Am J Ophthalmol 2006;142:147. [PMID: 16815265]

Gupta V, Gupta A, Rao NA: Intraocular tuberculosis—an update. Surv Ophthalmol 2007;52:561. [PMID: 18029267]

Hayreh SS, Podhajsky PA, Zimmerman MB: Branch retinal artery occlusion: natural history of visual outcome. Ophthalmology 2009;116:1188. [PMID: 19376586]

Hayreh SS, Podhajsky PA, Zimmerman MB: Retinal artery occlusion associated: systemic and ophthalmic abnormalities. Ophthalmology 2009;116:1928. [PMID: 19577305]

Herbort CP et al: International criteria for the diagnosis of ocular sarcoidosis: results of the first international Workshop on Ocular Sarcoidosis (IWOS). Ocul Immunol Inflamm 2009;17:160. [PMID: 19585358]

Holland GN: AIDS and ophthalmology: the first quarter century. Am J Ophthalmol 2008;145:397. [PMID: 18282490]

Hong MC et al: Ocular uveitis as the initial presentation of syphilis. J Chin Med Assoc 2007;70:274. [PMID: 17631463]

Imrie FR, Dick AD: Biologics in the treatment of uveitis. Curr Opin Ophthalmol 2007;18:481. [PMID: 18163000]

Jabs DA et al: Longitudinal study of the ocular complications of AIDS: 1. Ocular diagnoses at enrollment. Ophthalmology 2007;114:780. [PMID: 17258320]

Jabs DA et al: Longitudinal study of the ocular complications of AIDS: 2. Ocular examination results at enrollment. Ophthalmology 2007;114:787. [PMID: 17210182]

Kawaguchi T, Spencer DB, Mochizuki M: Therapy for acute retinal necrosis. Semin Ophthalmol 2008;23:285. [PMID: 18584565]

Kempen JH et al: Long-term risk of malignancy among patients treated with immunosuppressive agents for ocular inflammation: a critical assessment of the evidence. Am J Ophthalmol 2008;146:802. [PMID: 18579112]

Khanna A et al: Pattern of ocular manifestations in patients with sarcoidosis in developing countries. Acta Ophthalmol Scand 2007;85:609. [PMID: 17651463]

Kunkel J et al: Ocular syphilis-indicator of previously unknown HIV-infection. J Infect 2009;58:32. [PMID: 19081634]

Lam FC, Law A, Wykes W: Herpes zoster ophthalmicus. BMJ 2009;339:457. [PMID: 19679612]

Liesegang TJ: Herpes zoster ophthalmicus natural history, risk factors, clinical presentation, and morbidity. Ophthalmology 2008;115:S3. [PMID: 18243930]

Li Q et al: Antiviral treatment for preventing postherpetic neuralgia. Cochrane Database Syst Rev 2009;(2):CD006866. [PMID: 19370655]

Lloyd MJ, Fraunfelder FW: Drug-induced optic neuropathies. Drugs Today 2007;43:827. [PMID: 18174968]

Lowery AJ, Kerin MJ: Graves' ophthalmopathy: the case for thyroid surgery. Surgeon 2009;7:290. [PMID: 19848063]

Masharani U, Rushakoff RJ: Update on systemic management of diabetes. Int Ophthalmol Clin 2009;49:13. [PMID: 19349784]

Mendes D et al: Behçet's disease–a contemporary review. J Autoimmun 2009;32:178. [PMID: 19324519]

Pakrou N, Selva D, Leibovitch I: Wegener's granulomatosis: ophthalmic manifestations and management. Semin Arthritis Rheum 2006;35:284. [PMID: 16616151]

Pasadhika S et al: Azathioprine for ocular inflammatory diseases. Am J Ophthalmo. 2009;148:500. [PMID: 19570522]

Pineles SL, Arnold AC: Giant cell arteritis. Int Ophthalmol Clin 2007;47:105. [PMID: 18049284]

Pujari SS et al: Cyclophosphamide for ocular inflammatory diseases. Ophthalmology 2010;117:356. [PMID: 19969366]

Suvajac G et al: Ocular manifestations in antiphospholipid syndrome. Autoimmun Rev 2007;6:409. [PMID: 17537387]

Rudkin AK, Lee AW, Chen CS: Vascular risk factors for central retinal artery occlusion. Eye 2010;24:678. [PMID: 19521436]

Santaella RM, Fraunfelder FW: Ocular adverse effects associated with systemic medications: recognition and management. Drugs 2007;67:75. [PMID: 17209665]

Sikdera S, Weinberg RS: Thyroid eye disease: pathogenesis and treatment. Ophthalmologica 2010;224:199. [PMID: 19940525]

Stiebel-Kalish H et al: Treatment modalities for Graves' ophthalmopathy: systematic review and metaanalysis. J Clin Endocrinol Metab 2009;94:2708. [PMID: 19491222]

Subramanian PS, Williams ZR: Arteriovenous malformations and carotid-cavernous fistulae. Int Ophthalmol Clin 2009;49:81. [PMID: 19584623]

Suvajac G, Stojanovich L, Milenkovich S: Ocular manifestations in antiphospholipid syndrome. Autoimmun Rev 2007;6:409. [PMID: 17537387]

Uretsky S: Surgical interventions for idiopathic intracranial hypertension. Curr Opin Ophthalmol 2009;20:451. [PMID: 19687737]

Usui Y, Goto H: Overview and diagnosis of acute retinal necrosis syndrome. Semin Ophthalmol 2008;23:275. [PMID: 18584564]

Vannucchi G et al: Graves' orbitopathy activation after radioactive iodine therapy with and without steroid prophylaxis. J Clin Endocrinol Metab 2009;94:3381. [PMID: 19567525]

Wong TY, Mitchell P: The eye in hypertension. Lancet 2007;369:425. [PMID: 17276782]

Wong TY et al. Rates of progression in diabetic retinopathy during different time periods: a systematic review and meta-analysis. Diabetes Care 2009;32:2307. [PMID: 19940227]

Yau JW et al: Retinal vein occlusion: an approach to diagnosis, systemic risk factors and management. Intern Med J 2008;38:904. [PMID: 19120547]

Zeboulon N, Douados M, Gossec L: Prevalence and characteristics of uveitis in spondyloarthropathies: a systematic literature review. Ann Rheum Dis 2008;67:955. [PMID: 17962239]

Zierhut M et al: MMF and eye disease. Lupus 2005;14:s50. [PMID: 1580393]

Immunologic Diseases of the Eye

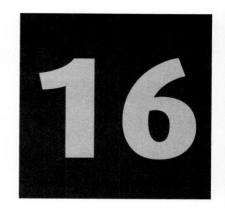

Toby Y.B. Chan, MD, and
William G. Hodge, MD, MPH, PhD, FRCSC

Ocular manifestations are a common feature of immunologic diseases even though, paradoxically, the eye is also a site of immune privilege. The propensity for immunologic disease to affect the eye derives from a number of factors, including the highly vascular nature of the uvea, the tendency for immune complexes to be deposited in various ocular tissues, and the exposure of the mucous membrane of the conjunctiva to environmental allergens. Inflammatory eye disorders are more obvious (and often more painful) than those of other organs, such as the thyroid or the kidney.

Immunologic diseases of the eye can be grossly divided into two major categories: antibody-mediated and cell-mediated diseases. As is the case in other organs, there is ample opportunity for the interaction of these two systems in the eye.

ANTIBODY-DEPENDENT & ANTIBODY-MEDIATED DISEASES

Before it can be concluded that a disease of the eye is antibody-dependent, the following criteria must be satisfied:

1. There must be evidence of specific antibody in the patient's serum or plasma cells.
2. The antigen must be identified and, if feasible, characterized.
3. The same antigen must be shown to produce an immunologic response in the eye of an experimental animal, and the pathologic changes produced in the experimental animal must be similar to those observed in the human disease.
4. It must be possible to produce similar lesions in animals passively sensitized with serum from an affected animal upon challenge with the specific antigen.

Unless all of the above criteria are satisfied, the disease may be thought of as *possibly* antibody-dependent.

In such circumstances, the disease can be regarded as antibody-mediated if only one of the following criteria is met:

1. If antibody to an antigen is present in higher quantities in the ocular fluids than in the serum (after adjustments have been made for the total amounts of immunoglobulins in each fluid).
2. If abnormal accumulations of plasma cells are present in the ocular lesion.
3. If abnormal accumulations of immunoglobulins are present at the site of the disease.
4. If complement is fixed by immunoglobulins at the site of the disease.
5. If an accumulation of eosinophils is present at the site of the disease.
6. If the ocular disease is associated with an inflammatory disease elsewhere in the body for which antibody dependency has been proved or strongly suggested.

HAY FEVER CONJUNCTIVITIS (SEE ALSO CHAPTER 5)

This disease is characterized by edema and hyperemia of the conjunctiva and lids (Figure 16–1) and by itching, which is always present, and tearing. There is often an associated itching sensation in the nose as well as rhinorrhea. The conjunctiva appears pale and boggy because of the intense edema, which is often rapid in onset. There may be a distinct seasonal incidence, patients being able to establish the onset of their symptoms at precisely the same time each year. These times usually correspond to the release of pollens by specific grasses, trees, or weeds.

▶ Immunologic Pathogenesis

Hay fever conjunctivitis is one of the few inflammatory eye disorders for which antibody dependence has been definitely

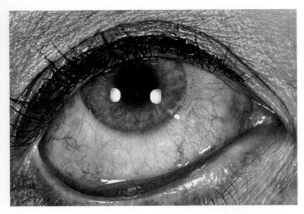

▲ **Figure 16–1.** Hay fever conjunctivitis. Note edema and hyperemia of the conjunctiva. (Courtesy of M Allansmith and B McClellan.)

established. It is recognized as a form of atopic disease with an implied hereditary susceptibility. IgE (reaginic antibody) is attached to mast cells lying beneath the conjunctival epithelium. Contact of the offending antigen with IgE triggers the release of vasoactive substances, principally leukotrienes and histamine, which results in vasodilation and chemosis.

The role of circulating antibody to ragweed pollen in the pathogenesis of hay fever conjunctivitis has been demonstrated by passively transferring serum from a hypersensitive person to a nonsensitive one. When exposed to the offending pollen, the previously nonsensitive individual reacted with the typical signs of hay fever conjunctivitis.

▶ Immunologic Diagnosis

Victims of hay fever conjunctivitis show many eosinophils in Giemsa-stained scrapings of conjunctival epithelium, and this is the test most commonly used to confirm the diagnosis. They show the immediate type of response, with wheal and flare, when tested by scratch tests of the skin with extracts of pollen or other offending antigens. Biopsies of the skin test sites have occasionally shown the full-blown picture of an Arthus reaction, with deposition of immune complexes in the walls of the dermal vessels. Passive cutaneous anaphylaxis can also be used to demonstrate the presence of circulating antibody.

▶ Immunologic Treatment

Immunotherapy with gradually increasing doses of sublingual or subcutaneously injected pollen extracts or other suspected allergens appears to reduce the severity of allergic disease in some individuals. The mechanism is presumed to be production of blocking antibodies in response to the injection of small, graded doses of the antigen. Despite some benefit in the treatment of respiratory allergies, immunotherapy does not seem to be effective in treating hay fever

conjunctivitis. As well, acute anaphylactoid reactions have occasionally resulted from overzealous immunotherapy. Topical antihistamines and mast cell stabilizers are the mainstay of treatment. Occasionally, mild nonpenetrating corticosteroids may be used in recalcitrant cases.

Other forms of treatment are discussed in Chapter 5.

VERNAL CONJUNCTIVITIS & ATOPIC KERATOCONJUNCTIVITIS (SEE ALSO CHAPTER 5)

These two diseases also belong to the group of atopic disorders. Both are characterized by itching and lacrimation of the eyes but are more chronic than hay fever conjunctivitis. Furthermore, both ultimately result in structural modifications of the lids and conjunctiva, especially atopic keratoconjunctivitis.

Vernal conjunctivitis characteristically affects children and adolescents; the incidence decreases sharply after the second decade of life. Like hay fever conjunctivitis, vernal conjunctivitis occurs only in the warm months of the year. Most patients live in hot, dry climates. The disease characteristically produces giant ("cobblestone") papillae of the tarsal conjunctiva (Figure 16–2). The keratinized epithelium from these papillae may abrade the underlying cornea, giving rise to complaints of foreign body sensation or even producing frank epithelial loss ("shield ulcer"). Alternatively, in some individuals, this disease affects the limbal region, producing a characteristic gelatinous thickening of the limbal conjunctiva, often associated with white accumulations of eosinophils and desquamated epithelial cells ("Horner-Trantas dots").

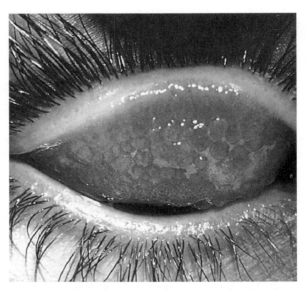

▲ **Figure 16–2.** Giant papillae ("cobblestones") in the tarsal conjunctiva of a patient with vernal conjunctivitis.

Atopic keratoconjunctivitis affects individuals of all ages and has no specific seasonal incidence. The skin of the lids has a characteristic dry, scaly appearance. The conjunctiva is pale and boggy. Both the conjunctiva and the cornea may develop scarring in the later stages of the disease. Staphylococcal blepharitis, manifested by scales and crusts on the lids, commonly complicates this disease. These patients are also more prone to herpes simplex ocular infections, cataract, and retinal detachment.

Although vernal and atopic disease may lie along a disease spectrum, often the two disorders can be differentiated. Atopic disease tends to occur in older patients, and there is little or no seasonal exacerbation. The papillae in atopic disease are smaller than in vernal disease and are as often found on the lower palpebral conjunctiva as the upper. Furthermore, corneal vascularization and conjunctival scarring are much more common in atopic disease. Finally, in atopic disease, eosinophils on smears are less numerous and less often degranulated.

▶ Immunologic Pathogenesis

Reaginic antibody (IgE) is fixed to subepithelial mast cells in both of these conditions. Contact between the offending antigen and IgE is thought to trigger degranulation of the mast cell, which in turn allows for the release of vasoactive amines in the tissues. It is unlikely, however, that antibody action alone is responsible, since—at least in the case of papillae of vernal conjunctivitis—there is heavy papillary infiltration by mononuclear cells. Furthermore, hay fever and asthma occur much more frequently in patients with vernal conjunctivitis and atopic keratoconjunctivitis than in the general population. These and other findings suggest that T-cell dysregulation also plays a role in the pathogenesis of vernal and atopic conjunctivitis.

▶ Immunologic Diagnosis

Patients with atopic keratoconjunctivitis and vernal conjunctivitis generally show large numbers of eosinophils in conjunctival scrapings. Skin testing with food extracts, pollens, and various other antigens reveals a wheal-and-flare type of reaction within 1 hour after testing, but the significance of these reactions is not established. Furthermore, the exact identities of the inciting antigens in these cases are usually unknown.

▶ Immunologic Treatment

Avoidance of allergens (if known) is helpful; such objects as duck feathers, animal danders, and certain food proteins (egg albumin and others) are possible offenders. Specific allergens have been especially difficult to demonstrate in the case of vernal disease, although some workers feel that such substances as rye grass pollens may play a causative role. Installation of air conditioning in the home or relocation to a cool, moist climate is useful in vernal conjunctivitis.

Other treatments are discussed in Chapter 5.

JOINT DISEASES AFFECTING THE EYE

The diseases in this category vary greatly in their clinical manifestations depending on the specific disease entity and the age of the patient. **Uveitis and scleritis** (Chapter 7) are the principal ocular manifestations associated with joint diseases.

Rheumatoid arthritis of adult onset may be accompanied by acute scleritis (Figure 16–3) or episcleritis but very rarely by uveitis (see also Chapter 7). The oligoarticular subgroup of **juvenile idiopathic arthritis**, which more commonly affects females with positive antinuclear antibodies, is commonly accompanied by iridocyclitis of one or both eyes (see Chapters 7, 15, and 17).

Ankylosing spondylitis affects males more frequently than females, and the onset is in the second to sixth decades. It may be accompanied by iridocyclitis of acute onset, often with fibrin in the anterior chamber (Figure 16–4).

Reactive arthritis (Reiter's syndrome) affects men more frequently than women. The first attack of ocular inflammation usually consists of a self-limited papillary conjunctivitis. It follows, at a highly variable interval, the onset of nonspecific urethritis and the appearance of inflammation in one or more of the weight-bearing joints. Subsequent attacks of ocular inflammation may consist of acute iridocyclitis of one or both eyes, occasionally with hypopyon (Figure 16–5).

▶ Immunologic Pathogenesis

Rheumatoid factor, an IgM autoantibody directed against the patient's own IgG, may play a major role in the pathogenesis of rheumatoid arthritis. The union of IgM antibody with IgG is followed by fixation of complement at the tissue site and the attraction of leukocytes and platelets to this area. An occlusive vasculitis, resulting from this chain of events, is thought to be the cause of rheumatoid nodule formation in the sclera as well as elsewhere in the body. The

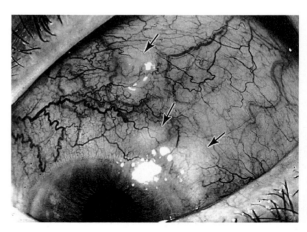

▲ **Figure 16–3.** Scleral nodules (arrows) in a patient with rheumatoid arthritis. (Courtesy of S Kimura.)

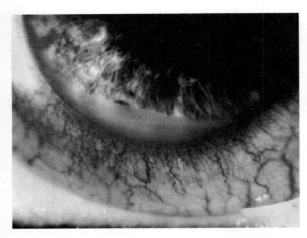

▲ **Figure 16–4.** Acute iridocyclitis in a patient with ankylosing spondylitis. Note fibrin clot in anterior chamber.

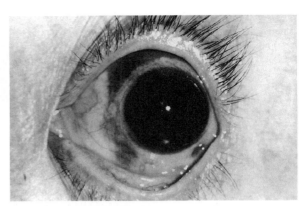

▲ **Figure 16–6.** Scleral thinning in a patient with rheumatoid arthritis. Note dark color of the underlying uvea.

occlusion of vessels supplying nutrients to the sclera is thought to be responsible for the "melting away" of the scleral collagen that is so characteristic of rheumatoid arthritis (Figure 16–6).

While this explanation may suffice for rheumatoid arthritis, patients with the ocular complications of juvenile idiopathic arthritis, ankylosing spondylitis, and reactive arthritis usually have negative tests for rheumatoid factor, so other explanations must be sought.

Outside the eyeball itself, the lacrimal gland has been shown to be under attack by circulating antibodies. Destruction of acinar cells within the gland and invasion of the lacrimal gland (as well as the salivary glands) by mononuclear cells result in decreased tear secretion. The combination of dry eyes (keratoconjunctivitis sicca) and dry mouth (xerostomia) is known as **Sjögren's syndrome** (see Chapter 15).

A growing body of evidence indicates that the immunogenetic background of certain patients accounts for the expression of their ocular inflammatory disease in specific ways. Analysis of the HLA antigen system shows that the incidence of HLA-B27 is significantly greater in patients with ankylosing spondylitis and reactive arthritis than could be expected by chance alone. It is not known how this antigen controls specific inflammatory responses. Other well-established HLA disease associations include HLA-A11 in sympathetic ophthalmia, HLA-A29 in birdshot choroidopathy, HLA-B51 in Behçet's syndrome, and HLA-B7 in macular histoplasmosis. However, it remains unclear whether these HLA associations are indicative of causation or merely markers for other cosegregating genes that are responsible for disease.

▶ Immunologic Diagnosis

Rheumatoid factor can be detected in the serum by several standard tests involving the agglutination of IgG-coated erythrocytes or latex particles. Unfortunately, the test for rheumatoid factor is not positive in the majority of isolated rheumatoid afflictions of the eye.

The HLA types of individuals suspected of having ankylosing spondylitis and related diseases can be determined. HLA-B27 is associated with ankylosing spondylitis and reactive arthritis. X-ray of the sacroiliac area is a valuable screening procedure that may show evidence of spondylitis prior to the onset of low back pain in patients with the characteristic form of iridocyclitis.

OTHER ANTIBODY-MEDIATED EYE DISEASES (SEE ALSO CHAPTER 15)

The following antibody-mediated diseases are infrequently encountered by the practicing ophthalmologist.

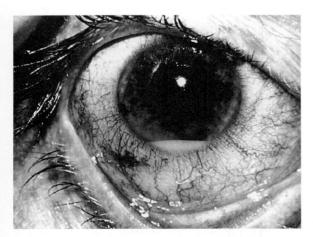

▲ **Figure 16–5.** Acute iridocyclitis with hypopyon in a patient with reactive arthritis (Reiter's syndrome).

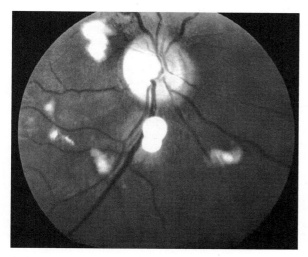

▲ **Figure 16–7.** Cotton-wool spots in the retina of a patient with systemic lupus erythematosus.

Systemic lupus erythematosus, associated with the presence of circulating antibodies to DNA, produces an occlusive vasculitis of the nerve fiber layer of the retina, manifesting as retinal cotton-wool spots (Figure 16–7).

Pemphigus vulgaris produces painful intraepithelial bullae of the conjunctiva. It is associated with the presence of circulating antibodies to an intercellular antigen located between the deeper cells of the conjunctival epithelium.

Cicatricial pemphigoid is characterized by subepithelial bullae of the conjunctiva. In the chronic stages of this disease, cicatricial contraction of the conjunctiva may result in severe dryness of the eyes, scarring of the cornea, and ultimately, blindness. Pemphigoid is associated with local deposits of tissue antibodies directed against one or more antigens located in the basement membrane of the epithelium. Systemic immunosuppressive treatment is often needed in the progressive stages of this disease.

Lens-induced uveitis is a rare condition that may be associated with circulating antibodies to lens proteins. It is seen in individuals whose lens capsules have become permeable to these proteins as a result of trauma or other disease (see Chapter 7). It is believed that the anatomy of the lens sequesters lens antigens during immune system maturation, thereby preventing the development of tolerance.

▼ CELL-MEDIATED DISEASES

This group of diseases appears to be associated with cell-mediated immunity or delayed hypersensitivity. Various structures of the eye are invaded by mononuclear cells, principally lymphocytes and macrophages, in response to one or more chronic antigenic stimuli. In the case of chronic infections such as tuberculosis, leprosy, toxoplasmosis, and herpes simplex, the antigenic stimulus has clearly been identified as an infectious agent in the ocular tissue. Such infections are often associated with delayed skin test reactivity following the intradermal injection of an extract of the organism.

More intriguing but less well understood are the granulomatous diseases of the eye, for which no infectious cause has been found. Such diseases are thought to represent cell-mediated, possibly autoimmune processes, but their origin remains obscure.

Stevens–Johnson syndrome and **toxic epidermal necrolysis**, the more extensive variant of the same disease, which are most commonly incited by drugs such as sulfonamides but mycoplasma or viral infections may be responsible, and **erythema multiforme**, which is usually precipitated by acute infection, most often recurrent herpes simplex virus infection, cause skin and mucous membrane lesions, the latter possibly leading to cicatrizing conjunctivitis, with the potential for severe corneal dryness and scarring. The pathogenesis in all three entities is cell-mediated cytotoxicity, primarily directed against keratinocytes.

OCULAR SARCOIDOSIS

Ocular sarcoidosis is characterized by a panuveitis with occasional inflammatory involvement of the optic nerve, conjunctiva, and retinal blood vessels (see Chapters 7 and 15).

▶ Immunologic Pathogenesis

Although many infectious or allergic causes of sarcoidosis have been suggested, none has been confirmed. Noncaseating granulomas are seen in the uvea, optic nerve, conjunctiva, and adnexal structures of the eye as well as elsewhere in the body. The presence of macrophages and giant cells suggests that particulate matter is being phagocytosed. Some studies have suggested that mycobacterial infection is an etiological factor.

Patients with sarcoidosis are usually anergic to extracts of the common microbial antigens, such as those of mumps, trichophyton, candida, and *Mycobacterium tuberculosis*. As in other lymphoproliferative disorders, such as Hodgkin's disease and chronic lymphocytic leukemia, this may represent suppression of T-cell activity such that the normal delayed hypersensitivity responses to common antigens cannot take place. Meanwhile, circulating immunoglobulins are usually detectable in the serum at higher than normal levels.

▶ Immunologic Diagnosis

There is no specific test but the strongest diagnostic evidence is the presence of noncaseating granulomas, such as in a biopsy of a conjunctival nodule, skin lesion, or enlarged lacrimal gland or lymph node, or in samples obtained at bronchoscopy. Chest x-ray abnormalities, usually bilateral hilar lymphadenopathy, are frequent and often direct further investigation. Gallium scan may also be positive. Negative skin tests to a battery of antigens to which the patient is known to have been exposed, for instance tuberculin, are highly suggestive Serum angiotensin-converting enzyme (ACE) is often elevated but this is more useful for monitoring disease activity than diagnosis.

▶ Treatment

See Chapter 15.

SYMPATHETIC OPHTHALMIA & VOGT–KOYANAGI–HARADA SYNDROME

These two disorders are discussed together because they have certain common clinical features. Both are thought to represent autoimmune phenomena affecting pigmented structures of the eye and skin, and both may give rise to meningeal symptoms.

▶ Clinical Features

Sympathetic ophthalmia is an inflammation in the second eye after the other has been damaged by penetrating injury. In most cases, some portion of the uvea of the injured eye has been exposed to the atmosphere for at least 1 hour. The uninjured or "sympathizing" eye develops minor signs of anterior uveitis after a period ranging from 2 weeks to many years. However, the vast majority of cases occur within 1 year. As a result of ciliary body inflammation, floating spots and loss of the power of accommodation are among the earliest symptoms. The disease may progress to severe iridocyclitis with pain and photophobia. Usually, however, the eye remains relatively painless while the inflammatory disease spreads around the entire uvea. The retina usually remains uninvolved except for perivascular cuffing of the retinal vessels with inflammatory cells. There may be choroidal lesions, representing the macroscopic manifestation of Dalen–Fuchs nodules (see later in the chapter). Optic nerve swelling and secondary glaucoma may occur. The disease may be accompanied by vitiligo (patchy depigmentation of the skin) and poliosis (whitening) of the eyelashes. For unknown reasons, the incidence of this disease has decreased markedly over the last several decades.

Vogt–Koyanagi–Harada syndrome consists of inflammation of the uvea of one or both eyes characterized by acute iridocyclitis, patchy choroiditis, and serous detachment of the retina (see Chapter 15). It usually begins with an acute febrile episode with headache, dysacusis, and occasionally vertigo. Patchy loss or whitening of scalp hair is described in the first few months of the disease. Vitiligo and poliosis are commonly present but are not essential for the diagnosis. Although the initial iridocyclitis may subside quickly, the course of the posterior disease is often indolent, with long-standing serous detachment of the retina and significant visual impairment.

▶ Immunologic Pathogenesis

In both sympathetic ophthalmia and Vogt–Koyanagi–Harada syndrome, a delayed hypersensitivity to melanin-containing structures, in the eye, skin, and hair, is provoked. Soluble materials from the outer segments of the photoreceptor layer of the retina (retinal S-antigens) have been incriminated as possible autoantigens. Patients with Vogt–Koyanagi–Harada syndrome are usually of Southeast Asian ancestry, which suggests an immunogenetic predisposition to the disease.

Histologic sections of the traumatized eye from a patient with sympathetic ophthalmia may show uniform infiltration of most of the uvea by lymphocytes, epithelioid cells, and giant cells. The overlying retina is characteristically intact, but nests of epithelioid cells may protrude through the pigment epithelium of the retina, giving rise to **Dalen–Fuchs nodules.** The inflammation may destroy the architecture of the entire uvea, leaving an atrophic, shrunken globe.

▶ Immunologic Diagnosis

Skin tests with soluble extracts of human or bovine uveal tissue are said to elicit delayed hypersensitivity responses in these patients. Several investigators have shown that cultured lymphocytes from patients with these two diseases undergo transformation to lymphoblasts in vitro when extracts of uvea or rod outer segments are added to the culture medium. Circulating antibodies to uveal antigens have been found in patients with these diseases, but such antibodies are to be found in any patient with long-standing uveitis, including those suffering from several infectious entities. The spinal fluid of patients with Vogt–Koyanagi–Harada syndrome may show increased numbers of mononuclear cells and elevated protein in the early stages. Treatment of both conditions requires at least systemic steroids and often oral immunosuppressive therapy.

OTHER DISEASES OF CELL-MEDIATED IMMUNITY

Giant cell arteritis (temporal arteritis) (see Chapter 15) may have disastrous effects on the eye. The condition presents in elderly individuals usually with headache and numerous systemic complaints, including polymyalgia rheumatica. Ocular complications include anterior ischemic optic neuropathy and central retinal artery occlusion. Such patients have an elevated sedimentation rate. Biopsy of the temporal artery reveals extensive infiltration of the vessel wall with giant cells and mononuclear cells.

Polyarteritis nodosa (see Chapter 15) is a vasculitis that predominantly affects small- to medium-sized vessels. It can affect both the anterior and posterior segments of the eye. The corneas of such patients may show peripheral thinning and cellular infiltration. The retinal and ciliary vessels reveal extensive necrotizing inflammation characterized by eosinophil, plasma cell, and lymphocyte infiltration.

Wegener's granulomatosis is another systemic vasculitis with potential ocular manifestations. In this disorder, necrotizing granulomatous inflammation primarily involves the upper respiratory tract and kidneys. Ophthalmic involvement usually consists of peripheral ulcerative keratitis and scleritis, but retinal vasculitis can occur. The presence of cytoplasmic pattern of antineutrophil cytoplasmic antibodies (C-ANCA) is helpful in making the diagnosis.

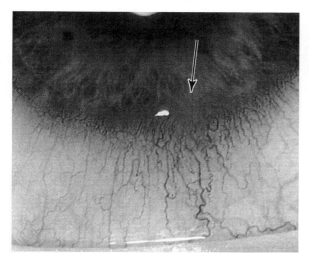

▲ **Figure 16–8.** Phlyctenule **(arrow)** at the margin of the cornea. (Courtesy of P Thygeson.)

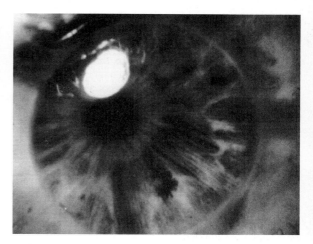

▲ **Figure 16–9.** A cornea severely scarred by chronic atopic keratoconjunctivitis, into which a central graft of clear cornea has been placed. Note how distinctly the iris landmarks are seen through the transparent graft. (Reproduced, with permission, from Parslow TG et al [editors]: Medical Immunology, 10th ed. McGraw-Hill, 2001.)

Behçet's disease (see Chapter 15) has an uncertain place in the classification of immunologic disorders. It is characterized by recurrent iridocyclitis with hypopyon and occlusive vasculitis of the retinal vessels. Although it has many of the features of a delayed hypersensitivity disease, dramatic alterations of serum complement levels at the very beginning of an attack suggest an immune complex disorder. Furthermore, high levels of circulating immune complexes have recently been detected in patients with this disease. Most patients with eye symptoms are positive for HLA-B51, a subtype of HLA-B5, and are of eastern Mediterranean or Southeast Asian ancestry.

Contact dermatitis of the eyelids represents a significant although minor disease caused by delayed hypersensitivity. Topical medications such as brimonidine and atropine, eye drop preservatives, perfumed cosmetics, materials contained in plastic spectacle frames, and other locally applied agents may act as the sensitizing hapten. The lower lid is more extensively involved than the upper lid when the sensitizing agent is applied in drop form. Periorbital involvement with erythematous, vesicular, pruritic lesions of the skin is characteristic.

Phlyctenular keratoconjunctivitis (Figure 16–8) represents a delayed hypersensitivity response to certain microbial antigens, principally those of *M tuberculosis* and *Staphylococcus aureus* (see Chapters 5 and 6).

▼ CORNEAL GRAFT REACTIONS (FIGURE 16–9)

Blindness due to opacity or distortion of the central portion of the cornea is a remediable disease. If all other structures of the eye are intact, a patient whose vision is impaired solely by corneal opacity can expect great improvement from a graft of clear cornea into the diseased area (see Chapter 6). Trauma,

including chemical burns, is one of the most common causes of central corneal opacity. Others include scars from herpetic keratitis, endothelial cell dysfunction with chronic corneal edema (including pseudophakic bullous keratopathy and Fuchs' dystrophy), keratoconus, and opacities from previous graft failures. All of these conditions represent indications for corneal grafts, provided the patient's eye is no longer inflamed and the opacity has been allowed maximal time to undergo spontaneous resolution (usually 6–12 months). Over 40,000 corneal grafts are performed in the United States annually, of which 90% can be expected to produce a beneficial result.

The cornea was one of the first human tissues to be successfully grafted. The fact that recipients of corneal grafts generally tolerate them well can be attributed to (1) the absence of blood vessels or lymphatics in the normal cornea; (2) the paucity of antigen-presenting cells; (3) expression of Fas ligand by corneal endothelial and epithelial cells, which induces apoptosis of inflammatory cells; and (4) anterior chamber acquired immune deviation (ACAID). The latter is a series of unique immunologic properties of the anterior chamber, conferring on the graft area the status of immune privilege. Local constitutive expression of transforming growth factor (TGF)-β plays a central role in ACAID by downregulating delayed type hypersensitivity reactions. Reactions to corneal grafts do occur, however, particularly in individuals whose own corneas have been damaged by previous inflammatory disease. Such corneas may have developed both lymphatics and blood vessels and may possess greater numbers of antigen-presenting cells, thus providing afferent and efferent channels for immunologic reactions in the engrafted cornea. Graft rejection is a major cause of corneal graft failure.

Although attempts have been made to transplant corneas from other species into human eyes (xenografts), particularly in countries where human material is not available for religious reasons, most corneal grafts have been taken from human eyes (allografts). Except in the case of identical twins, such grafts always represent the implantation of foreign tissue into a donor site; thus, the chance for a graft rejection due to an immune response to foreign antigens is virtually always present.

The cornea is a three-layered structure composed of a surface epithelium, an oligocellular collagenous stroma, and a single-cell–layered endothelium. Although the surface epithelium may be sloughed and later replaced by the recipient's epithelium, certain elements of the stroma and all of the donor's endothelium remain in place for the rest of the patient's life. This has been firmly established by sex chromosome markers in corneal cells when donor and recipient were of opposite sexes.

A number of foreign elements exist in corneal grafts that might stimulate the immune system of the host to reject this tissue. In addition to the structural cells and proteins mentioned above, the corneal stroma is regularly perfused with IgG and serum albumin from the donor, although none of the other blood proteins are present—or only small amounts. While these serum proteins of donor origin rapidly diffuse into the recipient stroma and are thus removed from the graft site, they are theoretically immunogenic.

Overall, the endothelium is more important than the epithelium or stroma in stimulating corneal graft rejection. Whenever possible, corneal graft surgery is limited to lamellar keratoplasty, in which the epithelium and stroma but not the endothelium are transplanted, but this does not totally prevent graft rejection.

HLA incompatibility between donor and recipient has been shown by several authors to be significant in determining graft survival, particularly when the corneal bed is vascularized. It is known that most cells of the body possess these HLA antigens, including the endothelial cells of the corneal graft and certain stromal cells (keratocytes). The epithelium has been shown to possess a non-HLA antigen that diffuses into the anterior third of the stroma. Thus, while much foreign antigen may be eliminated by purposeful removal of the epithelium at the time of grafting, that amount of antigen which has already diffused into the stroma is automatically carried over into the recipient.

Despite numerous analytic studies supporting the role of HLA incompatibility in corneal graft rejection, a multicenter clinical trial found no use in HLA typing high-risk grafts. In this study, ABO blood typing did provide a slight protective effect in high-risk cases. More recent studies have shown the potential benefit on corneal graft survival of HLA triplet string-matching systems, originally developed for renal transplantation.

Both humoral and cellular mechanisms have been implicated in corneal graft reactions. It is likely that early graft rejections (2–4 weeks from surgery) are cell-mediated reactions. Cytotoxic lymphocytes have been found in the limbal area and stroma of affected individuals, and phase microscopy in vivo has revealed an actual attack on the grafted endothelial cells by these lymphocytes. However, CD8 T-cell knockout mice have been shown to mount vigorous rejection responses, with delayed type hypersensitivity inflammatory cells predominating, thus, indicating that cytolytic T-cells may not be essential in graft rejection. Lymphocytes mediating rejection generally move inward from the periphery of the cornea, making what is known as a "rejection line" as they move centrally. The donor cornea becomes edematous as the endothelium becomes compromised by an accumulation of lymphoid cells.

Late rejection of a corneal graft may occur several weeks to many months after implantation of donor tissue into the recipient eye. Such reactions may be antibody-mediated, since cytotoxic antibodies have been isolated from the serum of patients with a history of multiple graft reactions in vascularized corneal beds. These antibody reactions are complement-dependent and attract polymorphonuclear leukocytes, which may form dense rings in the cornea at the sites of maximum deposition of immune complexes. In experimental animals, similar reactions have been produced by corneal xenografts, but the intensity of the reaction can be markedly reduced either by decomplementing the animal or by reducing its leukocyte population through mechlorethamine therapy.

▶ Treatment

The mainstay of the treatment of corneal graft reactions is corticosteroid therapy. This medication is generally given in the form of frequently applied eye drops (eg, 1% prednisolone acetate every hour) until the clinical signs abate. These clinical signs consist of conjunctival hyperemia in the perilimbal region, a cloudy cornea, cells and protein in the anterior chamber, and keratic precipitates on the corneal endothelium. The earlier treatment is applied, the more effective it is likely to be. Some cases may require systemic or periocular corticosteroids in addition to local eye drop therapy. High-dose intravenous steroids may also be efficacious if used sooner than 8 days after onset of the rejection period. Occasionally, vascularization and opacification of the cornea occur so rapidly as to make corticosteroid therapy useless, but even the most hopeless-appearing graft reactions have occasionally been reversed by corticosteroid therapy. Oral cyclosporine has been used successfully in the treatment of corneal graft rejection, and some benefit may be derived from cyclosporine eye drops.

Patients known to have rejected many previous corneal grafts or at high risk of rejection for other reasons are managed somewhat differently, particularly if disease affects their only remaining eye. Some surgeons may choose to find a close HLA match between donor and recipient. Pretreatment of the recipient with immunosuppressive agents such as azathioprine, cyclosporine, or, most recently, mycophenolate mofetil has also been resorted to in some cases.

RECENT DEVELOPMENTS IN IMMUNOTHERAPY

While the initiators of ocular inflammatory diseases remain in many cases the subject of active speculation, the complex signals that mediate the inflammatory response are rapidly being elucidated. Of paramount importance in many systemic and ocular inflammatory conditions are T-cell-mediated immune reactions and cytokines. Therapies directed against T-cells and cytokines (immunosuppressants and biologic response modifiers) are now in clinical use.

Immunosuppressants

These include antimetabolites (azathioprine, methotrexate, and mycophenolate mofetil), T-cell inhibitors (cyclosporine and tacrolimus), and alkylating agents (cyclophosphamide and chlorambucil). T-cell inhibitors, for instance, were found to be useful in treating allergic eye disease and dry eyes. The treating physician must be familiar with the ocular and systemic side effects of these medications, which are discussed in Chapter 15.

Biologic Response Modifiers

These include antibodies against cytokines or cytokine receptors. Anti-TNFα agents (infliximab, adalimumab and etanercept), successful in treating rheumatoid arthritis, have shown promising results in the control of uveitis. Daclizumab, a monoclonal antibody against CD25 subunit of IL-2 receptor on T cells, is clinically effective in controlling certain types of uveitis. Rituximab (chimeric monoclonal antibody against CD20 on B cells) reduces inflammation in Graves' ophthalmopathy and Wegener's granulomatosis. Other antibodies, such as anti-IL-12/23 and anti-IL-17, have been effective in treating Crohn's disease and rheumatoid arthritis. Their clinical efficacy in ocular immunologic diseases has yet to be determined. Apart from antibodies, interferon-α2a, a cytokine released in viral infections, has achieved remission of Behcet's disease and other forms of uveitis.

Modes of Delivery

In order to enhance anti-inflammatory effect on the eye and to minimize systemic side effects, alternative modes of delivery of these agents (apart from oral or intravenous) have also been studied. A topical anti-TNFα antibody, ESBA105, is being investigated for its feasibility in treating ocular inflammation. Intraocular methotrexate has shown vision improvement and reduction of macular edema in uveitic patients.

Sustained implants of immunosuppressants, as well as intraocular viral and nonviral gene therapies that deliver anticytokine agents, are being investigated in animal studies.

Despite advances in the understanding of immunoregulatory mechanisms, the perfect immunotherapy agent remains to be discovered. With further discovery of the roles of individual components in immunologic pathways, it will be possible to improve the treatment of immunologic diseases of the eye.

REFERENCES

Andreoli CM, Foster CS: Vogt–Koyanagi–Harada disease. Int Ophthalmol Clin 2006;46:111. [PMID: 16770158]

Bielory L, Friedlaender MH: Allergic conjunctivitis. Immunol Allergy Clin North Am 2008;28.43. [PMID; 18282545]

Bohringer D et al: Beneficial effect of matching at the HLA-A and -B amino-acid triplet level on rejection-free clear graft survival in penetrating keratoplasty. Transplantation 2004;77:417. [PMID: 14966417]

Borchers AT et al: Stevens–Johnson syndrome and toxic epidermal necrolysis. Autoimmun Rev 2008;7:598. [PMID: 18603022]

Butrus S, Portela R: Ocular allergy: diagnosis and treatment. Ophthalmol Clin North Am 2005;18:485. [PMID: 16314214]

Chang JH, McCluskey PJ, Wakefield D: Acute anterior uveitis and HLA-B27. Surv Ophthalmol 2005;50:364. [PMID: 15967191]

Coster DJ, Williams KA: The impact of corneal allograft rejection on the long-term outcome of corneal transplantation. Am J Ophthalmol 2005;140:1112. [PMID: 16376660]

Dahl R et al: Efficacy and safety of sublingual immunotherapy with grass allergen tablets for seasonal allergic rhinoconjunctivitis. J Allergy Clin Immunol 2006;118:434. [PMID: 16890769]

Damico FM, Kiss S, Young LH: Vogt–Koyanagi–Harada disease. Semin Ophthalmol 2005;20:183. [PMID: 16282153]

Frew AJ et al: Efficacy and safety of specific immunotherapy with SQ allergen extract in treatment-resistant seasonal allergic rhinoconjunctivitis. J Allergy Clin Immunol 2006;117:319. [PMID: 16461133]

Hingorani M, Lightman S: Ocular cicatricial pemphigoid. Curr Opin Allergy Clin Immunol 2006;6:373. [PMID: 16954792]

Jap A, Chee SP: Immunosuppressive therapy for ocular diseases. Curr Opin Ophthalmol 2008;19:535. [PMID: 18854699]

Jun J, Bielory L, Raizman MB: Vernal conjunctivitis. Immunology Allergy Clin North Am 2008;28:59. [PMID: 18282546]

Koh MJ, Tay YK: An update on Stevens–Johnson syndrome and toxic epidermal necrolysis in children. Curr Opin Pediatr 2009;21:505. [PMID: 19474732]

Kumar S: Vernal keratoconjunctivitis. Acta Ophthalmol 2009;87:133. [PMID: 18786127]

Leonardi a et al: Case series of 406 vernal keratoconjunctivitis patients: a demographic and epidemiological study. Acta Ophthalmol Scand 2006;84:406. [PMID: 16704708]

Mannon PJ et al: Anti-interleukin-12 antibody for active Crohn's disease. N Engl J Med 2004;351(20):2069. [PMID: 15537905]

Niederkorn JY et al: CD4+ T-cell–independent rejection of corneal allografts. Transplantation 2006;81:1171. [PMID: 16641604]

Niederkorn JY et al: Differential roles of CD8+ and CD8− T lymphocytes in corneal allograft rejection in 'high-risk' hosts. Am J Transplant 2006;6:705. [PMID: 16539627]

Onal S et al: Rituximab for remission induction in a patient with relapsing necrotizing scleritis associated with limited Wegener's granulomatosis. Ocul Immunol Inflamm 2008;16(5):230. [PMID: 19065418]

Ottiger M et al: Efficient intraocular penetration of topical anti-TNF-alpha single-chain antibody (ESBA105) to anterior and posterior segment without penetration enhancer. Invest Ophthalmol Vis Sci 2009;50(2):779. [PMID: 18757511]

Paredes I, Ahmed M, Foster CS: Immunomodulatory therapy for Vogt–Koyanagi–Harada patients as first-line therapy. Ocul Immunol Inflamm 2006;14:87. [PMID: 16597537]

Randleman JB, Stulting RD: Prevention and treatment of corneal graft rejection: current practice patterns (2004). Cornea 2006;25:286. [PMID: 16633028]

Rosenbaum JT: An algorithm for the systemic evaluation of patients with uveitis: guidelines for the consultant. Semin Arthritis Rheum 1990;19:248. [PMID: 2181671]

Schwartzman S, Fleischmann R, Morgan GJ Jr: Do anti-TNF agents have equal efficacy in patients with rheumatoid arthritis? Arthritis Res Ther 2004;6(Suppl 2):S3. [PMID: 15228615]

Sopo SM et al: Sublingual immunotherapy in asthma and rhinoconjunctivitis: systematic review of pediatric literature. Arch Dis Child 2004;89:620. [PMID: 15210490]

Suhler EB et al: A prospective trial of infliximab therapy for refractory uveitis: preliminary safety and efficacy outcomes. Arch Ophthalmol 2005;123:903. [PMID: 16009830]

Taylor SR et al: Intraocular methotrexate in the treatment of uveitis and uveitic cystoid macular edema. Ophthalmology 2009;116(4):797. [PMID: 19344827]

Tsai ML et al: Suppression of experimental uveitis by a recombinant adeno-associated virus vector encoding interleukin-1 receptor antagonist. Mol Vis 2009;15:1542. [PMID: 19693263]

van den Berg WB, Miossec P: IL-17 as a future therapeutic target for rheumatoid arthritis. Nat Rev Rheumatol 2009;5(10):549. [PMID: 19798029]

Watson SL, Tuft SJ, Dart JK: Patterns of rejection after deep lamellar keratoplasty. Ophthalmology 2006;113:556. [PMID: 16581417]

Special Subjects of Pediatric Interest

17

Douglas R. Fredrick, MD

Pediatric ophthalmology offers particular challenges to the ophthalmologist, pediatrician, and family physician. Symptoms are often nonspecific, and the usual examination techniques require modification. Development of the visual system is still occurring during the first decade of life, with the potential for amblyopia even in response to relatively mild ocular disease. Because the development of the eye often reflects organ and tissue development of the body as a whole, many congenital somatic defects are mirrored in the eye. Collaboration with pediatricians, neurologists, and other health workers is essential in managing these conditions. Similar collaboration is required in assessing the educational needs of any child with poor vision.

Details of the embryology and the normal postnatal growth and development of the eye are discussed in Chapter 1.

NEONATAL OCULAR EXAMINATION

All infants should have their eyes examined as a part of the newborn physical examination, and the practitioner should look for the presence of a normal red reflex in both eyes, normal external ocular anatomy, and symmetry between the eyes. A careful eye examination soon after birth may reveal congenital abnormalities that suggest the presence of abnormalities elsewhere in the body and the need for further investigations. A pediatric examination table is presented in Table 17–1.

The instruments required for the ocular examination of the newborn are a good hand light, direct and indirect ophthalmoscopes, a loupe for magnification, and occasionally a portable slitlamp. Phenylephrine 2.5% and cyclopentolate 1% or tropicamide 1% are generally safe for pupillary dilation in full-term neonates, although even these concentrations may have adverse effects on blood pressure and gastrointestinal function in premature neonates and those with lightly pigmented eyes; in these instances the combination of cyclopentolate 0.2% and phenylephrine 1% (Cyclomydril) should be used to dilate the pupils.

Subjective response testing is limited to observing the following response to a visual target, the most effective being a human face. Visual fixation and following movements can be demonstrated in most newborn babies; however, some infants do not demonstrate consistent fixation behavior until 2 months of age. Following movements in the first 2 months of life can be coarse and jerky and should not be expected to resemble the smooth pursuit movements of older children and adults.

► External Inspection

The eyelids are inspected for growths, deformities, lid notches, and symmetric movement with opening and closing of the eyes. The absolute and relative size of the eyeballs is noted, as well as position and alignment. The size and luster of the corneas are noted, and the anterior chambers are examined for clarity and iris configuration. The size, position, and light reaction of the pupils are also noted. The pupils are normally relatively dilated until 29 weeks of gestation, at which time the pupillary light response first becomes apparent. The light response is not a reliable test until 32 weeks of gestation. Anisocoria of 0.5 mm can be seen in as many as 20% of neonates. It is important to carefully examine the pupils of any infant with ptosis, looking for anisocoria, as Horner's syndrome, while usually benign, can be due to neuroblastoma and the ophthalmologist can play a pivotal role in making the timely diagnosis.

► Ophthalmoscopic Examination

With undilated pupils, some information can be obtained by use of the ophthalmoscope in a dimly lighted room but ideally all newborns should be examined with an ophthalmoscope through dilated pupils. Ophthalmoscopic examination will demonstrate any corneal, lens, or vitreous opacities as well as abnormalities in the fundus. In premature infants, remnants of the tunica vasculosa lentis are frequently visible, either in front of the lens, behind the lens, or in both positions. The remnants are usually regressed by

Table 17–1. Pediatric Eye Examination Schedule

Neonatal Examination

External eye examination and confirmation of presence of red reflex. In infants requiring examination for retinopathy of prematurity (ROP) or with abnormal red reflex, dilate eyes with phenylephrine 2.5% and cyclopentolate 1% or tropicamide 1% in each eye instilled 1 hour prior to examination. (Cyclopentolate 0.2% and phenylephrine 1% combination [Cyclomydril] is used in babies with lightly pigmented eyes and premature neonates.) Special attention should be paid to the optic disks and maculas; detailed examination of the peripheral retinas is not necessary unless the baby is at risk for ROP.

Age 6 months

Test ocular fixation and ocular movements. Look for strabismus.

Age 4 years

Test visual acuity with Snellen letters, HOTV matching optotypes, or Lea symbols. Visual acuity should be normal (20/20-20/30).

Age 5-16 years

Test visual acuity at age 5. If normal, test visual acuity with the Snellen chart every 2 years until age 16. Color vision should be tested at ages 8-12. No other routine eye examination (eg, ophthalmoscopy) is necessary if visual acuity is normal and the eyes appear normal upon inspection.

the time the infant has reached term, but rarely they remain permanently and appear as a complete or partial "cobweb" in the pupil. At other times, remnants of the primitive hyaloid system fail to absorb completely, leaving either a cone on the optic disk that projects into the vitreous—Bergmeister's papilla—or a gliotic tuft on the posterior lens capsule called Mittendorf's dot.

Physiologic cupping of the disk is usually not seen in premature infants and is rarely seen at term; if seen then, it is usually very slight. In such cases the optic disk will appear gray, resembling optic nerve atrophy. This relative pallor, however, gradually changes to the normal adult pink color at about 2 years of age. Preretinal and intraretinal hemorrhages have been reported in 30%–45% of newborns, usually clearing completely within a few weeks and leaving no permanent visual dysfunction.

OCULAR EXAMINATION OF INFANTS & YOUNG CHILDREN

▶ Tests for Visual Acuity

In the early years, visual acuity should be assessed as part of each general "well child" examination. It is best not to wait until the child is old enough to respond to visual charts, since these may not furnish accurate information until school age.

During the first 3–4 years, estimations of vision rely greatly on observation and reports about the child's behavior both at play and during interactions with parents and with other children. Unfortunately, at this age, seemingly normal visual performance is possible with relatively poor vision, and obviously abnormal performance probably reflects extremely poor acuity. The influence of visual impairment on motor and social development must always be borne in mind. The pupillary responses to light are a gross test of visual function and are reliable only for ruling out complete dysfunction of the anterior visual or efferent pupillary pathways. The ability to fixate and follow a target is much more informative. The target must be appropriate to the age of the child. Binocular following and converging reflexes are best examined first to establish the child's cooperation. Each eye should then be tested separately, preferably with occlusion of the fellow eye by an adhesive patch. Comparison of the performance of the two eyes will give useful information about their relative acuities. Resistance to occlusion of one eye strongly suggests it is the preferred eye, and therefore that the fellow eye must have comparatively poor vision. In cases of latent nystagmus—nystagmus increasing with occlusion of one eye—the child is likely to resent occlusion of each eye because of the effect such nystagmus has on visual acuity. Manifest nystagmus may be indicative of an anterior visual pathway disorder or other central nervous system disease until these have been excluded. (Further discussion of the assessment of nystagmus is given in Chapter 14.)

After 3 months of age, the presence of strabismus, detected by examining the relative position of the corneal light reflections, must also be regarded as indicative of poor vision in the deviated eye, particularly if this eye does not take up or is slow to take up fixation of a light upon occlusion of the fellow eye. (Further discussion of the assessment of strabismus is given in Chapter 12.)

These inferences about the status of the developing sensory systems can now be augmented by the quantitative techniques of optokinetic nystagmus, forced-choice preferential looking methods, and visually evoked responses (see Chapter 2). Although visually evoked potentials have suggested that normal adult visual acuity is attained before 2 years of age, this is probably an overestimate and it is likely that 3–4 years of age is a more accurate estimate (Table 17–2). Forced-choice preferential looking methods have gained increasing popularity as a reliable and relatively easy assessment of visual acuity in

Table 17–2. Development of Visual Acuity (Approximate)

Age	Visual Acuity
2 months	20/400
6 months	20/100
1 year	20/50
3 years	20/20

preverbal children, even in the very young. This technique does, however, have a tendency to overestimate visual acuity in amblyopes.

From about age 4 on, it becomes possible to elicit subjective responses by use of the illiterate "E" chart, child recognition figures, Lea figures, or HOTV cards. Usually, at the first- or second-grade level, the regular Snellen chart may be employed. Stereoacuity can be shown to develop in most infants beginning at 3 months of age, but clinical testing is not generally possible until 3–4 years of age. Absence of stereopsis, as judged with the Random Dot "E" test or the Titmus stereo test, is suggestive of strabismus or amblyopia and should prompt further investigation.

▶ Refraction

Objective refraction is an important part of the pediatric ophthalmic examination, especially if there is any suggestion of poor vision or strabismus. In young children, this should be performed under cycloplegia in order to overcome the child's tendency to accommodate. In most circumstances, cyclopentolate 1% drops applied twice—separated by an interval of 5 minutes—30 minutes prior to examination will provide sufficient cycloplegia, but atropine cycloplegia may be required if convergent strabismus is present or the eyes are heavily pigmented. Because atropine drops can be associated with systemic side effects, atropine 1% ophthalmic ointment applied once daily for 2 or 3 days prior to examination is the recommended regimen. The parents should be warned of the symptoms of atropine toxicity—fever, flushed face, and rapid pulse—and the necessity for discontinuing treatment, cooling the child with sponge bathing, and, in severe cases, seeking urgent medical assistance. Cycloplegic refraction provides the additional advantage of good mydriasis to facilitate examination of the fundus.

About 80% of children between the ages of 2 and 6 years are hyperopic, 5% are myopic, and 15% are emmetropic. About 10% have refractive errors that require correction before age 7 or 8. Myopia often develops between ages 6 and 9 and increases throughout adolescence, with the greatest change at the time of puberty. Astigmatism is relatively common in babies but decreases in prevalence during the first few years of life. Thereafter, it remains relatively constant in prevalence and degree throughout life. Asymmetric refractive error can lead to (anisometropic) amblyopia, which is detected only by assessing visual acuity.

▶ Anterior & Posterior Segment Examination

Further examination needs to be tailored to each child's age and ability to cooperate. Anterior segment examination in the young child relies mainly on the use of a hand light and magnifying loupe, but slitlamp examination is often possible in babies with the cooperation of the mother and in young children with appropriate encouragement. Measurement of intraocular pressure and gonioscopy are more of a problem and frequently necessitate examination under anesthesia. Fundus examination relies on good mydriasis. It is generally easier in neonates and babies than in young children because they can be restrained easily by being wrapped in a blanket and examination is often easily accomplished by allowing the infant to feed or nurse during the examination, at which time it is often possible to obtain intraocular pressure measurements as well as examine the eye thoroughly.

The foveal light reflection is absent in infants. Instead, the macula has a bright "mother-of-pearl" appearance with a suggestion of elevation. This is more pronounced in heavily pigmented infants. At 3–4 months of age, the macula becomes slightly concave and the foveal light reflection appears.

The peripheral fundus in the infant is gray, in contrast to the orange-red fundus of the adult. In white infants, the pigmentation is more pronounced near the posterior pole and gradually fades to almost white at the periphery. In more heavily pigmented infants, there is more pigment in the fundus, and a gray-blue sheen is seen throughout the periphery. In white infants, a white periphery is normal and should not be confused with retinoblastoma. During the next several months, pigment continues to be deposited in the retina, and usually at about 2 years of age, the adult color is evident.

CONGENITAL OCULAR ABNORMALITIES

Congenital defects of the ocular structures fall into two main categories: (1) developmental anomalies, of which genetic defects are an important cause; and (2) tissue reactions to intrauterine insults (infections, drugs, etc).

▶ Congenital Abnormalities of the Globe

Failure of formation of the optic vesicle results in **anophthalmos.** Failure of invagination leads to a **congenital cystic eye.** Failure of optic vesicle/fissure closure produces **colobomas of the iris, retina, and/or choroid. Cryptophthalmos** occurs when the eyelids fail to separate.

Abnormally small eyes can be divided into **nanophthalmos,** in which function is normal, and **microphthalmos,** in which function is abnormal and there may be other ocular abnormalities such as cataract, coloboma, or congenital cyst.

▶ Lid Abnormalities

Congenital ptosis is commonly due to dystrophy of the levator muscle of the upper lid (see Chapter 4). Other causes are congenital Horner's syndrome and congenital third nerve palsy. Severe ptosis can lead to unilateral astigmatism or visual deprivation, and thus cause amblyopia.

Palpebral coloboma is a cleft of either the upper or lower eyelid due to incomplete fusion of fetal maxillary processes. Large defects require early repair to avoid corneal ulceration due to exposure. Congenital eyelid colobomas are commonly seen in association with craniofacial disorders such as Goldenhar's syndrome.

Corneal Abnormalities

Congenital opacification of the cornea may be partial or complete, and causes include congenital glaucoma, forceps injuries at birth, faulty development of the corneal endothelium, developmental anterior segment abnormalities with persistent corneal-lens attachments, intrauterine inflammation, interstitial keratitis, and mucopolysaccharide depositions of the cornea as in Hurler's syndrome. The most frequent cause of opaque corneas in infants and young children is congenital glaucoma, in which the eye is often larger than normal (buphthalmos). Forceps injuries at birth may cause extensive corneal opacities with edema as a result of rupture of Descemet's membrane. These usually clear spontaneously but frequently induce anisometropic amblyopia. Megalocornea is an enlarged cornea with normal clarity and function, usually transmitted as an X-linked recessive trait. It must be differentiated from congenital glaucoma. There are usually no associated defects.

Iris & Pupillary Defects

Misplaced or ectopic pupils (corectopia) are occasionally observed. The usual displacement is upward and laterally (temporally) from the center of the cornea. Such displacement is occasionally associated with ectopic lens, congenital glaucoma, or microcornea. Multiple pupils are known as **polycoria. Coloboma of the iris** indicates incomplete closure of the fetal ocular cleft and usually occurs inferiorly and nasally. A coloboma of the iris may be associated with coloboma of the lens, choroid, and optic nerve, and involvement of these structures can be associated with profound visual loss. **Aniridia** (absence of the iris) is a rare abnormality, frequently associated with secondary glaucoma (see Chapter 11) and usually due to an autosomal dominant hereditary pattern. There is a significant association between sporadic aniridia and Wilms' tumor. Frequent abdominal examinations with periodic renal ultrasonography should be performed to detect Wilms' tumor at an early treatable stage. All children with aniridia should receive genetic testing, as identification of deletions will determine whether they have a low or high risk of developing Wilms' tumor.

The color of the iris is determined largely by heredity. Abnormalities in color include **albinism,** due to the absence of normal pigmentation of the ocular structures and frequently associated with poor visual acuity and nystagmus; and **heterochromia,** which is a difference in color in the two eyes that may be a primary developmental defect with no functional loss, due to congenital Horner's syndrome or secondary to an inflammatory process.

Lens Abnormalities

The lens abnormalities most frequently noted are cataracts (also see Chapter 8), although there may be faulty development, forming colobomas, or subluxation, as seen in Marfan's syndrome.

Any lens opacity that is present at birth is a congenital cataract, regardless of whether or not it interferes with visual acuity. Congenital cataracts are often associated with other conditions. Maternal rubella during the first trimester of pregnancy is a common cause of congenital cataract in emerging countries but less common in developed nations. Other congenital cataracts have a hereditary background, with autosomal dominant transmission being the most common cause of hereditary cataracts in developed countries.

Congenital lenticular opacities may occur at any time during formation of the lens, and the stage during which the opacity started to develop is often measurable by the depth of the opacity. The innermost fetal nucleus of the lens forms early in embryonic life and is surrounded by the embryonic nucleus. During adult life, further growth in the lens is peripheral and subcapsular.

If the opacity is small enough so that it does not occlude the pupil, adequate visual acuity is attained by focusing around the opacity. If the pupillary opening is entirely occluded, however, normal sight does not develop, and visual deprivation may lead to nystagmus and profound irreversible amblyopia. Good visual results have been reported with both unilateral and bilateral cataracts treated by early surgery and prompt correction of aphakia and amblyopia therapy. Aphakic correction is with extended-wear contact lenses with the power changed frequently to maintain optimal correction as the globe grows and the refractive status changes, or by implantation of an intraocular lens but determining the appropriate power is difficult.

A common management problem in congenital cataracts is the associated amblyopia. Whether this can be dealt with adequately is the major determinant in deciding whether early surgery for monocular congenital cataract is justified. In the case of bilateral congenital cataracts, the time interval between operating on the two eyes must be as short as possible if amblyopia in the second eye is to be avoided. If early surgery is to be undertaken for congenital cataracts, it is best done within the first 2 months of life, and early referral to an ophthalmologist is essential.

Developmental Anomalies of the Anterior Segment

Failure of migration or subsequent development of neural crest cells produces abnormalities involving the anterior chamber angle, iris, cornea, and lens. Mutations of the PAX6 gene cause many of these developmental anomalies of the eye, such as **Axenfeld–Rieger syndrome,** and **Peter's anomaly.** Glaucoma is a major clinical problem that often requires surgical intervention, as good control of intraocular pressure is required before considering corneal transplantation.

Congenital Glaucoma

Congenital glaucoma (see Chapter 11) may occur alone or in association with many other congenital lesions. Early recognition is essential to prevent permanent blindness. Involvement is often bilateral. The most striking symptom is extreme photophobia. Early signs are corneal haze or opacity, increased corneal diameter, and increased intraocular pressure. Since the outer coats of the eyeball are not as rigid in the child, the increased intraocular pressure expands the corneal and scleral tissues, producing an eye that is larger than normal (buphthalmos). The major differential diagnoses are forceps injuries at birth, developmental anomalies of the cornea or anterior segment, and mucopolysaccharidoses such as Hurler's syndrome. All of these cause corneal clouding, but none produce enlargement of the globe. Useful vision may be preserved by early diagnosis and medical and surgical treatment by an ophthalmologist.

Vitreous Abnormalities

Remnants of the hyaloid artery may be seen on the posterior surface of the lens (Mittendorf's dot) or on the optic disk (Bergmeister's papilla). Persistent hyperplastic primary vitreous is an important cause of leukocoria that must be differentiated from retinoblastoma, congenital cataract, and retinopathy of prematurity.

Choroid & Retina

Choroidal colobomas, usually in the lower nasal region and sometimes involving the iris and all or part of the optic nerve, are often associated with syndromes such as CHARGE, Aicardi's, and Goldenhar's (hemifacial microsomia). Posterior polar chorioretinal scarring is often caused by toxoplasmosis or other maternally acquired intrauterine infections.

Optic Nerve

Congenital anomalies of the optic nerve are relatively common. They are usually benign, such as minor abnormalities of the retinal vessels at the nerve head and tilted disks due to an oblique entrance of the nerve into the globe, but they may be associated with severe visual loss in the case of optic nerve hypoplasia or the rare central coloboma of the disk (morning glory syndrome) (See also Chapter 14).

Optic nerve hypoplasia is a nonprogressive congenital abnormality of one or both optic nerves in which the number of axons in the involved nerve is reduced. Previously regarded as rare, it is now recognized to be a major cause of visual loss in children. The degree of visual impairment varies from normal acuity with a wide variety of visual field defects to no perception of light. Clinical diagnosis is hampered by the difficulties of examining young children and the subtlety of the clinical signs. In more marked cases, the optic disk is obviously small and the circumpapillary halo of the normal-sized scleral canal produces the characteristic "double ring sign." In other cases, the hypoplasia may be only segmental and much more difficult to detect.

Optic nerve hypoplasia is frequently associated with midline deformities, including absence of the septum pellucidum, agenesis of the corpus callosum, dysplasia of the third ventricle, pituitary and hypothalamic dysfunction, and midline facial abnormalities. Jaundice and hypoglycemia in the neonatal period and growth retardation, hypothyroidism, and diabetes insipidus during childhood are important clinical effects of the resultant endocrine disturbances. More severe intracranial abnormalities such as anencephaly and porencephaly also occur. Endocrine and neuroradiographic investigations should be undertaken in all patients with optic nerve hypoplasia.

Visual performance in children with optic nerve hypoplasia occasionally may be improved by occlusion therapy. Conversely, optic nerve hypoplasia is an important cause of poor vision that does not normalize with occlusion therapy in children with or without strabismus. A number of patients with optic nerve hypoplasia are not diagnosed until adult life because of the subtlety of the optic nerve abnormality.

Extraocular Dermoids

Congenital rests of surface ectodermal tissues may lead to formation of dermoids that occur frequently in the extraocular structures. These dermoids occur most commonly superolaterally, arising from the frontozygomatic suture.

Congenital Nasolacrimal Duct Obstruction

Canalization of the distal nasolacrimal duct normally occurs before birth or during the first month of life, and as many as 30% of infants will have epiphora during this time. Approximately 6% have more prolonged symptoms, of which the majority will also resolve aided by lacrimal sac massage and treatment of episodes of conjunctivitis with topical antibiotics. Nasolacrimal probing is usually curative in the remainder and is best deferred until about 1 year of age. In the event of acute dacryocystitis, earlier probing is often indicated. In a few cases, temporary intubation and/or balloon catheter dilation of the lacrimal system, or lacrimal surgery is required. The possibility of more extensive congenital nasolacrimal anomalies should be borne in mind in patients with craniofacial anomalies. Epiphora may also be due to inflammatory anterior segment disease, lid abnormalities, and congenital glaucoma.

Orbital Abnormalities

Craniofacial dysostosis (Crouzon's disease) is a rare hereditary deformity due to an autosomal dominant gene, characterized by exophthalmos, hypoplasia of the maxilla, enlargement of the nasal bones, abnormal increase in the space between the eyes (ocular hypertelorism), optic atrophy, and bony abnormalities of the region of the perilongitudinal sinus. The palpebral fissures slant downward (in contrast to the upward slant of Down's syndrome). Strabismus is also present. The strabismus is secondary to both structural anomalies of the muscles and orbital angle anomalies.

Various congenital abnormalities of skull development—due to premature closure of the skull sutures—are associated with deformities of the orbits and ocular complications resembling those associated with Crouzon's disease. Examples are oxycephaly and coronal synostosis.

INVESTIGATION OF THE BLIND BABY WITH NORMAL OCULAR & NEUROLOGIC EXAMINATION

An important part of pediatric ophthalmology is the investigation of infants with poor visual performance for which clinical examination reveals no ocular or neurologic cause. This presumes that defects such as optic nerve hypoplasia, albinism, and high refractive errors have been excluded. The important conditions to be considered are Leber's congenital amaurosis, cortical blindness, cone dystrophy, ocular motor apraxia, and delayed visual maturation.

Leber's congenital amaurosis—as distinct from Leber's hereditary optic neuropathy—and **cone dystrophy** are congenital retinal dystrophies that cause poor vision in infants who present with large amplitude nystagmus and poor visual fixation. These infants will frequently demonstrate eye pressing behavior, the oculo-digital sign, which is quite specific for congenital retinal disorders. Diagnosis is confirmed by electroretinography. **Cerebral (cortical) visual impairment**, a common cause of vision impairment in premature infants and infants who sustained perinatal hypoxic-ischemic encephalopathy, is the leading cause of infantile blindness in developed countries. Diagnosis is confirmed by neuroimaging and clinical history. In ocular motor apraxia, a defect in initiation of horizontal saccades gives the impression of visual unresponsiveness, although the visual pathways are normal. Affected children develop characteristic compensatory head movements to overcome the eye movement disorder. Delayed visual maturation is a rare condition in which vision does not develop until after 2 months of age. In some cases, there may be associated ocular and neurologic abnormalities that limit final visual performance, but normal vision is attained in those in which it is an isolated condition.

POSTNATAL PROBLEMS

The most common ocular disorders of children are external infections of the conjunctiva and eyelids (bacterial conjunctivitis, hordeola, blepharitis), amblyopia, strabismus, ocular foreign bodies, allergic reactions of the conjunctiva and eyelids, and refractive errors. Since it is more difficult to elicit an accurate history of causative factors and subjective complaints in children, it is not uncommon to overlook significant ocular disorders (especially in very young children). Aside from the altered frequency of occurrence of the types of ocular disorders, the causes, manifestations, and treatment of eye disorders are about the same for children as for adults. Certain special problems encountered more frequently in infants and children are discussed below.

▶ Ophthalmia Neonatorum (Conjunctivitis of the Newborn)

Conjunctivitis of the newborn may be of chemical, bacterial, chlamydial, or viral origin. Differentiation is sometimes possible according to the timing of presentation, but appropriate smears and cultures are essential. Antenatal diagnosis and treatment of maternal genital infections should prevent many cases of neonatal conjunctivitis. The presence of active maternal genital herpes at the time of delivery may be an indication for elective cesarean section (see Chapter 20).

A. Conjunctivitis due to Chlamydial Infection

Chlamydia is now the most common identifiable infectious cause of neonatal conjunctivitis in the United States. Inclusion blennorrhea due to chlamydial infection typically has its onset between the fifth and fourteenth days; the presence of characteristic inclusion bodies in the epithelial cells of a conjunctival smear confirms the diagnosis. Direct immunofluorescent antibody staining of conjunctival scrapings is a highly sensitive and specific diagnostic test and polymerase chain reaction is now clinically available. Systemic therapy with erythromycin is more effective than topical therapy and aids in the eradication of concurrent nasopharyngeal carriage, which may predispose to the development of pneumonitis.

B. Conjunctivitis due to Bacterial Infection

Bacterial conjunctivitis, usually due to *Staphylococcus aureus,* haemophilus species, *Streptococcus pneumoniae, Streptococcus faecalis, Neisseria gonorrhoeae,* or pseudomonas species—the last two being the most serious because of potential corneal damage—presents between the second and fifth days after birth. Provisional identification of the causative organism may be made from conjunctival smears. Gonococcal conjunctivitis necessitates parenteral therapy with ceftriaxone, or cefotaxime if there is hyperbilirubinemia. In all cases due to chlamydial or gonococcal infection, both parents should also be given systemic treatment. Other types of bacterial conjunctivitis require topical instillation of antibacterial agents, such as sodium sulfacetamide, bacitracin, or polymixin-trimethoprim, as soon as results of smears are known. It is imperative that the infant be tested and treated for all other sexually transmitted diseases and that the mother and all sexual partners receive notification and treatment.

C. Conjunctivitis due to Viral Infection

Herpes simplex virus produces characteristic giant cells and viral inclusions on cytologic examination. Herpetic keratitis occurring in children younger than 6 months necessitates admission to the hospital for lumbar puncture with PCR evaluation to determine whether there is CNS systemic infection and whether systemic therapy is needed. Herpetic keratoconjunctivitis usually resolves spontaneously but may require antiviral therapy, particularly when associated with disseminated infection that occurs chiefly in atopic individuals.

Uveitis in Childhood

Inflammatory eye disease is relatively uncommon in children, but there are a number of important syndromes. The conditions that are seen in the same form as in adults are acute nongranulomatous anterior uveitis associated with the HLA-B27 spondylarthritides, intermediate uveitis, Fuchs' uveitis syndrome, and idiopathic anterior uveitis. These are treated in the same way as in adults, but with care in the use of systemic steroids because of their effects on growth. Uveitis in association with juvenile idiopathic arthritis is generally asymptomatic in its early stages and if undetected may produce severe loss of vision due to glaucoma, cataract, or band keratopathy. Regular ophthalmic screening of children with oligoarticular disease, which generally occurs in girls with positive antinuclear antibodies, is essential. Long-term use of topical steroids and mydriatic/cycloplegic agents is often effective in controlling the uveitis but some patients will require systemic immunosuppression, including with agents other than steroids. (See also Chapters 7 and 15.)

Retinopathy of Prematurity

Retinopathy of prematurity has been estimated to result in 550 new cases of infant blindness each year in the United States. Improved neonatal care may reduce the percentage of babies affected but has also greatly increased the total number at risk. Laser ablation of the immature retina delivered by a head-mounted indirect ophthalmoscope diode or argon laser is now recommended treatment for severe active disease.

Retinal vascularization proceeds centrifugally from the optic nerve, beginning at the fourth month of gestation. Retinal vessels normally reach the nasal ora serrata at 8 months and the temporal ora serrata at 9 months. Retinopathy of prematurity develops if this process is disturbed. It is usually bilateral but often asymmetric. The active phase involves changes at the junction of vascularized and avascular retina, initially as an obvious demarcation line (stage 1), followed by formation of a distinct ridge (stage 2), then extraretinal fibrovascular proliferation (stage 3). Even among patients with stage 3 disease, there is a high incidence of spontaneous regression. Consideration is also given to the location of the changes with respect to distance from the optic disk (zone I or II), the extent of the disease in clock hours, and the presence of venous dilation and arterial tortuosity in the posterior segment ("plus" disease). The cicatricial phase (stages 4 and 5) is defined by increasingly severe retinal detachment, which results in profound vision impairment even with vitreoretinal surgery.

The major risk factors for retinopathy of prematurity are decreasing gestational age and decreasing birth weight. Although recognition of the causative role of supplemental oxygen and its restriction seems to have reduced the incidence of retinopathy of prematurity, other factors contribute to the onset and severity of the disease. Associated risk factors include acidosis, apnea, patent ductus arteriosus, septicemia, blood transfusions, and intraventricular hemorrhage.

It is recommended that all babies younger than 30 weeks gestational age, or a birth weight of 1500 g or less, and those that receive prolonged supplemental oxygen therapy undergo repeated screening for retinopathy of prematurity. As many as 60% of such babies will develop the disease, even if only in its early stages. Screening should begin at 2–4 weeks after birth and continue until the retina is fully vascularized, the retinal changes have undergone spontaneous resolution, or appropriate treatment has been given. Pupillary dilation is achieved with Cyclomydril (cyclopentolate 0.2% and phenylephrine 1%). The timing of laser ablation therapy has changed in the past decade, with the most recent recommendations resulting from the Early Treatment of Retinopathy of Prematurity Study, which recommends treatment for infants with stage 2 disease with vascular tortuosity and engorgement (plus disease) because of significantly reduced risk of poor visual and structural outcomes. Such treatment should be carried out with the assistance of an experienced neonatologist and under careful monitoring because of the risks of serious systemic complications, including respiratory and cardio-respiratory arrest.

Vitrectomy and lensectomy may be beneficial in cicatricial disease, but probably should be reserved for babies with severe disease in both eyes.

See also Chapter 10 and discussion of oxygen toxicity in Chapter 15.

Leukocoria (White Pupil)

Parents will occasionally see, or identify on photographs as absence of the "red-eye" effect, a white spot through the infant's pupil (leukocoria). Although retinoblastoma must be ruled out, the opacity is more often due to cataract, retinopathy of prematurity, persistent hyper-plastic primary vitreous, or refractive error in the case of absence of the red-eye effect in photographs. Any child who presents with the complaint of leukocoria must be seen urgently to assure that vision and life-threatening conditions are diagnosed and treated promptly.

Retinoblastoma

This rare malignant tumor of childhood is fatal if untreated. In 90% of cases, the diagnosis is made before the end of the third year. In about 30% of cases, retinoblastoma is bilateral. Development of the tumor is thought to occur because of the loss—from both members of the chromosome pair—of the normally protective dominant allele at a single locus within chromosomal band 13q14. This gene is normally responsible for production of a nuclear phosphoprotein with DNA binding activity. Loss of the allele is caused by mutations, either in the somatic retinal cells alone (nonheritable retinoblastoma) or in the germ-line cells as well (heritable retinoblastoma). In heritable retinoblastoma, the genetic predisposition is inherited as an autosomal dominant trait; children of survivors have a nearly 50% chance of having the disease; and the tumor is more apt to be bilateral and multifocal. Unaffected parents who have produced one child with retinoblastoma run a 4%–7% risk of having a subsequent child with the disease. Recent sequencing of the retinoblastoma gene locus now allows more specific genetic counseling and identification of individuals carrying the mutation. In sporadic cases, the tumor is usually not discovered until it has advanced far enough to produce an opaque pupil. Infants and children with presenting symptoms of strabismus should be examined carefully to rule out retinoblastoma, since a deviating eye may be the first sign of the tumor. In children of families affected by familial retinoblastoma, regular screening until the individual has been shown by genetic testing not to be at risk is important in the early detection of tumors (see also Chapter 18). Treatment of retinoblastoma now largely avoids enucleation, unless there is very extensive ocular disease or regional extraocular extension, and relies upon local obliterative therapy, supplemented if necessary by intravenous or possibly intra-arterial chemotherapy, and avoidance of external beam radiotherapy (see Chapter 10).

▶ Strabismus

Strabismus is present in about 2% of children. Its early recognition is often the responsibility of the pediatrician or the family physician. Occasionally, childhood strabismus has neurologic significance. The idea that a child may outgrow crossed eyes should be discouraged. Any child with evidence of strabismus after 3 months of age must be referred as soon as possible for ophthalmologic assessment. Neglect in the treatment of strabismus may lead to undesirable cosmetic effects, psychic trauma, and amblyopia. Strabismus is covered in Chapter 12.

▶ Amblyopia

Amblyopia is decreased visual acuity of one eye in the absence of sufficient organic eye disease to explain the level of vision.

Normal anatomic development of the retina and visual cortex is determined by postnatal visual experience. Visual deprivation due to any cause, congenital or acquired, during the critical period of development (probably lasting up to age 8 in humans) prevents the establishment of normal vision in the involved eye. Reversal of this effect becomes increasingly difficult with increasing age of the child. Early suspicion and prompt referral for treatment of the underlying condition are important in preventing amblyopia.

The most common causes of amblyopia are strabismus, in which the image from the deviated eye is suppressed to prevent diplopia, and anisometropia, in which an inability to focus the eyes simultaneously causes suppression of the image of one eye. High degrees of hypermetropia or astigmatism, in which both eyes may become amblyopic because of failure to form a focused image in either eye, are less common causes of amblyopia. All of these conditions are treatable if detected early in life and if the patient is compliant with treatment recommendations. Treatment of amblyopia involves appropriate correction of refractive error and then, if necessary, initiating occlusion therapy (patching) of the sound eye several hours a day, or the use of atropine penalization (pharmacologic blurring of the sound eye) daily for several weeks. No matter what the therapy instituted, visual acuity of both eyes must be monitored.

Since poor visual function in a young child may go unnoticed, routine screening by the age of 4 years is advocated to detect decreased visual acuity or the presence of amblyogenic factors (strabismus, anisometropia) (see Chapter 20).

▶ Child Abuse (Shaken Baby Syndrome)

Child abuse is an increasingly recognized cause of childhood trauma. Making the diagnosis is essential if affected children are to be appropriately protected, but wrong diagnosis must also be avoided if families are not to be unjustly treated.

In the shaken baby syndrome, external signs of head injury are absent, but intraretinal, preretinal, and vitreous hemorrhages are common. They are often accompanied by intracranial hemorrhage and may be indicative of the presence of cerebral injury, even if computed tomography is normal. Retinal hemorrhages in children less than 3 years of age without external evidence of head injury is strongly suggestive of child abuse, as long as other causes such as blood dyscrasia have been excluded.

Blunt trauma to the head and eyes is a more readily recognized form of child abuse. Ocular manifestations include subconjunctival hemorrhage, hyphema, cataract, lens subluxation, glaucoma; retinal, vitreous, intrascleral, and optic nerve hemorrhages; and papilledema.

Victims of child abuse may present initially to ophthalmologists, and the diagnosis must be kept in mind. Ophthalmologists may also provide evidence of injuries to the head and eyes in children presenting with unexplained injuries to other parts of the body. The ophthalmologist should work in close collaboration with the pediatrician to ensure that all other potential causes of hemorrhage have been evaluated and to document all other injuries of the child.

▶ Learning Disabilities & Dyslexia

Ophthalmologists are often asked to evaluate children with suspected learning disabilities in order to rule out ocular disorders. Dyslexia is the most common type of learning disability and is characterized by the inability to develop good reading and writing skills. Affected children are usually of normal intelligence and have no associated physical or visual abnormalities. Parents and educators sometimes attribute learning disabilities to visual perceptual abnormalities, but most of these affected children have no visual or ocular impairment. It is believed that dyslexia is caused by a specific defect of information processing in the central nervous system. The diagnosis of learning disabilities can be readily made by education specialists, and treatment is often effective in ameliorating this condition. When asked to evaluate a child with a learning disorder, the ophthalmologist should perform a complete examination and treat any refractive, strabismic, or amblyopic conditions identified. It is important to advise the parents that ocular or visual abnormalities generally do not lead to learning disabilities, and special educational programs may be necessary to treat these children. "Vision training," "visual therapy," and "perceptual training" programs have not been evaluated in a scientifically controlled, randomized, or prospective fashion, and thus their efficacy has not been proved. Ophthalmologists should provide indicated care of ocular problems and refer patients to appropriate educational programs for diagnosis and treatment of learning disabilities.

REFERENCES

Ahmed E, Loewenstein J: Leber congenital amaurosis: disease, genetics and therapy. Semin Ophthalmol 2008;23:39. [PMID: 18214790]

Allen RJ, Speedwell L, Russell-Eggitt I: Long-term visual outcome after extraction of unilateral congenital cataracts. Eye 2009 Dec 18. [Epub ahead of print] [PMID: 20019767]

American Academy of Pediatrics, et al: Joint statement--Learning disabilities, dyslexia, and vision. Pediatrics 2009;124:837. [PMID: 19651597]

Bothun ED: Ten critical diagnoses not to miss on a pediatric eye screening. Minn Med 2009;92:34. [PMID: 19653470]

Casady DR et al: Stepwise treatment paradigm for congenital nasolacrimal duct obstruction. Ophthal Plast Reconstr Surg 2006;22:243. [PMID: 16855492]

Ciralsky J, Colby K: Congenital corneal opacities: a review with a focus on genetics. Semin Ophthalmol 2007;22:241. [PMID: 18097987]

Cools G et al: Literature review on preschool vision screening. Bull Soc Belge Ophthalmol 2009;313:49. [PMID: 20108573]

Creavin AL, Brown RD: Ophthalmic abnormalities in children with Down syndrome. J Pediatr Ophthalmol Strabismus 2009;46:76. [PMID: 19343968]

Curcoy AI et al: Do retinal haemorrhages occur in infants with convulsions? Arch Dis Child 2009;94:873. [PMID: 19666457]

Davitt BV, Wallace DK: Plus disease. Surv Ophthalmol 2009;54:663. [PMID: 19665743]

Day S, Menke AM, Abbott RL: Retinopathy of prematurity malpractice claims: the Ophthalmic Mutual Insurance Company experience. Arch Ophthalmol 2009;127:794. [PMID: 19506200]

Donnelly UM, Stewart NM, Hollinger M: Prevalence and outcomes of childhood visual disorders. Ophthalmic Epidemiol 2005;12:243. [PMID: 16033745]

Early Treatment for Retinopathy of Prematurity Cooperative Group: Revised indications for the treatment of retinopathy of prematurity: results of the early treatment for retinopathy of prematurity randomized trial. Arch Ophthalmol 2003;121:1684. [PMID: 14662586]

Golnik KC: Cavitary anomalies of the optic disc: neurologic significance. Curr Neurol Neruosci Rep 2008;8:409. [PMID: 18713577]

Good WV: Early Treatment for Retinopathy of Prematurity Cooperative Group: final results of the Early Treatment for Retinopathy of Prematurity (ETROP) randomized trial. Trans Am Ophthalmol Sci 2004;102:233. [PMID: 15747762]

Gopal L: A clinical and optical coherence tomography study of choroidal colobomas. Curr Opin Ophthalmol 2008;19:248. [PMID: 18408502]

Groenewoud JH et al: Rotterdam Amblyopia Screening Effectiveness Study: detection and causes of amblyopia in a large birth cohort. Invest Ophthalmol Vis Sci 2010 Jan 20. [Epub ahead of print] [PMID: 20089868]

Guercio JR, Martyn LJ: Congenital malformations of the eye and orbit. Otolaryngol Clin North Am 2007;40:113. [PMID: 17346564]

Hejtmancik JF: Congenital cataracts and their molecular genetics. Semin Cell Dev Biol 2008;19:134. [PMID: 18035564]

Hubbard GB 3rd: Surgical management of retinopathy of prematurity. Curr Opin Ophthalmol 2008;19:384. [PMID: 18772670]

Infant Aphakia Treatment Study Group: The infant aphakia treatment study: design and clinical measures at enrolment. Arch Ophthalmol 2010;128:21. [PMID: 20065212]

Lee BJ, Traboulsi EI: Update on the morning glory disc anomaly. Ophthalmic Genet 2008;29:47. [PMID: 18484308]

Levin AV: Retinal hemorrhages: advances in understanding. Pediatr Clin North Am 2009;56:333. [PMID: 19358919]

Lim M et al: Development of visual acuity in children with cerebral visual impairment. Arch Ophthalmol 2005;123:1215. [PMID: 16157801]

Lin AA, Buckley EG: Update on pediatric cataract surgery and intraocular lens implantation. Curr Opin Ophthalmol 2010;21:55. [PMID: 19855277]

Lin P, O'Brein JM: Frontiers in the management of retinoblastoma. Am J Ophthalmol 2009;148:192. [PMID: 19477707]

Maguire S et al: Which clinical features distinguish inflicted from non-inflicted brain injury? A systematic review. Arch Dis Child 2009;94:860. [PMID: 19531526]

Matschke J, Püschel K, Glatzel M: Ocular pathology in shaken baby syndrome and other forms of infantile non-accidental head injury. Int J Legal Med 2009;123:189. [PMID: 18936952]

McClatchey SK, Hofmeister EM: The optics of aphakic and pseudophakic eyes in childhood. Surv Ophthalmol 2010;55:174. [PMID: 19786290]

Ospina LH: Cortical visual impairment. Pediatr Rev 2009;30:e81. [PMID: 19884281]

Pediatric Eye Disease Investigator Group: Primary treatment of nasolacrimal duct obstruction with probing in children younger than 4 years. Ophthalmology 2008;115:577. [PMID: 17996306]

Pediatric Eye Disease Investigator Group: Primary treatment of nasolacrimal duct obstruction with nasolacrimal duct intubation in children younger than 4 years of age. J AAPOS 2008;12:445. [PMID: 18595756]

Pediatric Eye Disease Investigator Group: Primary treatment of nasolacrimal duct obstruction with balloon catheter dilation in children younger than 4 years of age. J AAPOS 2008;12:451. [PMID: 18929305]

Ragge NK, Subak-Sharpe ID, Collin JR: A practical guide to the management of anophthalmia and microphthalmia. Eye 2007;21:1290. [PMID: 17914432]

Repka MX et al: Balloon catheter dilation and nasolacrimal duct intubation for treatment of nasolacrimal duct obstruction after failed probing. Arch Ophthalmol 2009;127:633. [PMID: 19433712]

Scheiman MM et al: Patching versus atropine to treat amblyopia in children aged 7 to 12 years: a randomized trial. Arch Ophthalmol 2008;126:1634. [PMID: 19064841]

Section on Ophthalmology, American Academy of Pediatrics et al: Screening examination of premature infants for retinopathy of prematurity. Pediatrics 2006;117:572. [PMID: 16452383]

Sharma SM, Dick AD, Ramanan AV: Non-infectious pediatric uveitis: an update on immunomodulatory management. Pediatr Drugs 2009;11:229. [19566107]

Sylvester CL: Retinopathy of prematurity. Semin Ophthalmol 2008;23:318. [PMID: 19085434]

Taylor D: Developmental abnormalities of the optic nerve and chiasm. Eye 2007;21:1271. [PMID: 17914430]

Zetterström C, Kugelberg M: Paediatric cataract surgery. Acta Ophthalmol Scand 2007;85:698. [PMID: 17944624]

Ophthalmic Genetics

James J. Augsburger, MD, and Zélia M. Corrêa, MD, PhD

18

Ophthalmic genetics is concerned with the genetic contribution to ophthalmic disease, including determination of patterns and risks of inheritance, as well as diagnosis, prognosis, and development of treatments for genetic abnormalities. Information on the genetics of particular inherited diseases and the availability of genetic testing are available from various internet websites, including those maintained by the National Center for Biotechnology Information [www.ncbi.nlm.nih.gov] and the Gene Test Organization [www.genetest.org].

PATTERNS OF INHERITANCE

▶ Abnormalities of Nuclear or Mitochondrial DNA

A great number of disorders with ophthalmic manifestations are transmitted in characteristic hereditary patterns through many generations, generally being attributable to deletions, mutations, and/or duplications of small segments of specific chromosomes of nuclear DNA or the circular DNA of mitochondria. **Autosomal dominant disorders** include neurofibromatosis type 1, tuberous sclerosis, Best vitelliform macular dystrophy, von Hippel–Lindau disease, autosomal dominant optic atrophy, most cases of multifocal retinoblastoma, and some cases of retinitis pigmentosa. **Autosomal recessive disorders** include oculocutaenous albinism, gyrate atrophy, xeroderma pigmentosum, and some cases of retinitis pigmentosa. **X-linked recessive disorders** include red-green color blindness, X-linked retinoschisis, ocular albinism, Norrie disease, some cases of retinitis pigmentosa, and most cases of choroideremia. **Matrilineal inheritance** is characteristic of abnormalities of mitochondrial DNA, such as the point mutations that cause Leber's hereditary optic neuropathy (LHON). Other mitochondrial disorders, in which the characteristic ophthalmic manifestations are chronic progressive external ophthalmoplegia (CPEO) and pigmentary retinopathy, may also be caused by point mutations of mitochondrial DNA, but also may be caused by large deletions of mitochondrial DNA such as in the Kearns–Sayre syndrome, or mutations of nuclear DNA causing abnormalities of mitochondrial function and inherited with an autosomal dominant or autosomal recessive pattern.

Some abnormalities of nuclear or mitochondrial DNA, for example in some mitochondrial disorders, are rarely transmitted through more than one generation, because the severity of the disorder resulting from a small or more extensive genetic defect limits lifespan or reproductive capability. Occasionally, disease due to a genetic abnormality is not transmitted because the genetic abnormality is confined to somatic cells without being present in the germ cells, for example, most cases of unifocal retinoblastoma (see Chapter 10).

▶ Chromosomal Abnormalities

In most disorders with ophthalmic manifestations that clearly have a genetic basis but are rarely transmitted through more than one generation, the genetic abnormality is a major or complete loss or duplication of one or more chromosomes involving numerous genes. Due to the absence of half the normal complement of genes associated with a particular chromosome in cases with complete chromosomal deletions and to the presence of 50% more than the normal complement of genes associated with a particular chromosome in cases with complete chromosomal duplications, affected individuals characteristically have multiple morphological abnormalities, frequently prompting chromosomal analysis during infancy or early childhood. They are frequently sterile or unsuccessful in reproducing. In most cases, the abnormal complement of chromosomes can be identified by karyotyping.

Chromosomal disorders with ophthalmic manifestations include:

1. **Trisomy syndromes**
   - Trisomy 13 (Patau's syndrome)—commonly associated with microophthalmia, uveal colobomas, and congenital cataract.

- Trisomy 18 (Edward's syndrome)—commonly associated with hypertelorism, hypoplastic supraorbital ridges, and anomalies of eyelids.
- Trisomy 21 (Down's syndrome)—commonly associated with epicanthal folds, iris hypoplasia, and keratoconus.
- XXY trisomy (Klinefelter's syndrome)—characterized by epicanthal folds, hypertelorism, and upward slant of palpebral fissures.

2. **Monosomy syndrome**
- Monosomy X (Turner's syndrome)—commonly associated with congenital ptosis, strabismus, and cataracts.

3. **Partial chromosomal deletion or duplication syndromes**
- Chromosome 13q deletion syndrome—commonly associated with hypertelorism, epicanthal folds, and retinoblastoma.
- Chromosome 11p deletion syndrome—commonly associated with congenital aniridia.

▶ Polygenic and Multifactorial Inheritance

Some ophthalmic diseases, including age-related macular degeneration (AMD) and primary open-angle glaucoma, appear to be inherited with a polygenic and multifactorial pattern. No simple transmission pattern can be identified, but the disease prevalence in family members is substantially greater than expected on the basis of chance. Associations with mutations of several different genes have been identified, for example involving the complement pathway in AMD (see Chapter 10), and interaction between these genetic abnormalities and environmental conditions appear to affect disease characteristics such as age at clinical onset, severity at initial detection, rapidity of progression, and ultimate outcome.

GENETIC DIAGNOSIS

The principal uses of ophthalmic genetic diagnosis are:

1. Identification of an inherited disease in affected individuals, to establish diagnosis, provide prognosis, recommend any treatment, and offer genetic counseling with respect to transmission of the genetic abnormality and development of the disease in their existing or future offspring.
2. Identification of clinically unaffected carriers of an inherited disease, to advise on likelihood of developing the disease, including the advisability of periodic screening for conditions that benefit from pre-symptomatic treatment, and to offer genetic counseling, including estimation of risks of transmission of the genetic abnormality and development of the disease in their offspring.

In practice, the clinician must first either

1. recognize a familial inheritance pattern for an ophthalmic disease, disorder, or abnormality in more than one generation or branch of a family, or

2. diagnose in one or more members of the same generation of a family an ophthalmic disease, condition, or abnormality that is known to be transmitted genetically in at least some families.

▶ Recognition of Familial Inheritance Pattern

Once a familial inheritance pattern is suspected, a genetic counselor is usually involved to:

1. Investigate the family pedigree, identify the likely inheritance pattern of the disease, and suggest and arrange for familial genetic testing for the disorder.
2. Determine which family members, whether already affected, likely to develop the disease, or who will never be affected, who are carriers and can transmit the disease to their offspring, and advise the family as a whole and individual family members about the genetic findings and their implications for future offspring.

The results can then be used by unaffected carriers in family planning, or to justify early genetic and clinical evaluation of any future offspring for evidence of the disease or genetic susceptibility to it. In potentially fatal diseases for which effective treatment is available in the early stages, differentiation by genetic testing between individuals who are and individuals who are not predisposed to develop the disease assists targeting of screening programs. For instance, frequent ophthalmic examinations under general anesthesia to detect newly emerging retinal tumors in infants at risk of familial retinoblastoma is more readily justifiable when genetic testing has established disease susceptibility and can be avoided in infants shown not to be at risk.

▶ Diagnosis of a Genetically Transmitted Condition

Following clinical diagnosis in one or more members of the same generation of a family of an ophthalmic disease, condition, or abnormality known to be transmitted genetically in at least some families and for which genetic testing is currently available (eg, Norrie disease and Leber's hereditary optic neuropathy), testing of the affected individual(s) and their parents and siblings can be performed to establish a genetic diagnosis. If a relevant genetic abnormality is identified in an affected family member but not in any other family members, it is likely to be due to a new mutation. In contrast, if neither the affected individual nor any first-degree relative has a relevant genetic abnormality, either the clinical diagnosis is incorrect or an unknown genetic abnormality is responsible.

The family pedigree can help confirm or refute a clinical diagnosis. For example Leber's hereditary optic neuropathy (LHON) has a matrilineal pattern of inheritance because it is caused by a mutation of mitochondrial DNA and only maternal not paternal mitochondrial DNA is transmitted, that is, the mutation is transmitted from carrier mothers, whether affected or not, to all their children but it is not transmitted from carrier fathers, whether affected or not, to any of their children. Thus, a clinical diagnosis of LHON would need to be reconsidered if an affected individual is found to have an affected father, or if an affected male is found to have affected children. (An unusual feature of LHON, which does not occur in other diseases due to mutations of mitochondrial DNA, is that carrier males are about 5 times more likely to be affected than carrier females. This is thought to be due to an X-linked modifier gene determining risk of visual loss in carriers.)

With an X-linked recessive pattern of inheritance, males, because they have only one X chromosome, are much more commonly affected than females. Affected males do not transmit the disease to their sons but all their daughters will be carriers. 50% of sons of carrier females are affected and 50% of their daughters are carriers. Although women rarely fully manifest the disease, which would require both X chromosomes to be mutant, due to X chromosome inactivation (Lyon hypothesis) some cells will manifest the abnormal phenotype, such that the female carrier state may be detectable clinically, for example, limited fundal abnormalities in ocular albinism, and X-linked recessive retinitis pigmentosa.

With autosomal recessive or autosomal dominant inheritance, males and females are equally affected. With autosomal recessive inheritance, overall 25% of siblings are affected. More than one sibling being affected in the absence of any affected individuals in the preceding generations, affected individuals in collateral branches of the same family, and consanguinity are suggestive. Direct transmission over 2 or more generations and about 50% of family members being affected are characteristic of autosomal dominant inheritance. Variable **expression** in autosomal dominant disease refers to different severity of disease amongst affected individuals, such as in neurofibromatosis type 1. **Anticipation** means increasing severity of disease with succeeding generations, and is typically seen in diseases caused by duplications of triplet base pairs of DNA, as in Huntington's disease, with the number of mutant copies increasing from generation to generation. **Penetrance** refers to whether carriers manifest disease. Autosomal dominant inheritance with reduced penetrance may be confused with autosomal recessive inheritance. **Codominant inheritance** refers to autosomal dominant disease in which the heterozygote state has a distinct phenotype from the homozygote state, for example the difference between sickle cell trait and sickle cell anemia.

GENETIC PROGNOSTICATION

Genetic prognostication refers to the use of genetic information to predict a patient's prognosis. In ophthalmology, genetic information is increasingly being used to predict the severity of visual loss in hereditary degenerative retinal diseases, and the probability of metastasis in patients with primary uveal melanoma.

▶ Predicting Prognosis in Hereditary Retinal Disease

Retinitis pigmentosa is the clinical manifestation of numerous genetic abnormalities, with autosomal dominant, autosomal recessive, or X-linked recessive patterns of inheritance. Individuals from a particular family, thus sharing the same genetic abnormality (genotype), tend to have the same clinical manifestations (phenotype) (eg, age when visual symptoms are first recognized, severity of visual field loss at initial detection, rate of progression following initial symptoms, and ultimate level of visual loss) but different from members of another family with a different genetic abnormality. It is increasingly becoming possible to define the correlation between genotype and phenotype in the different genetic subtypes of retinitis pigmentosa. Similarly, the autosomal dominant disorder von Hippel–Lindau disease has genetic subgroups with substantially different risk of developing renal cell carcinoma.

▶ Predicting Risk of Metastatis in Primary Uveal Melanoma

Most primary uveal melanomas that ultimately metastasize exhibit monosomy 3 (deletion of one chromosome 3) or a characteristic gene expression profile (Class 2) within the tumor cells, and patients in whom either abnormality is detected, such as in a biopsy, enucleation, or resection specimen, should be regarded as being at high risk of metastatic disease and encouraged to participate in clinical trials attempting to identify interventions that prevent or delay its occurrence (see www.clinicaltrials.gov).

GENE THERAPY

Gene therapy refers to treatment to eliminate or ameliorate the effects of loss (deletion) or functional inactivation of one or a few adjacent genes, by inserting segments of replacement DNA into diseased cells in the hope that they will be incorporated and re-establish expression of the defective genes. Gene therapy for ocular disorders is still in its infancy, and only a few prospective Phase I trials are in progress. Good safety profile of viral vector gene transfer into target tissues, limited visual recovery in some eyes of patients with retinitis pigmentosa and Leber's hereditary optic neuropathy, and improvement in genetic corneal disorders have been reported (see www.clinicaltrials.gov).

REFERENCES

Bollinger K, Traboulsi EI: Molecular genetics for the pediatric ophthalmologist. J Pediatr Ophthalmol Strabismus 2007;44:209. [PMID: 17694825]

Bonaldi L, Midena E, Filippi B et al: FISH analysis of chromosomes 3 and 6 on fine needle aspiration biopsy samples identifies distinct subgroups of uveal melanomas. J Cancer Res Clin Oncol 2008;134:1123. [PMID: 18386059]

Chung DC, Lee V, Maguire AM: Recent advances in ocular gene therapy. Curr Opin Ophthalmol 2009;20:377. [PMID: 19667988]

Chung DC, Traboulsi EI: Leber congenial amaurosis: clinical correlations with genotypes, gene therapy trials update, and future directions. J AAPOS 2009;13:587. [PMID: 20006823]

Colella P, Colungo G, Auricchio A: Ocular gene therapy: current progress and future prospects. Trends Mol Med 2009;15:23–31. [PMID: 19097940]

Damato B, Coupland SE: Translating uveal melanoma cytogenetics into clinical care. Arch Ophthalmol 2009;127:423. [PMID: 19365018]

Drack AV, Lambert SR, Stone EM: From the laboratory to the clinic: molecular genetic testing in pediatric ophthalmology. Am J Ophthalmol 2010;149:10. [PMID: 20103038]

Fan BJ, Tam PO, Choy KW et al: Molecular diagnostics of genetic eye diseases. Clin Biochem 2006;39:231. [PMID: 16412407]

Harbour JW: Molecular prognostic testing and individualized patient care in uveal melanoma. Am J Ophthalmol 2009;148:823. [PMID: 19800609]

Hewitt AW, Craig JE, Mackey DA: Complex genetics of complex traits: the case of primary open angle glaucoma. Clin Experiment Ophthalmol 2006;34:472. [PMID: 16872346]

Mastrangelo D, De Francesco S, Di Leonardo A et al: The retinoblastoma paradigm revisited. Med Sci Monit 2008;14:RA231. [PMID: 19043380]

Michaelides M, Hardcastle AJ, Hunt DM, Moore AT: Progressive cone and cone-rod dystrophies: phenotypes and underlying molecular genetic basis. Surv Ophthammol 2006;51:232. [PMID: 16644365]

Onken MD, Worley LA, Davila RM et al: Prognostic testing in uveal melanoma by transciptomic profiling of fine needle biopsy specimens. J Mol Diagn 2006;8:567. [PMID: 17332290]

Onken MD, Worley LA, Ehlers JP, Harbour JW: Gene expression profiling in uveal melanoma reveals two molecular classes and predicts metastatic death. Cancer Res 2004;64:7205. [PMID: 15492234]

Petrausch U, Martus P, Tönnies H et al: Significance of gene expression analysis in uveal melanoma in comparison to standard risk factors for risk assessment of subsequent metastases. Eye 2008;22:997. [PMID: 17384575]

Shankar SP, Fingert JH, Carelli V et al: Evidence of a novel x-linked modifier locus for Leber hereditary optic neuropathy. Ophthalmic Genet 2008;29:17. [PMID: 18363168]

Shildkrot Y, Wilson MW: Update on posterior uveal melanoma: treatment of the eye and emerging strategies in the prognosis and treatment of metastatic disease. Curr Opin Ophthalmol 2009;20:504. [PMID: 19644367]

Simonelli F, Maguire AM, Testa F et al: Gene therapy for Leber's congenital amaurosis is safe and effective through 1.5 years after vector administration. Mol Ther 2010;18:643. [PMID: 19953081]

Simunovic MP: Colour vision deficiency. Eye 2010;24:747. [PMID: 19927164]

Sutherland JE, Day MA: Genetic counseling and genetic testing in ophthalmology. Curr Opin Ophthalmol 2009;20:343. [PMID: 19620864]

Swaroop A, Branham KE, Chen W, Abecasis G: Genetic susceptibility to age-related macular degeneration: a paradigm for dissecting complex disease traits. Hum Mol Genet 2007;16 Spec No. 2: R174. [PMID: 17911160]

Tschentscher F, Hüsing J, Hölter T et al: Tumor classification based on gene expression profiling shows that uveal melanomas with and without monosomy 3 represent two distinct entities. Cancer Res 2003;63:2578. [PMID: 12750282]

Yen MY, Wang AG, Wei YH: Leber's hereditary optic neuropathy: a multifactorial disease. Prog Ret Eye Res 2006;25:381. [PMID: 16829155]

Williams KA, Coster DJ: Gene therapy for diseases of the cornea – a review. Clin Experiment Ophthalmol 2010;38:93. [PMID: 19958372]

Worley LA, Onken MD, Person E et al: Transcriptomic versus chromosomal prognostic markers and clinical outcome in uveal melanoma. Clin Cancer Res 2007;13:1466. [PMID: 17332290]

Wu DM, Khanna H, Atmaca-Sonmez P et al: Long-term follow-up of a family with dominant X-linked retinitis pigmentosa. Eye 2010;24:764. [PMID: 19893586]

Ophthalmic Trauma

James J. Augsburger, MD, and
Zélia M. Corrêa, MD, PhD

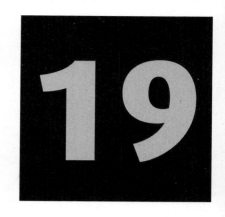

Ophthalmic trauma occurs in many settings and manifests in many ways, with widely different degrees of severity. It can result in a broad range of permanent problems, including mild to total visual loss in one or both eyes, temporary or persistent diplopia, minor to severe cosmetic abnormalities of the eyes and face, and ocular or periocular pain.

INITIAL EVALUATION

Patients with ophthalmic trauma may be of any age and either sex, and may have any extent of preexistent abnormality of the eyes, eyelids, or orbits. Their injuries may be confined to the eyes or associated with facial, head, or other potentially life-threatening injuries. Commonly the patients are fully conscious and aware of their circumstances and surroundings, but they may be affected by drugs, alcohol, or psychiatric disease. In cases of severe trauma with head injury, including when elective sedation and ventilation have been undertaken to manage cerebral injury, or when sedation has been required for other reasons, such as intubation and ventilation for airway compromise in facial injuries or severe chest injury, they may be unconscious and unresponsive.

Initial evaluation of a patient with ophthalmic trauma is frequently undertaken by a paramedic at the scene of the incident, or in an emergency room by a triage nurse or physician, who primarily is responsible for assessing the injured person's overall condition, identifying any potentially life-threatening problems that require priority treatment. Once the management of any immediately life-threatening injuries has been determined, and the patient's general condition has been stabilized, the ophthalmic injuries can be assessed, either by emergency room staff or an ophthalmologist depending upon the circumstances.

▶ History

It is essential to establish as precisely as possible the circumstances and mechanism of injury and any preexisting ophthalmic abnormality, not only to optimize the ophthalmic care but also in case of subsequent legal action for personal injury. Surprisingly frequently the crucial history of hammering metal on metal, from which penetrating injury needs to be assumed until proven otherwise, is missed. Particularly if the patient is unconscious or unable to provide enough information, persons present at the time of the injury or when the patient was found, including paramedics, should be questioned about the circumstances, and family members or friends should be asked about any preexisting ophthalmic condition.

Cooperative patients should be questioned about any subjective change in vision of either eye, pain, including foreign body sensation that would suggest ocular surface abnormality including corneal or subtarsal foreign body, or corneal abrasion, and tetanus immunization status, which might also be obtainable from a family member, especially for children.

▶ Examination

Although it is vitally important to obtain as much information as possible about vision, ocular motility, pupillary function, and any structural damage to the eyes and periocular tissues, it is crucial that examination does not exacerbate any ocular damage, a particular example being pressure on the globe to open swollen eyelids causing extrusion of intraocular contents when there is an open globe injury. Emergency room staff should not hesitate to seek assistance from an ophthalmologist. If an open globe injury is suspected, the eye should be protected by an eye shield to avoid inadvertent pressure on the globe. In some cases of severe trauma, it is quickly apparent that little can be achieved without examination under anesthesia, although even then assessment, if possible, should include measurement of vision and assessment of pupillary function.

An important general rule is that whenever possible the first step in assessment of ophthalmic trauma is to assess vision in each eye, preferably using a Snellen or other vision testing chart. It is important to bear in mind that the patient may have broken or lost glasses or contact lenses as a result of the trauma, such that pinhole testing to overcome refractive

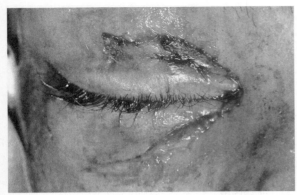

A

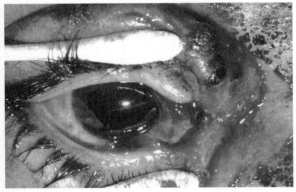

B

▲ **Figure 19–1.** Eyelid laceration with concurrent open globe injury. **A:** Rather innocuous-appearing V-shaped eyelid laceration involving the upper and lower lids and medial canthal skin. **B:** Total dark red hyphema and hemorrhagic chemosis are evident when the lids are separated. Note also that laceration extends through both lacrimal canaliculi. See color insert.

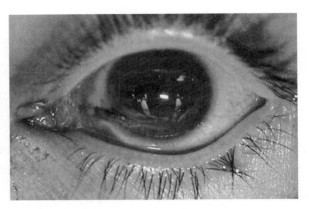

▲ **Figure 19–2.** Corneoscleral laceration inferonasally with pupil displaced toward the laceration and iris incarcerated in wound. See color insert.

error may be important. Visual acuity less than counting fingers, not explained by refractive error or preexisting abnormality, is a strong indication of severe globe injury.

The periocular tissues are examined for any obvious abnormalities, particular attention being paid to eyelid wounds involving the margin or lacrimal canaliculi (Figure 19–1), both requiring management by an ophthalmologist, and proptosis, which may be due to orbital hemorrhage, air (orbital emphysema that characteristically causes crepitus) from a paranasal sinus fracture, infection (orbital cellulitis) including abscess formation, or carotid artery-cavernous sinus fistula.

The globes are then examined, including for subconjunctival hemorrhage, corneal, conjunctival, or scleral wound, corneal clarity, corneal foreign body, hyphema, and whether the eye is deformed due to low intraocular pressure suggestive

of globe rupture. If there is eyelid swelling but no evidence of globe laceration or rupture, the eyelids may need to be gently separated avoiding pressure on the globes. Examination of the pupils is important, not least whether they can be clearly visualized or the view is impaired suggesting corneal or anterior segment damage. Abnormalities of pupil shape are important clues to severe globe injury, including corneal or corneo-scleral laceration (Figure 19–2), globe rupture, or severe blunt anterior segment trauma. A dilated unreactive pupil may be due to third nerve palsy when there has been head injury, and a relative afferent pupillary defect (RAPD) is an important sign of optic nerve damage. The latter is particularly relevant to assessment of unconscious patients with mid-facial trauma possibly resulting in optic nerve damage in the region of the optic canal, with or without associated fracture.

Assessment of ocular motility not only provides information about injury to the bony orbit, typically blow-out fracture of the floor or medial orbital wall, and orbital soft tissues, but also about intracranial damage, including skull base fracture resulting in sixth nerve palsy or more extensive limitation of eye movements due to carotid artery-cavernous sinus fistula, in which case there will also be proptosis and usually a bruit that can be heard by the patient as well as by listening with a stethoscope over the orbit or temple.

Ophthalmoscopy provides assessment of the clarity of the ocular media, which will be impaired by corneal damage, hyphema (anterior chamber hemorrhage), lens damage, or vitreous hemorrhage, the last being an important clue to scleral laceration or globe rupture. The fundi are examined for retinal or optic nerve abnormalities such as hemorrhages, retinal edema or detachment, and optic nerve avulsion—characteristically occurring after rapid rotation of the globe such as from a finger being forcibly poked into the eye, as well as choroidal rupture. Whether it is appropriate to dilate the pupils for fundal examination will depend upon what ocular damage has already been identified and the patient's neurological status.

Slitlamp examination facilitates assessment of the anterior and posterior segments, as well as allowing measurement of intraocular pressure, although this can also be assessed by digital pressure, assuming that corneal or scleral laceration and globe rupture have been adequately excluded, or with the portable Perkins tonometer or Tonopen.

Partly because its superior 3-dimensional capabilities improve localization, orbital CT generally has superseded plain x-rays for suspected metallic intraocular or orbital foreign body, MRI being specifically contraindicated. CT can also detect some glass foreign bodies but it frequently fails to identify wooden foreign bodies, for which MRI or ultrasound is preferable and which commonly lead to orbital infection. CT has increasingly been used to detect globe rupture and is the preferred modality for identification of orbital fractures, although MRI may be preferable for the assessment of associated soft tissue changes, including infection, either orbital or intracranial.

In all cases of ophthalmic trauma, it is important to fully examine uninjured eyes, in part to ensure that there is no undiagnosed preexisting abnormality. In all cases of perforating ocular or periocular trauma, adequate tetanus immunization needs to be ensured.

EMERGENCY TREATMENTS

First aid and emergency hospital treatment can make a vital contribution to improving outcome from ophthalmic trauma.

▶ Chemical Injury

If there is a history of chemical injury from assault with alkali or acid or airbag injury; splashing of battery acid, cleaning solution, or chemicals either industrial or domestic; spraying of pesticide or chemical dust; or foreign bodies containing noxious substances, such as lime within cement or plaster; and initial examination shows no evidence of open globe injury, prior to any further assessment the ocular surface immediately should be copiously irrigated with tap water or, if available, sterile isotonic saline solution at the scene of the injury and in the emergency room. Administration of topical anesthetic drops and insertion of an eyelid speculum may be required to perform irrigation effectively and for removal of any retained foreign bodies. Identification of the relevant chemical is helpful. Alkalis continue to cause damage to the conjunctiva and cornea long after the injury is sustained, and thus irrigation of the eye should continue for a prolonged period (more than half an hour) in most such cases. In contrast, acids tend to form a barrier of precipitated necrotic tissue that limits penetration and deep tissue damage (as long as the offending chemical is washed away), such that irrigation need not continue for as long.

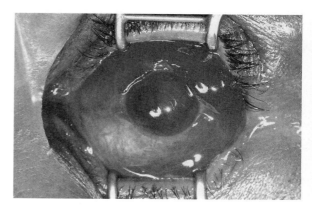

▲ **Figure 19–3.** Massive hemorrhagic chemosis following severe blunt ocular trauma. A globe rupture in the superonasal quadrant was confirmed by surgical exploration.

▶ Open Globe Injury

Corneal laceration may be obvious, or inferred from displacement of the pupil toward the wound, flat anterior chamber, hyphema, or uveal prolapse (Figure 19–2). Similar abnormalities, as well as hemorrhagic chemosis, softening and possible collapse of the eye, and vitreous hemorrhage, occur in **scleral laceration**, which should be particularly suspected if there is deep eyelid laceration (Figure 19–1), and **globe rupture** due to blunt ocular trauma (Figures 19–3 and 19–4). Whenever there is evidence or suspicion of open globe injury, the eye is protected with an eye shield, not least to prevent the patient from causing further injury by rubbing the eye and to alert

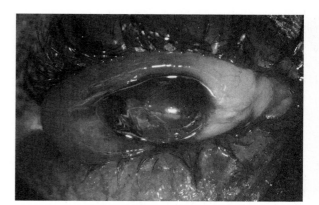

▲ **Figure 19–4.** Pellet gun injury to the right eye resulting in open globe injury. Note massive hemorrhagic chemosis, irregular corneal shape, distorted pupil, and dark brown iris tissue incarcerated into limbal wound. See color insert.

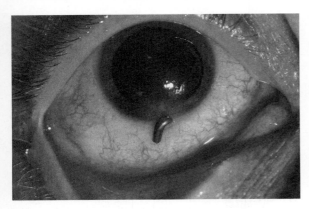

▲ **Figure 19–5.** Perforating ocular laceration with retained foreign body, the tip of the metallic foreign body protruding from the eye at the limbus.

other staff to the need to avoid manipulation of the eye. Analgesia and possibly antiemetic medication, to reduce the chance of vomiting, are administered.

▶ Foreign Body

A foreign body injury should be suspected whenever there is a history of explosion, gunshot wound, striking of metal upon metal, metal grinding, or a sharp object hitting the eye. If there is evidence or suspicion of a perforating ocular laceration (Figures 19–1 and 19–2), or signs of an orbital injury, CT orbits should be performed to identify and localize any foreign body unless one is already apparent (Figure 19–5). Ocular examination should identify any corneal foreign body or abrasion, if necessary aided by instillation of fluorescein (Figure 19–6). Particularly if there is curvilinear fluorescein staining of the superior cornea or persisting foreign body, the upper eyelid should be everted to identify any subtarsal foreign body (see Chapter 2).

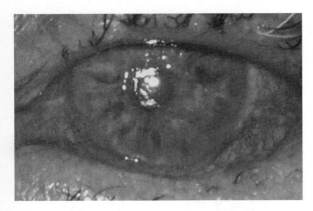

▲ **Figure 19–6.** Corneal abrasion stained with fluorescein. See color insert.

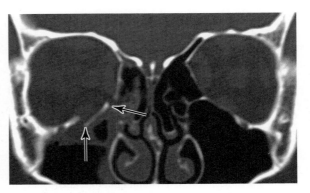

▲ **Figure 19–7.** Coronal CT scan of orbits showing right orbital floor fracture (arrows).

▶ Orbital Injury

Enophthalmos, step defect on palpation of the orbital rim, massive orbital swelling, orbital crepitus, ocular motility defects, or profound visual impairment in the absence of direct ocular injuries consistent with that visual loss, should prompt CT orbits to detect rim, wall, or apex fractures (Figure 19–7), displaced bone fragments, air, hemorrhage, infection, or foreign bodies.

▼ CATEGORIES OF OPHTHALMIC TRAUMA

Ophthalmic trauma can be divided into mechanical, chemical, thermal, and electromagnetic injuries.

MECHANICAL INJURIES

Mechanical ophthalmic trauma may be produced by objects that are blunt, sharp, or a combination of the two, and can be categorized into closed and open globe injuries, eyelid wounds, and orbital injuries, but these may co-exist, in which case coordination of management with maxillo-facial surgeons is important.

1. CLOSED GLOBE INJURIES

Corneal abrasion, which is one of the most common ophthalmic injuries encountered in an urgent care or emergency room setting, occurs when the corneal epithelium is disrupted, usually by a tangential impact such as from a fingernail or edge of a piece of paper. The patient typically complains of severe discomfort with foreign body sensation, profuse tearing, inability to keep the eyelids open, and impaired vision. If initial examination shows no obvious corneal laceration, topical anesthetic drops can be instilled, usually resulting in rapid reduction in discomfort and easier examination. Instillation of fluorescein highlights the corneal epithelial defect, which is usually in the inferior cornea, by staining the exposed basement membrane

(Figure 19–6). If instead, there is curvilinear staining of the superior cornea, a subtarsal foreign body should be suspected (see later in the chapter).

Corneal abrasion is treated by instillation of an antibacterial ointment and patching of the eye. The patient is instructed to remove the patch, and apply antibacterial ointment and another patch, 2 to 4 times daily until the eye is comfortable. The patient can be reexamined periodically during the healing period to ensure that microbial infection has not developed, and certainly should be reexamined if symptoms do not settle within a few days or increase. Under no circumstance should topical anesthetic drops be provided or prescribed for the patient's use, because they delay corneal epithelial healing, mask progression of disease, and if used for a prolonged period can cause a persistent neurotrophic corneal epithelial defect.

Corneal foreign body occurs when a small particle, usually with sharp rather than smooth edges, strikes the eye with insufficient momentum to cause it to pass completely through the cornea but sufficient for it become embedded within it. Alternatively, the particle may become embedded in the conjunctival surface of the upper eyelid (**subtarsal foreign body**). Symptoms are similar to those of a corneal abrasion, but usually not as severe and with predominance of foreign body sensation with eye opening and closing. Depending on its size, color, and transparency, metal being easier to detect than untinted glass, a corneal foreign body may be visible on diffuse flashlight examination of the ocular surface (Figure 19–8), but slitlamp examination is definitive. If examination is negative, the upper eyelid should be everted to detect any subtarsal foreign body (see Chapter 2), which usually can be removed by wiping the conjunctival surface with a sterile cotton bud, the only other required treatment being a single instillation of antibacterial ointment.

Emergency room staff trained in slitlamp examination can remove corneal foreign bodies, otherwise the patient should be referred to an ophthalmologist. The cornea should be anesthetized with topical anesthetic drops. Before attempting to remove a corneal foreign body, it must be confirmed by slitlamp examination that it is superficial and does not extend completely through the cornea, in which case removal should be performed by an ophthalmologist, generally in an operating room with an operating microscope so that tissue glue can be applied or sutures inserted if necessary. A superficial corneal foreign body can usually be removed at the slitlamp, using the tip of a sterile (18 or 21 gauge) needle. Iron or copper foreign bodies usually produce a ring of chemical tissue staining ("**rust ring**"), which can be scraped off with the needle tip or removed with a burr tip on a battery-operated drill. Following removal of a corneal foreign body, antibacterial ointment is instilled and the eye is patched. The patient is instructed to remove the patch, and apply antibacterial ointment and another patch, 2 to 4 times daily until the corneal epithelial defect has healed. The patient should be reexamined periodically during the healing period to ensure that microbial infection of the defect has not developed.

Subconjunctival hemorrhage of limited extent is common after ocular or orbital blunt injury (Figure 19–9). Extensive hemorrhagic chemosis, especially if the eye is soft or collapsed indicating low intraocular pressure, is strongly suggestive of globe rupture (Figures 19–3 and 19–4), and urgent surgical exploration is required (see later in the chapter).

Most **conjunctival lacerations** and **partial-thickness corneal,** and/or **scleral lacerations** can be managed like a corneal abrasion. Following slitlamp examination to ensure that any corneal or sclera laceration is not full-thickness, antibacterial ointment is instilled and the eye is patched. The patient is instructed to remove the patch, and apply additional antibacterial ointment and patch the eye 2 to 4 times daily until the laceration has healed. The patient should be reexamined periodically during the healing period to ensure that microbial infection of the wound has not developed.

Traumatic iritis frequently develops after closed globe injury. Symptoms include pain, especially in bright light,

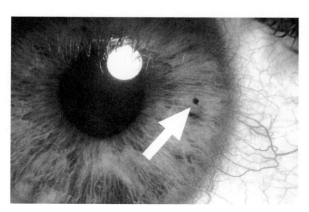

▲ **Figure 19–8.** Metallic corneal foreign body appearing as dark brown speck on the cornea (arrow). See color insert.

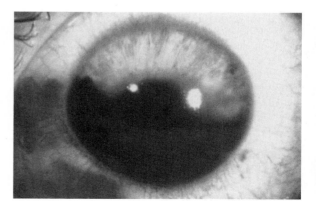

▲ **Figure 19–9.** Post-traumatic hyphema and associated subconjunctival hemorrhage.

blurred vision, and tenderness of the globe. Slitlamp examination reveals inflammatory cells and flare in the anterior chamber, and finely dispersed cellular keratic precipitates on the corneal endothelium. There may be a (Vossius) ring of dark brown iris pigment on the anterior lens capsule. Posterior synechiae and peripheral anterior synechiae may develop. Treatment consists of cycloplegic mydriatic drops (eg, cyclopentolate 1% or atropine 1% twice a day) and topical corticosteroid drops (eg, dexamethasone 0.1%) 2 to 4 times a day until the intraocular inflammation subsides.

Traumatic **hyphema** (anterior chamber hemorrhage) (Figure 19–9) reflects damage to iris blood vessels, and may be associated with iridodialysis or cyclodialysis (see later in the chapter). It should always raise concern about open globe injury (Figure 19–1). It may be short-lived and resolve spontaneously, but it can be complicated by secondary glaucoma and corneal blood staining, particularly if there is recurrence of hemorrhage. Depending on the extent of the hyphema and the severity of any other ocular damage, treatment ranges from restriction of activities to reduce the risk of rebleeding until the hyphema has resolved, to hospitalization with medical therapy (topical, oral, or even intravenous) to control intraocular pressure, and possibly anterior chamber washout. Oral aminocaproic acid reduces the risk of rebleeding. Aspirin and non-steroidal anti-inflammatory drugs (NSAIDS) should be avoided. The consequences of hyphema are more serious in sickle cell disease.

The concussive shock wave of blunt ocular trauma can result in small radial tears in the iris sphincter muscle at the pupillary margin (**iris sphincter ruptures**), localized or extensive circumferential tearing of the iris at the iridociliary junction (**iridodialysis**), or even a localized or extensive circumferential separation of the peripheral iris and ciliary body from the sclera at and behind the scleral spur (**cyclodialysis**). Such defects may not be apparent initially if accompanied by hyphema. Because cyclodialysis allows increased drainage of aqueous into the suprachoroidal space, it frequently results in low intraocular pressure (**hypotony**). Ultrasound biomicroscopy is useful for identifying cyclodialysis and associated ciliochoroidal effusion in hypotonous eyes.

Traumatic **anterior chamber angle recession** is circumferentially oriented tearing of the trabecular meshwork tissue. It is also frequently accompanied by hyphema and may not be evident until any blood clears from the anterior chamber. It may be detectable by gonioscopy or ultrasound biomicroscopy. It is important that eyes that have sustained significant blunt trauma, particularly if there has been hyphema, undergo gonioscopy to detect angle recession because its presence provides information on the likelihood of subsequent glaucoma, which may occur from structural damage and/or impairment of trabecular meshwork function.

Traumatic **lens dislocation** (subluxation) due to damage to the zonules may manifest as instability of the crystalline lens (phakodonesis), often more evident on slitlamp examination as abnormal quivering movements of the iris (iridodenesis) on rapid rotation of the globe, or prolapse of vitreous into the anterior chamber. The entire lens may be dislocated posteriorly into the vitreous or (rarely) anteriorly into the anterior chamber. Lens dislocation may be associated with subsequent development of glaucoma, largely reflecting the severity of the ocular trauma resulting in trabecular meshwork damage but also possibly due to blockage of flow of aqueous through the pupil (pupillary block).

Cataract may be a delayed consequence of blunt ocular trauma and usually can be managed with conventional surgical techniques with insertion of a posterior chamber intraocular lens, but the surgery may be complicated by lens instability due to zonular damage. An uncommon entity is traumatic posterior lens capsule rupture, usually requiring early surgery with specialized techniques.

Commotio retinae is a characteristic pattern of retinal whitening that occurs after severe closed globe ocular contusion. It generally develops 180° opposite the site of impact, the shock wave travelling posteriorly in the eye to strike the fundus (contrecoup injury). The retinal whitening typically appears within 24 hours and gradually fades over several days to weeks. If the macula is affected, visual acuity may be profoundly reduced.

Choroidal rupture is tearing of the retinal pigment epithelium, characteristically in a crescentic or curvilinear shape orientated tangentially to the optic disc margin, after closed globe ocular contusion (see Chapter 10). Involvement of the central macula, which commonly occurs, usually results in profound and permanent reduction of visual acuity. There is also a risk of subsequent choroidal neovascularization, but this is usually amenable to treatment.

Full-thickness macular hole (Figure 19–10) may follow severe closed globe contusion injury in which the shock wave

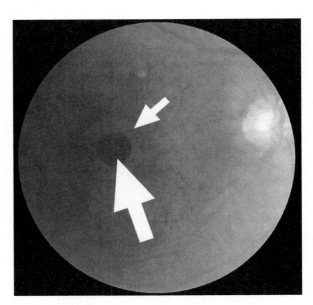

▲ **Figure 19–10.** Post-traumatic macular hole **(larger arrow)** with surrounding serous subretinal fluid **(smaller arrow).** See color insert.

is transmitted directly to the fovea. The hole usually develops acutely as separation of vitreous adherent to the macula pulls off an operculum of full-thickness retina in the foveal region. The hole can sometimes be closed by vitreo-retinal surgery, but visual acuity frequently does not improve.

Closed globe ocular injuries frequently result in **vitreous hemorrhage**, which may be mild to severe. The usual mechanism is partial to complete posterior vitreous detachment with tearing of superficial retinal blood vessels in areas of particularly firm vitreo-retinal adhesion. As long as there is no retinal tear, the intravitreal blood usually clears spontaneously within a few weeks to months. If the retina is torn, **retinal detachment** frequently develops, requiring surgical reattachment that commonly necessitates vitrectomy.

2. OPEN GLOBE INJURIES

Open globe injuries are characterized by full-thickness wound of the cornea and/or sclera, resulting in exposure or extrusion of intraocular contents. They are divided into **perforating ocular lacerations** and **globe ruptures**.

A. Perforating Ocular Lacerations

A perforating ocular laceration (penetrating ocular trauma) may be caused by a sharp object that enters the globe and

a. is then instantaneously or subsequently withdrawn prior to the patient's presentation, such as glass, wire, or the blade of a knife or scissors, that is, single wound without a retained intraocular foreign body,

b. passes completely through it and then lodges in the orbit, such as a metallic foreign body, or then is withdrawn, such as a hypodermic needle for administration of local anesthetic injection for cataract surgery, that is, separate entry and exit wounds (double ocular perforation) without a retained intraocular foreign body, or

c. remains completely or partially inside the globe, that is, retained intraocular foreign body.

Ocular lacerations without a retained intraocular foreign body (Figures 19–1 and 19–2) represent the most common type of open globe injury encountered in most trauma centers. As discussed above, as soon as the laceration is recognized, the injured eye is protected with an eye shield; analgesia, and possibly antiemetic medication to reduce the chance of vomiting, and if necessary tetanus toxoid, are administered; and orbital CT scan is performed to exclude any ocular or orbital foreign body and to provide further information about the extent of damage to the globe. Systemic antibiotics are administered if there is involvement of the sclera, or extensive anterior segment damage.

Urgent exploration under anesthesia (usually general but possibly local supplemented if necessary with intravenous sedation) is then undertaken. (Double ocular perforation with a hypodermic needle may be self-sealing and not require urgent exploration, but later may require vitreo-retinal surgery to manage retinal complications or remove vitreous hemorrhage.)

Whenever possible, it is crucial that the full extent of the wound is determined; if necessary, by opening the conjunctiva through 360° and detachment of rectus muscles, because failure to identify and close the ends of the wound will usually lead to postoperative hypotony and increases the risk of endophthalmitis. Once the wound has been fully exposed, any prolapsed uveal tissue and retina are identified, with a view during closure of the laceration to replacing (repositing) them within the globe, as long as they are not dirty, dessicated, or necrotic, in which case the externalized portions are abscissed. Prolapsed vitreous is abscissed. The crystalline lens may be intact, absent, or damaged, the last possibly requiring aspiration of lens material or deferral of specific treatment until a later procedure (see later in the chapter).

The laceration is sutured as accurately as possible, with particular attention to the limbus if it is involved and to avoidance of sutures being placed across the visual axis of the cornea, as well as avoidance of incarceration of corneal or conjunctival epithelium. Corneal lacerations are usually closed using 10–0 nylon sutures with buried knots, scleral lacerations with 8–0 or 9–0 nylon sutures, and conjunctival wounds with absorbable 7–0 or 8–0 sutures. At the end of the repair, the wound should be watertight. If the globe is soft, sterile isotonic saline solution is injected into the anterior chamber or vitreous cavity to restore the ocular shape and volume. Subconjunctival antibiotic is administered, or if there is involvement of the posterior segment, particularly if the mechanism of injury suggests a high risk of infection or presentation was delayed, intravitreal antibiotic may be administered. A sterile eye patch and protective eye shield are applied.

On the following day, topical antibiotic, steroid and cycloplegic/mydriatic are started. The patient should be reexamined frequently to identify wound leaks, corneal ulceration, intraocular infection (endophthalmitis), recurrent intraocular bleeding, hypotony, or ocular hypertension that may require additional interventions. Many eyes with a scleral wound require vitreo-retinal surgery because of retinal complications, usually related to incarceration of vitreous into the wound and the development of vitreo-retinal traction. Corneal scarring may require penetrating keratoplasty (corneal transplantation), assuming that other complications such as glaucoma or retinal damage have not rendered it inappropriate.

If exploration shows so much damage that suturing of the globe is not feasible (eg, in some gunshot wounds and shrapnel injuries), primary removal of the globe is probably appropriate. Traditionally enucleation rather than evisceration is advised to maximize removal of uveal tissue, and thus reduce the risk of sympathetic ophthalmia (see Chapter 7), but studies indicate that there is no difference in risk and evisceration is associated with fewer complications. Similarly, in eyes that have undergone primary repair but have no perception of light, the conventional treatment is enucleation

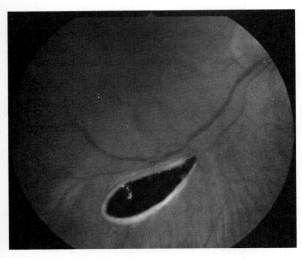

▲ Figure 19–11. Metallic foreign body lying on the surface of the retina.

within 10 days of the initial injury to reduce the risk of sympathetic ophthalmia, but the availability of effective treatments for sympathetic ophthalmia and its rarity, the better cosmetic outcome if the globe is retained, and the possibility of recovery of vision following vitreo-retinal surgery, have led to a questioning of this approach.

Ocular lacerations associated with one or more retained foreign bodies (eg, an embedded fishhook, a sliver of glass, a portion of the casing of an exploded firework, or a metallic fragment generated by striking metal on metal) (Figure 19–11) must be managed on an individual basis, taking into account the type of foreign body, its size, its anatomic location, the extent and severity of the globe laceration, and availability of surgical expertise and instrumentation such as for vitrectomy. Foreign bodies that project partly in and partly out of the eye (eg, an embedded fishhook or wire) (Figure 19–5), can usually be removed during the primary surgery. For foreign bodies that are completely inside the eye and cannot be visualized adequately intraoperatively, for instance because of intraocular blood or lens opacity, or cannot be removed successfully without strong probability of avoidable additional intraocular damage, for instance because of lack of appropriate expertise or instrumentation, generally attempted removal should be deferred until a subsequent procedure. Whereas magnets were previously used to remove magnetic intraocular foreign bodies, removal with forceps, which can also be used for non-magnetic foreign bodies, is now preferred. High-velocity metallic foreign bodies are usually sterile with a low risk of endophthalmitis, whereas other foreign bodies, particularly wooden, are associated with higher risk of endophthalmitis, and intravitreal antibiotics may be administered at the time of the initial and/or subsequent surgery.

In many cases of corneal or corneoscleral laceration, the lens is retained but its anterior capsule is damaged, leading to hydration of lens matter that will usually progress over the ensuing days and caused marked intraocular inflammation. Occasionally, it is possible or necessary to aspirate the lens matter at the time of initial repair, but frequently it is deferred until a second operation, when there is more information about the extent of ocular damage, including whether vitreo-retinal surgery is required, and there is likely to be better visualization of the anterior segment. Whether an intraocular lens can be inserted will depend upon several factors, including whether sufficient posterior capsule has been retained and how much iris has been lost.

In some instances of corneal or corneoscleral laceration, the crystalline lens is extruded from the eye. The expulsed lens may be identified or its absence noted during surgery, but in most cases the eye is found to be aphakic at postoperative slitlamp or ultrasound examination.

B. Globe Ruptures

Globe rupture refers to a breach of the integrity of the globe due to forceful indentation by blunt trauma, such as from a punch, particularly if the assailant is wearing a bulky ring. Relatively common sites are the limbus, the sclera beneath the insertion of the extraocular muscles (especially in the superonasal quadrant), and at prior incision sites (eg, at the interface between donor and recipient cornea following penetrating keratoplasty). Globe rupture should be suspected in any blunt ocular trauma associated with massive hemorrhagic chemosis, especially if the eye is soft or collapsed indicating low intraocular pressure (Figures 19–3 and 19–4). Whenever globe rupture is suspected, urgent surgical exploration is required. The pre-, per- and postoperative management is broadly the same as for perforating ocular laceration without foreign body, except that preoperative CT scan may not be deemed necessary if the history clearly does not suggest a risk of intraocular foreign body.

3. EYELID WOUNDS

Lacerations and tears of the eyelids are a common type of ophthalmic injury, occurring in a wide variety of situations, such as automobile accidents, fights, impacts by blunt or sharp projectiles, falls, animal bites, and explosions. The most important step in management is thorough examination to determine the precise location, depth, and extent of the wound, whether there is embedded foreign material, and to detect all relevant associated ocular and orbital injuries, including involvement of the lacrimal drainage system. Whenever there is a full-thickness eyelid laceration, the possibility of open globe injury must be borne in mind (Figures 19–1 and 19–12).

All wounds need to be thoroughly debrided, with removal of as much foreign material as possible. Prophylactic systemic antibiotics should be considered for animal bites and

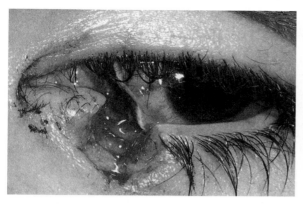

▲ **Figure 19–12.** Full-thickness laceration of medial left lower eyelid involving the margin with underlying scleral laceration with uveal prolapse.

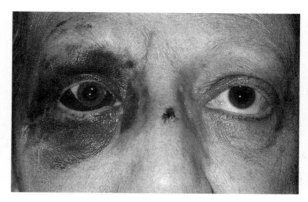

▲ **Figure 19–13.** Prominent right eyelid ecchymosis and subconjunctival hemorrhage due to blunt trauma suffered in a fall.

dirty wounds, particularly if there is a delayed presentation. Superficial wounds that do not involve the eyelid margin or medial canthal region should be repaired in the same way as skin wounds elsewhere. Full-thickness wounds that involve the eyelid margin require specialist repair to ensure correct realignment of the tarsal plate, mucocutaneous junction, and lash line. Involvement of the medial canthal region warrants microsurgical exploration, to allow repair of torn or lacerated lacrimal canaliculi, commonly by insertion of a lacrimal stent, and reconstruction of the medial canthal tendon, to reduce the likelihood of epiphora and to limit cosmetic abnormality.

4. ORBITAL INJURIES

Contusion of the orbital soft tissues, resulting from blunt injury such as from a punch, batted baseball, or fall, may be associated with eyelid wounds, ocular injuries, or orbital fractures. The most common manifestation is orbital swelling, possibly with proptosis, and eyelid ecchymosis (Figure 19–13). There may be limitation of eye movements. If there is severe proptosis with corneal exposure or visual loss due to optic nerve compression, usually due to **orbital hemorrhage**, lateral canthotomy and cantholysis may be performed as an emergency procedure. Orbital CT can also be undertaken to identify whether there is an orbital hematoma suitable for surgical evacuation. If there is no corneal exposure or optic nerve compression, no treatment except analgesics and cold compresses is usually needed.

Orbital fractures (Figure 19–7) are a common consequence of mechanical trauma, with involvement of one or more of the bony walls and/or the anterior rim, possibly extending to a tripod fracture involving the zygoma (malar eminence) or even a Le Fort II or III fracture, by a combination of shock waves and shearing forces. Clinical signs include orbital swelling and eyelid ecchymosis, depression of the

malar eminence, step-off defect on palpation of the orbital rim, numbness in the distribution of the infraorbital nerve that traverses the orbital floor, crepitus on palpation indicating the presence of intraorbital air, enophthalmos but this may not be present initially if there is orbital soft tissue swelling, and restricted ocular motility. Orbital CT provides confirmation. Mid-facial or head trauma, such as from automobile accidents or severe falls or assaults, that results in orbital fracture is commonly associated with other fractures of the face or of the vault or base of the skull. Appropriate further imaging should be undertaken to identify such fractures, as well as potentially life-threatening intracranial or other injuries, and consultation obtained from neurosurgeons and maxillo-facial surgeons as necessary.

Most orbital rim and wall fractures do not require immediate surgical repair. Exceptions are orbital wall fractures with entrapment of an extraocular muscle that is complicated by recurring profound bradycardia (due to a persistent oculocardiac reflex from the entrapped muscle), the trap-door variety of orbital floor fracture that usually occurs in children and may be accompanied by nausea and vomiting, and possibly profound acute visual loss due to a bone fragment impinging on the optic nerve in the posterior orbit or optic canal, but the benefit from surgical exploration in this situation is not well established. Otherwise, surgery can usually be delayed for one to two weeks to allow the soft tissue swelling to diminish, determination whether surgery is required, and management of any globe injuries. The indications for repair of orbital floor fractures are enophthalmos, extensive fracture that is likely to result in the development of enophthalmos, and troublesome diplopia due to entrapment of orbital soft tissue, possibly including the inferior rectus muscle, which is not spontaneously improving. Repair is accomplished by elevating the periosteum over the defect, freeing entrapped tissue, removing or replacing displaced fragments of bone, and closing the defect such as with an alloplastic plate. Further surgery may be needed to manage persisting strabismus or ptosis, the latter usually being due to damage to the levator muscle. Displaced zygomatic arch fractures generally require surgery.

Some eyelid wounds extend deep into the orbit, resulting in damage to the extraocular muscles, lacrimal gland, orbital blood vessels and nerves, and possibly the optic nerve. Most fully embedded orbital foreign bodies, except perhaps those that are known to have been grossly contaminated or composed of organic material such as wood, do not need to be removed, unless they result in orbital infection.

Optic nerve injury (see Chapter 14) may occur in orbital wounds, including local anesthetic injections for ocular surgery, or indirectly following blunt trauma to the forehead without fracture due to transmission of shock waves to the orbital apex, but most commonly occurs with severe head or facial injury with fracture involving the optic canal or posterior orbit. Although in the last situation high-dose systemic steroid therapy and optic canal decompression have been advocated, there is little evidence that either is beneficial. Surgery may be indicated for orbital hemorrhage. Optic nerve avulsion characteristically occurs after abrupt rotation of the globe, such as from the eye being poked forcibly with a finger and has a poor prognosis with no effective treatment.

CHEMICAL INJURIES

Chemical injuries warrant emergent copious irrigation of the ocular surface to remove any residual chemical and prevent avoidable additional ocular damage (see earlier in the chapter). According to the severity of ocular surface damage as judged by the severity of epithelial loss, corneal stromal opacity, and limbal ischemia, treatment then may include

a. topical antibiotic to prevent infection whilst there is a corneal epithelial defect,

b. topical cycloplegic/mydriatic to reduce discomfort,

c. topical steroid therapy to reduce ocular surface and intraocular inflammation,

d. ascorbate (vitamin C) topically (10% 4 times a day) and orally (1 g per day) to prevent collagen lysis.

e. potassium citrate topically (10% 4 times a day) to chleate calcium, thus reducing inflammatory cell activity,

f. oral doxyxcycline (100 mg twice a day) to reduce inflammation and prevent corneal melting,

g. topical lubricants to prevent drying, and

h. oral acetazolamide (250 mg up to 4 times a day) to treat raised intraocular pressure.

Severe damage to the eyelids may result in necrosis and sloughing. Tissue contracture may lead to ectropion, entropion, or lagophthalmos. Treatment for chemical injuries of the eyelids is similar to that recommended for thermal burns (see later in the chapter).

Persisting corneal epithelial defects, with the potential for superadded infection, and corneal scarring with vascularization are usually secondary to damage to limbal stem cells, but tear deficiency due to conjunctival damage involving the accessory lacrimal glands and goblet cells, and trichiasis due to eyelid scarring may contribute. Achieving corneal epithelialization is important because it suppresses inflammation and halts corneal melting. It may require insertion of a bandage contact lens, botulinum toxin-induced ptosis, eyelid surgery including tarsorrhaphy, or amniotic membrane graft.

Once the ocular status has been stabilized following a severe chemical injury, limbal stem cell transplantation, preferably using donor tissue from the other eye but otherwise needing cadaveric donor tissue, may be beneficial particularly prior to consideration of penetrating keratoplasty, which has a high risk of failure and requires optimization of the condition of the ocular surface. In severely damaged eyes not suitable for ocular surface reconstruction, the only available option to restore vision may be implantation of a keratoprosthesis.

THERMAL INJURIES

Thermal burns of the eyelids, such as from fires and explosions, manifest initially as redness and swelling of the skin with blistering and charring in severe cases. Topical antibiotic ointment is applied regularly to keep the tissues lubricated and prevent secondary infection. In deep burns, ectropion and lid retraction start to develop within a few days. In severe cases, tarsorrhaphies and skin grafts are needed to prevent corneal exposure and ulceration. Repeated procedures over weeks to months are frequently required.

Thermal burns to the globe are much less frequent, but unsuccessful treatment of eyelid damage may lead to corneal and conjunctival exposure and drying, leading to corneal ulceration, infection and even perforation, with the possibility of permanent blindness.

ELECTROMAGNETIC INJURIES

The most common electromagnetic injury to the eye is ultraviolet radiation-induced damage to the corneal and conjunctival epithelium from arc welding, use of a sunbed, or prolonged exposure to sunlight reflected off snow, water, or white sand, without the use of appropriate eye protection. The eye typically becomes scratchy and painful several hours after exposure, with profuse tearing. Slitlamp examination, following instillation of fluorescein, to confirm the diagnosis is usually possible after administration of topical anesthetic drops. Treatment is similar to that described above for corneal abrasions but routine re-examination is not usually required. Topical anesthetic drops for the patient's use must not be provided or prescribed.

Radiation-induced damage may occur when the radiation field of external beam radiation includes the eyelids. In most cases, redness of the eyelid skin develops within 1–2 weeks of the start of treatment and persists for several weeks following its conclusion. The usual treatment is topical antibiotic or corticosteroid ointment until the redness resolves.

IMPORTANT SEQUELAE OF OPHTHALMIC TRAUMA

Ophthalmic trauma in its various forms is frequently complicated by sequelae, including corneal and eyelid scarring, retinal detachment, glaucoma, and intraocular hemorrhage.

Ocular hypotony, generally accepted to mean intraocular pressure less than 6 mm Hg, results in infolding of the cornea, diffuse corneal and uveal thickening, and macular edema, all of which can cause mild to profound visual impairment. It may be due to fistula including unrecognized globe rupture, serous ciliochoroidal effusion, cyclodialysis, ciliary body failure, retinal detachment, or chronic intraocular inflammation. Intractable hypotony usually leads to a blind shrunken eye (phthisis bulbi).

Microbial infection is a serious and potentially blinding complication of many ocular injuries. It may be limited to the cornea following partial or full-thickness corneal or corneoscleral laceration, or may extend to involve the whole globe (endophthalmitis) or the whole orbit (panophthalmitis). Infection is more likely when the injury was caused by a grossly contaminated object or there is a retained wooden foreign body.

Corneal blood staining occurs when there is extensive hyphema and substantial elevation of intraocular pressure. Blood cells are forced into the stroma of the cornea by the high intraocular pressure, and hemosiderin pigment is deposited in the corneal stroma as the blood cells disintegrate, giving the cornea a reddish brown color in a discoid distribution that is most pronounced centrally and inferiorly. Once the hyphema resolves and intraocular pressure returns to normal with or without treatment, the corneal blood staining slowly disappears over many months. While this is a tolerable problem for most adults, it is a potential cause of amblyopia in young children.

Retained iron intraocular foreign body that is not recognized or removed, leads to deposition of iron pigment within many intraocular tissues (**ocular siderosis**), including the cornea, lens, and retina, resulting in rusty to greenish discoloration that is most evident in the iris and associated with loss of pupillary function. Retained copper intraocular foreign body similarly leads to deposition of copper salts (**ocular chalcosis**), particularly in Descemet's membrane, lens capsule, and retina. In either case, if the foreign body is not removed, vision can be lost due to retinal toxicity and electroretinography is usually diagnostic.

Sympathetic ophthalmia is an uncommon uveitis in which one eye is traumatized but granulomatous intraocular inflammation eventually develops in both eyes (see Chapter 7). The disorder is most commonly associated with extensive corneoscleral lacerations complicated by incarceration of uveal tissue in the wound, but it may occur after elective uncomplicated intraocular surgery. Inflammation in the traumatized (inciting) eye usually begins shortly following the injury, but inflammation in the fellow (sympathizing) eye may begin as early as 1–2 weeks after the trauma or as long as several years later, with the possibility of profound visual loss in both eyes. Generally the intraocular inflammation can be controlled with preservation of good vision by topical, periocular, and if necessary systemic corticosteroids or other immunosuppressant therapy. Removal of a traumatized eye within 10 days of the initial injury is thought to reduce the risk of sympathetic ophthalmia.

Following orbital injuries, some patients will experience persistent double vision (**diplopia**) due to entrapment of tissue in an orbital floor fracture, or neural or muscular damage. In most cases of entrapment with troublesome diplopia that is not spontaneously improving, surgical repair of the fracture with release of the entrapped tissue is performed 1 to 2 weeks after the initial injury, thus allowing some of the acute swelling to subside. Extraocular muscle surgery may be appropriate in patients unsuitable for surgery or when diplopia persists following orbital surgery.

Injuries to the lacrimal canaliculi and fractures of the facial bones damaging the nasolacrimal duct can result in chronic bothersome **epiphora** (overflow of tears onto the face due to lack or substantially reduced drainage of tears through the nasolacrimal system). Lacrimal surgery may be beneficial.

Severe injuries caused by explosions, gunshots, and severe thermal or chemical burns can result in profound facial disfigurement. Ophthalmologists need to recognize the psychological impact of such disfigurement and work with maxillo-facial surgeons, plastic surgeons, and other reconstructive specialists, including ocular prosthetists, to optimize the cosmetic outcome.

REFERENCES

Al-Mezaine HS, Osman EA, Kangave D , Abu El-Asrar AM: Risk factors for culture-positive endophthalmitis after repair of open globe injuries. Eur J Ophthalmol 2010;20:201. [PMID: 19882538]

Atkins EJ, Newman NJ, Biousse V: Post-traumatic visual loss. Rev Neurol Dis 2008;5:73. [PMID: 18669739]

Belli E, Matteini C, Mazzone N: Evolution in diagnosis and repairing of orbital medial wall fractures. J Craniofac Surg 2009;20:191. [PMID: 19165024]

Bord SP, Linden J: Trauma to the globe and orbit. Emerg Med Clin North Am 2008;26:97. [PMID: 18249259]

Castellarin AA, Pieramici DJ: Open globe management. Compr Ophthalmol Update 2007;8:111. [PMID: 17651540]

Castiblanco CP, Adelman RA: Sympathetic ophthalmia. Graefes Arch Clin Exp Ophthalmol 2009;247:289. [PMID: 18795315]

Chi MJ, Ku M, Shin KH, Baek S: An analysis of 733 surgically treated blowout fractures. Ophthalmologica 2010;224:167. [PMID: 19776656]

Close JK, Shiels WE 2nd, Foster JA et al: Percutaneous ultrasound-guided intraorbital foreign body removal. Ophthal Plast Reconstr Surg 2009;25:335. [PMID: 19617806]

Cole P, Kaufman Y, Hollier L: Principles of facial trauma: orbital fracture management. J Craniofac Surg 2009;20:101. [PMID: 19165002]

Colyer MH, Weber ED, Weichel ED et al: Delayed intraocular foreign body removal without endophthalmitis during Operations Iraqi Freedom and Enduring Freedom. Ophthalmology 2007;114:1439. [PMID: 17331579]

Ehlers JP, Kunimoto DY, Ittoop S et al: Metallic intraocular foreign bodies: characteristics, interventions, and prognostic factors for visual outcome and globe survival. Am J Ophthalmol 2008;146:427. [PMID: 18614135]

Fish R, Davidson RS: Management of ocular thermal and chemical injuries, including amniotic membrane therapy. Curr Opin Ophthalmol 2010 May 12. [Epub ahead of print] [PMID: 20467317]

Gerbino G, Roccia F, Bianchi FA, Zavattero E: Surgical management of orbital trapdoor fracture in a pediatric population. J Oral Maxillofac Surg 2010 Apr 8. [Epub ahead of print] [PMID: 20381939]

Gosse EM, Ferguson AW, Lymburn EG, Gilmour C, MacEwen CJ: Blow-out fractures: patterns of ocular motility and effect of surgical repair. Br J Oral Maxillofac Surg 2010;48:40. [PMID: 19716636]

Harissi-Dagher M, Dohlman CH: The Boston keratoprosthesis in severe ocular trauma. Can J Ophthalmol 2008;43:165. [PMID: 18347618]

Heidari E, Taheri N: Surgical treatment of severely traumatized eyes with no light perception. Retina 2010;30:294. [PMID: 19952999]

Jamal BT, Pfahler SM, Lane KA et al: Ophthalmic injuries in patients with zygomaticomaxillary complex fractures requiring surgical repair. J Oral Maxillofac Surg 2009;67:986. [PMID: 19375007]

Khodabukus R, Tallouzi M: Chemical eye injuries 1: presentation, clinical features, treatment and prognosis. Nurs Times 2009;105:28. [PMID: 19624054]

Kubal WS: Imaging of orbital trauma. Radiographics 2008;28:1729. [PMID: 18936032]

Lakshmanan A, Bala S, Belfer KF: Intraorbital organic foreign body – a diagnostic challenge. Orbit 2008;2008;27:131. [PMID: 18415875]

Malhotra R, Sheikh I, Dheansa B: The management of eyelid burns. Surv Ophthalmol 2009;54:356. [PMID: 19422964]

Mansouri M, Faghihi H, Hajizadeh F, et al: Epidemiology of open-globe injuries in Iran: analysis of 2,340 cases in 5 years (report no. 1). Retina 2009;29:1141. [PMID: 19536042]

Mowat L, Chambers C: Ocular morbidity of traumatic hyphema in a Jamaican hospital. Eur J Ophthalmol 2010;20:584. [PMID: 19967662]

Naik MN, Kelapure A, Rath S, Honavar SG: Management of canalicular lacerations: epidemiological aspects and experience with Mini-Monoka monocanalicular stent. Am J Ophthalmol 2008;145:375. [PMID: 18061134]

Rodrigues Z: Irrigation of the eye after alkaline and acidic burns. Emerg Nurs 2009;17:26. [PMID: 20043429]

Salehi-Had H, Andreoli CM, Andreoli MT, Kloek CE, Mukai S: Visual outcomes of vitreoretinal surgery in eyes with severe open-globe injury presenting with no-light-perception vision. Graefes Arch Clin Exp Ophthalmol 2009;247:477. [PMID: 19172288]

Savar A, Andreoli MT, Kloek CE, Andreoli CM: Enucleation for open globe injury. Am J Ophthalmol 2009;147:595. [PMID: 19181305]

Spector J, Fernandez WG: Chemical, thermal, and biological ocular exposures. Emerg Med Clin North Am 2008;26:125. [PMID: 18249260]

Tuft SJ, Shortt AJ: Surgical rehabilitation following severe ocular burns. Eye 2009;23:1966. [PMID: 19169226]

Weichel ED, Colyer MH, Bautista C, Bower KS, French LM: Traumatic brain injury associated with combat ocular trauma. J Head Trauma Rehabil 2009;24:41. [PMID: 19158595]

Yang CS, Lu CK, Lee FL, et al: Treatment and outcome of traumatic endophthalmitis in open globe injury with retained intraocular foreign body. Ophthalmologica 2010;224:79. [PMID: 19707031]

Yeh S, Colyer MH, Weichel ED: Current trends in the management of intraocular foreign bodies. Curr Opin Ophthalmol 2008;19:225. [PMID: 18408498]

Yeniad B, canturk S, Esin Ozdemir F, Alparsian N, Akarcay K: Toxic keratopathy due to abuse of topical anesthetic drugs. Cutan Ocul Toxicol 2010;29:105. [PMID: 20236030]

Yu-Wai-Man P, Griffiths PG: Steroids for traumatic optic neuropathy. Cochrane Database Syst Rev 2007;4:CD006032. [PMID: 17943877]

Zhang Y, Zhang MN, Jiang CH, Yao Y, Zhang K: Endophthalmitis following open globe injury. Br J Ophthalmol 2010;94:111. [PMID: 19692359]

Causes and Prevention of Vision Loss

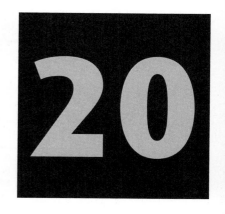

Adnan Pirbhai, MD, Shefalee Shukla Kent, MD,
and William G. Hodge, MD, PhD, FRCSC

This chapter addresses vision loss as a worldwide health problem, providing information on causes, with data on prevalence, and measures to prevent it. All of the disorders that may cause vision loss are discussed more fully in other chapters.

20.I Causes of Vision Loss

Adnan Pirbhai, MD and William G. Hodge, MD, PhD, FRCSC

DEFINITIONS

Vision loss has significant consequences. Differentiating between different degrees of vision loss is important, because the demands for medical, social, and rehabilitative interventions vary.

Vision loss has been defined in many different ways, determined by the intended purpose but resulting in many terms that may not be consistent with one another. Whereas to the lay person it implies complete loss of vision, the term "blindness" is often used for individuals who have significant and useful residual vision, an extreme example being the use of the term "color blindness" for individuals with mild color vision deficiency. "Industrial blindness," a term from the early 19th century, may be used to describe the impact on employability. "Automobile blindness" may be used to indicate that the individual does not meet the requirements for a driver's license. "Legal blindness" is used in the United States for those who meet various legal requirements for benefits.

An important challenge is categorizing the broad range of vision loss. The eighth revision of the International Classification of Diseases (ICD-8) recognizes only two categories of vision: *Sighted* and *Blind*. In the 1970s the International Council of Ophthalmology (ICO) worked with the World Health Organization (WHO) to define three major categories in the US adaptation of the ninth revision

(ICD-9-CM): *Normal Vision, Low Vision,* and *Blindness*. ICD-9 and ICD-10 do not utilize the first category.

The ICD major categories are now used in almost all population surveys, with the WHO definitions (ICD-9/ICD-10) usually having been used for surveys aimed at the detection of eye disease. Low vision is defined as *best-corrected* visual acuity less than 20/70 (6/18, 0.3) but equal to or better than 20/400 (3/60, 0.05) and blindness is defined as visual acuity less than 20/400, or maximum diameter of visual field 20° or less in the better eye. To describe how people live their lives, the WHO has subsequently recommended categorization according to visual acuity with *presenting* correction, that is, using whatever correction the subject has. This definition acknowledges the importance of uncorrected (or under-corrected) refractive error as a cause of vision loss worldwide and almost doubles the number of people counted as having vision loss.

In the United States and Canada, legal blindness is defined as best-corrected visual acuity equal to or less than 20/200 (6/60, 0.1), which corresponds with the ICD-8 criteria, or maximum diameter of visual field less than 20° in the better eye. Low vision has been defined as best-corrected visual acuity worse than 20/40 (6/12, 0.5) but better than 20/200 (6/60, 0.1). Across Europe the visual acuity criterion for registration as blind (or certification as severely sight impaired) varies, being less than 20/200 (6/60, 0.1) in the Republic of

Table 20–1. Various Definitions of Vision Loss

Visual Acuity			Functional ranges	USA, ICD-8	WHO – ICD-9, ICD-10	ICD-9-CM (USA)	England, Wales	Scotland
Decimal	US	6 m	recommended by the ICO					
1.6	20/12.5	6/3.8	Range of normal vision	Legally sighted	No code	(Near-) normal vision		
1.25	20/16	6/4.8						
1.0	**20/20**	**6/6**						
0.8	20/25	6/7.5						
0.63	20/32	6/9.5	Mild vision loss					
0.5	20/40	6/12						
0.4	20/50	6/15						
0.32	20/63	6/19						
0.25	20/80	6/24	Moderate vision loss		Low vision			Partially sighted
0.20	20/100	6/30						
0.16	20/125	6/38						
0.125	20/160	6/48						
0.10	**20/200**	**6/60**	Severe vision loss			Low vision	Partially sighted	
0.08	20/250	6/75						
0.063	20/320	6/95						
0.05	20/400	6/120						
0.04	20/500	6/150	Profound vision loss	Legally blind	Blindness		Blind	Blind
0.03	20/630	6/190						
0.025	20/800	6/240						
0.02	20/1000	6/300						
0.016	20/1250	6/380	Near-total vision loss			(Near-) blindness		
0.0125	20/1600	6/480						
0.01	**20/2000**	**6/600**						
---	---	---						
No light perception (NLP)			**Total loss**					

Ireland and Scotland, less than 20/400 (6/120, 0.05) in England, Wales, and Italy, and less than 20/1000 (6/300) in Germany. There is also a partially sighted (sight-impaired or significant visual impairment) category, for example in England and Wales being between 20/200 (6/60, 0.1) and 20/400 (6/120, 0.05) and in Scotland being worse than 20/60 (6/18, 0.33) but equal to or better than 20/200 (6/60, 0.1).

Table 20–1 shows the comparison between the ICD-8, ICD-9, ICD-9-CM, and ICD-10 major categories, the recommendations of the ICO and, as examples of variations within Europe, the criteria for registration in England, Wales, and Scotland. The differences emphasize the importance of knowing which definition was used whenever statistics about vision loss are compared. It should be noted that the ICO's category of "Profound Vision Loss" is classified as blindness in ICD-9 but as (profound) low vision in ICD-9-CM to indicate that there still is useful residual vision.

▶ Driving Privileges

In the United States the visual requirements for driving vary from state to state for both private and commercial drivers. 20/40 best-corrected visual acuity with both eyes is the most common requirement for private drivers, but some accept less. These requirements set a safety margin between letter chart performance in the office and on-the-road performance under adverse conditions. The requirements for commercial drivers are often more stringent, not because they drive in a different visual environment, but because a wider safety margin is deemed desirable. In Canada, the legal limit for driving for private drivers is best-corrected visual acuity with both eyes 20/50 (6/15) or better and a continuous field of vision horizontally no less than 120° and vertically 15° above and below central fixation, and with no evidence of diplopia within the central 40° of fixation.

Responsible health professionals are legally obligated to report patients failing these requirements to the Ministry of Transportation. There are published vision standards for pilots and for admission to service academies.

PREVALENCE

Historically, prevalence studies on blindness were varied and inconsistent, making it difficult to compare reports from different parts of the world. Comparable data has become available from nearly every WHO member state allowing attempts at more accurate comparison of worldwide statistics. In a 2004 WHO report summarizing available population-based studies, the worldwide prevalence of profound vision loss (WHO blindness) was estimated to be 0.57%, and the worldwide prevalence of moderate low vision (WHO low vision) was estimated to be 2%. The prevalence of profound vision loss ranged from 0.2%–0.3% in developed countries in American, European, and the Western Pacific regions, to 1% in developing countries in the regions of Southeast Asia, the Eastern Mediterranean, and Africa. Prevalence of low vision largely followed these regional trends.

Approximately 314 million people worldwide are visually impaired from various causes (including uncorrected refractive error), 65 million of whom have profound vision loss. Population-based studies indicate that the global prevalence of vision loss has been declining since the early 1990s, with less vision loss from infectious diseases such as trachoma but increasing vision loss from conditions related to aging, such as cataract and age-related macular degeneration. Accordingly, the majority of the visually impaired are older (82% over the age of 50) but also poor, with close to 90% of the world's visually impaired living in low and middle-income countries. Vision loss is additionally clustered into disadvantaged communities in rural areas and urban slums, where the risk of profound vision loss is 10–40 times higher than in the industrially developed regions of Europe and America. Women are at much higher risk of vision loss, population-based surveys estimating that 64% of those with vision loss worldwide are women. There are approximately 1.5 million children with profound vision loss in the world, with an annual incidence of 500,000 and 40% of cases being due to causes that are considered avoidable.

CAUSES

Although the ICD-9 definition of visual impairment is based on *best-corrected* visual acuity, nearly 153 million people worldwide have impaired vision (<20/60 to 20/200 in the better eye) due to *uncorrected refractive error*. It is estimated that over 12 million children (between the ages of 5 and 15) with impaired vision could have normal vision with correction of refractive error alone.

Overall, the leading causes of profound vision loss in the world, in order of decreasing prevalence, are cataract, uncorrected refractive error, glaucoma, and age-related macular

Table 20–2. Causes as a Percentage of Total World Blindness (WHO definition) in 2004

Cause	Percentage of Total Worldwide Blindness
Cataract	39.1
Uncorrected refractive error	18.2
Glaucoma	10.1
Age-related macular degeneration	7.1
Corneal opacities	4.2
Diabetic retinopathy	3.9
Childhood blindness	3.2
Trachoma	2.9
Oncocerciasis	0.7
Other	10.6

Data taken from Resnikoff S, Pascolini D et al. Global magnitude of visual impairment caused by uncorrected refractive errors in 2004. Bull World Health Org 2008;86:63-70.

degeneration (Table 20–2). Other major causes include corneal scarring, diabetic retinopathy, and trauma, the last being the most common cause of monocular profound vision loss globally. Vision loss caused by infectious diseases is decreasing due to improvements in public health. Trachoma affects 40 million people today, compared to 360 million in 1985.

Across the world, the relative prevalence of the different causes of vision loss is influenced by the level of social development and local geography. In developing countries, cataract is the leading cause, with glaucoma, trachoma, leprosy, onchocerciasis, and xerophthalmia also being important. Corneal scarring is a significant cause of monocular vision loss in the developing world, accounting for 850,000 cases of corneal profound vision loss per year in India alone. In more developed countries, vision loss is to a great extent related to the aging process. Although cataract is still an important cause of vision loss, the leading causes of profound vision loss in North America and other developed countries are age-related macular degeneration, diabetic retinopathy, and glaucoma. Other causes are herpes simplex keratitis, retinal detachment, retinal vascular disorders, and inherited retinal degenerative disorders.

With regards to global vision loss in children, retinal diseases such as retinopathy of prematurity (ROP) account for 29%, corneal scarring, predominantly due to xerophthalmia, rubella, and infection, accounts for 21%, and congenital disorders (including cataract, glaucoma, and structural abnormalities of the globe) accounts for 14%. Differences again exist when comparing the relative causes in developed and developing countries. In developed countries, the major causes are ROP, cataract, hereditary disease of the retina, diseases of the central nervous system (including hypoxic injury to the visual pathway), congenital malformations of the globe (microphthalmos, anophthalmos, and optic nerve hypoplasia), and nystagmus. The major causes in developing countries are corneal scarring, trachoma, genetic diseases, and cataract.

▶ Cataract

Close to 40% of profound vision loss worldwide can be attributed to cataract. In many parts of the developing world, the facilities available for treating cataract are grossly inadequate, hardly sufficient to cope with new cases and completely inadequate for dealing with the backlog of existing cases, currently estimated to be 10 million.

It is not fully understood why the frequency of cataract varies so greatly in different geographic areas, although exposure to ultraviolet radiation and recurrent episodes of dehydration, often occurring in severe diarrheal diseases, are thought to be important. With decreasing mortality rates and changing demographics, age-related causes of vision loss, including cataract, are expected to continue to rise. Worldwide, approximately 17 million people are currently blind from cataract. By 2020, this number is expected to reach 40 million. Although no current medical treatments exist to delay the development of cataract, it is estimated that a 10-year delay in cataract formation would reduce the number of individuals requiring surgery by 45%. Until an effective treatment that can prevent or delay cataract formation is devised, it will remain a leading cause of vision loss and will become an increasingly important global public health concern.

▶ Uncorrected Refractive Error

When included in the global statistics, uncorrected refractive error accounts for over 18% of profound vision loss, with a much larger percentage of moderate and severe vision loss, affecting approximately 8 million people with 1 million in India alone. It is clearly avoidable and should be easy to correct, provision of corrective lenses being the most cost-effective means of addressing a massive global health problem. However, uncorrected refractive error remains a major cause of vision loss throughout the world, even in developed countries such as the United States but particularly in developing countries where limited access to eye care professionals, low prevalence of eye health-seeking behavior, and low affordability of corrective lenses remain major problems. In children, ineffective screening also contributes.

▶ Glaucoma

The incidence of vision loss due to glaucoma has decreased in recent years as a result of earlier detection, improved medical and surgical treatment, and a greater awareness and understanding of the disorder by the lay population. However, in many developing countries, glaucoma remains the second most common cause of vision loss after cataract. This is especially the case in West Africa, where untreated open-angle glaucoma is extremely common. In China and Southeast Asia, there appears to be a preponderance of narrow-angle glaucoma. Glaucoma now blinds 6 million individuals worldwide, and a simple easy method of detecting patients at risk still does not exist. Treatment is also a major problem because of the poor compliance of most patients for taking daily eye drops. A simple but safe surgical procedure may ultimately be the only solution for reducing the needless burden of vision loss from this disease. More research in this area is essential.

▶ Trachoma

Trachoma causes bilateral keratoconjunctivitis, generally in childhood that leads in adulthood to corneal scarring, which, when severe, causes vision loss. About 40 million people have trachoma, most of them in Africa, the Middle East, and Asia. It can be treated with various antibiotics, including tetracyclines and erythromycin, but azithromycin is proving to be the drug of choice. The number of individuals with profound vision loss from trachoma has dropped from 6 million to 1.3 million, which is a tribute to current WHO-supervised treatment programs and the effectiveness of azithromycin. However, to eliminate the disease will depend on global implementation of WHO's SAFE strategy (Surgery for trichiasis, Antibiotic treatment, Face washing, and Environmental changes such as latrine building). Prevention of spread of infection will require provision of proper sanitary facilities, including clean water for drinking and washing, waste disposal, fly control, and behavioral change in hygiene.

▶ Onchocerciasis

Onchocerciasis is transmitted by bites of the blackfly, which breeds in clear running streams (hence the name river blindness). It is endemic in the greater part of tropical Africa and Central and South America. The most heavily infested zone is the Volta River basin, which extends over parts of Dahomey, Ghana, Ivory Coast, Mali, Niger, Togo, and Upper Volta. Worldwide, 15–20 million people are affected by onchocerciasis, with 20% of individuals in hyperendemic areas blinded by the disease.

The major ophthalmic manifestations of onchocerciasis are keratitis, uveitis, retinochoroiditis, and optic atrophy. The disease is prevented by insect eradication and personal protection by screening. Treatment with ivermectin is extremely effective in killing the microfilaria and sterilizing the adult females residing in nodules in the body. The effect of the mass distribution of ivermectin in areas where onchocerciasis is endemic is a public health success story. Like leprosy, onchocerciasis is definitely decreasing in its importance as a worldwide cause of vision loss because of successful treatment programs.

Other Causes

Age-related macular degeneration, diabetic retinopathy, and corneal disorders are discussed elsewhere in this and other chapters (see Chapters 6, 10, and 15).

Leprosy (Hansen's disease) affects 14 million people in the world and has a higher percentage of ocular involvement than any other systemic disease. Up to 10% of leprosy patients are blind or visually impaired from the disease. The social stigma attached to leprosy has greatly hindered its treatment, but there are now highly effective chemotherapeutic agents that in most cases eradicate the infection. Effective treatment programs using triple drug therapy (dapsone, clofazamine, and rifampin) have markedly reduced the number of cases of leprosy worldwide as well as prevented the deformity and morbidity associated with the disease.

Xerophthalmia, due to hypovitaminosis A, is estimated to affect 5 million children each year. 500,000 develop corneal involvement, half of whom develop profound vision loss. It is a common cause of vision loss in infants, particularly in India, Bangladesh, Indonesia, and the Philippines. Clinically, there is xerosis of the conjunctiva with characteristic Bitot's spots and softening of the cornea (keratomalacia), which may lead to corneal perforation. Protein malnutrition exacerbates the condition and renders it refractory to treatment. Affected infants often do not reach adulthood, dying from malnutrition, pneumonia, or diarrhea. Xerophthalmia can be prevented by general dietary improvement or vitamin A supplementation. If the problems of distribution and administration were solved, the cost of a quantity of the vitamin sufficient to prevent vision loss in 1000 infants would be only about $25. Measles immunization is also important because of the close association of measles epidemics with the blinding complications of xerophthalmia.

Hereditary conditions are important causes of vision loss but should gradually decrease in incidence in response to the efforts of genetic counselors to increase public awareness of the preventable nature of these disorders.

20.2 Prevention of Vision Loss

Shefalee Shukla Kent, MD and William G. Hodge, MD, PhD, FRCSC

Preventive medicine is increasingly important in attempts to fulfill society's expectations of modern medicine with the resources available. Although prevention is a logical approach to the solution of many problems in all branches of medicine, in practice there are a number of hurdles to be overcome. For any particular condition, it is essential that individuals at risk be easily identified. If their identification requires population screening, the screening process should be easy to perform, accurate, and reliable. Preventive measures must be both effective and acceptable to the target population. Unwarranted interference with the at-risk individual's lifestyle only leads to poor compliance. Legislation may be required for certain measures but may engender resentment when it is felt to infringe on personal liberty. For preventive medicine to be successful, there must be cooperation among all segments of society—not just the medical community—in identifying problem areas, establishing workable solutions, and disseminating information. The successes that have been achieved in occupational health are an example of what can be accomplished if a consensus of opinion is established.

In ophthalmology, the major avenues for preventive medicine are ocular injuries and infections, genetic and systemic diseases with ocular involvement, and ocular diseases in which the early treatable stages are often unrecognized or ignored.

PREVENTION OF OCULAR INJURIES

Ocular injuries are a very preventable cause of vision loss because simple preventive measures are often available. Injuries can vary from closed globe, such as blunt trauma or chemical injuries, to open globe injuries including rupture, perforation, and penetration (see Chapter 19). WHO statistics show that over 55 million eye injuries occur each year. 1.6 million people are rendered blind, 2.3 million develop bilateral low vision and 19 million have monocular blindness or low vision. The United States Eye Injury Register (USEIR) statistics show that over 57% of the injuries occur in people under 30 years of age, the percentage being even higher in work-related injuries.

Occupational Injuries

Approximately 30% of all eye patients presenting to emergency departments have ocular trauma. Eye injuries remain a significant risk to worker health, especially among individuals in jobs requiring intensive manual labor.

Many manufacturing processes pose a particular threat to the eye. Grinding or drilling commonly propels small fragments of metal into the environment at high velocity, and these missiles can easily lodge on the cornea or penetrate the globe through the cornea or sclera. Tools with sharp ends, such as screwdrivers, are also commonly involved in producing penetrating ocular injuries. Welding arcs produce ultraviolet radiation that may cause epithelial keratitis ("arc eye"). Industrial chemicals—particularly those containing high concentrations of alkali or acid—can rapidly produce severe ocular damage that is often bilateral and associated with a poor visual outcome.

New legislation, increased worker training, particularly targeting groups most at risk, provision of effective eye protection equipment, and development of a culture of safety in the workplace, have led to a decline in eye injuries. Workers must be properly trained in the use of tools, machinery, and chemicals. Safety guards must be fitted to all machinery, and safety goggles must be worn whenever the worker is doing hazardous work or is in the workplace area where such hazards exist. It is surprising how many workers assume that they are no longer at risk of injury when they are not themselves performing hazardous tasks even though they are in the vicinity of work being performed by others.

The growing interest in "do-it-yourself" projects in the home exposes many more individuals to the risks of ocular injury from machinery, tools, and chemicals. Education of the public to recognize and minimize such risks, which may not be obvious to the ordinary householder or hobbyist, is particularly important.

Early recognition and urgent expert ophthalmologic assessment of any injuries sustained is essential. In the case of chemical injuries, immediate copious lavage of the eyes with sterile water, saline if available, or tap water for at least 5 minutes is the most important method of limiting the damage incurred. Neglect of penetrating injuries or corneal foreign bodies markedly increases the potential for long-term morbidity. Obtaining an accurate history is crucial in identifying the possibility of a penetrating injury. This is particularly true when medical help is sought some time after the injury and the patient may not realize the importance of a seemingly minor episode of trauma. Any worker who presents with unexplained visual loss or intraocular inflammation must be carefully questioned about the possibility of recent ocular injuries and the possibility of an occult intraocular foreign body borne in mind.

Chronic exposure to ultraviolet light or ionizing radiation, such as from improperly screened nuclear materials or in radiology departments, can lead to early and rapid cataract and care must be taken to monitor and decrease exposure. In one study, the prevalence of cataract was 64% in radiology technicians, 16% in radiologists, 10% in respiratory physicians, and 2% in nuclear medicine department staff, with an overall relative risk of 5 compared to unexposed health care workers.

▶ Non-Occupational Injuries

The marked reduction in the incidence of severe ocular and facial damage associated with car windshield injuries as a result of legislation requiring the wearing of seat belts is a testament to the effectiveness of such legislation. Similar attempts to reduce the incidence of injuries from fireworks by limiting their availability have not yet been as successful.

Various sports are notorious for the high incidence of severe injuries to the eye, for example, blunt injuries such as in racquetball, baseball, basketball, soccer, and boxing or penetrating injuries such as in ice hockey. Injuries range from minor, including corneal abrasion and superficial foreign bodies, to more severe, including hyphema, orbital fracture, and globe rupture. The availability of toughened plastic protective glasses—which can be fitted with refractive correction if required—is a major advance in preventing such injuries.

A large number of ocular injuries are suffered in the home. Corks from bottles of champagne or other sparkling wines can produce severe blunt injuries, and explosion of any bottle containing carbonated beverages may lead to penetrating eye injuries from glass fragments. Unless adequately supervised, children using pencils, scissors, or air guns, including BB guns, may sustain or cause serious penetrating injuries.

Unfortunately, a significant proportion of serious ocular trauma results from violent assaults, notably those involving firearms or broken glass. Prevention requires a reduction in the frequency of such incidents and use of plastic rather than glass containers. In countries that have recently endured the ravages of war, unexploded bombs and land mines are a major cause of corneal vision loss in children.

Acute keratitis from **ultraviolet irradiation,** such as seen after exposure to a welding arc, may also occur during skiing if protective goggles are not worn. People wearing contact lenses and with previous history of eye diseases are more vulnerable. Prevention of the keratitis is best achieved with sunglasses with sidepieces and goggles with polarized or photochromic lenses. The role of long-term exposure to ultraviolet light in the etiology of cataract and age-related macular degeneration is still debated. Since the cornea and crystalline lens are effective barriers to the transmission of ultraviolet light—becoming even more effective with age in the case of the crystalline lens—it is hardly surprising that the development of age-related macular degeneration in phakic individuals has not been shown to be related to ultraviolet exposure, and thus is not preventable by the use of sunglasses. The effect of ultraviolet light on the maculas of the increasing numbers of pseudophakic individuals has yet to be fully assessed. Largely on empirical grounds, ultraviolet filters have been incorporated into many of the intraocular lenses implanted. Individuals without such filters in their intraocular lenses or who are aphakic have been encouraged to incorporate ultraviolet filters in their spectacle lenses or wear appropriate sunglasses whenever possible. There is substantial evidence linking ultraviolet exposure to the development of cataract. However, since ultraviolet exposure occurs from the time of birth, the benefit of regular use of ultraviolet filters in spectacle lenses or sunglasses as a preventive measure has not been demonstrated. The role of ultraviolet light exposure in the etiology of certain corneal disorders—particularly pterygium—and of basal cell carcinoma and melanoma of the eyelids is much more widely accepted. Education of the public about the dangers of skin cancer following prolonged sun exposure is very important. Ultraviolet-blocking skin creams should not be used around the eyes, and for that reason reliance must be placed on avoiding unnecessary exposure to the sun or the use of sunglasses. In patients with xeroderma pigmentosum, the eyelids and bulbar conjunctiva frequently develop carcinomas and melanomas, and their development can be minimized, if not prevented entirely, by protective lenses.

Solar retinitis (eclipse retinopathy) is a specific type of radiation injury that usually occurs after solar eclipses as a result of direct observation of the sun without an adequate filter. Under normal circumstances, sun-gazing is difficult because of the glare, but cases have been reported in young people who have suffered self-inflicted macular damage by deliberate sun-gazing, perhaps while under the influence of drugs.

The optical system of the eye behaves as a strong magnifying lens, focusing the light onto a small spot on the macula, usually in one eye only, and producing a thermal burn. The resulting edema of the retinal tissue may clear with minimal loss of function, or it may cause significant atrophy of the tissue and produce a defect that is visible ophthalmoscopically. A permanent central scotoma then results. Eclipse retinopathy can easily be prevented by the use of adequate filters when observing eclipses, but the surest way to prevent it is to watch the eclipse on television.

Similar to eclipse retinopathy is the iatrogenic retinal damage that may occur from use of the operating microscope and indirect ophthalmoscope (photic retinopathy). The risk of damage from the operating microscope can be reduced by the use of filters to block both ultraviolet light and the blue portion of the visible spectrum, light barriers such as an opaque disk placed on the cornea, or air injected into the anterior chamber.

PREVENTION OF ACQUIRED OCULAR INFECTION

Infections are a major cause of preventable ocular morbidity. Preventive measures are based on maintenance of the integrity of the normal barriers to infection and the avoidance of inoculation with pathogenic organisms. The pathogenicity of various organisms and the size of the inoculum required to establish infection vary enormously according to the state of the eye. A compromised eye is highly susceptible to infection. Nevertheless, there are bacteria that penetrate despite having normal barriers intact. For instance, *Corynebacterium diphtheriae, Acanthamoeba, Haemophilus aegyptius, Neissera gonorrhea* and *meningitidis, Listeria, Shigella,* and *Serratia* are bacteria that can penetrate despite a normal intact corneal epithelium.

The major barrier to exogenous ocular infection is the epithelium of the cornea and conjunctiva. This can be damaged directly by trauma, including surgical trauma and contact lens wear, or by the secondary effects of other abnormalities of the outer eye, such as lid abnormalities or tear deficiency. In all such situations, particular care must be taken to avoid or recognize secondary infection in its earliest stages.

In the presence of a corneal or conjunctival epithelial defect, particularly when there is an associated full-thickness wound of the cornea or sclera—for example, following penetrating trauma or intraocular surgery—it is essential to use prophylactic antibiotic therapy and most importantly to make certain that any drops or ointments are sterile. Accidental epithelial injury should be avoided whenever possible, particularly in compromised eyes, for example, dry eyes, eyes with corneal exposure due to exophthalmos or abnormal eyelid function such as produced by facial nerve paralysis or ectropion, and eyes with reduced corneal sensation. The classic situation is the combination of fifth and seventh nerve dysfunction such as which occurs with cerebellopontine angle tumors, producing a dry, anesthetic eye with poor eyelid closure. Any comatose patient is also at risk of corneal exposure, and prophylactic ocular lubrication and possibly horizontal eyelid taping should be undertaken.

Any unnecessary exposure of the eye to pathogenic organisms should be avoided, but it becomes critical in certain situations. During intraocular surgery, the normal barriers to infection are circumvented, and meticulous attention must be paid to avoiding contamination of the eye with organisms. The ocular environment must be assessed preoperatively to identify and treat any sources of pathogenic organisms. These include colonization or infection of the lacrimal sac, the lid margins, which are frequently colonized by *Staphylococcus epidermidis*—a major cause of endophthalmitis after cataract surgery, the conjunctiva, and the cornea. Considerations may need to be given to other sites of bacterial colonization or infection, such as the bladder, throat, nose, and skin. In emergency situations, it may only be possible to identify such sources and use prophylactic antibiotic therapy to reduce the chances of subsequent infection, whereas for elective surgery, more definitive therapy to eradicate or minimize the pathogenic organisms should be possible. In patients with no identifiable external ocular disease, immediately preoperative instillation of povidone-iodine into the conjunctival sac has been shown to be beneficial, and postoperative antibiotics are presumed to be important. Intraocular injection of cefuroxime at the conclusion of cataract surgery reduces the risk of postoperative endophthalmitis, but the correct formulation must be used to avoid corneal damage. Whether inclusion of antibiotic, such as vancomycin, in the infusion fluid during cataract surgery is appropriate continues to be debated. Sterility must be ensured of the operative field, instruments, intraocular and topical medications and other fluids introduced into the eye. During the postoperative period, sterile medications must be used and contact with other patients with established ocular infections avoided.

Contact lens wear is strongly associated with suppurative keratitis due to the combination of an abnormal load of pathogenic organisms and probable recurrent minor trauma to the corneal epithelium. The incidence of suppurative keratitis is particularly high with soft lenses, especially with extended wear. Overnight wear increases the risk by 5 times compared to daily wear with regular replacement. It is apparent that many people wearing contact lenses for cosmetic reasons are not aware of the risks involved. Whereas it may be reasonable to face the risks of infection with extended-wear soft lenses in elderly aphakes who are dependent on contact lenses for refractive correction and cannot cope with daily wear lenses—or in patients with highly compromised eyes that are symptomatic from bullous keratopathy—the arguments in favor of extended-wear soft lenses for refractive correction in patients with low refractive errors are less strong. A number of patients in this latter group start off their contact lens career using extended-wear disposable lenses, which is of course an attractive arrangement because it dispenses with the need for lens cleaning and the associated paraphernalia, but this practice is likely to require an unwelcome sacrifice of safety for convenience. Contact lens wear exposes the eye to an abnormal load of pathogenic organisms, which have been shown to adhere with particular tenacity to soft lenses, unless the user is absolutely meticulous about contact lens hygiene. The use of preservative-free solutions, multipurpose solutions, and no rub formulas may have increased the chances of suppurative keratitis by providing less antimicrobial activity. Epidemics of *Fusarium* and *Acanthamoeba keratitis* have been related to particular contact lens solutions.

All contact lens wearers must be apprised of the relative risk of suppurative keratitis, and the need for meticulous contact lens hygiene and avoidance of overnight wear or continuing to use lenses beyond their disposal time. Many do not realize that many ocular infections are contracted in swimming pools and hot tubs, with chlorine levels not being adequate to kill protozoa like Acanthamoeba, such that contact lenses should be removed. All should be advised to keep a pair of spectacles available so that contact lens wear be discontinued immediately whenever an eye becomes uncomfortable or inflamed. If ocular discomfort or inflammation persists, the wearer should seek ophthalmologic advice without delay.

In developing countries where contact lens wear is uncommon, the greatest risk factor for corneal ulceration is trauma, usually experienced in the course of everyday agricultural activities. These undocumented abrasions are now recognized as the cause of a "silent epidemic" of corneal ulceration that is a major cause of monocular vision loss in those regions. Studies in India have shown that both bacterial and fungal ulcers that occur after corneal abrasion can be prevented by the application of an antibiotic ointment three times a day for 3 days in the injured eye. The biological mechanism for fungal ulcer prevention by an antibiotic is not readily understood.

Neonatal conjunctivitis (see Chapter 17) is a good example of exposure to a heavy load of pathogenic organisms with the added inherent susceptibility of the poorly developed immune mechanisms of the neonatal eye. The major organisms that may produce neonatal conjunctivitis are *N gonorrhoeae*, chlamydiae, herpes simplex, *Staphylococcus aureus*, haemophilus species, and *Streptococcus pneumoniae*. Exposure to these organisms occurs during passage down the birth canal. It should be possible to prevent neonatal conjunctivitis by treating mothers harboring these organisms prior to delivery, and this has been achieved for the bacteria, including chlamydia. The alternative approach is the routine ocular prophylaxis of neonates. This started with the silver nitrate prophylaxis of Credé and has been superseded in a number of centers by topical erythromycin in view of the predominance of chlamydial neonatal conjunctivitis. Neonatal gonococcal infection can rapidly lead to corneal perforation such that urgent treatment with intravenous ceftriaxone is important.

PREVENTION OF IATROGENIC OCULAR AND NON-OCULAR INFECTION

Ophthalmologists have been clearly implicated in the transmission of infectious eye disease. Outbreaks of **epidemic keratoconjunctivitis** have been traced to contamination within the hospital or ophthalmologist's office. The adenovirus is transmitted via hands, a tonometer, or solutions contaminated by droppers accidentally rubbed against the infected conjunctiva or lid margin of a patient. Contaminated ophthalmic solutions have also been the source of infection in bacterial corneal ulcers and endophthalmitis following intraocular surgery. Spread of infection can be reduced by infection control policies. A study from the United Kingdom demonstrated a reduction in the proportion of adenovirus infections that were hospital-acquired from 48.4% to 22.7% at 12 months and 3.4% at 24 months after new infection control policy, including separate waiting and examination areas and expediting examination of suspected cases. *Pseudomonas aeruginosa* used to be a common contaminant of ophthalmic solutions, particularly fluorescein. Instillation of contaminated fluorescein solution to delineate corneal epithelial defects (eg, after removal of a corneal foreign body) may result in severe pseudomonal keratitis and, frequently, loss of the eye.

The ophthalmologist should be alert to the possibility of transmission by ophthalmic instruments, or in donor cornea or sclera, of agents responsible for non-ocular infection, including hepatitis B virus, human immunodeficiency virus (HIV), and prions. Applanation tonometer tips may be adequately sterilized with respect to many infectious agents, including hepatitis B virus, HIV, herpes simplex virus, and adenovirus, by wiping with 70% isopropyl alcohol swabs and then allowing the instrument to dry by evaporation. It is imperative that the tonometer tip be completely dry before use on the next patient or corneal epithelial damage will result. However, this method of sterilization is probably not effective against prions, for which immersion in hypochlorite, which is less practical and more likely to damage the tonometer tip and result in corneal injury, is required. In this case, the tonometer tip should be rinsed in tap water and dried before use. Immersion in hypochlorite at the end of each working day and after examination of high-risk patients is a possible compromise. Many ophthalmologists have changed to routine or as required use of disposable tonometer tips, which provide reliable results. The noncontact tonometer is recommended for reducing the risks of disease transmission, but it may generate an aerosol spray that endangers the individual operating the tonometer. Goldmann three-mirror and similar contact lenses used for patient examination are also susceptible to damage from immersion in hypochlorite and use of disposables is not always feasible. Corneal and scleral donors must be adequately screened for transmissible infections.

Ophthalmologists and their staffs must maintain the highest level of personal hygiene at all times and must use standard sterile technique when appropriate, keeping in mind the possibility of contamination of any solution brought into contact with the eye.

Hands play a major role in the transmission of infection. They should be washed or disinfected (eg, with isopropyl alcohol) before and after the examination of every patient, especially if an ocular infection is thought to be present.

PREVENTION OF OCULAR DAMAGE DUE TO CONGENITAL INFECTIONS

Viral disease of the mother with resultant embryopathy may lead in the offspring to microphthalmos, retinopathy, infantile glaucoma, iridocyclitis, cataract, uveal tract coloboma, amblyopia, strabismus, nystagmus etc, and prevention may in some cases be possible. Two viruses, rubella and cytomegalovirus, can be extremely damaging to the infant, and one of them—rubella virus—can be prevented by vaccination. Once a common childhood disease, rubella led to lifelong immunity. Now vaccination is universal in developed countries but not in developing countries, such that rubella has essentially been eradicated in the developed world but still poses a risk in the developing world. If a mother contracts rubella during early pregnancy, she should be informed of the likelihood of ocular and other abnormalities in her baby, and the arguments for and against abortion should be presented. Unfortunately, cytomegalovirus (CMV) continues to be a serious and unsolved threat, potentially causing life- and sight-threatening systemic and ocular complications. No protective vaccine is available, although one is under study. At present, early diagnosis and treatment with intravenous and intravitreal ganciclovir is the best way to prevent complications.

Toxoplasmosis is another important cause of congenital infection, leading to (1) chorioretinitis, which may be apparent at birth or may remain subclinical until reactivation occurs later in life; (2) cerebral or cerebellar calcification; (3) hydrocephalus; and, occasionally, (4) more severe central nervous system abnormalities. Unless the mother is immunocompromised, fetal infection occurs only if she acquires primary infection during pregnancy, with a 40% risk of transmission to the fetus. Maternal infection can be prevented by eating only meat that is well cooked, by washing vegetables and fruits, and by wearing gloves when disposing of cat litter or working in the garden so that contact with viable oocysts and tissue cysts is avoided. It has been shown that if acute maternal infection during pregnancy can be identified—such as with the serial serologic tests that are required by law in France and Austria—appropriate antibiotic treatment as early as the 15th week of gestation in those pregnancies allowed to proceed, with adjustments according to whether fetal infection is also present, reduces the incidence of congenital infection and improves the clinical outcome in fetuses that are infected.

Herpes simplex 2 (HSV 2) infection is a sexually transmitted disease, with a 50% risk of transmission to the neonate if the mother has active cervitis at the time of delivery. Women who acquire HSV 2 as a primary infection in the second half of pregnancy, rather than prior to pregnancy, are at greatest risk of transmitting the virus. An additional risk factor for neonatal HSV infection is the use of a fetal-scalp electrode. HSV 2 infection not only causes ocular disease (vesicular eyelid lesions, conjunctivitis, keratitis, cataract, or retinochoroiditis) but also disseminated infection, which has 75% mortality.

If primary genital infection is acquired during the first two trimesters, repeated viral cultures of genital secretions should be carried out from the 32nd week of gestation. If two consecutive cultures are negative and there are no active herpetic genital lesions at the time of delivery, it is safe to perform a vaginal delivery. If primary genital infection is acquired during the third trimester of pregnancy, guidelines are unclear but the current recommendation is to perform elective cesarean section.

Pregnant women with a first clinical episode or recurrent infection, particularly within a few weeks of delivery, may be treated with acyclovir or valacyclovir. Neither drug is approved for treatment of pregnant women. No increase in fetal abnormalities has been attributed so far to such treatment.

PREVENTION OF GENETIC DISEASES WITH OCULAR INVOLVEMENT

There are now genetic counseling centers in many medical centers, and the genetic nature of many disorders that affect the eye is recognized and their transmission better understood. If there is a relevant personal or family history, for example of retinitis pigmentosa, retinoblastoma, or neurofibromatosis, in collaboration with pediatricians and other health care workers, the ophthalmologist may recommend genetic counseling for couples contemplating children, particularly if they are related in the case of recessively inherited disease.

Prenatal diagnosis, with the option of abortion if the diagnosis is made sufficiently early, is available for an increasing number of conditions. Postnatal screening to facilitate early diagnosis is also important when there is a relevant family history. For example, children at risk of retinoblastoma should be examined every 6 months until the age of 5 or 6, or until genetic testing has been performed.

PREVENTION OF OCULAR DAMAGE DUE TO SYSTEMIC DISEASES

It is important for non-ophthalmologic practitioners, particularly internists, general practitioners, and pediatricians, to be aware of the systemic diseases that have avoidable ophthalmic consequences.

Diabetic retinopathy is the most common cause of blindness developing between ages 20 and 64 in developed countries. Treatment is available to prevent such vision loss, but for best effect it must be administered before visual loss has occurred, that is, diabetics must undergo regular fundal examination and be referred whenever treatment is indicated (see later in the chapter). As or even more important is prevention of development of diabetic retinopathy, which is dependent upon optimization of blood sugar, blood pressure, serum lipids, and renal function.

Even in the United States, where it should now be all but unknown, occasional cases of **vitamin A deficiency**, potentially leading to visual loss due to retinal, predominantly rod photoreceptor, dysfunction or due to xerophthalmia with associated corneal disease (keratomalacia) still occur, and in developing countries, where nutrition is often poor, xerophthalmia is still common. Worldwide, the usual cause of vitamin deficiency is poor diet associated with poverty (see earlier in the chapter). Other causes are poor absorption from the gastrointestinal tract due to gastrointestinal disease, bowel resection, or bariatric surgery, weight-reducing diets, dietary management of food allergy, and chronic alcoholism. Because of the ocular manifestations (night blindness, Bitot's spots, and a lackluster corneal epithelium), the ophthalmologist may be the first to recognize vitamin A deficiency. Early recognition and treatment can prevent loss of vision. Treatment of the acute condition may require large intramuscular doses of vitamin A followed by corrective diet and careful analysis of all possible causes. Individuals at risk of deficiency, such as due to severe gastrointestinal disease or following bowel resection or bariatric surgery, should be prescribed prophylactic vitamin A supplementation.

PREVENTION OF VISUAL LOSS DUE TO DRUGS

It is the ophthalmologist's responsibility to prevent visual loss or major ocular disability from drugs used to treat eye diseases. Topical **corticosteroids** predispose to bacterial keratitis and exacerbate herpes simplex keratitis. Long-term use of topical, oral or inhaled corticosteroids may lead to open-angle glaucoma and posterior subcapsular cataract. **Topical**

anesthetics should never be prescribed or made available for long-term use because severe corneal ulceration and scarring may result. **Preservatives** in eye drops are commonly the cause of allergic reactions and, with long-term use, may cause a cicatrizing conjunctivitis similar to cicatricial pemphigoid (see Chapter 5).

Many drugs used **systemically** have serious ocular side effects, for example, Stevens–Johnson syndrome (erythema multiforme), angle-closure glaucoma, optic neuropathy, and retinopathy (see Chapter 22). For this reason, the ophthalmologist must take a careful history of the patient's use of drugs as part of the initial examination.

EARLY DETECTION OF TREATABLE OCULAR DISEASE

Early diagnosis and treatment markedly improves the visual outcome of many ophthalmic conditions. For some, such as suppurative keratitis, acute angle-closure glaucoma, neovascular age-related macular degeneration, retinal detachment, and giant cell arteritis, the crucial factor is the recognition by health care workers and advice to patients of the importance of seeking ophthalmological assessment as soon as visual symptoms occur. For other conditions, the early stages of the disease, when treatment might be most effective, are asymptomatic and routine screening of individuals at risk may be indicated, but it needs to be established that screening is effective both in terms of cost and its impact on the course of disease. For example, routine screening for sickle cell retinopathy is not indicated because detection of asymptomatic disease does not improve the long-term outcome.

▶ Primary Open-Angle Glaucoma

Primary open-angle glaucoma is a major cause of preventable vision loss worldwide, particularly among individuals of African or Caribbean racial origin. About 2 million Americans have the disease, although half are undiagnosed. The prevalence of primary open-angle glaucoma increases from 0.1% for those aged 40–49 to 5% for those over age 75. Symptoms do not usually occur until there is advanced visual field loss. For treatment to be effective, the disease must be detected at a much earlier stage. Screening programs are hampered by the high prevalence of raised intraocular pressure in the absence of glaucomatous visual field loss (ocular hypertension), which is 10 times more common than primary open-angle glaucoma, the high frequency of normal intraocular pressure on a single reading in untreated open-angle glaucoma, and the complexities of screening for optic disk or visual field abnormalities. Nevertheless, the best means of detecting primary open-angle glaucoma early is annual tonometry and optic disk assessment of adult first-degree relatives of affected individuals with referral to an ophthalmologist of all those with relevant abnormalities.. Examination of all individuals over age 50 every 3–5 years may also be worthwhile, particularly in high-risk populations.

Diabetic Retinopathy

As already discussed (see earlier in the chapter), in developed countries diabetic retinopathy is the leading cause of new blindness among adults aged 20–65 years. It is present in about 40% of diagnosed diabetic patients and its prevalence is particularly increasing in individuals aged 65 years or older. Retinopathy increases in prevalence and severity with increasing duration and poorer control of diabetes. In type 1 diabetes, retinopathy is not detectable for at least 3 years after diagnosis. In type 2 diabetes, retinopathy is present in up to 20% of patients at diagnosis and may be the presenting feature. Diabetic retinopathy is broadly classified as **nonproliferative**, comprising **background retinopathy** and **maculopathy**, or **proliferative,** characterized by formation of retinal new vessels. Maculopathy and proliferative retinopathy may coexist, particularly in severe disease. To reduce the risk of permanent visual loss, the main abnormalities to which screening programs are directed are new vessel formation, particularly on the optic disk, and exudates around the macula. Screening programs generally rely upon review of at least annual fundal photographs following pupil dilation, with referral to an ophthalmologist when vision-threatening abnormalities are detected. More frequent screening is needed during pregnancy. Any diabetic developing visual loss should be referred for ophthalmic assessment. (The management of diabetic retinopathy is discussed further in Chapters 10 and 15.)

Retinopathy of Prematurity

Retinopathy of prematurity is the consequence of disturbance of the retinal vascularization that normally occurs during the latter half of pregnancy, for which the main risk factors are decreasing gestational age and decreasing birth weight. It has been estimated to result in 550 new cases of infant blindness each year in the United States (see Chapter 17). In many cases, retinopathy of premature regresses spontaneously but laser treatment for sever active disease is beneficial. It is recommended that all babies younger than 30 weeks gestational age or with a birth weight 1500 g or less, and those that receive supplemental oxygen therapy, undergo regular screening from 2–4 weeks after birth until the retina is fully vascularized in both eyes, any retinopathy of prematurity has regressed, or until any necessary treatment has been completed.

Amblyopia ("Lazy Eye")

Amblyopia literally means poor vision but is generally used to mean reduced visual acuity in excess of that explained by structural ocular or visual pathway disease. Central vision develops from birth to age 8, after which time further development is unlikely to occur. The formation of the necessary neural structures and connections for development of central vision is dependent upon normal visual experience. The common entities preventing this are **strabismus,** impairing binocular function by causing double vision and visual confusion,

and unequal refractive error (**anisometropia**), either hyperopia or astigmatism, causing a less well-focused retinal image in one eye as well as disrupting binocular function, The consequence is preferential development of central vision in the fixing eye in the case of strabismus and the eye with less refractive error in the case of anisometropia, and impaired central vision (amblyopia) in the fellow eye. Media opacity, such as congenital cataract, marked refractive error, hyperopia or astigmatism, or severe ptosis, can also result in amblyopia.

Amblyopia is treated by correction of any refractive error or other cause and then, if required, patching (occlusion) or blurring of vision with atropine (penalization) of the dominant eye (see Chapters 12 and 17). A crucial determinant of treatment success is age at which the amblyopia is first detected and treated.

Routine neonatal examinations should include assessment of red reflex to identify media opacity. Routine examination of infants by family physicians or pediatricians should also include screening for strabismus. Any child observed to have strabismus after the age of 3 months should be seen by an ophthalmologist. All preschool children should have their visual acuity tested. **Photorefraction**, which relies upon assessment of the red reflex from each eye, is useful in screening for anisometropia, ametropia, astigmatism, and strabismus in preschool children.

Parents should be made aware of the importance of reporting strabismus, abnormal ocular appearance, or poor visual performance, particularly if there is a relevant family history. Visual acuity testing can be performed at home with the illiterate "E" chart, which is sometimes known as the "Home Eye Test." Abnormalities of the red reflex on photographs may alert parents to ocular abnormalities.

Juvenile Idiopathic Arthritis

Uveitis associated with oligoarticular juvenile idiopathic arthritis, which generally occurs in girls with positive antinuclear antibodies, is generally asymptomatic in its early stages and often remains undetected until severe loss of vision due to glaucoma, cataract, or band keratopathy has already occurred. Regular ophthalmic screening every 6 months should take place.

REFERENCES

Causes of Vision Loss

Abdull MM et al: Causes of blindness and visual impairment in Nigeria: The Nigeria National Blindness and Visual Impairment Survey. Invest Ophthalmol Vis Sci 2009;50:4114. [PMID: 19387071]

Abou-Gareeb I et al: Gender and blindness: a meta-analysis of population-based prevalence surveys. Ophthalmic Epidemiol 2001;8(1):39–56.

Abraham AG et al: The new epidemiology of cataract. Ophthalmol Clin North Am 2006;19:415. [PMID: 17067897]

Christian P: Recommendations for indicators: night blindness during pregnancy—a simple tool to assess vitamin A deficiency in a population. J Nutr 2002;132:284S. [PMID: 12221265]

Cook C: Glaucoma in Africa: size of the problem and possible solutions. J Glaucoma 2009;18:124. [PMID: 19225348]

Dandona L et al: What is the global burden of visual impairment? BMC Med 2006;4:6. [PMID: 16539747]

Foster A et al: The impact of Vision 2020 on global blindness. Eye 2005;19:1133. [PMID: 16304595]

Gritz D et al: The antioxidants in prevention of cataracts (APC) study: Effects of antioxidant supplements on cataract progression in South India. Br J Ophthalmol 2006;90:847. [PMID: 16556618]

Harper K et al: Low vision service models in Alberta: innovation, collaboration, and future opportunities. Can J Ophthalmol 2006;41:373. [PMID: 16767196]

Hatt S et al: Screening for prevention of optic nerve damage due to chronic open-angle glaucoma. Cochrane Database Syst Rev 2006;4:CD006129. [PMID: 17054274]

Ho VH et al: Social economic development in the prevention of global blindness. Br J Ophthalmol 2001;85:653. [PMID: 11371481]

Hogeweg M et al: Prevention of blindness in leprosy and the role of the Vision 2020 Programme. Eye 2005;19:1099. [PMID: 16304590]

Iwase A et al: Prevalence and causes of low vision and blindness in a Japanese adult population: the Tajimi study. Ophthalmology 2006;113:1354. [PMID: 16877074]

Kelliher C, Kenny D, O'Brien C: Trends in blind registration in the adult population of the Republic of Ireland 1996–2003. Br J Ophthalmol 2006;90:367. [PMMID: 16488964]

Knauer C, Pfeiffer N: Blindness in Germany – today and in 2030. Ophthalmologe 2006;103:735. [PMID: 16924449]

Kyari F et al: Prevalence of blindness and visual impairment in Nigeria: The National Blindness and Visual Impairment Study. Invest Ophthalmol Vis Sci 2009;50:2033. [PMID: 19117917]

Lapointe ML: Services available to sight-impaired and legally blind patients in Ontario: The Ontario model. Can J Ophthalmol 2006;41:367. [PMID: 16767194]

Limburg H et al: Review of recent surveys on blindness and visual impairment in Latin America. Br J Ophthalmol 2008;92:315. [PMID: 18211928]

Lindfield R et al: Outcome of cataract surgery at one year in Kenya, the Philippines and Bangladesh. Br J Ophthalmol 2009;93:875. [PMID: 19211611]

Maberley DA et al: The prevalence of low vision and blindness in Canada. Eye 2006;20:341. [PMID: 15905873]

Maberley DA et al: The prevalence of low vision and blindness in a Canadian inner city. Eye 2007;21:528. [PMID: 16456592]

Maida JM, Mathers K, Alley CL: Pediatric ophthalmology in the developing world. Curr Opin Ophthalmol 2008;19:403. [PMID: 18772673]

MD Support. State Vision Screening and Standards for License to Drive. Available at: http://www.mdsupport.org/library/drivingrequirements.html, accessed Ferbuary 19, 2010.

Mariotti SP et al: Trachoma: global magnitude of a preventable cause of blindness. Br J Ophthalmol 2009;94:563. [PMID: 19098034]

Resnikoff S et al: Blindness prevention programmes: past, present, and future. Bull World Health Organ 2001;79:222. [PMID: 11285666]

Resnikoff S et al: Global data on visual impairment in the year 2002. Bull World Health Org 2004;82:844.

Resnikoff S, et al: Global magnitude of visual impairment cause by uncorrected refractive error in 2004. Bull World Health Org 2008:86;63. [PMID: 18235892]

Thylefors B. Epidemiological patterns of ocular trauma. Aust N Z J Ophthalmol. 1992; 20: 95. [PMID: 1389141]

Thylefors B et al: Towards the elimination of onchocerciasis. Ann Trop Med Parasitol 2006;100:733. [PMID: 17227651]

Vision standards and low-vision aids. In: PDR for Ophthalmic Medicines. 37th ed. Montvale, NJ: Thomson Reuters: 2008:30–32. (Vision standards in the United States for commercial drivers, pilots, and admission to service academies)

Vitale S et al: Prevalence of visual impairment in the United States. JAMA 2006;295:2158. [PMID: 16684986]

West KP Jr: Vitamin A deficiency disorders in children and women. Food Nutr Bull 2003;24:S78. [PMID: 17016949]

Whitcher JP et al: Corneal blindness: a global perspective. Bull World Health Organ 2001;79:214. [PMID: 11285665]

Whitcher JP et al: Prevention of corneal ulceration in the developing world. Int Ophthalmol Clin 2002;42:71. [PMID: 12189616]

Wong TY et al: The epidemiology of age related eye diseases in Asia. Br J Ophthalmol 2006;90:506. [PMID: 16547337]

World Health Organization: Magnitude and causes of visual impairment [fact sheet No. 282]. Available at: http://www.who.int/mediacentre/factsheets/fs282/en. Published November 2004; accessed November 2, 2009

World Health Organization: International Statistical Classification of Diseases and Related Health Problems, 10th Revision (ICD-10). Available at: http://apps.who.int/classifications/apps/icd/icd10online, accessed February 19, 2010.

World Health Organization: Change to the Definition of Blindness. Available at: http://www.who.int/blindness/Change%20the%20Definition%20of%20Blindness.pdf, accessed February 19, 2010.

Yorston D: The Global initiative – VISION 2020: the right to sight: childhood blindness. J Comm Eye Health 1999;12(31):44–45

Prevention of Visual Loss

American Academy of Pediatrics; Section on Ophthalmology; American Association for Pediatric Ophthalmology and Strabismus; American Academy of Ophthalmology; American Association of Certified Orthoptists: Red reflex examination in neonates, infants, and children. Paediatrics 2008;122:1401. [PMID: 19047263]

Anzivino E et al: Herpes simplex virus infection in pregnancy and in neonate: status of art of epidemiology, diagnosis, therapy and prevention. Virol J 2009;6:40. [PMID: 19348670]

Atkinson J et al: Infant hyperopia: detection, distribution, changes and correlates-outcomes from the Cambridge infant screening programs. Optom Vis Sci 2007;84:88. [PMID: 17299337]

Bhatnagar A et al: Diabetic retinopathy in pregnancy. Curr Diabetes Rev 2009;5:151. [PMID: 19689249]

Bhogal G et al: Penetrating ocular injuries in the home. J Public Health (Oxf) 2007;1:72. [PMID: 17090631]

Brophy M et al: Pediatric eye injury-related hospitalizations in the United States. Pediatrics 2006;117:e1263. [PMID: 16740824]

Bullock JD: Root cause analysis of the fusarium keratitis epidemic of 2004–2006 and prescriptions for preventing future epidemics. Trans Am Ophthalmol Soc 2009;107:194. [PMID: 20126495]

Chang DC et al: Multistate outbreak of Fusarium keratitis associated with a use of a contact lens solution. JAMA 2006;296:953. [PMID: 16926355]

Corrales G et al: Eye trauma in boxing. Clin Sports Med 2009;28:591. [PMID: 19819404]

Dart JK et al: Risk factors for microbial keratitis with contemporary contact lenses: a case-control study. Ophthalmology 2008; 115:1647. [PMID: 18597850]

Dart JK et al: Identification and control of nosocomial adenovirus keratoconjunctivitis in an ophthalmic department. Br J Ophthalmol 2009;93:18.[PMID: 18697812]

Ellerton JA et al: Eye problems in mountain and remote areas: prevention and onsite treatment—official recommendations of the International Commission for Mountain Emergency Medicine ICAR MEDCOM. Wilderness Environ Med 2009;20:169. [PMID: 19594215]

Endophthalmitis Study Group: Prophylaxis of postoperative endophthalmitis following cataract surgery: results of the ESCRS multicenter study and identification of risk factors. J Cataract Refract Surg 2007;33:978. [PMID: 17531690]

Gaujoux T et al: Outbreak of contact lens-related Fusarium keratitis in France. Cornea 2008;27:1018. [PMID: 18812765]

Genuth S: Insights from the diabetes control and complications trial/epidemiology of diabetes interventions and complications study on the use of intensive glycemic treatment to reduce the risk of complications of type 1 diabetes. Endoc Pract 2006;12 Suppl 1:34. [PMID: 16627378]

Greven CM et al: Circumstance and outcome of ocular paintball injuries. Am J Ophthalmol 2006;141:393. [PMID: 16458707]

Hazin R, Hendrick AM, Kahook MY: Primary open-angle glaucoma: diagnostic approaches and management. J Natl Med Assoc 2009;10:46. [PMID: 19245072]

Hecker S: Major cause of vision loss in children can go undetected. Early diagnosis and treatment of amblyopia can reverse damaging effects. Insight 2008;33:38. [PMID: 18853732]

Heimmel MR et al: Ocular injuries in basketball and baseball: what are the risks and how can we prevent them? Curr Sports Med Rep 2008;7:284. [PMID: 18772689]

Holmes JM et al: Amblyopia. Lancet 2006;367:1343. [PMID: 16631913]

Ikeda N et al: Alkali burns of the eye: effect of immediate copious irrigation with tap water on their severity. Ophthalmologica 2006;220:225. [PMID: 16785752]

Kersey JP et al: Corticosteroid-induced glaucoma: a review of the literature. Eye 2006;20:407. [PMID: 15877093]

Krishnaiah S et al: Ocular trauma in a rural population of Southern India: the Andhra Pradesh Eye Disease Study. Ophthalmology 2006;113:1159. [PMID: 16815400]

Kuhn F et al: Epidemiology of blinding trauma in the United States Eye Injury Registry. Ophthalmic Epidemiol 2006;13:209. [PMID: 16854775]

McCall BP et al: Occupational eye injury and risk reduction: Kentucky workers' compensation claim analysis 1994–2003. Inj Prev 2009;15:176. [PMID: 19494097]

Mets MB et al: Eye manifestations of intrauterine infections and their impact on childhood blindness. Surv Ophthalmol 2008;53:95. [PMID: 18348876]

Milacic S: Risk of occupational radiation-induced cataract in medical workers. Med Lav 2009;100:178.[PMID: 19601402]

Nootheti S et al: Risk of cataracts and glaucoma with inhaled steroid use in children. Compr Ophthalmol Update 2006;7:31. [PMID: 16630414]

Patel A, Hammersmith K: Contact lens-related microbial keratitis: recent outbreaks. Curr Opin Ophthalmol 2008;19:302. [PMID: 18545011]

Paulus YM et al: Diabetic retinopathy: a growing concern in an aging population. Geriatrics 2009;64:16. [PMID: 19256582]

Powell C, Hart SR: Vision screening for amblyopia in childhood. Cochrane Database Syst Rev 2009;3:CD005020. [PMID: 19588363]

Prásil P: Current options for the diagnosis and therapy of toxoplasmosis in HIV-negative patients. Klin Mikrobiol Infekc Lek 2009;15:83. [PMID: 19637138]

Robinson JL et al: Prevention of congenital rubella syndrome: what makes sense in 2006? Epidemiol Rev 2006;28:81. [PMID: 16775038]

Rodriguez-Fontal M et al. Metabolic control and diabetic retinopathy. Curr Diabetes Rev 2009;51:3. [PMID: 19199891]

Santaella RM et al: Ocular adverse effects associated with systemic medications: recognition and management. Drugs 2007;67:75. [PMID: 17209665]

Saw SM et al: Risk factors for contact-lens-related fusarium keratitis: a case-control study in Singapore. Arch Ophthalmol 2007;125:611. [PMID: 17502498]

Shah A et al: Educational interventions for the prevention of eye injuries. Cochrane Database Syst Rev 2009;(4):CD006527. [PMID: 19821372]

Sharifi E, Proco TC, Naseri A: Cost-effectiveness analysis of intracameral cefuroxime use for prophylaxis of endophthalmitis after cataract surgery. Ophthalmology 2009;116:1887. [PMID: 19560825]

Srinivasan M et al: Corneal ulceration in South East Asia III: prevention of fungal keratitis at the village level in South India using topical antibiotics. Br J Ophthalmol 2006;90:1472. [PMID: 16916874]

Spurling G et al: Retinopathy – screening recommendations. Aust Fam Physician 2009;38:780. [PMID: 19893816]

Teed RG et al: Amblyopia therapy in children identified by photoscreening. Ophthalmology 2010;117:159. [PMID: 19896190]

Thompson GJ et al: Occupational eye injuries: a continuing problem. Occup Med 2009;59:123. [PMID: 19129239]

Verani JR et al: National outbreak of Acanthamoeba keratitis associated with use of a contact lens solution, United States. Emerg Infect Dis 2009;15:1236. [PMID: 19751585]

Vistamehr S et al: Glaucoma screening in a high-risk population. J Glaucoma 2006;15:534. [PMID: 17106368]

Vyas U et al: Magnitude and determinants of ocular morbidities among persons with diabetes in a project in Ahmedabad, India. Diabetes Technol Ther 2009;11:601. [PMID: 19764840]

Whitcher JP et al: Corneal blindness: a global prospective. Bull World Health Organ 2001;79:214. [PMID: 11285665]

Yip TP et al: Incidence of neonatal chlamydial conjunctivitis and its association with nasopharyngeal colonisation in a Hong Kong hospital, assessed by polymerase chain reaction. Hong Kong Med J 2007;13:22. [PMID: 17277388]

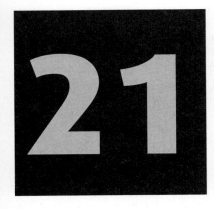

Optics & Refraction

Paul Riordan-Eva, FRCOphth

The correct interpretation of visual information depends on the eye's ability to focus incoming rays of light on the retina. An understanding of this process and how it is influenced by normal variations or ocular disease is essential to the successful use of any optical aid, for example, glasses, contact lenses, intraocular lenses, or low-vision aids. To achieve this understanding, it is necessary to master the concepts of geometric optics, which define the effect on light rays as they pass through different surfaces and media.

GEOMETRIC OPTICS

▶ Speed, Frequency, & Wavelength of Light

Speed, frequency, and wavelength of light are related by the following expression:

$$\text{Frequency} = \frac{\text{Speed}}{\text{Wavelength}}$$

In different optical media, speed and wavelength of light change, but frequency is constant. Color depends on frequency, so that the color of a ray of light is not altered as it passes through optical media except by selective nontransmittance or fluorescence. The optical characteristics of a substance can only be defined with respect to clearly specified frequencies of light. A substance to be used for lenses to refract visible light is usually tested with the yellow sodium light (D line) and the blue (F line) and the red (C line) of a rarefied hydrogen discharge tube.

In a vacuum, the speed of all frequencies of light is the same, that is, 299,792.46 kilometers per second (186,282.40 statute miles per second). Since the frequency of the yellow D line is approximately 5.085×10^{14} Hz, the wavelength of this line in a vacuum is 0.5896 μm. Similarly, the wavelengths in a vacuum of the blue F and red C lines are 0.4861 and 0.6563 μm, respectively.

▶ Index of Refraction

If the speed of a light ray is altered by a change in the optical medium, refraction of the ray will also occur (Figure 21–1). The effect of an optical substance on the speed of light is expressed as its index of refraction, n. The higher the index, the slower the speed and the greater the effect on refraction.

In a vacuum, n has the value 1.00000. The **absolute index of refraction** of a substance is the ratio of the speed of light in a vacuum to the speed of light in the substance. The **relative index of refraction** of a substance is calculated with reference to the speed of light in air. The absolute index of refraction of air varies with the temperature, pressure, and humidity of the air and the frequency of the light, but it is about 1.00032. In optics, n is assumed to be relative to air unless specified as absolute.

▶ Thermal Coefficient of Index of Refraction

The index of refraction changes with the temperature of the medium—it is higher when the substance is colder. This lability of n to temperature is different for different substances. The change in n per degree Celsius for the following substances (all to be multiplied by 10^{-7}) is as follows: glass, 1; fluorite, 10; plastic, 140; water, aqueous, and vitreous, 185. This makes plastic undesirable for precision optical devices. (Plastic also has 8 times the thermal expansion of glass.) Water lenses date back to antiquity but generally are not practical because of problems with thermal instability, evaporation, freezing, and susceptibility to contamination; but in the eye, these objections all but disappear, making the fluid lenses of the eye acceptable.

▶ Dispersion of Light

In a vacuum, the speed of all frequencies of light is the same; thus, the index of refraction is also the same for all colors (1.00000). In all substances, n is different for each color or frequency, being larger at the blue end and smaller at the red

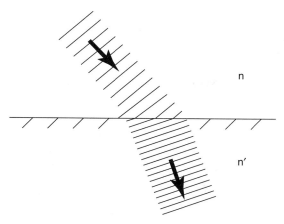

▲ Figure 21–1. Refraction of light as it enters a transparent medium of higher refractive index n′.

Table 21–1. Indices of Refraction and Dispersion Values of Some Substances of Ophthalmologic Interest

Substance (20 °C unless noted)	Indices of Refraction (n_D)	Dispersion Values (V)
Water	1.33299	
Water 37 °C	1.33093	55.6
Sea water	1.344	
Sea water, 11,000 m depth	1.361	
Polymethylmethacrylate	1.49166	57.37
Polymethylmethacrylate 37 °C	1.48928	
Acrylonitrile styrene copolymer	1.56735	34.87
Polystyrene	1.59027	30.92
Fluorite	1.4338	95.2
Spectacle crown glass	1.523	58.8
Flint glass	1.617	36.6
Aqueous and vitreous 37°C	1.3337	55.6
Hydroxyethylmethacrylate (HEMA)	1.43	
Cellulose acetate butyrate (CAB)	1.47	
Silicone	1.439	

end of the spectrum. This difference can be quantified as the dispersion value, V:

$$V = \frac{n_D - 1}{n_F - n_C},$$

where n_D, n_F, and n_C are the indices of refraction for the yellow sodium line and the blue and the red hydrogen lines.

The higher the value of V, the lesser the dispersion of colors. Table 21–1 gives the indices of refraction and some dispersion values for substances of ophthalmologic interest.

▶ Transmittance of Light

Optical materials vary in their transmittance or transparency to different frequencies. Some "transparent" materials such as glass are almost opaque to ultraviolet light. Red glass would be almost opaque to the green frequency. Optical media must be selected according to the specific wavelength of light with which they are to be used.

▶ Laws of Reflection & Refraction

The laws of reflection and refraction were formulated in 1621 by the Dutch astronomer and mathematician Willebrod Snell at the University of Leyden. These laws, together with Fermat's principle, form the basis of applied geometric optics. They can all be stated as follows (Figure 21–2):

1. Incident, reflected, and refracted rays all reside in a plane known as the plane of incidence, which is normal (at a right angle) to the interface.
2. For reflection, relative to the normal, the angles of reflection and incidence are equal.
3. For refraction, the product of the index of refraction of the medium of the incident ray and the sine of the angle of incidence of the incident ray is equal to the product of the same terms of the refracted ray (designated by a prime): n sin I = n′ sin I′ (Snell's law).
4. A ray of light passing from one point to another follows the path that takes the least time to negotiate (Fermat's principle). Optical path length is the index of refraction times the actual path length.

▶ Critical Angle & Total Reflection

In the example of refraction in Figure 21–2, the arriving ray is in the less-dense medium (air) and is refracted toward the normal within the denser medium (glass). Conversely, if the arriving ray were in the denser medium, it would be refracted away from the normal. In this situation, as the angle of incidence is increased, the critical angle is reached when the light is totally reflected (total internal reflection) and the sine of the incident ray in the denser medium reaches the value n′/n. This is one method used to determine the index of refraction. For water, with an index of refraction of 1.330, the critical angle has the sine of 1/1.330, or 48.75° (Figure 21–3).

Total internal reflection obeys the laws of regular reflection, allowing perfect reflection without coatings and being used extensively in fiberoptics.

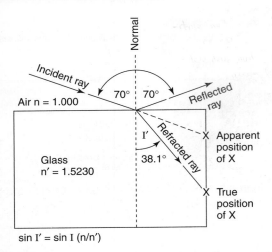

▲ **Figure 21–2.** Examples of the laws of reflection and refraction.

In Figure 21–3, the shaded area is not directly visible from the surface, explaining why visualization of the anterior chamber angle of the eye requires a gonioscopy lens (see Chapter 2). The index of refraction of the aqueous, not the index of refraction of the tears or cornea, is the determining factor in this context.

CALCULATIONS USED IN OPTICS

There are two approaches to the application of the principles of geometric optics to single lenses or to compound lens systems. **Trigonometric ray tracing** is the more valid and

exact approach, as it makes no assumptions other than those already determined by the laws of refraction. The **algebraic method** is a system based on a number of assumptions that greatly simplify calculation of the effects of various lens systems but also limit accuracy to an ever-increasing extent as the lens systems become more complex. The algebraic method cannot be relied on for accurate results, particularly in the assessment of the optical effects of contact lenses, intraocular lenses, and keratorefractive procedures.

Certain considerations are universal to optical calculations whatever method is used. For any optical system, the object and its image are said to lie in **conjugate planes.** If the object were to be placed in the plane of its own image, the optical system would produce its new image in the original object plane. Thus, the effects of any optical system will be the same for whichever direction light travels through the system. Each optical system has an infinite number of pairs of conjugate planes. Corresponding points on conjugate planes are known as **conjugate points.**

▶ Trigonometric Ray Tracing

The trigonometric method of ray tracing consists of mathematically plotting the course of certain specified rays through the lens systems. The three rays most frequently traced are shown in Figure 21–4. They are named according to their positions relative to the first refracting surface. The marginal ray enters at the margin of the lens, the paraxial ray very near the optical axis (center of the lens), and the zonal ray in the portion of the lens where the average luminous flux of light passes through the lens. At each refracting surface, the change in direction of each of these rays is calculated according to the principles of Snell's law. This requires knowledge of the radius of curvature of the surface, the index of refraction of the medium on each side of the refracting surface, and the distance to the next surface. Elementary trigonometry is the only

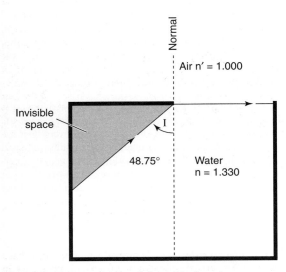

▲ **Figure 21–3.** Example of the critical angle.

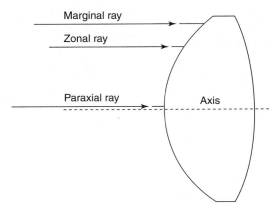

▲ **Figure 21–4.** Illustration of 3 rays traced in trigonometric ray tracing.

mathematical skill necessary for such calculations, although a programmable calculator greatly assists with the number of such calculations that have to be carried out.

Trigonometric ray tracing provides an exact determination of the point of focus and information on the quality of the image formed by a lens system. The difference between the back focal lengths (distance along the optical axis from the last refracting surface to the point of focus) of the marginal and paraxial rays is a measure of the "spread of focus," thus indicating the degree of **spherical aberration** (see later in the chapter). Similarly, if rays of different color (frequency), with their different indices of refraction in each medium, are traced through the system, the degree of **chromatic aberration** (see later in the chapter) will be determined. The optical pathway is the sum of the actual distance a ray passes through the substances multiplied by the index of refraction in the various substances through which it passes. How closely the optical pathways of the marginal and paraxial rays match determines the brightness and contrast of the final image.

Trigonometric ray tracing permits determination of the performance of each refracting surface relative to the contribution to the final image. For example, it is easily shown that a planoconvex intraocular lens gives a better image with the convex surface forward and the flat surface closer to the retina. The point of focus often requires—and is easily adjusted by—postoperative refraction. However, the distorted image caused by selecting an intraocular lens of improper shape cannot be repaired by refraction. Suitability in this respect must be achieved by proper preoperative lens design, and this can only be achieved by calculation using the trigonometric method of ray tracing.

Graphic ray tracing is a system comparable to trigonometric ray tracing that uses drawings to determine the optical properties of lens systems; it should not be confused with the method of "ray tracing" described in several books, in which tracings of an image are based on (a derivation of the algebraic method of optical calculations discussed below).

▶ Algebraic Method

Carl Friedrich Gauss (1777–1855) is responsible for refining a method of optical calculations that dispensed with the sines and cosines of the trigonometric method. This assumed that the lenses are "infinitely thin," placed close together, and of small diameter, such that any angle will be so small that the size of the angle measured in radians will have the same value as the sine of the angle and that the sine and the tangent of the angle can be assumed to be the same. The results are the **thin lens equations** used by opticians to calculate curves for lenses. "Fudge factors" derived from experience are then necessary to correct for the inaccuracies of these equations.

Use of the algebraic method depends on certain definitions. The position of the lens, reduced to a single line, is the **principal plane,** which intersects the optical axis at the **nodal point** (optical center). The **primary focal point (F)** is that

$$\text{Lens power} \cong \frac{1}{\text{Focal length}} \cong \frac{1}{\text{Distance of image}} - \frac{1}{\text{Distance of object}}$$

$$\text{Lens power} \cong (n-1)\frac{1}{\text{Front surface radius}} - \frac{1}{\text{Back surface radius}}$$

$$\frac{\text{Size of image}}{\text{Distance of image}} \cong \frac{\text{Size of object}}{\text{Distance of object}}$$

$$\text{Magnification} = \frac{\text{Size of image}}{\text{Size of object}} \cong \frac{\text{Distance of image}}{\text{Distance of object}}$$

Power for Several Lenses Combined
$$\text{Total power} \cong \text{Power}_1 + \text{Power}_2 + \text{Power}_3, \text{ etc}$$

▲ **Figure 21–5.** Algebraic thin lens approximations. All lengths in meters.

point along the optical axis where an object must be placed to form an image at infinity. The **secondary focal point (F′)** is that point along the optical axis where parallel incident rays are brought to a focus. If the medium on either side of the lens is of the same refractive index, the distance between the nodal point and each of the focal points, the **focal length,** is the same.

Figure 21–5 shows some of the important thin lens equations.

The **diopter (D)** is a measure of lens power derived from the algebraic method of optical calculations. It is defined as the reciprocal of the focal length of a lens in air measured in meters. Diopters are additive, but only for low-power lenses. The result of combining lenses of high power varies greatly with their thickness and the separation distance. High-power lenses must be described by three values: (1) radii of curvature, (2) index of refraction, and (3) thickness.

In Gaussian optics, a thick lens is treated as if there are two nodal points and two principal planes (n and n′ and H and H′ in Figure 21–6). The nodal points lie on the principal planes only if the refractive medium is the same on either side of the lens. The true focal lengths are measured from the principal planes to the focal points, but the front and back focal lengths—essential to the prescription of corrective lenses—are measured from the respective surfaces of the lens to the focal points. The reciprocal of the back focal length corresponds to the back vertex power as measured with a lensometer.

For making high plus contact lenses or thick-spectacle lenses, according to the algebraic method the equation for lens power in diopters is:

$$\text{Power} \cong \frac{1}{F} \cong (n-1)\left[\frac{1}{r_1} - \frac{1}{r_2} - \frac{(n-1)d}{nr_1r_2}\right],$$

where F = focal length, r_1 = front surface radius, r_2 = back surface radius, and d = thickness of lens, all measured in meters, and n = refractive index.

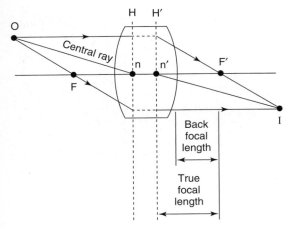

▲ Figure 21–6. Description of a thick lens in Gaussian optics.

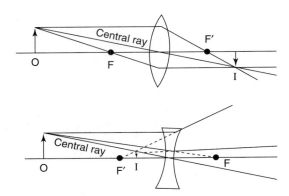

▲ Figure 21–7. Ray tracing through plus and minus lenses.

For contact lenses, a derivation of the thin-lens equations is presently used to relate dioptric power to radius of curvature:

$$\text{Power} \approx \frac{(n-1)}{r} \approx \frac{1.3375-1}{r} \approx \frac{337.5}{r_{mm}} \text{ and } r_{mm} \approx \frac{337.5}{\text{Power}}$$

n of "cornea" is for this purpose assumed to be 1.3375. r_{mm} = radius in millimeters. These equations are only approximations.

The ray tracing method commonly described in ophthalmic optics texts is a graphic representation of the algebraic system of optical calculations—in contrast to true graphic ray tracing, which is a graphic representation of the trigonometric system. Rays are traced through the optical system to connect conjugate points. The positions of the conjugate planes are derived mathematically from the thin lens equations. The size and orientation of the object are then determined by tracing the central ray, which passes straight through the tip of the image, the nodal point of the lens (without being refracted), and the tip of the object. The rays that traverse the focal points of the lens are derived by extrapolation (Figure 21–7).

For multiple lens systems, the conjugate planes and the path of the central ray are determined for each lens in succession, producing an image that becomes the object for the next lens until the size and orientation of the final image is located. In the case of a thick lens, refraction occurs at the principal planes of the lens, the position of rays being translated from one principal plane to another without any change in their vertical separation from the optical axis (Figure 21–6). The central ray passes from the tip of the object to the first nodal point and then emerges from the second nodal point parallel to its original direction to reach the tip of the image. When the media on either side of the lens have different refractive indices, the nodal points do not coincide with the principal planes.

Magnification

Linear magnification is the ratio of the height of the image to the height of the object. For an infinitely thin lens in air—as assumed by the algebraic method of optical calculation—this ratio is equal to the ratio of the distance of the image to the distance of the object. For real lens systems, such as those of the eye, a more complex equation including the index of refraction of the initial and final media must be used. Trigonometric ray tracing quickly provides other information necessary for the calculation.

Change of Vertex Distance

If the vertex distance (the distance from the eye) of a lens of given power is altered, the effective power of the lens will also change. To calculate a new lens that will have the same effect at the new distance, a derivation of the thin lens equations can be used:

$$\text{Power}_2 \approx \frac{1}{\dfrac{1}{\text{Power}_1}-(D_1-D_2)}$$

where Power_1 and Power_2 are the old and new lens powers and D_1 and D_2 are the old and new vertex distances.

Example 1: A + 13 diopter lens at 11 mm (0.011 m) is to be replaced by a lens at 9 mm (0.009).

$$\text{Power}_2 \cong \frac{1}{\dfrac{1}{13}-(0.011-0.009)} \cong 13.347\,\text{diopters}$$

Example 2: Same lens to be replaced by a contact lens $(D_2 = 0)$.

$$\text{Power}_2 \cong \frac{1}{\dfrac{1}{13}-(0.01)} \cong 15.169\,\text{diopters}$$

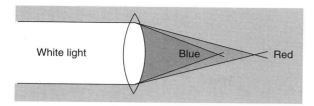

White light | Blue | Red

▲ **Figure 21–8.** Chromatic aberration of lenses.

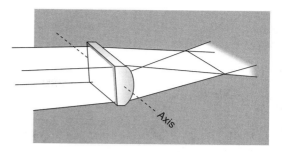

Axis

▲ **Figure 21–10.** A planocylindrical lens with axis in the horizontal meridian.

This vertex equation is also an approximation and should not be used for intraocular lens calculations, but it is useful for conversion from spectacle to contact lens powers.

▶ **Aberrations of Spherical Lenses**

Spherical lenses are subject to a number of aberrations that reduce the quality of image produced. The variation of refractive index with frequency of light (dispersion) results in greater refraction of blue than red light (**chromatic aberration**) (Figure 21–8). Marginal rays are refracted more than paraxial rays, producing **spherical aberration** (Figure 21–9). **Coma,** a characteristic comet-shaped blur, is the result of spherical aberration of light originating away from the optical axis of the lens. When light traverses a spherical lens obliquely, there is an additional cylindrical lens effect—**astigmatism of oblique incidence. Curvature of field** is the production of a curved image from a flat object. Prismatic effects of the lens periphery also cause image distortion. Achromatic lenses may be made by cementing together plus and minus lenses of different refractive indices. The nonchromatic aberrations are overcome by combining or shaping lenses to reduce the power of the lens periphery, by restricting the area of the lens used to the paraxial zones, and by use of meniscus lenses.

▶ **Cylindrical Lenses**

A **planocylindrical lens** (Figure 21–10) has one flat surface and one cylindrical surface, producing a lens with no optical power in the meridian of its axis and maximum power in the meridian 90° away from the axis meridian. The total effect is the formation of a line image, parallel to the axis of the lens, from a point object. The orientation of a planocylindrical lens is specified by the meridian of its axis. The ophthalmic convention for specifying the orientation of the axis of a cylindrical lens is shown in Figure 21–11. Zero begins nasally in the right lens and temporally in the left lens and proceeds in a counterclockwise direction to 180°.

In a **spherocylindrical** lens, the cylindrical surface is curved in two meridians but not to the same extent. In ophthalmic lenses, these principal meridians are at 90° to each other. The effect of a spherocylindrical lens on a point object is to produce a geometric figure known as the **conoid of Sturm** (Figure 21–12), consisting of two focal lines separated by the interval of Sturm. The position of the focal lines relative to the lens is determined by the power of the two meridians and their orientation by the angle between the meridians.

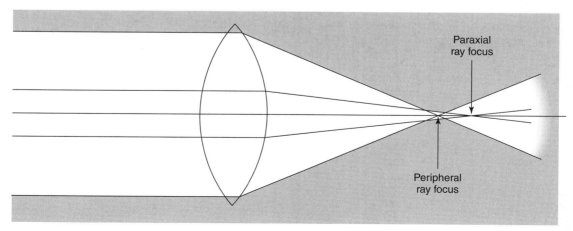

Paraxial
ray focus

Peripheral
ray focus

▲ **Figure 21–9.** Spherical aberration of a biconvex lens.

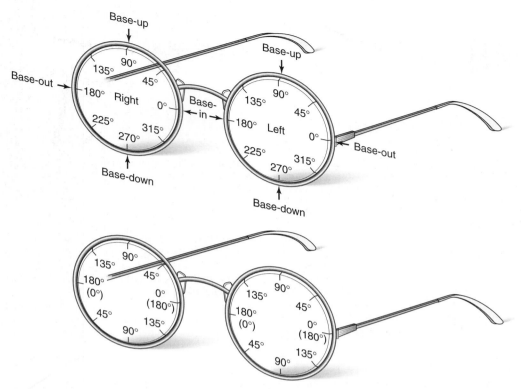

▲ **Figure 21–11.** **Top:** Illustration of prism base notation. **Bottom:** Illustration of cylinder axis notation.

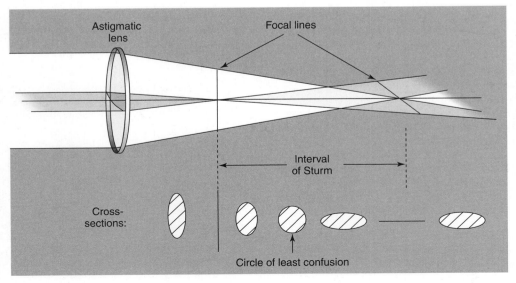

▲ **Figure 21–12.** The conoid of Sturm, formed by light refracted by an astigmatic lens.

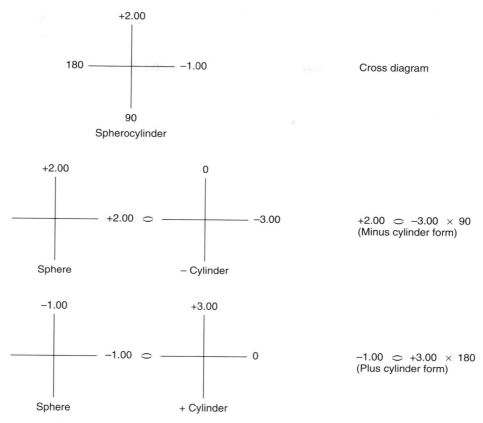

▲ **Figure 21–13.** Cross diagram and equivalent combinations, including longhand notations, for a spherocylindrical lens.

Cross-sections through the conoid of Sturm reveal lines at the focal lines and generally ellipses elsewhere. In one position, the cross-section will be a circle that represents the **circle of least confusion.**

A spherocylindrical lens can be thought of as a combination of a spherical lens and a planocylindrical lens. It can then be specified by the orientation of principal meridians and the power acting in each (Figure 21–13). In a cross diagram, the arms are drawn parallel to the principal meridians and labeled with the relevant power. In longhand notation, the cylinder is specified by the orientation of its axis, which is 90° away from the meridian of maximum power.

Writing prescriptions for spherocylindrical lenses uses longhand notation, and the lens can be specified in either plus or minus cylinder form (Figure 21–13). The procedure for transposing between these forms is as follows: (1) algebraically sum the original sphere and cylinder; (2) reverse the sign of the cylinder; and (3) change the axis of the cylinder by 90°.

If their principal meridians correspond, combinations of spherocylindrical lenses can be summed mathematically. Otherwise, trigonometric formulas are required. Alternatively, the power of such combinations can be determined by placing them together in a lensometer. The principal meridians of any such combination will be 90° apart.

▶ **Prisms**

A prism consists of a transparent material with nonparallel flat surfaces. In cross-section, it has an apex and a base. The prism is specified by its power and the orientation of its base.

A prism refracts light toward its base, whereas an object seen through a prism appears deviated toward the apex of the prism. The amount of deviation varies according to the tilt of the prism, that is, the angle of incidence of the light. For glass prisms, calibration is performed in the **Prentice position,** in which the incident light is perpendicular to the face of the prism (Figure 21–14). For plastic prisms and in general optics, a prism is calibrated in the **position of minimum deviation,** in which the amount of refraction at the two surfaces of the prisms is equal (Figure 21–14). When prisms are used in clinical practice, these orientations must be adhered to for accurate results.

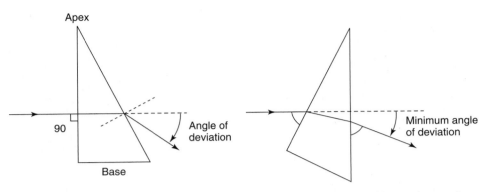

▲ **Figure 21–14.** Calibration of prisms. Glass prisms and spectacle prisms are calibrated according to the Prentice position, whereas plastic prisms are calibrated according to the position of minimum deviation.

For a glass prism in the Prentice position, the incident rays are not refracted at the first surface because they are perpendicular to one another (Figure 21–15). At the second surface, the angle of incidence is the same as the apex angle of the prism (A). If I′ is the angle of the final refracted ray, from Snell's law, sin I′ = (n/n′) sin A, n being the refractive index of the prism and n′ the refractive index of the surrounding medium. For example, if the prism is of glass with n = 1.523 and A = 30°, then sin I′ is 1.523 × 0.5, or 0.7615. I′ is 49.6°. The angle of deviation is I′ − A, or 19.6°.

The power of a prism is measured in prism diopters (PD). One prism diopter deviates an image 1 cm at 1 m (Figure 21–16). The arc tangent of 1/100 is 0.57°. Therefore, 1 PD produces an angle of deviation of almost one-half degree. The "rule of thumb" is that a prism of 2 PD produces an angle of deviation of 1°, but this cannot be applied to prisms of more than 100 PD.

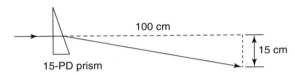

▲ **Figure 21–16.** Power of a prism in prism diopters.

Prisms are used in ophthalmology both to measure and to treat heterotropia and heterophoria. The orientation of a prism's base is indicated by its direction, usually descriptively, that is, "base-up right eye," "base-down left eye," "base-in" or "base-out," or occasionally by a mathematical system (Figure 21–11).

Fresnel prisms are lightweight plastic prisms consisting of narrow, parallel strips of prism with the same apex angle as the desired single prism (Figure 21–17). They are available as press-on prisms for attachment to the back of spectacle lenses, providing an easily adjusted temporary prismatic correction that is less heavy than conventional glass prisms.

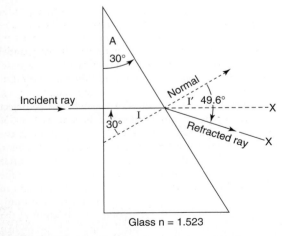

▲ **Figure 21–15.** Example of the prism as used in ophthalmology.

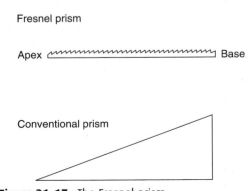

▲ **Figure 21–17.** The Fresnel prism.

Their disadvantages are the image degradation due to light scatter and dirt within the grooves.

Prismatic Effect of Spherical Lenses

Spherical lenses have increasing prismatic power as the light path moves away from the optical center of the lens. The amount of prism power can be calculated from Prentice's rule, which states that the prism power in prism diopters is equal to the dioptric power of the lens in diopters multiplied by the displacement from the optical center in centimeters. For example, at 0.5 cm away from the optical center of a 6-diopter lens, the prismatic power is 3 PD. Plus lenses produce prism power with the base oriented toward the optical center of the lens, and minus lenses produce prism power with the base oriented away from their optical center.

The prismatic effect of spherical lenses is an important consideration in the correction of anisometropia. Appropriate spectacle lenses may produce significant vertical prismatic deviation when the peripheral portions of the lenses are used. This occurs mainly when the patient attempts to read. The prismatic effect can be overcome by adopting a chin-down position, thus using the optical centers of the lenses once again, by grinding of a compensatory prism into the reading segment of the glasses (**slab-off prism**) or by changing to contact lenses.

If a prism needs to be incorporated into a patient's spectacle correction, such as in the control of hypertropia, it may be achieved by decentration of the spherical lens rather than by addition of a prism to the spherical component.

Rapid Detection of Lens Characteristics

The nature of a spherical lens may be rapidly detected by looking through it 0.5 m (20 in) or so from the eye and moving the lens at right angles to the visual axis. The image seen through a minus (concave) lens will tend to move *with* the lens. The same test with a plus (convex) lens causes the image to tend to move *away from* the direction of motion. This effect is due to the prismatic effect of the periphery of the lens. The power of the lens can be approximated by neutralization of these movements by lenses of known power. A cylindrical lens shows changing distortion of the image when the lens is rotated about the visual axis. (Spherical lenses do not.) The orientations of the lens in which the image is clearest indicate the principal meridians. The power in each of the principal meridians can then be determined by the method described above for spherical lenses. A prism is recognized by deviation of the image as the static lens is viewed through its center.

OPTICS & THE EYE

Many attempts have been made to simplify the optical system of the human eye, particularly using the thick lens equations of the algebraic method of optical calculations.

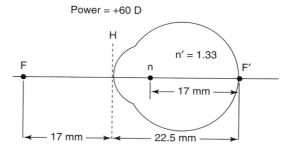

▲ Figure 21–18. The reduced schematic eye.

Much has been made of the concept that the image on the retina is formed by two lens elements, the cornea contributing about 43 D and the lens the remaining 19 D, but this is a gross oversimplification. The **schematic eye of Gullstrand** and its reduced form (Figure 21–18) are models from which mathematical values for the optical characteristics of the eye were derived. For instance, in the reduced schematic eye, the cornea is assumed to be the only refracting surface, the principal plane (H) being placed at its apex and a single nodal point (n) at its center of curvature. The globe has an axial length of 22.5 mm, and the refractive index of the eye is said to be 1.33. Unfortunately, these numbers have become accepted by many as true physiologic values rather than as the convenient mathematically derived values they really are. The refractive index of aqueous is about 1.3337 (for the sodium D line at 37 °C).

Trigonometric ray tracing demonstrates that the optical system of the human eye is more accurately conceptualized as a three-lens system: the aqueous lens, the crystalline lens, and the vitreous lens (Figure 21–19). Contrary to popular belief, the cornea itself has almost no power of refraction in the optical system but is important only in shaping the anterior curve of the aqueous lens. The crystalline lens is an interesting optical component because its index of refraction varies throughout its thickness rather than being constant, as assumed in most optical calculations. The vitreous lens is particularly important because of its major effect on magnification.

Reassessment of models for the optical system of the human eye is essential now that much of ophthalmic surgery, whether it is cataract surgery, keratorefractive procedures, or vitreous surgery, produces profound effects on individual components of the system. Gullstrand's models, in which the system is assumed to function as an integrated unit, cannot be applied under such circumstances.

Accommodation

The eye changes refractive power to focus on near objects by a process called accommodation. Study of Purkinje images, which are reflections from various optical surfaces in the eye, has shown that accommodation results from changes in the crystalline lens. Contraction of the ciliary muscle results in

Prior to "assembly"

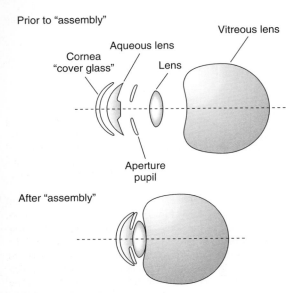

After "assembly"

▲ **Figure 21–19.** The optical system of the eye, illustrating the three-lens concept.

thickening and increased curvature of the lens, probably due to relaxation of the lens capsule.

Visual Acuity

Assessment of visual acuity with the Snellen chart is described in Chapter 2. The average resolving power of the normal human eye is 1 minute of arc. Since the Snellen letters are made from squares of 5×5 units (Figure 21–20), the 20/20-size letter has a visual angle of 5 minutes of arc at 20 ft. This is equivalent to 8.7 mm (0.35 in) width and height. The eye

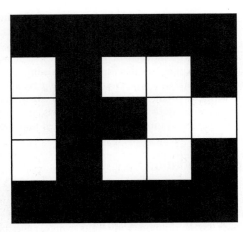

▲ **Figure 21–20.** Snellen block E.

minifies an image at 20 ft by about 350 times. Therefore, the size of the 20/20 letter on the retina is 0.025-mm high and wide. This is equivalent to a resolution capacity of 100 lines per millimeter. For a 6-mm pupil and light of wavelength 0.56 μm (in air), the absolute theoretic limit would be 345 lines per millimeter.

REFRACTIVE ERRORS

Emmetropia is absence of refractive error, and **ametropia** is the presence of refractive error.

▶ Presbyopia

The loss of accommodation that comes with aging to all people is called presbyopia (Table 21–2). A person with emmetropic eyes (no refractive error) will begin to notice inability to read small print or discriminate fine close objects at about age 44–46. This is worse in dim light and usually worse early in the morning or when the subject is fatigued. These symptoms increase until about age 55, when they stabilize but persist.

Presbyopia is corrected by use of a plus lens to make up for the lost automatic focusing power of the lens. The plus lens may be used in several ways. Reading glasses have the near correction in the entire aperture of the glasses, making them fine for reading but blurred for distant objects. Half-glasses can be worn to abate this nuisance by leaving the top open and uncorrected for distance vision. Bifocals do the same but allow correction of other refractive errors. Trifocals correct for distance vision by the top segment, the middle distance by the middle section, and the near distance by the lower segment. Progressive power (varifocal) lenses similarly correct for far, middle, and near distances but by progressive change in lens power rather than stepped changes.

▶ Myopia

When the image of distant objects focuses in front of the retina in the unaccommodated eye, the eye is myopic, or

Table 21–2. Table of Accommodation

Age (Years)	Mean Accommodation (Diopters)
8	13.8
25	9.9
35	7.3
40	5.8
45	3.6
50	1.9
55	1.3

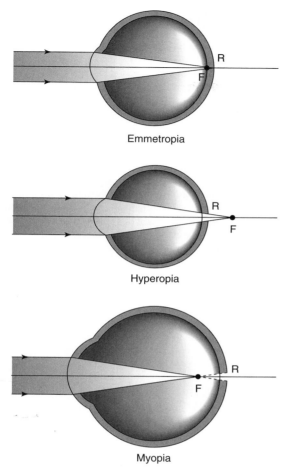

Emmetropia

Hyperopia

Myopia

▲ Figure 21–21. Spherical refractive errors as determined by the position of the secondary focal point with respect to the retina.

susceptibility to degenerative retinal changes, including retinal detachment.

Concave spherical (minus) lenses are used to correct the image in myopia. These lenses move the image back to the retina.

▶ Hyperopia

Hyperopia (hypermetropia, farsightedness) is the state in which the unaccommodated eye would focus the image behind the retina (Figure 21–21). It may be due to reduced axial length (axial hyperopia), as occurs in certain congenital disorders, or reduced refractive error (refractive hyperopia), as exemplified by aphakia.

Hyperopia is a more difficult concept to explain than myopia. The term "farsighted" contributes to the difficulty, as does the prevalent misconception among laymen that presbyopia is farsightedness and that one who sees well far away is farsighted. If hyperopia is not too great, a young person may obtain a sharp distant image by accommodating, as a normal eye would to read. The young hyperopic person may also make a sharp near image by accommodating more—or much more than one without hyperopia. This extra effort may result in eye fatigue that is more severe for near work. The degree of hyperopia a person may have without symptoms is variable. However, the amount decreases with age as presbyopia (decrease in ability to accommodate) increases. Three diopters of hyperopia might be tolerated in a teenager but will require glasses later, even though the hyperopia has not increased. If the hyperopia is too high, the eye may be unable to correct the image by accommodation. The hyperopia that cannot be corrected by accommodation is termed manifest hyperopia. This is one of the causes of deprivation amblyopia in children and can be bilateral. There is a reflex correlation between accommodation and convergence of the two eyes. Hyperopia is therefore a frequent cause of esotropia (crossed eyes) and monocular amblyopia (see Chapter 12).

▶ Latent Hyperopia

As explained above, a prepresbyopic person with hyperopia may obtain a clear retinal image by accommodation. The degree of hyperopia overcome by accommodation is known as latent hyperopia. It is detected by refraction after instillation of cycloplegic drops, which determines the sum of both manifest and latent hyperopia. Refraction with a cycloplegic is very important in young patients who complain of eyestrain when reading and is vital in esotropia, where full correction of hyperopia may achieve a cure.

Remember that a moderately "farsighted" person may see well for near or far when young. However, as presbyopia comes on, the hyperope first has trouble with close work—and at an earlier age than the nonhyperope. Finally, the hyperope has blurred vision for near *and far* and requires glasses for both near and far.

nearsighted (Figure 21–21). If the eye is longer than average, the error is called axial myopia. (For each additional millimeter of axial length, the eye is approximately 3 diopters more myopic.) If the refractive elements are more refractive than average, the error is called curvature myopia or refractive myopia. As the object is brought closer than 6 m, the image moves closer to the retina and comes into sharper focus. The point reached where the image is most sharply focused on the retina is called the "far point." One may estimate the extent of myopia by calculating the reciprocal of the far point. Thus, a far point of 0.25 m would suggest a 4-diopter minus lens correction for distance. The myopic person has the advantage of being able to read at the far point without glasses even at the age of presbyopia. A high degree of myopia results in greater

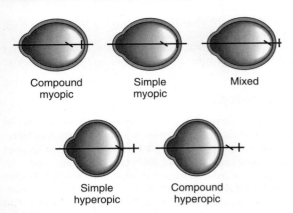

▲ Figure 21–22. Types of regular astigmatism as determined by the positions of the two local lines with respect to the retina.

▶ Astigmatism

In astigmatism, the eye produces an image with multiple focal points or lines. In **regular astigmatism,** there are two principal meridians, with constant power and orientation across the pupillary aperture, resulting in two focal lines. The astigmatism is then further defined according to the position of these focal lines with respect to the retina (Figure 21–22). When the principal meridians are at right angles and their axes lie within 20° of the horizontal and vertical, the astigmatism is subdivided into **astigmatism with the rule,** in which the greater refractive power is in the vertical meridian, and **astigmatism against the rule,** in which the greater refractive power is in the horizontal meridian. Astigmatism with the rule is more commonly found in younger patients, and astigmatism against the rule more commonly in older patients (Figure 21–23). **Oblique astigmatism** is regular astigmatism in which the principal meridians do not lie within 20° of the horizontal and vertical. In **irregular astigmatism,** the power or orientation of the principal meridians changes across the pupillary aperture.

The usual cause of astigmatism, particularly irregular astigmatism, is abnormalities of corneal shape. The crystalline lens may also contribute. In contact lens terminology, lenticular astigmatism is called residual astigmatism because it is not corrected by a spherical hard contact lens, which does correct corneal astigmatism.

Regular astigmatism often can be corrected with cylindrical lenses, frequently in combination with spherical lenses, or sometimes more effectively by altering corneal shape with rigid contact lenses, which are usually the only optical means of managing irregular astigmatism. Because the brain is capable of adapting to the visual distortion of an uncorrected astigmatic error, new glasses that do correct the error may cause temporary disorientation, particularly an apparent slanting of images.

▶ Natural History of Refractive Errors

Most babies are slightly hyperopic, mean refractive error at birth being 0.5 D. The hyperopia slowly decreases, with a slight acceleration in the teens, to approach emmetropia. The corneal curvature is much steeper (6.59-mm radius) at birth and flattens to nearly the adult curvature (7.71 mm) by about 1 year. The lens is much more spherical at birth and reaches adult conformation at about 6 years. The mean axial length is short at birth (16.6 mm), lengthens rapidly in the first 2 or 3 years (to 21.8 mm), then moderately (0.4 mm per year) until age 6, and then slowly (about 1 mm total) to stability (24 mm) at about 10 or 15 years. Presbyopia becomes manifest in the fifth decade.

Refractive errors are inherited. The mode of inheritance is complex, as it involves so many variables. Refractive error, although inherited, need not be present at birth any more than

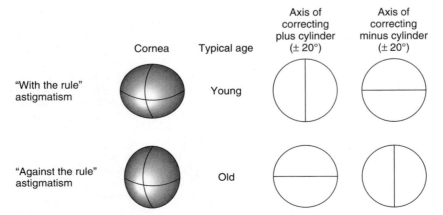

▲ Figure 21–23. Types of astigmatism as determined by the orientation of the principal meridians and the orientation of the correcting cylinder axis.

tallness, which is also inherited, need be present at birth. For example, a child who reaches emmetropia at age 10 years will probably soon become myopic. Myopia usually increases during the teens. Factors influencing progression of myopia are poorly defined but probably include close work. Optical and pharmacological treatments to retard progression of myopia in children have not yet been shown to have long-term benefit.

▶ Anisometropia

Anisometropia is a difference in refractive error between the two eyes. It is a major cause of amblyopia because the eyes cannot accommodate independently and the more hyperopic eye is chronically blurred. Refractive correction of anisometropia is complicated by differences in size of the retinal images (**aniseikonia**) and oculomotor imbalance due to the different degree of prismatic power of the periphery of the two corrective lenses. Aniseikonia is predominantly a problem of monocular aphakia. Spectacle correction produces a difference in retinal image size of approximately 25%, which is rarely tolerable. Contact lens correction reduces the difference in image size to approximately 6%, which can be tolerated. Intraocular lenses produce a difference of less than 1%.

▶ Correction of Refractive Errors

A. Spectacle Lenses

Spectacles continue to be the safest method of refractive correction. To reduce nonchromatic aberrations, the lenses are made in meniscus form (corrected curves) and tilted forward (pantascopic tilt).

B. Contact Lenses

The first contact lenses were glass fluid-filled scleral lenses. These were difficult to wear for extended periods and caused corneal edema and much ocular discomfort. Hard corneal lenses, made of polymethylmethacrylate, were the first really successful contact lenses and gained wide acceptance for cosmetic replacement of glasses. Subsequent developments include gas-permeable lenses, made of cellulose acetate butyrate, silicone, or various silicone and plastic polymers, and soft contact lenses, made of various hydrogel plastics, all of which provide increased comfort but greater risk of serious complications.

Rigid (hard and gas-permeable) lenses correct refractive errors by changing the curvature of the anterior surface of the eye. The total refractive power consists of the power induced by the back curvature of the lens, the base curve, together with the actual power of the lens due to the difference between its front and back curvatures. Only the second is dependent on the refractive index of the contact lens material. Rigid lenses overcome corneal astigmatism, including irregular astigmatism, by modifying the anterior surface of the eye into a truly spherical shape.

Soft contact lenses, particularly the more flexible forms, adopt the shape of the patient's cornea. Thus, their refractive power resides only in the difference between their front and back curvature, and they correct little corneal astigmatism unless a cylindrical correction is incorporated to make a toric lens.

Contact lens base curves are selected according to corneal curvature, as determined by keratometry or trial fittings. The front curvature is then calculated from the results of overrefraction with a trial contact lens, or from the patient's spectacle refraction as corrected for the corneal plane.

Rigid contact lenses are specifically indicated for the correction of irregular astigmatism, such as in keratoconus. Soft contact lenses are used for the treatment of corneal surface disorders, but for control of symptoms rather than for refractive reasons. All forms of contact lenses are used in the refractive correction of aphakia, particularly in overcoming the aniseikonia of monocular aphakia, and the correction of high myopia, in which they produce a much better visual image than spectacles. However, the vast majority of contact lenses worn are for cosmetic correction of low refractive errors. This has important implications for the risks that can be reasonably accepted in the use of contact lenses. (Further discussion of therapeutic and cosmetic contact lens use, and the associated complications, is given in Chapter 6.)

C. Keratorefractive Surgery

Keratorefractive surgery encompasses a range of methods for changing the curvature of the anterior surface of the eye. The expected refractive effect is generally derived from empirical results of similar procedures in other patients and not based on mathematical optical calculations. Further discussion of the methods and outcome of keratorefractive procedures is included in Chapter 6.

D. Intraocular Lenses

Implantation of an intraocular lens has become the preferred method of refractive correction for aphakia, usually being undertaken at the time of cataract surgery but sometimes deferred in complicated cases. A large number of designs are available, foldable lenses, made of silicone or hydrogel plastics, which can be inserted into the eye through a small incision, generally being preferred when available and applicable, but rigid lenses, most commonly consisting of an optic made of polymethylmethacrylate and loops (haptics) made of the same material or polypropylene, also still being used. The safest position for an intraocular lens is within an intact capsular bag following extracapsular surgery.

Intraocular lens power was usually determined by the empirical regression method of analyzing experience with lenses of one style in many patients, from which was derived a mathematical formula based on a constant for the particular lens (A), average keratometer readings (K), and axial length in millimeters (L). A simple example is the **SRK (Sanders–Retzlaff–Kraff) equation:**

$$\text{Power IOL} = A - 2.5L - 0.9K$$

A derivation is the SRK II formula. However, regression formulas are now rarely used. Theoretic formulas utilizing a lens constant, keratometer readings, and axial length, together with estimated anterior chamber depth following surgery, include the SRK/T, Haigis, Holladay, and Hoffer Q formulas. Unfortunately, none of these formulas are based on trigonometric ray tracing methods, which do accurately predict the correct power of intraocular lens for an individual patient. However, satisfactory results are generally obtained with selection of the most reliable formula for the particular axial length. Hoffer Q is indicated for short eyes (axial length less than 22 mm), Holladay for relatively long eyes (axial length 24.6–26 mm), and Haigis or SRK/T for especially long eyes (axial length greater than 26 mm). Because there is a tendency to underestimate the required power in eyes that have previously undergone keratorefractive surgery, calculation of the correct intraocular lens is much more difficult in such cases but is assisted by knowledge of refractive error and keratometer readings prior to the refractive surgery.

An additional (piggyback) intraocular lens is sometimes implanted to correct residual refractive error. Intraocular lenses are occasionally inserted without removal of the crystalline lens (phakic intraocular lens) for treatment of refractive error in young individuals without cataract and prior to onset of presbyopia.

E. Clear Lens Extraction for Myopia

Extraction of noncataractous lenses may be undertaken for the refractive correction of moderate to high myopia, with reported outcomes comparable to those achieved with laser keratorefractive surgery. The operative and postoperative complications of intraocular surgery, particularly in high myopia, need to be borne in mind.

METHODS OF REFRACTION

Determination of a patient's refractive correction can be achieved by objective or subjective means and is best accomplished by a combination of the two methods where possible.

▶ Objective Refraction

Objective refraction is performed by retinoscopy, in which a streak of light, known as the **intercept,** is projected into the patient's eye to produce a similarly shaped reflex, the **retinoscopic reflex,** in the pupil (Figure 21–24). Parallel alignment of the intercept and the retinoscopic reflex indicates the presence of only a spherical error, or an additional cylindrical error in which the intercept coincides

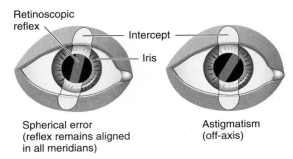

▲ **Figure 21–24.** The retinoscopic reflex.

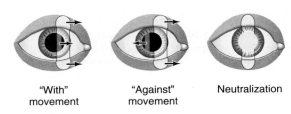

▲ **Figure 21–25.** Movement of the retinoscopic reflex.

with one of the principal meridians. Rotation of the projected streak will determine which of these applies and the location of the other principal meridian in the case of a cylindrical error.

The intercept is then swept across the patient's pupil, and the effect on the retinoscopic reflex is noted (Figure 21–25). If it moves in the same direction (**with movement**), plus lenses are placed before the patient's eye; and if it moves in the opposite direction (**against movement**), minus lenses are added—until the pupillary reflex fills the whole pupillary aperture and no movement is detected (**point of neutralization**). When the point of neutralization has been reached, the patient's refractive error has been corrected with an additional correction related to the distance between the patient and examiner (**working distance**). Spherical power equal to the reciprocal of the working distance (measured in meters) is subtracted to compensate for this additional correction and obtain the patient's refractive correction. The working distance is usually 2/3 m, and the correction to be subtracted for the working distance thus is usually 1.5 D.

Automated refractors are available to rapidly determine the objective refraction, but they are not useful in young children or in adults with significant anterior segment disease.

▶ Subjective Refraction

In cooperative patients, subjective refraction produces more accurate results than objective refraction. It relies on the patient's response to alterations in lens power and orientation, using objective refraction or the patient's current refractive correction as the starting point.

The spherical correction is checked by small changes, initially increasing the plus power so as to overcome any accommodative effort, until the clearest image is obtained. The duochrome test of black letters on red and green backgrounds uses the normal chromatic aberration of the eye to refine spherical correction. When the black letters of the two halves of the chart are equally clear, the end point has been reached.

A **cross cylinder** consists of two planocylindrical lenses of equal power but opposite sign superimposed such that their axes of refractive power lie at right angles to one another. This is equivalent to a spherocylindrical lens in which the power of the cylinder is twice the power of the sphere and of the opposite sign. The cross cylinder allows rapid small changes in the axis and power of a cylindrical correction.

▶ Cycloplegic Refraction

In the determination of full hyperopic refractive correction, either in the management of childhood esotropia or the assessment of eyestrain in adult hyperopes, it is necessary to overcome accommodation. This can usually be achieved in adults by fogging techniques in which plus lenses are used to overcome accommodative effort. But otherwise—and always in children—accommodation has to be relaxed by cycloplegic drugs. Cyclopentolate 1%, 1 drop instilled twice 30 minutes prior to refraction, may be sufficient, but atropine 0.5% or 1% ointment, applied twice a day for 3 days, may be necessary in children with dark irides and in the initial assessment of accommodative esotropia. Parents should be warned of the symptoms of atropine toxicity (fever, flushed face, and rapid pulse) and the necessity for discontinuing treatment, cooling the child with sponge bathing, and—in severe cases—seeking urgent medical assistance.

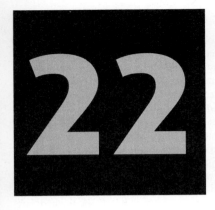

Ophthalmic Therapeutics

Allan J. Flach, PharmD, MD, and
Frederick W. Fraunfelder, MD

22.1 Commonly Used Eye Medications

Allan J. Flach, PharmD, MD

The following is intended to serve as a concise formulary of commonly used ophthalmic drugs. Product leaflets, package inserts, and standard pharmacology and toxicology texts should be consulted for more detailed information.

TOPICAL ANESTHETICS

Topical anesthetics are useful for diagnostic and therapeutic procedures, including tonometry, removal of foreign bodies or sutures, gonioscopy, corneal or conjunctival scraping, and minor surgical operations on the cornea and conjunctiva. Cataract (phacoemulsification) surgery is increasingly being carried out under topical anesthesia, supplemented if necessary by (intracameral) injection of local anesthetic into the anterior chamber (see later in the chapter), or oral or intravenous sedation. One or two instillations of topical anesthetic are usually sufficient, but the dosage may be repeated during the procedure.

Proparacaine, tetracaine, and benoxinate are the most commonly used topical anesthetics. For practical purposes, they can be said to have equivalent anesthetic potency. Lidocaine 3.5% gel (Akten) and cocaine 1%–4% solution are also used for topical anesthesia.

Note: *Topical anesthetics should never be prescribed for home use,* since prolonged application may cause corneal complications and mask serious ocular disease.

▶ Proparacaine (Proxymetacaine) Hydrochloride (Ophthaine, Others)

Preparation: Solution, 0.5%. A combined preparation of proparacaine and fluorescein is available as Fluoracaine.

Dosage: 1 drop and repeat as necessary.

Onset and duration of action: Anesthesia begins within 20 seconds and lasts 10–15 minutes.

Comment: Least irritating of the topical anesthetics and most suitable for corneal scraping for microbiological cultures.

▶ Tetracaine Hydrochloride (Pontocaine)

Preparations: Solution, 0.5% and ointment, 0.5%.

Dosage: 1 drop and repeat as necessary.

Onset and duration of action: Anesthesia occurs within 1 minute and lasts for 15–20 minutes.

Comment: Stings considerably on instillation.

▶ Benoxinate Hydrochloride

Preparation (as Fluress): Solution, 0.4%.

Dosage: 1 drop and repeat as necessary.

Onset and duration of action: Anesthesia begins within 1 or 2 minutes and lasts for 10–15 minutes.

Comment: Benoxinate 0.4% and fluorescein 0.25% (Flurate, Fluress) may be used prior to applanation tonometry.

LOCAL ANESTHETICS FOR INJECTION

Lidocaine, procaine, and mepivacaine are commonly used local anesthetics for eye surgery. Longer-acting agents such as bupivacaine and etidocaine are often mixed with other local anesthetics to prolong the duration of effect. Local anesthetics are extremely safe when used with discretion, but the physician must be aware of the potential systemic toxic action when rapid absorption occurs from the site of the injection, with excessive dosage, or following inadvertent intravascular injection.

The addition of hyaluronidase encourages spreading of the anesthetic and shortens the onset to as little as 1 minute. For these reasons, hyaluronidase is commonly used in peribulbar injections prior to cataract extraction. Injectable anesthetics are used by ophthalmologists most commonly in older patients, who may be susceptible to cardiac arrhythmias; therefore, l-epinephrine should not be used in concentrations greater than 1:200,000.

Lidocaine (Lignocaine) Hydrochloride (Xylocaine)

Owing to its rapid onset and longer action (1–2 hours), lidocaine has become the most commonly used local anesthetic. It is approximately twice as potent as procaine. Up to 30 mL of 1% solution, without epinephrine, may be used safely. In cataract surgery, 10 mL is usually sufficient for peribulbar or sub-Tenon's injections. The maximal safe dose is 4.5 mg/kg without epinephrine and 7 mg/kg with epinephrine. Intracameral preservative-free lidocaine 1% solution is employed for anesthesia in cataract surgery.

Procaine Hydrochloride (Novocaine)

Preparations: Solution, 1%, 2%, and 10%.

Dosage: Approximately 50 mL of a 1% solution can be injected without causing systemic effects. The maximal safe dose is 10 mg/kg.

Duration of action: 45–60 minutes.

Mepivacaine Hydrochloride (Carbocaine, Others)

Preparations: Solution, 1%, 1.5%, 2%, and 3%.

Dosage: Infiltration and nerve block, up to 20 mL of 1% or 2% solution.

Duration of action: Approximately 2 hours.

Comment: Carbocaine is similar to lidocaine in potency. It is usually used in patients who are allergic to lidocaine. The maximum safe dose is 7 mg/kg.

Bupivacaine Hydrochloride (Marcaine, Sensorcaine)

Preparations: Solution, 0.25%, 0.5%, and 0.75%.

Dosage: The 0.75% solution has been used most frequently in ophthalmology. The maximal safe dose in an adult is 250 mg with epinephrine and 200 mg without epinephrine. Bupivacaine is frequently mixed with an equal amount of lidocaine.

Onset and duration of action: The onset of action is slower than that of lidocaine, but it persists much longer (up to 6–10 hours).

Etidocaine Hydrochloride (Duranest)

Preparations: Solution, 1% and 1.5%.

Dosage: The maximal safe dose of etidocaine is 4 mg/kg without epinephrine and 5.5 mg/kg with epinephrine. This agent is frequently mixed with lidocaine for local anesthesia in ophthalmic surgery.

Onset and duration of action: The onset of action is slower than that of lidocaine, but more rapid than that of bupivacaine. The duration of action is approximately twice as long as that of lidocaine (4–8 hours).

MYDRIATICS & CYCLOPLEGICS

Mydriatics and cycloplegics both dilate the pupil. In addition, cycloplegics cause paralysis of accommodation (patient unable to see near objects, for example, printed words). They are commonly used drugs in ophthalmology, singly and in combination. Their prime uses are (1) for dilating the pupils to facilitate ophthalmoscopy; (2) for paralyzing the muscles of accommodation, particularly in young patients, as an aid in refraction; and (3) for dilating the pupil and paralyzing the muscles of accommodation in uveitis to prevent synechia formation and relieve pain and photophobia. Since mydriatics and cycloplegics both dilate the pupil, they should be used with extreme caution in eyes with narrow anterior chamber angles since either a mydriatic or a cycloplegic can cause angle-closure glaucoma in such eyes.

1. MYDRIATICS (SYMPATHOMIMETICS)

Phenylephrine is a mydriatic with no cycloplegic effect.

Phenylephrine Hydrochloride (Neo-Synephrine, Others)

Preparations: Solution, 0.12%, 2.5%, and 10%.

Dosage: 1 drop and repeat in 5–10 minutes.

Onset and duration of action: The effect usually occurs within 30 minutes after instillation and lasts 2–3 hours.

Comment: Phenylephrine is used both singly and with cycloplegics to facilitate ophthalmoscopy, in treatment of uveitis, and to dilate the pupil prior to cataract surgery. The 10% solution should not be used in newborn infants, in cardiac patients, or in patients receiving reserpine, guanethidine, or tricyclic antidepressants, because of increased susceptibility to the vasopressor effects.

2. CYCLOPLEGICS (PARASYMPATHOLYTICS)

Atropine Sulfate

Preparations: Solution, 0.5%–3%; ointment, 0.5% and 1%.

Dosage: For refraction in children, instill 1 drop of 0.25%–0.5% solution in each eye twice a day for 1 or 2 days before the examination and then 1 hour before the examination; ointment, ¼-in ribbon twice a day for 2 days prior to examination.

Onset and duration of action: The onset of action is within 30–40 minutes. A maximal effect is reached in about 2 hours. The effect lasts for up to 2 weeks in a normal eye, but in the presence of acute inflammation, the drug must be instilled 2 or 3 times daily to maintain its effect.

Toxicity: Atropine drops must be used with caution to avoid toxic reactions resulting from systemic absorption. Restlessness and excited behavior with dryness and flushing of the skin of the face, dry mouth, fever, inhibition of sweating, and tachycardia are prominent toxic symptoms, particularly in young children.

Comment: Atropine is an effective and long-acting cycloplegic. In addition to its use for cycloplegia in children, atropine is applied topically 2 or 3 times daily in the treatment of iritis. It is also used to maintain a dilated pupil after intraocular surgical procedures.

Scopolamine Hydrobromide

Preparation: Solution, 0.25%.

Dosage: 1 drop 2 or 3 times daily.

Onset and duration of action: Cycloplegia occurs in about 40 minutes and lasts for 3–5 days when scopolamine is used as an aid to refraction in normal eyes. The duration of action is much shorter in inflamed eyes.

Toxicity: Scopolamine occasionally causes dizziness and disorientation, mainly in older people.

Comment: Scopolamine is an effective cycloplegic. It is used in the treatment of uveitis, in refraction of children, and postoperatively.

Homatropine Hydrobromide

Preparations: Solution, 2% and 5%.

Dosage: For refraction, 1 drop in each eye and repeat 2 or 3 times at intervals of 10–15 minutes.

Onset and duration of action: Maximal cycloplegic effect lasts for about 3 hours, but complete recovery time is about 36–48 hours. In certain cases, the shorter action is an advantage over scopolamine and atropine.

Toxicity: Sensitivity and side effects associated with the topical instillation of homatropine are rare.

Comment: Homatropine is an effective cycloplegic often used in the treatment of uveitis.

Cyclopentolate Hydrochloride (Cyclogyl, Others)

Preparations: Solution, 0.5%, 1%, and 2%.

Dosage: For refraction, 1 drop in each eye and repeat after 10 minutes.

Onset and duration of action: The onset of dilatation and cycloplegia is within 30–60 minutes. The duration of action is less than 24 hours. Comment: Cyclopentolate is more popular than homatropine and scopolamine in refraction because of its shorter duration of action. Occasionally, neurotoxicity may occur, manifested by incoherence, visual hallucinations, slurred speech, and ataxia. These reactions are more common in children.

Tropicamide (Mydriacyl, Others)

Preparations: Solution, 0.5% and 1%; 0.25% with 1% hydroxamphetamine hydrobromide (Paremyd).

Dosage: 1 drop of 1% solution 2 or 3 times at 5-minute intervals.

Onset and duration of action: The time required to reach the maximal cycloplegic effect is usually 20–25 minutes, and the duration of this effect is only 15–20 minutes; therefore, the timing of the examination after instilling tropicamide is important. Complete recovery requires 5–6 hours.

Comment: Tropicamide is an effective mydriatic with weak cycloplegic action and is therefore most useful for ophthalmoscopy.

Cyclopentolate Hydrochloride- Phenylephrine Hydrochloride (Cyclomydril)

Preparations: Solution, 0.2% cyclopentolate hydrochloride and 1% phenylephrine hydrochloride.

Dosage: 1 drop every 5–10 minutes for 2 or 3 doses. Pressure should be applied over the nasolacrimal sac after drop instillation to minimize systemic absorption.

Onset and duration of action: Mydriasis and some cycloplegia occur within the first 3–6 minutes. The duration of action is usually less than 24 hours. This drug combination is of particular value for pupillary dilation in examination of premature and small infants.

DRUGS USED IN THE TREATMENT OF GLAUCOMA

The dose and frequency of administration of therapy should be individualized according to measurements of intraocular pressure, the minimum treatment being used that sufficiently controls the intraocular pressure to adequately prevent optic nerve damage.

1. TOPICAL PROSTAGLANDIN ANALOGS

The prostaglandin analogs reduce intraocular pressure by increasing outflow of aqueous, mainly via the uveoscleral pathway. Each agent may be used alone or in combination with other types of glaucoma medication, but additive effect is more likely when used in conjunction with agents that reduce aqueous production.

Toxicity: All preparations are associated with increased brown pigmentation of the iris, eyelash growth, hyperpigmentation of periorbital skin, conjunctival hyperemia, punctate epithelial keratopathy, and foreign body sensation. In addition, they may aggravate ocular inflammation and have been associated with the development of cystoid macular edema.

▶ Latanoprost (Xalatan)

Preparation: Solution, 0.005%.

Dosage: 1 drop daily at night.

▶ Bimatoprost (Lumigan)

Preparation: Solution, 0.03%.

Dosage: 1 drop daily at night.

▶ Travoprost (Travatan)

Preparation: Solution, 0.004%.

Dosage: 1 drop daily.

▶ Tafluprost (Taflotan, Saflutan)

(Not available in the United States)

Preparation: Solution, 0.0015% (preservative-free)

Dosage: 1 drop daily at night.

▶ Unoprostone Isopropyl (Rescula)

(Not available in the United States)

Preparation: Solution, 0.15%.

Dosage: 2 drops daily.

2. TOPICAL BETA-ADRENERGIC RECEPTOR ANTAGONISTS (SYMPATHOLYTICS)

Beta-adrenergic blocking agents reduce intraocular pressure by suppressing aqueous production.

Toxicity: All preparations, particularly the non-selective agents, have the potential to cause adverse systemic effects (see discussion in separate section), especially bronchoconstriction and bradycardia but also depression, confusion, and fatigue. They are contraindicated in patients with obstructive airways disease, either asthma or chronic obstructive pulmonary disease (COPD), although betaxolol with its relative β_1 receptor selectivity is safer in this context, and in patients with cardiac conduction defects.

▶ Timolol Maleate (Timoptic; Timoptic XE, Timoptic GFS, Betimol)

Preparations: Solution, 0.25% and 0.5%; gel, 0.25% and 0.5%.

Dosage: 1 drop of 0.25% or 0.5% in each eye once or twice daily if needed. One drop of gel once daily.

Comment: Non-selective beta-blocker

▶ Levobunolol Hydrochloride (Betagan)

Preparations: Solution, 0.25% and 0.5%.

Dosage: 1 drop once or twice daily.

Comment: Non-selective beta-blocker, comparable in efficacy to timolol.

▶ Metipranolol Hydrochloride (OptiPranolol)

Preparation: Solution, 0.3%.

Dosage: 1 drop once or twice daily.

Comment: Non-selective beta-blocker, comparable in efficacy to timolol.

▶ Carteolol Hydrochloride (Ocupress)

Preparation: Solution, 1%.

Dosage: 1 drop once or twice daily.

Comment: Non-selective beta-blocker, comparable in efficacy to timolol.

▶ Betaxolol Hydrochloride (Betoptic; Betoptic S)

Preparations: Solution, 0.25% (Betoptic S) and 0.5%.

Dosage: 1 drop once or twice daily.

Comment: Betaxolol's relative β_1 receptor selectivity reduces the risk of pulmonary side effects, but it is less effective at reducing intraocular pressure than the non-selective beta-blockers.

3. TOPICAL ADRENERGIC RECEPTOR AGONISTS (SYMPATHOMIMETICS)

Sympathomimetic drugs, which reduce intraocular pressure by variable effects on production and drainage of aqueous, comprise the **α_2-adrenergic agonists** apraclonidine and brimonidine, and dipivefrin, a pro-drug of the **non-selective agonist** epinephrine.

▶ Apraclonidine Hydrochloride (Iopidine)

Apraclonidine hydrochloride is specifically indicated for prevention and management of intraocular pressure elevations after anterior segment laser procedures, and as adjunctive therapy in patients on maximally tolerated medical therapy who need further reduction of intraocular pressure. It lowers intraocular pressure by decreasing production of aqueous, the exact mechanism of which is not clearly understood, and may also improve aqueous outflow.

Preparation: Solution, 0.5% and 1%.

Dosage: 1 drop of 1% solution before anterior segment laser treatment and a second drop upon completion of the procedure. One drop of 0.5% solution 2 or 3 times a day as short-term adjunctive treatment in glaucoma uncontrolled by other medications.

Comment: Unlike clonidine, apraclonidine does not appear to penetrate blood–tissue barriers easily and produces few side effects. The reported systemic side effects include occasional decreases in diastolic blood pressure, bradycardia, and central nervous system symptoms of insomnia, irritability, and decreased libido. Ocular side effects include conjunctival blanching, upper lid elevation, mydriasis, and burning.

► Brimonidine Tartrate (Alphagan-P)

Brimonidine decreases aqueous production and perhaps also increases aqueous drainage through the uveoscleral pathway.

Preparation: Solution, 0.1 and 0.15%.

Dosage: 1 drop 2 or 3 times daily. May be used as monotherapy or in combination with other glaucoma medications. Frequently used as a replacement drug in patients unable to tolerate beta-blockers.

Toxicity: Brimonidine has only minimal effect on heart rate and blood pressure. Stinging on instillation, conjunctival hyperemia, and dry mouth are common side effects.

► Dipivefrin Hydrochloride (Propine)

Dipivefrin is an esterified form, of epinephrine, which is a non-selective adrenergic agonist that primarily acts by increasing outflow of aqueous but also decreases aqueous production with long-term use. Dipivefin is thought to pass more quickly through the cornea than epinephrine and then is rapidly hydrolyzed to it.

Preparation: Solution, 0.1%.

Dosage: 1 drop twice daily.

Comment: Epinephrine is no longer available for treatment of glaucoma. When it first became available, its advantages over pilocarpine (see later in the chapter) were longer duration of action (12–72 hours) and no miosis, which was especially important in patients with cataracts. However, at least 25% of patients developed local allergies, others complained of headache and heart palpitation, and the outcome of glaucoma drainage surgery was found to be compromised. Local adverse effects are less frequent with dipiverfrin.

4. TOPICAL CARBONIC ANHYDRASE INHIBITORS

Inhibition of carbonic anhydrase in the secretory epithelium of the ciliary body reduces production of aqueous.

The carbonic anhydrase inhibitors in use are sulfonamide derivatives.

Dorzolamide and brinzolamide can be used topically because they have sufficient corneal penetration to reach the ciliary body. They may be used as monotherapy but most frequently are used in combination with other glaucoma medications except for oral carbonic anhydrase inhibitors (see later in the chapter).

Toxicity: Local reactions include burning and stinging, superficial punctate keratopathy, and allergic reactions of the conjunctiva. Bitter after-taste is common. The systemic side effects associated with oral carbonic anhydrase agents are rare.

► Dorzolamide Hydrochloride (Trusopt)

Preparation: Solution, 2%.

Dosage: 1 drop 3 times daily when used alone or twice daily if being used in combination with other topical glaucoma treatment.

► Brinzolamide (Azopt)

Preparation: Suspension, 1%.

Dosage: 1 drop 3 times daily when used alone or twice daily if being used in combination with other topical glaucoma treatment.

5. TOPICAL DIRECT-ACTING CHOLINERGIC AGONISTS (PARASYMPATHOMIMETICS)

All parasympathomimetics decrease intraocular pressure by increasing the outflow of aqueous through the trabecular meshwork.

► Pilocarpine Hydrochloride & Nitrate

Preparations: Solution, 0.25%, 0.5%–6%, 8%, and 10%; gel, 4%. Also available in a sustained-release system (Ocusert).

Dosage: 1 drop up to 6 times a day; a ½-in strip of gel in lower conjunctival cul-de-sac at bedtime.

Comment: Pilocarpine should be avoided in eyes with active uveitis.

► Carbachol

Preparations: Solution, 0.75%, 1.5%, 2.25%, and 3%.

Dosage: 1 drop in each eye 3 or 4 times a day.

Comment: Carbachol is poorly absorbed through the cornea and usually is used if pilocarpine is ineffective. Its duration of action is 4–6 hours. If benzalkonium chloride is used as the vehicle, the penetration of carbachol is significantly increased. The pharmacodynamics of carbachol also include indirect activity.

6. TOPICAL INDIRECT-ACTING ANTICHOLINESTERASE AGENTS

▶ Physostigmine Salicylate & Sulfate (Eserine)

Preparations: Solution, 0.25%, and ointment, 0.25%.

Dosage: 1 drop 3 or 4 times a day or ¼-inch strip of ointment once or twice a day.

Comment: A high incidence of allergic reactions has limited the use of this old and seldom-used anti-glaucoma drug. It can be combined in the same solution with pilocarpine.

The following parasympathomimetics are strong and long-lasting and are used when other antiglaucoma medications fail to control the intraocular pressure. They are employed less frequently than in the past. The miosis produced is extreme; ciliary spasm and myopia are common. Local irritation is common, and phospholine iodide is believed to be cataractogenic in some patients. Pupillary block may occur. With the development of newer antiglaucoma medications, these agents rarely are used.

▶ Echothiophate Iodide (Phospholine Iodide)

Preparations: Solution, 0.03%, 0.06%, 0.125%, and 0.25%.

Dosage: 1 drop once or twice daily or less often, depending on the response.

Comment: Echothiophate iodide is a long-acting drug similar to isoflurophate with the advantages of being water-soluble and causing less local irritation. Systemic toxicity may occur in the form of cholinergic stimulation, including salivation, nausea, vomiting, and diarrhea. Ocular side effects include cataract formation, spasm of accommodation, and iris cyst formation.

▶ Demecarium Bromide (Humorsol)

Preparations: Solution, 0.125% and 0.25%.

Dosage: 1 drop once or twice a day.

Comment: Systemic toxicity similar to that associated with echothiophate iodide may occur.

7. TOPICAL COMBINATION PREPARATIONS

Increasing numbers of topical preparations combining pharmacologically different agents are being developed, mainly advocated to improve compliance but not necessarily resulting in as large a reduction in intraocular pressure as expected from summation of the effects of the individual agents administered separately. Most of them, except Cosopt, are not available in the United States. They include:

Azarga (brinzolamide 1% and timolol 0.5%), 1 drop twice daily.

Combigan (brimonidine 0.2% and timolol 0.5%), 1 drop twice daily.

Cosopt (dorzolamide 2% and timolol 0.5%), 1 drop twice daily.

Duotrav (travoprost 0.004% and timolol 0.5%), 1 drop once daily.

Ganfort (bimatoprost 0.03% and timolol 0.5%) 1 drop once daily.

Xalacom (latanoprost 0.005% and timolol 0.5%), 1 drop once daily in the morning.

8. SYSTEMIC CARBONIC ANHYDRASE INHIBITORS

Systemic administration of carbonic anhydrase inhibitors increases their efficacy, being able to reduce aqueous production by 40%–60%. It is used mainly when intraocular pressure cannot be controlled with topical therapy and in acute situations, including management of acute angle closure when parenteral therapy may be necessitated by vomiting as well as the urgency of the situation. The maximum effect occurs approximately 2 hours after oral administration, lasting 4–6 hours, and 20 minutes after intravenous administration.

Systemic administration is associated with several adverse effects including potassium depletion, particularly if the patient is also on diuretic therapy, acidosis, gastric distress, diarrhea, epidermal necrolysis, renal stone formation, shortness of breath, fatigue, and tingling of the extremities. Developments in topical medications and laser therapy for glaucoma have reduced the use of systemic carbonic anhydrase inhibitors.

▶ Acetazolamide (Diamox)

Preparations and dosages:

Oral: Tablets, 125 mg and 250 mg; give 125–250 mg 2 to 4 times a day (dosage not to exceed 1 g in 24 h). Sustained-release capsules, 500 mg; give 1 capsule once or twice a day.

Parenteral: May give 500-mg ampules intramuscularly or intravenously for short periods in patients who cannot tolerate the drug orally.

▶ Methazolamide (Neptazane)

Preparation: Tablets, 25 and 50 mg.

Dosage: 50–100 mg 2 or 3 times daily (total not to exceed 600 mg/d).

▶ Dichlorphenamide (Daranide)

Preparation: Tablets, 50 mg.

Dosage: Give a priming dose of 100–200 mg followed by 100 mg every 12 hours until the desired response is obtained. The usual maintenance dosage for glaucoma is 25–50 mg 3 or 4 times daily. The total daily dosage should not exceed 300 mg daily.

9. SYSTEMIC OSMOTIC AGENTS

Hyperosmotic agents such as urea, mannitol, and glycerin are used to reduce intraocular pressure by making the plasma hypertonic to aqueous. They are generally used in the management of acute (angle-closure) glaucoma and occasionally preoperatively.

▶ Glycerin (Osmoglyn)

Preparations and dosage: Glycerin is given orally usually as 50% solution with water, orange juice, or flavored normal saline solution over ice (1 mL of glycerin weighs 1.25 g). Dose is 1–1.5 g/kg.

Onset and duration of action: Maximal hypotensive effect occurs in 1 hour and lasts 4–5 hours.

Toxicity: Nausea, vomiting, and headache occasionally occur.

Comment: Oral administration and the absence of diuretic effect are significant advantages of glycerin over the other hyperosmotic agents.

▶ Isosorbide (Ismotic)

Preparation: 45% solution.

Dosage: 1.5 g/kg orally.

Onset and duration of action: Similar to glycerin.

Comment: Unlike glycerin, isosorbide does not produce calories or elevate blood sugar. Other side reactions are similar to glycerin. Each 220 mL of isosorbide contains 4.6 meq of sodium.

▶ Mannitol (Osmitrol)

Preparation: 5%–25% solution for injection.

Dosage: 1.5–2 g/kg intravenously, usually in 20% concentration.

Onset and duration of action: Maximal hypotensive effect occurs in about 1 hour and lasts 5–6 hours.

Comment: Problems with cardiovascular overload and pulmonary edema are more common with this agent because of the large fluid volumes required.

▶ Urea (Ureaphil)

Preparation: 30% solution of lyophilized urea in invert sugar.

Dosage: 1–1.5 g/kg intravenously.

Onset and duration of action: Maximal hypotensive effect occurs in about 1 hour and lasts 5–6 hours.

Toxicity: Accidental extravasation at the injection site may cause local reactions ranging from mild irritation to tissue necrosis.

TOPICAL CORTICOSTEROIDS

▶ Indications

Topical corticosteroid therapy is indicated for inflammatory conditions of the anterior segment of the globe. Some examples are allergic conjunctivitis, uveitis, episcleritis, scleritis, phlyctenulosis, superficial punctate keratitis, interstitial keratitis, vernal conjunctivitis, and postoperative inflammation.

▶ Administration & Dosage

Corticosteroids and their derivatives vary in their anti-inflammatory activity. The potency relative to hydrocortisone is 4 times for prednisolone and 25 times for dexamethasone and betamethasone. Adverse effects are not decreased with the higher-potency drugs even though the therapeutic dosage is lower.

The duration of treatment will vary according to the underlying disease process and may extend from a few days to several months. Initial therapy for a severely inflamed eye consists of instilling drops every 1 or 2 hours while awake. When a favorable response is observed, gradually reduce the dosage and discontinue as soon as possible.

Caution: Adverse effects of topical and periocular corticosteroid therapy are exacerbation or development of microbial keratitis, including reactivation of herpes simplex keratitis, ocular hypertension, including the risk of development of open-angle glaucoma, and rarely cataract formation. (These effects are produced to a lesser degree with systemic corticosteroid therapy, except for development of cataract, typically posterior subcapsular.) Any patient receiving topical corticosteroid therapy should be under the care of an ophthalmologist.

The following is a partial list of the available topical corticosteroids for ophthalmologic use:

Hydrocortisone ointment, 0.5%, 0.12%, 0.125%, and 1%.

Prednisolone acetate suspension, 0.125% and 1%.

Prednisolone sodium phosphate solution, 0.125% and 1%.

Dexamethasone sodium phosphate suspension 0.1%; ointment, 0.05%.

Medrysone suspension, 1%.

Fluorometholone suspension, 0.1% and 0.25%; ointment, 0.1%.

Rimexolone suspension, 1%.

Loteprednol etabonate suspension, 0.5%.

TOPICAL COMBINATION CORTICOSTEROID & ANTI-INFECTIVE AGENTS

There are numerous commercial products containing fixed-dose combinations of corticosteroid and one or more anti-infective agents. They are used by ophthalmologists chiefly to treat conditions in which both agents may be required, for example, marginal keratitis due to a combined staphylococcal infection and allergic reaction, blepharo-conjunctivitis, and phlyctenular keratoconjunctivitis. They are also used postoperatively.

These mixtures should not be used to treat conjunctivitis or blepharitis due to unknown causes. They should not be used as substitutes solely for anti-infective agents but only when a clear indication for corticosteroids exists as well. Mixtures of corticosteroid and anti-infective agents may cause all of the same complications that occur with the topical steroid preparations alone.

ORAL AND TOPICAL NONSTEROIDAL ANTI-INFLAMMATORY AGENTS (NSAIDS)

Oral NSAIDs—indomethacin 75 mg daily, flurbiprofen 150 mg daily, or ibuprofen 600 mg daily—are the first-line treatment for non-necrotizing scleritis. Gastric irritation and hemorrhage are a risk. Topical ophthalmic preparations of several NSAIDs provide ocular bioavailability with little toxicity. These agents act primarily by blocking prostaglandin synthesis through inhibition of cyclooxygenase, the enzyme catalyzing the conversion of arachidonic acid to prostaglandins. Some ophthalmologists use combinations of topical corticosteroids and NSAIDs to manage ocular inflammation.

Currently, flurbiprofen (Ocufen), 0.03%, and suprofen (Profenal), 1%, have been approved by the Food and Drug Administration (FDA) for inhibition of miosis during cataract surgery. Ketorolac (Acular), 0.5%, is approved for use in seasonal allergic conjunctivitis. Diclofenac (Voltaren), 0.1%, and ketorolac (Acular), 0.5%, were the first topically applied NSAIDs approved for treatment of postoperative inflammation following cataract surgery and for relief of pain and photophobia in patients undergoing laser corneal refractive surgery. In addition, two new topically applied NSAIDs, nepafenac suspension (Nevanac), 0.1%, and Bromfenac solution (Xibrom), 0.09%, are now commercially available. Another preparation, indomethacin suspension (Indocid), 1%, is not available in the United States. Although not approved by the FDA for this indication, topically applied NSAIDs are often used to prevent and treat cystoid macular edema following cataract surgery.

OTHER DRUGS USED IN THE TREATMENT OF ALLERGIC CONJUNCTIVITIS

▶ Cromolyn Sodium (Crolom)

Preparation: Solution, 4%.

Dosage: 1 drop 4 to 6 times a day.

Comment: Cromolyn is useful in the treatment of many types of allergic conjunctivitis. Response to therapy usually occurs within a few days but sometimes not until treatment is continued for several weeks. Cromolyn acts by inhibiting the release of histamine and slow-reacting substance of anaphylaxis (SRS-A) from mast cells. It is not useful in the treatment of acute symptoms.

▶ Ketotifen Fumarate (Zaditor)

Preparation: Solution, 0.025%.

Dosage: Twice daily.

Comment: Ketotifen has antihistamine and mast cell–stabilizing activity.

▶ Lodoxamide Tromethamine (Alomide)

Preparation: Solution, 0.1%.

Dosage: 1 drop 4 times a day.

Comment: Lodoxamide is a mast cell stabilizer that inhibits type 1 immediate hypersensitivity reactions. It is indicated in the treatment of allergic reactions of the external ocular tissues, including vernal conjunctivitis and vernal keratitis. As with cromolyn, a therapeutic response does not usually occur until after a few days of treatment.

▶ Nedocromil Sodium (Alocril)

Preparation: Solution, 2%.

Dosage: Twice daily.

Comment: Nedocromil has the rapid onset of an antihistamine and true mast cell–stabilizing activity.

▶ Olapatadine Hydrochloride

Preparations and dosages: Solution, 0.1% (Patanol) twice a day at intervals of 6–8 hours, 0.2% (Pataday) once daily.

Comment: Olapatadine has both antihistamine and mast cell–stabilizing actions.

▶ Levocabastine Hydrochloride (Livostin)

Preparation: Suspension, 0.05%.

Dosage: 1 drop 4 times a day (up to 2 weeks).

Comment: Levocabastine is a selective, potent histamine H1-receptor antagonist. It is useful in reducing acute symptoms of allergic conjunctivitis. Relief of symptoms occurs within minutes after application and lasts up to 2 hours.

▶ Azelastine Hydrochloride (Optivar)

Preparation: Solution, 0.5%.

Dosage: 1 drop 2 to 4 times daily (up to 6 weeks).

Comment: Azelastine is an antihistamine.

▶ Emedastine Difumarate (Emadine)

Preparation: Solution, 0.05%.

Dosage: 1 drop 4 times daily

Comment: Emedastine is an antihistamine.

Epinastine Hydrochloride (Elestat, Relestat)

Preparation: Solution, 0.05%

Dosage: 1 drop twice daily (up to 8 weeks).

Comment: Epinastine is an antihistamine.

Bepotastine Besilate (Bepreve)

Preparation: Solution, 1.5%.

Dosage: 1 drop twice daily.

Comment: Bepostastine is a histamine H1-receptor antagonist and is reported to have mast cell–stabilizing and eosinophil modulating/inhibiting activity.

Ketorolac Tromethamine (Acular)

Preparation: Solution, 0.5%.

Dosage: 1 drop 4 times daily.

Comment: This is the only cyclooxygenase inhibitor approved for allergy by the FDA.

Vasoconstrictors & Decongestants

There are many commercially available over-the-counter (OTC) ophthalmic vasoconstrictive agents. The active ingredients in these agents usually are either ephedrine 0.123%, naphazoline 0.012%–0.1%, phenylephrine 0.12%, or tetrahydrozoline 0.05%–0.15%.

These agents constrict the superficial vessels of the conjunctiva and relieve redness. They also relieve minor surface irritation and itching of the conjunctiva, which can represent a response to noxious or irritating agents such as smog, or swimming pool chlorine. Products also are available that contain an antihistamine, antazoline phosphate 0.25%–0.5%, or pheniramine maleate 0.3%.

TOPICAL IMMUNOMODULATOR

Cyclosporine (Restasis)

Preparation: Emulsion, 0.05%.

Dosage: 1 drop twice daily.

Comment: Cyclosporine suppresses T-cell activation by inhibiting calcineurin and is an effective systemic immunosuppressant, particularly used in transplant medicine. The topical ophthalmic formulation is approved by the FDA to treat dry eye disease, an inflammatory component to the underlying pathogenesis having been established, and increasingly is being tried for other ocular inflammatory diseases, including severe allergic disease, posterior blepharitis, and herpetic stromal keratitis, as well as in high-risk corneal graft patients. Few adverse effects have been reported in individuals treated for up to 4 years.

DRUGS USED IN THE TREATMENT OF OCULAR INFECTIONS

The adult doses of agents usually used to treat intraocular infections, such as exogenous or endogenous endophthalmitis due to bacteria or fungi and viral retinitis, are detailed in Table 22–1.

1. TOPICAL SULFONAMIDES

The sulfonamides are the most commonly used drugs in the treatment of bacterial conjunctivitis. Their advantages include (1) activity against both Gram-positive and Gram-negative organisms, (2) relatively low cost, (3) low allergenicity, and (4) the fact that their use is not complicated by secondary fungal infections, as sometimes occurs following prolonged use of antibiotics.

The most common sulfonamides employed are sulfacetamide sodium and sulfisoxazole.

Sulfacetamide Sodium (Various)

Preparations: Ophthalmic solution, 10%, 15%, and 30%; ointment, 10%.

Dosage: Instill 1 drop frequently, depending on the severity of the conjunctivitis.

Sulfisoxazole (Gantrisin)

Preparations: Ophthalmic solution, 4%; ointment, 4%.

Dosage: As for sulfacetamide sodium (above).

2. TOPICAL ANTIBIOTICS

Topical antibiotics are commonly used in the treatment of external ocular infection, including bacterial conjunctivitis, hordeola, marginal blepharitis, and bacterial corneal ulcers. The frequency of use is related to the severity of the condition. Bacitracin, neomycin, polymyxin, erythromycin, tetracycline, gentamicin, tobramycin, and the fluoroquniolones are the most commonly used commercially available products. They are used separately and in combination as solutions and as ointments. Formulations suitable for topical ophthalmic use of cephalosporins, such as cefazolin (5%) and ceftazidime (5%), as well as higher concentration (fortified) preparations of gentamicin (1.5%) and tobramycin (1.5%) can be obtained from compounding pharmacies.

As a general principle, topical use of antibiotics commonly used systemically should be avoided to reduce the risk of development of resistant organisms and because sensitization of the patient may interfere with future systemic use. However, clinical circumstances may necessitate their use. The availability for ophthalmic use of fluoroquinolones (ciprofloxacin, gatifloxacin, moxifloxacin, norfloxacin, and ofloxacin), with their efficacy against a wide variety of Gram-positive and Gram-negative ocular pathogens, including *Pseudomonas aeruginosa,* has made them the first

Table 22–1. Usual Adult Dose of Selected Antimicrobials for Intraocular Infection[1,2]

	Intravitreal Dose (0.1 mL)[3,4]	Subconjuctival Dose (0.5 mL)[3]	Oral or Intravenous Dose[3]
Acyclovir (Zovirax)			5–10 mg/kg IV every 8 h[5]
Amikacin (Amikin)	0.4 mg	25 mg	6 mg/kg IV every 12 h
Amphotericin B (Fungizone)	0.005–0.01 mg	1–2 mg	Varies (determined on case-by-case basis)
Cefamandole (Mandol)	1–2 mg	75 mg	1 g IV every 6–8 h[6]
Cefazolin (Ancef, Ketzol)	2.25 mg	100 mg	1–1.5 g IV every 6–8 h
Ceftazidime (Fortraz, others)	2 mg	100 mg	2 g IV every 12 h
Ceftriaxone (Rocephin)	1 mg		1–2 g IV once or twice a day
Cidofovir (Vistid)			5 mg/kg IV once weekly for 2 wk for induction therapy[7]
Ciprofloxacin			750 mg orally twice a day
Clindamycin (Cleocin)	0.5–1 mg	30 mg	600–900 mg IV every 8 h
Foscarnet (Foscavir)	1.2–2.4 mg		90 mg/kg IV every 12 h for induction therapy
Ganciclovir (Cytovene)	0.2–2 mg or 4.5 mg implant		5 mg/kg IV every 12 h for induction therapy[5]
Gentamicin (Garamycin, Jenamycin)	0.1–0.2 mg	20 mg	1 mg/kg IV every 8 h[6]
Methicillin (Staphcillin)	2 mg	100 mg	1–2 g IV every 6 h
Miconazole (Monistat)	0.025 mg	5 mg	200–600 mg IV every 8 h
Tobramycin (Nebcin)	0.5 mg	20 mg	1 mg/kg IV every 8 h[6]
Valacyclovir (Valtrex)			1–2 g orally 3 times daily[5]
Valganciclovir (Valcyte)			900 mg orally twice a day for induction therapy[5]
Vancomycin (Vancocin, others)	1 mg	25 mg	1 g IV every 12 h
Voriconazole (Vfend)	0.1 mg		6 mg/kg IV every 12 h for 2 doses then 4 mg/kg IV every 12 h

[1] Modified and reproduced, with permission, from Parke DW, Brinton GS: Endophthalmitis. In: *Infections of the Eye,* 2nd ed. Tabara KF, Hyndiuk RA (editors). Little Brown, 1996.
[2] Higher doses have been recommended in some cases. The doses listed here are considered appropriate by the present author based on drug-toxicity studies.
[3] Principal theory for microbial endophthalmitis is intravitreal, supplemented by subconjunctival and topical therapy especially if primary ocular surface infection. Systemic therapy does not appear to be of additional advantage in exogenous endophthalmitis following primary intraocular surgery but is indicated in endogenous endophthalmitis and for the treatment and prophylaxis of endophthalmitis complicating ocular trauma.
[4] Intravitreal antibiotic preparations should not contain preservatives.
[5] Renal excretion. Dose adjusted according to creatinine clearance.
[6] Nephrotoxic. Dose adjusted according to creatinine clearance and body weight.
[7] Nephrotoxic. Pretreatment with probenecid and adequate hydration required.

choice for treatment of corneal ulcers and resistant bacterial conjunctivitis.

Bacitracin

Preparation: Ointment, 500 U/g. Commercially available in combinations with polymyxin B.

Comment: Most Gram-positive organisms are sensitive to bacitracin. It is not used systemically because of its nephrotoxicity.

Neomycin

Preparations: Solution, 2.5 and 5 mg/mL; ointment, 3.5–5 mg/g. Commercially available in combinations with bacitracin and polymyxin B.

Dosage: Apply ointment or drops 3 or 4 times daily. Solutions containing 50–100 mg/mL have been used for corneal ulcers.

Comment: Effective against Gram-negative and Gram-positive organisms. Neomycin is usually combined with some other drug to widen its spectrum of activity. It is best known in ophthalmologic practice as Neosporin, both in ointment and solution form, in which it is combined with polymyxin and bacitracin. Contact skin sensitivity develops in 5% of patients if the drug is continued for longer than a week.

Polymyxin B

Preparations: Ointment, 10 000 U/g; suspension, 10 000 U/mL. Commercially available in combination with bacitracin and neomycin.

Comment: Effective against many Gram-negative organisms.

Erythromycin

Preparation: Ointment, 0.5%.

Comment: Particularly effective in staphylococcal conjunctivitis. It may be used instead of silver nitrate in prophylaxis of ophthalmia neonatorum.

Tetracyclines

Preparations: Suspension, 10 mg/mL; ointment, 10 mg/g.

Comment: Tetracycline, oxytetracycline, and chlortetracycline have limited uses in ophthalmology because their effectiveness is so often impaired by the development of resistant strains. Solutions of these compounds are unstable with the exception of Achromycin in sesame oil, which is widely used in the treatment of trachoma. Ointment may be used for prophylaxis of ophthalmia neonatorum.

Gentamicin (Garamycin, Genoptic, Gentacidin, Gentak)

Preparations: Solution, 3 mg/mL; ointment, 3 mg/g.

Comment: Gentamicin is widely accepted for use in serious ocular infections, especially corneal ulcers caused by Gram-negative organisms. It is also effective against many Gram-positive staphylococci but is not effective against streptococci. Many strains of bacteria resistant to gentamicin have developed.

Tobramycin (Tobrex, Aktop)

Preparations: Solution, 3 mg/mL; ointment, 3 mg/g.

Comment: Similar antimicrobial activity to gentamicin but more effective against streptococci. Best reserved for treatment of *Pseudomonas keratitis,* for which it is more effective.

Chloramphenicol (Chloromycetin, Chloroptic)

(Not available in the United States)

Preparations: Solution, 5 and 10 mg/mL; ointment, 10 mg/g.

Comment: Chloramphenicol is effective against a wide variety of Gram-positive and Gram-negative organisms. It rarely causes local sensitization, but cases of aplastic anemia have been associated with long-term therapy.

Ciprofloxacin (Ciloxan)

Preparation: Solution, 3 mg/mL.

Dosage: For treatment of conjunctivitis, 1 drop every 2–4 hours. For treatment of corneal ulcers, 1 drop every hour during the day and every 2 hours during the night for 48 hours, then gradually reducing.

Gatifloxacin (Zymar)

Preparation: Solution, 3 mg/mL.

Dosage: For conjunctivitis and corneal ulcers, same as that of ciprofloxacin.

Comment: This fourth-generation fluoroquinolone is more effective against a broader spectrum of Gram-positive bacteria and atypical mycobacteria than earlier fluoroquinolones.

Levofloxacin (Iquix, Oftaquix, Quixin)

Preparation: Solution, 5 mg/mL and 15 mg/mL.

Dosage: For conjunctivitis and corneal ulcers, same as that of ciprofloxacin.

Moxifloxacin (Vigamox)

Preparation: Solution, 5 mg/mL.

Dosage: For conjunctivitis and corneal ulcers, same as that of ciprofloxacin.

Comment: This fourth-generation fluoroquinolone is more effective against a broader spectrum of Gram-positive bacteria and atypical mycobacteria than earlier fluoroquinolones.

Norfloxacin (Chibroxin)

Preparation: Solution, 3 mg/mL.

Dosage: For conjunctivitis and corneal ulcers, same as that of ciprofloxacin.

Ofloxacin (Ocuflox)

Preparation: Solution, 3 mg/mL.

Dosage: For conjunctivitis and corneal ulcers, same as that of ciprofloxacin.

Fusidic Acid (Fucithalmic)

(Not available in the United States)

Preparation: Gel, 1%.

Dosage: Applied twice daily.

Comment: Popular for treatment of bacterial conjunctivitis because of twice-daily dosage.

3. COMBINATION ANTIBACTERIAL AGENTS

Several ophthalmic preparations are available that contain a mixture of antibiotics and bacteriostatic agents (Table 22–2).

4. TOPICAL ANTIFUNGAL AGENTS

Natamycin (Natacyn)

Preparation: Suspension, 5%.

Dosage: Instill 1 drop every 1–2 hours.

Comment: Effective against filamentary and yeast forms. Initial drug of choice for most mycotic corneal ulcers.

Nystatin (Mycostatin)

Nystatin is not available in ophthalmic ointment form, but the dermatologic preparation (100 000 U/g) is not irritating to ocular tissues and can be used in the treatment of fungal infection of the eye.

Table 22–2. Some Combination Antibiotic Preparations

Generic Name	Trade Name
Bacitracin and polymyxin B	Ak-Poly-Bac, Polycin-B, PolyTracin
Bacitracin (or gramicidin), neomycin, and polymyxin B	Various
Oxytetracycline and polymyxin B	Terramycin w/Polymyxin B, Terak
Polymyxin B and trimethoprim	Polytrim

Amphotericin B (Fungizone)

Amphotericin B is more effective than nystatin but not available in ophthalmic ointment form. The dermatologic preparation is highly irritating. A solution (1.5–8 mg/mL of distilled water in 5% dextrose) must be made up in the pharmacy from the powdered drug. Many patients have extreme ocular discomfort following application of this drug.

Miconazole (Monistat)

A 1% solution is available in the form of an intravenous preparation that may be instilled directly into the eye. The drug is not available in an ophthalmologic form.

Fluconazole (Diflucan)

An 0.2% parenteral preparation is available and may be instilled into the eye. No ophthalmologic product is available.

5. ANTIVIRAL AGENTS (ALSO SEE TABLE 22–1)

Idoxuridine (Herplex)

Preparations: Ophthalmic solution, 0.1%; ointment, 0.5%.

Dosage: 1 drop every hour during the day and every 2 hours at night. With improvement (as determined by fluorescein staining), the frequency of instillation is gradually reduced. The ointment may be used 4 to 6 times daily, or the solution may be used during the day and the ointment at bedtime.

Comment: Used in the treatment of herpes simplex keratitis. Epithelial infection usually improves within a few days. Therapy should be continued for 3 or 4 days after apparent healing. Many ophthalmologists still prefer to denude the affected corneal epithelium and not use idoxuridine.

Vidarabine (Vira-A)

Preparation: Ophthalmic ointment, 3%.

Dosage: In herpetic epithelial keratitis, apply 4 times daily for 7–10 days.

Comment: Vidarabine is effective against herpes simplex virus but not other RNA or DNA viruses. It is effective in some patients unresponsive to idoxuridine. Vidarabine interferes with viral DNA synthesis. The principal metabolite is arabinosylhypoxanthine (Ara-Hx). The drug is effective against herpetic corneal epithelial disease and has limited efficacy in stromal keratitis or uveitis. It may cause cellular toxicity and delay corneal regeneration. The cellular toxicity is less than that of idoxuridine.

Trifluridine (Viroptic)

Preparation: Solution, 1%.

Dosage: 1 drop every 2 hours (maximum total, 9 drops daily).

Comment: Acts by interfering with viral DNA synthesis. More soluble than either idoxuridine or vidarabine and probably more effective in stromal disease.

Acyclovir (Zovirax)

Preparations: Ointment, 3% (Not available in the United States); Tablets, 200, 400, and 800 mg.

Comment: Acyclovir is an antiviral agent with inhibitory activity against herpes simplex types 1 and 2, varicella-zoster virus, Epstein-Barr virus, and cytomegalovirus. It is phosphorylated initially by virus-specific thymidine kinase to acyclovir monophosphate and then by cellular kinases to acyclovir triphosphate, which inhibits viral DNA polymerase. Thus, there is a marked selectivity for virus-infected cells. Acyclovir has low toxicity. No commercial ophthalmic preparation is currently available in the United States; a topical product available for treatment of genital herpes should not be used in the eye. An oral preparation is available that may be used for treatment of selected herpes zoster ocular infections.

Ganciclovir (Vitrasert)

Preparation: Intravitreal implant, 4.5 mg.

Dosage: Replacement every 5–8 months as required.

Comment: The ganciclovir intravitreal insert allows treatment of cytomegalovirus retinitis without the adverse effects of systemic therapy.

DIAGNOSTIC DYE SOLUTIONS

Fluorescein Sodium

Preparations: Solution, 2%, in single-use disposable units; as sterile paper strips; as 10% sterile solution for intravenous use in fluorescein angiography.

Dosage: 1 drop.

Comment: Used as a diagnostic agent for detection of corneal epithelial defects, in applanation tonometry, and in fitting contact lenses.

Rose Bengal

Preparation: Solution, 1%, and strips, 1.3 mg.

Dosage: 1 drop.

Comment: Used in diagnosis of keratoconjunctivitis sicca; the mucous shreds and devitalized corneal epithelium stain with rose bengal.

TEAR REPLACEMENT & LUBRICATING AGENTS

Methylcellulose and related chemicals, polyvinyl alcohol and related chemicals, and gelatin are used in the formulation of artificial tears, ophthalmic lubricants, contact lens solutions, and gonioscopic lens solutions. These agents are particularly useful in the treatment of keratoconjunctivitis sicca (see Chapter 5).

To increase viscosity and prolong corneal contact time, methylcellulose is sometimes added to eye solutions (eg, pilocarpine). Preservative-free preparations are available for use in patients with sensitivities to these substances.

CORNEAL DEHYDRATING AGENTS

Dehydrating solutions and ointments applied topically to the eye reduce corneal edema by creating an osmotic gradient in which the tear film is made hypertonic to the corneal tissues. Temporary clearing of corneal edema results.

Preparations: Anhydrous glycerin solution (Ophthalgan); hypertonic sodium chloride 2% and 5% ointment and solution (Absorbonac, AkNaCl, Hypersal, Muro-128).

Dosage: 1 drop of solution or ¼-in strip of ointment to clear cornea. May be repeated every 3–4 hours.

TREATMENT OF NEOVASCULAR AGE-RELATED MACULAR DEGENERATION

Ranibizumab (Lucentis)

Preparation: Intravitreal injection, 0.5mg (0.05 mL).

Dosage: Monthly injection for 3 months then repeated according to disease activity.

Pegaptanib Sodium (Macugen)

Preparation: Intravitreal injection, 0.3mg (0.1mL).
Dosage: One injection every 6 weeks.

Bevacizumab (Avastin)

Comment: Off-label use of bevacizumab compounded to 1.25 mg in 0.05 mL is common.

22.2 Ocular & Systemic Side Effects of Drugs

Frederick W. Fraunfelder, MD

Ocular drugs can cause ocular or systemic reactions, and systemic medications may cause an adverse ocular reaction. Preservatives in topical ocular medications may also be associated with side effects. Tables 22–3 to 22–5 list possible ocular and systemic side effects of some ocular and systemic medications. This is not a complete listing. The reader is advised to consult product labels and the references at the end of this chapter.

SYSTEMIC SIDE EFFECTS OF TOPICAL BETA-BLOCKERS

Similar considerations should be applied to all topical ocular drugs, but beta-adrenoreceptor blocking drugs (beta-blockers) such as timolol particularly are known to cause systemic side effects. They are commonly used in the treatment of elevated intraocular pressure but have been associated with severe and sometimes fatal reactions. Plasma drug concentrations sufficient to cause systemic adrenoceptor blocking effects can occasionally result from topical ocular administration. When topical ocular timolol is administered in infants, blood levels are often more than 6 times what minimum therapeutic levels would be if the drug were given orally. If the lacrimal outflow system is functioning, an estimated 80% of a timolol eye drop is absorbed from the nasal mucosa and passes almost directly into the vascular system. This is called the first-order pass effect and is true for all drugs that can be easily absorbed through mucosal tissue in the head. The venous drainage is to the right atrium (first pass), and this blood containing the drug is pumped back to various target organs before returning to the left atrium (second pass). This blood containing the drug then reaches the liver or kidney, where it is detoxified. Therefore, a small amount applied to the nasal mucosa can result in therapeutic blood levels, whereas if given orally, its first pass includes absorption via the gastrointestinal tract and then the liver, where 80%–90% is detoxified before reaching the right atrium. In the United States, approximately 8% of the white population, 24% of the black population, and 1% of the Far Eastern population (Japanese, Chinese) lack the cytochrome P450 enzyme that metabolizes timolol. Therefore, some groups are at higher risk of developing systemic side effects.

Cardiopulmonary histories should be taken for candidates of beta-blocker glaucoma therapy. Pulmonary function studies should be considered in patients with bronchoconstrictive disease, and electrocardiograms should be ordered on selected patients with cardiac disease. Specifically, the precautions set forth in the package insert should be heeded carefully. Patients with known bronchial asthma, chronic respiratory or cardiovascular disease, or sinus bradycardia may need screening before using topical beta-blockers. The drugs should be used with caution in patients receiving other systemic beta-blocking agents. Although the β_1 receptor selectivity of betaxolol reduces the risk of pulmonary side effects, this is counterbalanced by its lesser efficacy at reducing intraocular pressure.

WAYS TO DIMINISH SYSTEMIC SIDE EFFECTS

One important principle in avoiding systemic side effects from topical ophthalmic medications is to prevent overdosing. The physician should prescribe the lowest concentration of medication that will be therapeutically effective. Only 1 drop of medication is needed at each dosage, since the volume the conjunctival sac can hold is much less than 1 drop. The proper method of topical administration of ophthalmic medication is as follows:

1. Position the patient with head tilted back.

2. Grasp the lower eyelid below the lashes and gently pull the lid away from the eye (Figure 22–1).

3. Instill 1 drop of medication into the inferior cul-de-sac nearest the involved area, taking care that the tip of the medication bottle does not touch the lashes or eyelids, thus avoiding contamination (Figure 22–2).

4. To deepen the inferior cul-de-sac, the lower eyelid should then be gently lifted upward to make contact with the upper lid as the eye looks down (Figure 22–3).

5. The eyelids should be kept closed for 3 minutes to prevent blinking, which pumps the drug into the nose and increases systemic absorption. The patient may be shown how to obstruct the lacrimal drainage system with firm pressure over the inner corner of the closed eyelids, and this may even be more important than lid closure (Figure 22–4).

6. Excess medication in the medial canthus should be blotted away before pressure is released or the eyelids opened. The patient receiving multiple topical medications should wait for 10 minutes between doses so that the first drug will not be washed out of the eye by the second.

NATIONAL REGISTRY OF DRUG-INDUCED OCULAR SIDE EFFECTS

The National Registry of Drug-Induced Ocular Side Effects (NRDIOSE) is a clearinghouse of drug information on ocular toxicology based at the Casey Eye Institute, Oregon Health and Science University. The principle underlying its

Table 22–3. Examples of Adverse Ocular Effects Secondary to Systemic Drugs

Drug	Adverse Effects	Drug	Adverse Effects
Acetazolamide	Epidermal necrolysis, myopia	Levonorgestrel	Pseudotumor cerebri
Amiodarone	Vortex keratopathy (Figure 15-40), thyroid ophthalmopathy (Figure 15-23), optic neuropathy	Linezolid	Optic neuropathy
		Methyldopa	Conjunctivitis
Amphetamines	Elevation of intraocular pressure	Minocycline	Papilledema
Anticholinergics	Angle-closure glaucoma, accommodative paresis, nystagmus, dry eyes	Morphine	Miosis
		Nalidixic acid	Papilledema
Barbiturates	Epidermal necrolysis, ptosis, optic atrophy	Naproxen	Corneal opacity
Beta-adrenoreceptor agonists	Angle-closure glaucoma	Oral contraceptives	Retinal vascular occlusion, optic neuropathy, papilledema
Bisphosphonates	Scleritis, episcleritis, uveitis	Paroxetine	Angle-closure glaucoma
Busulfan	Cataract	Penicillamine	Extraocular muscle paralysis, ptosis, optic neuritis
Cardiac glycosides	Retinal degeneration, changes in color vision	Phenothiazines	Conjunctival deposits, corneal opacity, oculogyric crisis, pigmentation of lens, retinal degeneration
Chloramphenicol	Optic neuropathy		
Chloroquine, hydroxychloroquine	Vortex keratopathy, retinal degeneration		
		Phenytoin	Nystagmus, extraocular muscle paralysis
Chlorpropamide	Epidermal necrolysis, corneal opacity, extraocular muscle paralysis	Quinacrine	Conjunctival deposits
Cisplatin	Optic neuropathy	Quinine	Retinal infarction
Clofazimine	Conjunctival deposits, corneal opacity	Retinoids	Papilledema
Corticosteriods	Elevation of intraocular pressure, cataract	Rifampin	Optic neuritis
Desferrioxmine	Retinopathy, optic neuropathy, lens opacities	Salicylates	Nystagmus, retinal hemorrhage
Diazepam	Nystagmus	Sildenafil	Blue-tinged vision, optic neuropathy
Disulfiram	Optic neuropathy	Statins	Diplopia, bleparoptosis, ophthalmoplegia
Doxycycline	Papilledema	Sulfonamides	Epidermal necrolysis, myopia
Ethambutol	Optic neuropathy	Tacrolimus	Optic neuropathy
Fluoroquinolones	Diplopia	Tamoxifen	Retinal and corneal deposits, optic neuropathy
Fluorouracil	Lacrimal obstruction	Tamsulosin	Complications during (floppy-iris syndrome) and after cataract surgery
Gold salts	Conjunctival deposits, corneal opacity, nystagmus, pigmentation of lens		
		Tetracyclines	Papilledema
Haloperidol	Cataract	Thioridazine	Corneal and lenticular pigmentation, retinal degeneration, oculogyric crisis
Hepatitis B vaccine	Uveitis		
Indomethacin	Corneal opacity	Topiramate	Angle-closure glaucoma, myopia
Interferon	Optic neuropathy	Tricyclic antidepressants	Angle-closure glaucoma, accommodative paresis
Isoniazid	Optic neuropathy		
Isotretinoin	Conjunctivitis, corneal opacity, papilledema, pseudotumor cerebri	Vigabatrin	Visual field constriction
		Vitamin A	Conjunctival deposits, papilledema
Ketamine	Nystagmus	Vitamin D	Conjunctival deposits, corneal opacity

Table 22–4. Examples of Adverse Systemic Effects of Topical Ocular Medications

Medication	Adverse Effects
Anesthetics, topical local Benoxinate, proparacaine, tetracaine	Allergic reactions, anaphylactic reactions, convulsions, faintness, hypotension, syncope
Antibiotics Chloramphenicol Sulfacetamide, sulfamethizole, sulfisoxazole Tetracycline	Bone marrow depression, including aplastic anemia; gastrointestinal symptoms Photosensitivity, epidermal necrolysis Photosensitivity, skin discoloration
Anticholinergics Atropine, homatropine, scopolamine, cyclopentolate, tropicamide	Confusion, dermatitis, dry mouth, excitement, fever, flushed skin, hallucinations, psychosis, tachycardia, thirst, amnesia, ataxia, convulsions, disorientation dysarthria
Anticholinesterases, long-acting Demecarium, echothiophate, isoflurophate	Abdominal cramps, diarrhea, fatigue, nausea, rhinorrhea, weight loss
Anticholinesterases, short-acting Neostigmine, physostigmine	Abdominal cramps, depigmentation, diarrhea, vomiting
Anti-inflammatory agents Corticosteroids	Exogenous Cushing's syndrome
Beta-adrenoceptor blocker Timolol, betaxolol, levobunolol, metipranolol, carteolol	Asthma, brachycardia, cardiac arrhythmia, confusion, depression, dizziness, dyspnea, hallucinations, impotence, myasthenia, psychosis
Parasympathomimetics Carbachol, pilocarpine	Abdominal cramps, diarrhea, hypotension, increased salivation, muscle tremors, nausea, respiratory distress, rhinorrhea, slurred speech, sweating, vomiting, weakness
Sympathomimetics Ephedrine, epinephrine, hydroxyamphetamine, phenylephrine	Cardiac arrhythmias, hypertension, palpitations, subarachnoid hemorrhage, tachycardia

Table 22–5. Examples of Adverse Ocular Effects of Topical Ocular Medications

Medication	Adverse Effects
Anesthetics, local Benoxinate, proparacaine, tetracaine	Allergic reactions, corneal opacity, decreased corneal wound healing
Antibiotics Tetracycline Neomycin	Allergic reactions, corneal discoloration Allergic reactions, follicular conjunctivitis, keratitis
Anticholinergics Cyclopentolate, tropicamide	Angle-closure glaucoma, blurred vision, photophobia
Anticholinesterases Demecarium, echothiophate, isoflurophate	Accommodative spasm, cataract, depigmentation of lids, iris cysts, lacrimal outflow obstruction
Anti-inflammatory agents Corticosteroids	Cataracts, corneal infection, decreased corneal wound healing, glaucoma

(continued)

Table 22–5. Examples of Adverse Ocular Effects of Topical Ocular Medications (*continued*)

Medication	Adverse Effects
Antiglaucoma medications Latanoprost, bimatoprost, travoprost	Increase iris pigment, increase length and darkening of eyelashes, new lashes, anterior uveitis
Antivirals Idoxuridine, trifluridine, vidarabine	Cicatricial pseudopemphigoid, keratitis, lacrimal outflow obstruction
Beta-adrenoceptor blocker Timolol	Blepharoconjunctivitis, corneal anesthesia, diplopia, dry eyes, keratitis, ptosis
Parasympathomimetic Pilocarpine	Accommodative spasm, cicatricial pseudopemphigoid, corneal haze (gel), myopia, retinal detachment
Preservatives Benzalkonium chloride, phenyl mercuric nitrate, thimerosal	Allergic reactions, corneal opacity, keratitis
Sympathomimetics Dipivefrin Epinephrine	Allergic reactions, angle-closure glaucoma, follicular conjunctivitis Cicatricial pseudopemphigoid, cystoid macular edema; discoloration of cornea, conjunctiva, and soft contact lens; lacrimal outflow obstruction

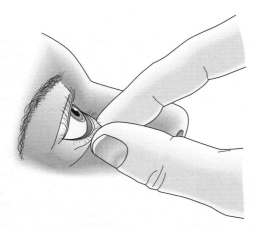

▲ **Figure 22–1.** With the patient's head tilted back, grasp the lower eyelid below the lashes and gently pull the lid away from the eye.

establishment is the assumption that the suspicions of practicing clinicians regarding possible ocular toxicity of drugs can be pooled to help detect significant adverse ocular side effects from these medications. Physicians who wish to report suspected adverse drug reactions or would like to receive references pertaining to the data in Tables 22–3 to 22–5 should make contact via www.eyedrugregistry.com, or call or fax the Casey Eye Institute, OHSU Foundation, Mailstop 45, PO Box 4000, Portland, OR 97208-9852 (Fax: 503-494-4286).

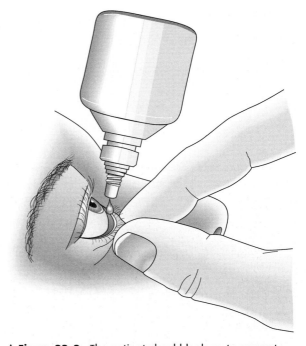

▲ **Figure 22–2.** The patient should look up to prevent the medication from first "hitting" the cornea, which stimulates tearing and dilutes the medication. One drop of solution or a "match head" amount of ointment should be placed in the inferior cul-de-sac, without touching the bottle to the lashes or eyelids (to prevent contamination).

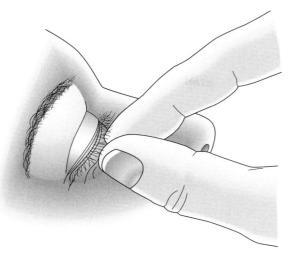

▲ **Figure 22–3.** While the patient is looking downward, gently lift the lower eyelid to make contact with the upper lid.

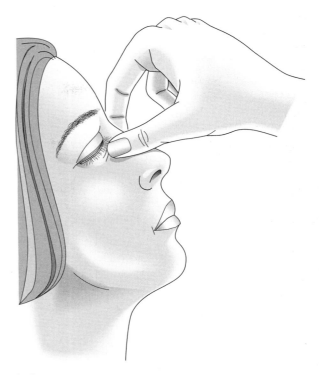

▲ **Figure 22–4.** For 2 minutes or more, firm pressure is maintained with the forefinger or thumb over the inner corner of the closed eyelids. Lid closure is more important than pressure over the lacrimal sac in decreasing systemic absorption. Any excess medication should be blotted away before pressure is released or the eye is opened.

REFERENCES

Commonly Used Eye Medications

Donnenfeld E, Pflugelder SC: Topical ophthalmic cyclosporine: pharmacology and clinical uses. Surv Ophthalmol 2009;54:321. [PMID: 19422961]

Ezra DG, Allan BDS: Topical anaesthesia alone versus topical anaesthesia with intracameral lidocaine for phacoemulsification. Cochrane Database Syst Rev 2007;18:CD005276. [PMID: 17636793]

Ezra DG, Nambiar A, Allan BD: Supplementary intracameral lidocaine for phacoemulsification under topical anaesthesia. A meta-analysis of randomized controlled trials. Ophthalmology 2008;115:455. [PMID:18061271]

Flach AJ: The importance of eyelid closure and nasolacrimal occlusion following ocular instillation of topical glaucoma medications and the need for the universal inclusion of one of these techniques in all patient treatments and clinical studies. Trans Amer Ophthalmol Soc 2009;106:138. [PMID: 19277229]

Flach AJ: Proposed mandate for instruction and labeling regarding the use of eye drops. Arch Ophthalmol 2009;127:1207. [PMID: 19752433]

Ho AL, Zakrzewski PA, Braga-Mele R: The effect of combined topical-intracameral anaesthesia on neuroleptic requirements during cataract surgery. Can J Ophthalmol 2010;45:52. [PMID: 20130711]

Kaiserman I, Fendyur A, Vinker S: Topical beta blockers in asthmatic patients – is it safe? Curr Eye Res 2009;34:517. [PMID: 19899964]

Kernt M, Kampik A: Endophthalmitis: pathogenesis, clinical presentation, management, and perspectives. Clin Ophthalmol 2010;4:121. [PMID: 20390032]

Kim SJ, Flach AJ, Jampol LM: Nonsteroidal anti-inflammatory drugs in ophthalmology. Surv Ophthalmol 2010;55:108. [PMID: 20159228]

Pelosini L, Treffene S, Hollick EJ: Antibacterial activity of preservative-free topical anesthetic drops in current use in ophthalmology departments. Cornea 2009;28:58. [PMID: 19092407]

Yeniad B, Canturk S, Esin Ozdemir F, Alparsian N, Akarcay K: Toxic keratopathy due to abuse of topical anesthetic drugs. Cutan Ocul Toxicol 2010;29:105. [PMID: 20236030]

Ocular & Systemic Side Effects of Drugs

Bell CM, Hatch WV, Fischer HD, et al: Association between tamsulosin and serious ophthalmic adverse events in older men following cataract surgery. JAMA 2009;301:1991. [PMID: 19454637]

Fraunfelder FT: *Drug-Induced Ocular Side Effects and Drug Interactions*, 5th ed. Butterworth & Heinemann, 2001.

Fraunfelder FT, Roy FH (editors): *Current Ocular Therapy*, 5th ed. Saunders, 2001.

Fraunfelder FW: Drug-induced ocular inflammatory diseases. Drugs Today 2007;43:117. [PMID: 17353948]

Fraunfelder FW, Fraunfelder FT: Evidence for a probable causal relationship between tretinoin, acitretin, and etretinate and intracranial hypertension. J Neuroophthalmol 2004;24:214. [PMID: 15348987]

Fraunfelder FW, Fraunfelder FT, Keates EU: Topiramate-associated acute, bilateral, secondary angle-closure glaucoma. Ophthalmology 2004;111:109. [PMID: 14711721]

Fraunfelder FW, Fraunfelder FT: Ocular side effects recently identified by the National Registry of Drug-Induced Ocular Side Effects. Ophthalmology 2004;111:1275. [PMID: 15234126]

Fraunfelder FW, Fraunfelder FT: Diplopia and fluoroquinolones. Ophthalmology 2009;116:1814. [PMID: 19643481]

Fraunfelder FW, Richards AB: Diplopia, blepharoptosis, and ophthalmoplegia and 3-hydroxy-3-methyl-glutaryl-CoA reductase inhibitor use. Ophthalmology 2008;115:2282. [PMID: 18930555]

Fraunfelder FW, Suhler EB, Fraunfelder FT: Hepatitis B vaccine and uveitis: an emerging hypothesis suggested from 32 case reports. Cutan Ocul Toxicol 2010;29:26. [PMID: 19947819]

French DD, Margo CE: Postmarketing surveillance rates of uveitis and scleritis with bisphosphonates among a national veteran cohort. Retina 2008;28:889. [PMID: 18536608]

Laties AM: Vision disorders and phosphodiesterase type 5 inhibitors: a review of the evidence to date. Drug Saf 2009;32:1. [PMID: 19132801]

Lloyd MJ, Fraunfelder FW: Drug-induced optic neuropathies. Drugs Today 2007;43:827. [PMID: 18174968]

Panday VA, Rhee DJ: Review of sulfonamiced-induced acute myopia and acute bilateral angle-closure glaucoma. Compr Ophthalmol Update 2007;8:271. [PMID: 18201514]

Lasers in Ophthalmology

23

N. Victor Chong, MD, FRCS, FRCOphth

Ophthalmology was the first medical specialty to utilize laser energy in patient treatment, and it still accounts for more laser operations than any other specialty.

The main use of ophthalmic lasers was to treat various intraocular conditions. The transparency of the optical media allows laser light to be focused upon the intraocular structures without the need for endoscopy. Lasers are now used in many other areas of ophthalmic practice, including refractive surgery, cosmetic eyelid surgery, and diagnostic imaging of ocular structures.

Because laser surgery irreversibly changes tissue, ocular laser surgery should be performed only by ophthalmologists with laser experience.

OCULAR LASER SYSTEMS

The word "laser" is an acronym for light amplification by stimulated emission of radiation. Most sources of visible light radiate energy at different wavelengths (ie, different colors) and at random time intervals (noncoherent). The unique properties of laser energy are monochromaticity (single wavelength), spatial coherence, and high density of electrons. These allow focusing of laser beams to extremely small spots with very high-energy densities.

A laser consists of a transparent crystal rod (solid-state laser), or a gas- or liquid-filled cavity (gas or fluid laser) constructed with a fully reflective mirror at one end and a partially reflective mirror at the other. Surrounding the rod or cavity is an optical or electrical source of energy that will raise the energy level of the atoms within the rod or cavity to a high and unstable level, a process known as population inversion. When the excited atoms spontaneously decay back to a lower-energy level, their excess energy is released in the form of light. This light can be emitted in any direction. In a laser cavity, however, light emitted along the long axis of the cavity can bounce back and forth between the mirrors, setting up a standing wave that stimulates the remaining excited atoms to release their energy into the standing wave, producing an intense beam of light that exits the cavity through the partially reflective mirror. All of the light produced has the same wavelength (monochromatic) and phase (coherent), with little tendency to spread out (low divergence). The laser light energy can be emitted continuously or in pulses, which may have pulse durations of nanoseconds or less.

MECHANISMS OF LASER EFFECTS

▶ Photocoagulation

The principal lasers used in ophthalmic therapy are the thermal lasers, in which tissue pigments absorb the light and convert it into heat, thus raising the target tissue temperature high enough to coagulate and denature the cellular components.

These lasers are used for retinal photocoagulation; for treatment of diabetic retinopathy (Figure 23–1), retinal vein occlusions, and retinopathy of prematurity; for sealing of retinal holes; for photocoagulation of the trabecular meshwork, iris, and ciliary body in the treatment of glaucoma; and for the treatment of both benign (eg, choroidal hemangioma) and malignant (eg, choroidal melanoma and retinoblastoma) intraocular tumors.

These laser photocoagulators operate in continuous mode or very rapidly pulsed (thermal) mode. The green argon laser has been the standard but others include the krypton red laser; the solid-state diode laser, producing a near-infrared wavelength; the tunable dye laser, producing wavelengths from green to red; the frequency-doubled Nd:YAG laser, producing green light; and the thermal mode Nd:YAG laser, producing infrared light. The diode laser can be programmed to deliver very short pulses of laser energy (micropulse). Each pulse consists of a short "on" mode, to deliver the energy, and a longer "off" mode, allowing cooling of the target tissue. The PASCAL (PAtterned SCAnning Laser) is a frequency-doubled Nd:YAG laser that produces patterns of burns, such as a 5×5 square grid of 25 burns of 0.02-seconds duration, reducing the duration and discomfort of the extensive treatment required for panretinal photocoagulation (PRP) (see later in the chapter). Because laser

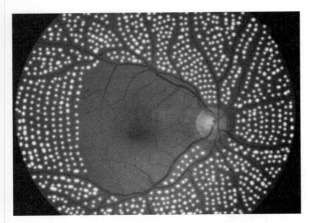

▲ **Figure 23-1.** Diagram of panretinal photocoagulation showing laser burns separated by 0.5–1 burn diameter, avoiding main blood vessels.

light is monochromatic, selective absorption by specific wavelengths makes it possible to target-specific tissues while sparing adjacent tissues (Table 23–1). Absorption of laser light by specific tissues can be enhanced by intravenous injection of absorbing dyes such as fluorescein for short-wavelength laser or indocyanine green for long-wavelength laser.

Photodisruption

Photodisruption lasers release a giant pulse of energy with a pulse duration of a few nanoseconds. When this pulse is focused to a 15–25 μm spot, so that the nearly instantaneous light pulse exceeds a critical level of energy density, "optical breakdown" occurs in which the temperature rises so high (about 10 000° K) that electrons are stripped from

Table 23-1. Energy Absorption by Different Tissues from Various Lasers

Laser	Wavelength (nm)	RPE	Blood	Xanthophyll[1]
Green	514	++++	++	+
Double frequency YAG	532	++++	++	+/−
Yellow	570	+++	++	−
Red	647	++	−	−
Diode	810	+	−	−

RPE = retinal pigment epithelium.
[1]Xanthophyll is a yellow macular pigment.

atoms, resulting in a physical state known as a plasma. This plasma expands with momentary pressures as high as 10 kilobars (150 000 psi), producing a cutting effect upon the ocular tissues. Because the initial plasma size is so small, it has little total energy and produces little effect away from the point of focus.

Photodisruptors are used for incision of posterior capsular thickening (posterior capsulotomy) or anterior capsular contraction following cataract surgery, peripheral laser iridotomy, and anterior laser vitreolysis. The principal laser of this class is the Q-switched neodymium:YAG laser.

The pulse duration of a femtosecond laser is even shorter, in the 10^{-15} second range. Produced by a solid-state neodymium:glass laser, the IntraLase is not absorbed by optically clear tissues. Thus, it is possible to focus it such as to produce precise cuts within the cornea, either as part of corneal refractive surgery or to assist in corneal dissection for penetrating or lamellar keratoplasty.

▶ Photo-Evaporation

The photo-evaporation laser produces a long-wavelength infrared heat beam that is absorbed by water, and therefore will not enter the interior of the eye.

These lasers are used for evaporating away surface lesions such as lid tumors, bloodless incisions in skin or sclera, contact photo-incision and photocoagulation within the eye delivered through special probes, controlled superficial skin burns that can tighten the eyelid skin for cosmetic improvement, and correction of hyperopia by altering the corneal surface.

This class of laser includes the carbon dioxide, erbium, and holmium lasers.

▶ Photodecomposition

Photodecomposition lasers produce very short-wavelength ultraviolet light that interacts with the chemical bonds of biologic materials, breaking the bonds and converting biologic polymers into small molecules that diffuse away. These lasers collectively are called excimer ("excited dimer") lasers because the cavity contains two gases, such as argon and fluorine, which react into unstable molecules, which then emit the laser light. They are used in correcting refractive errors by precisely recontouring the cornea (photorefractive keratectomy [PRK], laser in situ keratomileusis [LASIK], laser epithelial keratomileusis [LASEK], and epithelial LASIK [Epi-LASIK]), removing superficial corneal opacities resulting from injuries or dystrophies, and treating recurrent corneal erosions (phototherapeutic keratectomy [PTK]).

▶ Femtosecond Laser

The femtosecond laser is a focusable infrared (1053 nm) laser with femtosecond (10^{-15} seconds) pulses. By controlling the energy and firing pattern, tissue can be incised with minimal inflammation or collateral tissue damage, including very limited thermal damage to adjacent tissue. The cornea is transparent to the wavelength of the laser light so tissue can be precisely resected within the corneal substance. The femtosecond laser has been used for fashioning of stromal flaps for LASIK (IntraLASIK) and is being studied for other corneal procedures, including corneal grafting.

▼ THERAPEUTIC APPLICATIONS OF LASERS

DIABETIC RETINOPATHY

In nonproliferative diabetic retinopathy, vision may be impaired by macular edema and exudates resulting from breakdown of the inner blood–retinal barriers at the level of the retinal capillary endothelium. Many patients with long-term diabetes mellitus will gradually develop diffuse obliteration of the retinal microcirculation, especially of the capillaries, resulting in generalized retinal ischemia. This ischemic state leads to neovascularization of the retina and iris, at least partly mediated by diffusible vasoproliferative factors released from the ischemic retina into the ocular fluids. Untreated retinal neovascularization leads to vitreous hemorrhages and traction retinal detachment. Iris neovascularization leading to neovascular glaucoma is rare unless the patient has had vitreoretinal surgery. (The clinical features of diabetic retinopathy are more fully discussed in Chapter 10.)

Diabetic macular edema can be treated by focal or grid pattern laser photocoagulation, which principally acts by augmenting the function of the retinal pigment epithelium, rather than by direct closure of microaneurysms as previously suggested. Burns 50–100 μm in diameter are applied, avoiding the foveal avascular zone, which is approximately 500 μm in diameter. The areas of leakage to be treated can be identified by clinical examination (zones of retinal thickening), by fluorescein angiography (areas of discrete or diffuse fluorescein leakage and areas of capillary nonperfusion associated with retinal thickening), or now usually by optical coherence tomography (OCT). Burn intensity (laser power setting) depends on the laser used. Using a shorter-wavelength laser (green or yellow), a slight change in color is required. Using a longer-wavelength laser (diode), the burn should be almost invisible. Diode micropulse and argon green lasers are equally effective at reducing the edema, but laser scars are 8 times more likely to be visible after argon green laser and there is tendency to better visual outcome with diode micropulse laser, with which theoretically there is reduced likelihood of progressive expansion of the area of laser damage.

The most effective treatment for retinal and iris neovascularization is PRP, which usually consists of treating the entire retina except for the area within the temporal vascular arcades, with burns 200–500 μm in diameter separated by 0.5–1 burn diameter (Figure 23–1). PRP requires a total of at least 2000 and sometimes 6000 or more burns, usually delivered over two or more sessions spaced 1–2 weeks apart. Retrobulbar, peribulbar, or sub-Tenon anesthesia is some-times required, particularly if areas of the retina need to be treated again because of recalcitrant or recurrent neovascularization. Treatment is staged to reduce the incidence of uveitis, macular edema, exudative retinal detachment, and even shallowing of the anterior chamber with secondary angle closure. If there is significant macular edema, usually focal macular photocoagulation is performed before or together with PRP to avoid increase in edema. Intravitreal or orbital floor steroid (Triamcinolone) injection may prevent rebound macular edema after PRP. Currently it is restricted to patients requiring PRP and macular laser at the same time.

Adequate PRP is highly effective in producing regression of neovascularization. The exact mechanism of action has not been established, but reduction in the degree of retinal ischemia and production of diffusible vasostimulative substances are thought to be important. Reduction of ocular blood, suggesting reduction of oxygen demand in the retina, has been demonstrated after PRP. The type of laser used does not appear to influence the efficacy of PRP, but particular characteristics can be important in treatment, for example, the easier use of the diode infrared laser in the presence of vitreous hemorrhage and the more rapid laser delivery of the PASCAL.

PRP does not cause regression of the fibrosis associated with retinal neovascularization, which is responsible for tractional retinal detachment. Furthermore, PRP can be precluded by vitreous hemorrhage. Thus, PRP should be undertaken as soon as high-risk characteristics have developed. These include any new vessels on the disk with vitreous or preretinal hemorrhages, significant new vessels on the disk, and significant new vessels elsewhere with vitreous or preretinal hemorrhages.

Laser and other therapies are so effective in preventing blindness in diabetes that screening of asymptomatic diabetics for retinopathy is very worthwhile.

CENTRAL RETINAL VEIN OCCLUSION

Central retinal vein occlusion produces the classic fundus appearance of disk swelling, marked venous dilation, and almost confluent retinal hemorrhages (see Chapter 10). While these changes can progress to retinal neovascularization, vitreous hemorrhage, and fibrosis, a more common complication is the development of rubeosis iridis with neovascular glaucoma. If severe retinal ischemia is present on fluorescein angiography, there is a 60% chance of this complication. In neovascular glaucoma, substances produced by the ischemic retina diffuse forward and stimulate formation of a fibrovascular membrane that grows across the iris surface and covers the trabecular meshwork, resulting in glaucoma characterized by very high pressure, pain, and marked resistance to medical and surgical therapy, so that enucleation of the blind and painful eye may be required. PRP as described above for treatment of proliferative diabetic retinopathy—preferably with the krypton red or diode infrared laser to avoid preretinal fibrosis caused by heat absorption in the hemorrhages—can greatly reduce the incidence of neovascular glaucoma in ischemic central retinal vein occlusion. It is most effectively applied when iris neovascularization is present but before neovascular glaucoma has developed. However, in clinical practice, this timing can be difficult to achieve. Once neovascular glaucoma is present, adequate panretinal photocoagulation, possibly preceded by intra-vitreal injection of an anti-VEGF (Vascular Endothelial Growth Factor) agent, will usually cause regression of the anterior segment neovascularization, allowing the glaucoma to be controlled medically or by filtering surgery. Unfortunately, established neovascular glaucoma is often associated with corneal edema, miosis, or hyphema, so that PRP cannot be performed and only cyclophotocoagulation or enucleation can be used. For this reason, prophylactic PRP may be advisable in all cases of ischemic central retinal vein occlusion. A relative afferent pupillary defect, vision worse than 20/200, and multiple retinal cotton-wool spots are highly suggestive of ischemia severe enough to warrant prophylactic PRP. Electroretinography and fluorescein angiography provide further evidence when needed.

Laser treatment is ineffective for macular edema due to central retinal vein occlusion.

BRANCH RETINAL VEIN OCCLUSION

This condition varies from localized areas of venous congestion and hemorrhage to hemiretinal involvement from occlusion of the superior or inferior division of the central retinal vein (see Chapter 10). The principal complications are chronic macular edema (with or without exudates) and retinal neovascularization followed by vitreous hemorrhage. As the risk of neovascular glaucoma is extremely low, there is no evidence that prophylactic PRP is justified; however, if retinal neovascularization does develop, laser treatment should be performed promptly, preferably before vitreous hemorrhage occurs.

Focal and grid-pattern argon green laser photocoagulation, by obliterating areas of retinal leakage demonstrated by fluorescein angiography, is used to treat macular edema when vision is 20/40 or worse and 3 months have elapsed since the venous occlusion.

RETINAL TEARS

When a peripheral retinal tear occurs—usually due to posterior vitreous detachment causing vitreous traction—the patient often notices the sudden appearance of dot-like floaters. The tear can lead to retinal detachment, but if it is detected prior to the accumulation of subretinal fluid, it can be walled off by applying a double ring of laser burns around it to create an adhesion of the adjacent attached retina to the pigment epithelium. With modern contact lens, such as the Superquad 160, this can be achieved in most cases with a slitlamp laser delivery system. In the remaining few, indirect laser should be considered. Once retinal detachment has occurred, surgery is required. Prompt retinal examination through a dilated pupil is therefore indicated in any eye with sudden onset of floaters—particularly dot-like floaters suggesting red blood cells.

MACULAR DEGENERATION & RELATED DISEASES

Bruch's membrane forms a barrier layer between the retinal pigment epithelium and the choriocapillaris, which is the capillary layer of the choroid. If Bruch's membrane deteriorates or is damaged, choroidal neovascularization can grow through the break beneath the pigment epithelium, first causing exudative pigment epithelial detachment with distortion and edema of the overlying retina and later causing hemorrhage and fibrosis with destruction of retinal function in that area. The macula is particularly likely to develop Bruch membrane breaks and choroidal neovascularization, although these changes can occur anywhere in the fundus. The most frequent cause is age-related macular degeneration, which presents initially as asymptomatic yellowish deposits (drusen) in the macula. As the years advance, pigment epithelial atrophy and clumping are seen; finally, Bruch membrane breaks appear, leading to choroidal neovascularization, fibrosis, and loss of central vision. This condition is the leading cause of legal blindness in the developed world. Bruch membrane breaks and choroidal neovascularization can occur at sites of old chorioretinitis from childhood histoplasmosis, toxoplasmosis, and various other inflammatory disorders. They can develop from traumatic choroidal ruptures—even in children—and can occur in a host of hereditary diseases involving the retina.

Anti-VEGF therapy by repeated intra-vitreal injections has become the preferred treatment for choroidal neovascularization associated with age-related macular degeneration (neovascular AMD), particularly subfoveal disease (see Chapter 10). If choroidal neovascularization is located away from the central foveal area (extrafoveal), it can be destroyed by careful laser photocoagulation to preserve central vision. The yellow macular pigment (xanthophyll) strongly absorbs blue light, weakly absorbs green light, and does not absorb yellow, orange, or red light (Table 23–1). Hemoglobin strongly absorbs blue, green, yellow, and orange light but very weakly absorbs red light. Melanin absorbs all visible wavelengths. Selective absorption of laser energy is therefore possible. If the neovascular net has melanin pigment in it or is bleeding, then krypton red laser light allows deep penetration to the choriocapillaris without hemoglobin or xanthophyll absorption. If the net does not have much melanin and has not bled, argon green or dye laser yellow or orange will be absorbed by hemoglobin to coagulate the net but the scattered light will not be absorbed by xanthophyll. The whole area of choroidal neovascularization must be heavily treated (Figure 23–2).

Photodynamic therapy (PDT), in which an intravenous injection of a photosensitive dye (verteporfin), believed to localize within the choroidal neovascularization, is followed by treatment with a laser optimized for activation of the dye to cause thrombosis of the abnormal blood vessels, previously was the preferred treatment for subfoveal predominantly classic choroidal neovascularization associated with

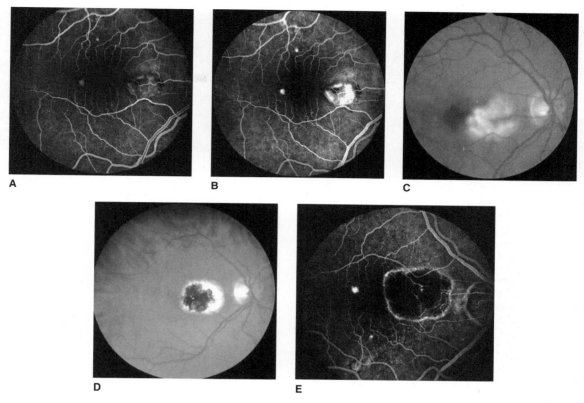

▲ Figure 23–2. Choroidal neovascularization. Fundus fluorescein angiogram in early venous (**A**) and late phase (**B**). **C:** Fundus color photograph immediately after laser therapy. Fundus color photograph (**D**) and fundus fluorescein angiogram (**E**) 6 months after laser therapy showing retinal scarring.

AMD With the development of anti-VEGF therapy, the role of PDT had greatly reduced in the management of choroidal neovascularization but remains useful under certain circumstances for other conditions.

GLAUCOMA

Treatment of open-angle glaucoma, angle-closure glaucoma, and glaucoma resistant to surgery has been radically altered by availability of effective laser techniques.

▶ Angle-Closure Glaucoma

In primary angle-closure glaucoma, aqueous flow through the pupil is blocked by contact of the lens with the posterior surface of the iris. The resulting pressure in the posterior chamber forces the peripheral iris forward into contact with the trabecular meshwork, blocking outflow and increasing intraocular pressure. While the classic dramatic acute glaucoma attack is usually considered the prototype of angle-closure glaucoma, acute attacks are actually very rare. Creeping or subacute angle-closure

glaucoma is far more common, especially in darkly pigmented eyes, and can occur with a normal central anterior chamber depth. Angle closure can be determined only by examining the anterior chamber angle by gonioscopy (see Chapters 2 and 11). Because angle closure is the most common type of glaucoma in Asian populations, it is probably the most common type of glaucoma worldwide. Surgical iridectomy was the standard treatment for angle-closure glaucoma for decades but carried the risks of hemorrhage, infection, anesthetic accidents, and even sympathetic ophthalmia.

Laser iridotomy was made more effective by the Abraham contact lens (with a 66-diopter focusing button) and the Wise iridotomy-sphincterotomy lens (103-diopter button) that increase energy density and improve visualization of the iris. With these high-energy densities, laser iridotomy (Figure 23–3) is often successful with either the argon laser or the Q-switched Nd:YAG laser, failing only when the cornea is so cloudy that the laser cannot be focused upon the iris. Alternative laser therapy may then be required (see later in the chapter).

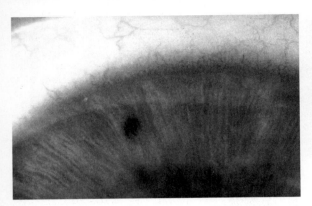

▲ **Figure 23-3.** Laser iridotomy for angle-closure glaucoma.

With the argon laser, the beam is focused through the iridotomy lens upon the far peripheral iris fibers, which are cut in a line parallel to the limbus by multiple shots at 0.01 or 0.02 seconds exposures and high-energy levels. With the Nd:YAG laser, iridotomy can be done through the iridotomy lens by a high-power single-point method using about 5–10 mJ per shot in a single-shot burst. The iridotomy can be enlarged by cutting the far peripheral iris fibers in a line parallel to the limbus with multiple shots at 1–2 mJ. The argon laser is preferable for dark brown, thick irides, which tend to bleed with the Nd:YAG laser, while light blue irides do not absorb argon laser energy well and are more easily perforated with the Nd:YAG laser. If both lasers are available, a very efficient method for thick brown irides is to cut the thick stroma with the argon laser and then remove strands and pigment with a few low-power Nd:YAG laser bursts. Because of its safety, laser iridotomy should be done not only for established angle-closure glaucoma but whenever progressive pupillary block is occurring, before irreversible damage from angle closure has occurred.

When the cornea is too cloudy to permit laser iridotomy for acute angle-closure glaucoma, argon laser peripheral iridoplasty can be attempted. To contract the iris stroma near the angle, a ring of contraction burns—low power (about 200 mW), long duration (0.5 seconds), and large spot size (500 μm)—is placed on the peripheral iris using the standard iridotomy lens. This mechanically pulls open the angle, thus lowering the intraocular pressure and allowing iridotomy to be performed. It has been shown to be as effective as medical therapy but sometimes causes discomfort. A combination of both laser and medical therapies is usually employed.

▶ Open-Angle Glaucoma

This is the most common type of glaucoma in Western countries and is characterized by painless gradual reduction in trabecular meshwork function with decreasing outflow, increasing intraocular pressure, progressive cupping of the

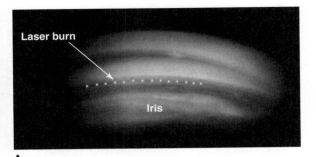

A

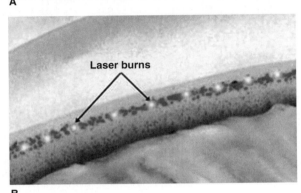

B

▲ **Figure 23-4.** Argon laser trabeculoplasty burns in the trabecular meshwork. **A:** Visualized by gonioscopy. **B:** Diagram.

optic nerve, and insidious loss of visual field, leading ultimately to blindness.

Topical medical therapy is the standard initial approach. If medical therapy is inadequate or unacceptable to the patient, argon or frequency-doubled Nd:YAG laser trabeculoplasty may be indicated (Figure 23–4). This consists of spacing 100 or more nonperforating laser burns 360° around the trabecular meshwork to shrink the collagen in the tissues of the trabecular ring, reducing the circumference, and therefore the diameter of the trabecular ring, thus pulling the trabecular layers apart with reopening of the intertrabecular spaces and of Schlemm's canal. Growth of new trabecular cells may also occur. Trabeculoplasty increases outflow and has no influence upon aqueous secretion.

The value of trabeculoplasty lies in reducing or avoiding medical therapy and postponing or avoiding the risks of drainage surgery. It seems to be most effective in patients with pseudoexfoliation and pigmentary glaucoma. In most other patients, the effect is relatively short-lived (1 or 2 years), but it may be preferable to trabeculectomy in black patients with advanced glaucoma. The main side effects are a rise in pressure for 1–4 hours in about one-third of eyes, usually preventable by pretreatment with apraclonidine drops, and a rise in pressure for 1–3 weeks in about 2% of treated eyes.

Initial treatment with 50 laser burns in 180° of the trabecular meshwork, followed by treatment to the other 180° at a later date if necessary, reduces the severity of these pressure rises. Subsequent loss of pressure control can be very sudden after trabeculoplasty, and thus requires more frequent follow-up than in patients stabilized on medical therapy.

Selective laser trabeculoplasty (SLT) delivers very high energy of extremely short duration, with minimal damage to the trabecular meshwork on histopathological studies. It is as effective as conventional trabeculoplasty but is easier to perform as the laser spot is larger and only needs to be aimed at the whole trabecular meshwork, and can be repeated.

► Cyclophotocoagulation

Glaucoma refractory to the usual operative procedures can often be controlled by direct destruction of the ciliary processes. This was first done by diathermy and later by cryosurgery. Cyclophotocoagulation through intact conjunctiva and sclera was originated by Beckman, using a high-energy ruby laser, but is currently performed by contact delivery through a fiberoptic probe with thermal-mode Nd:YAG laser or diode laser (Figure 23–5). Good control is usually obtained, but multiple treatments may be required. Side effects such as pain, inflammation, and reduction of vision are significantly less severe than with cryosurgery. Laser endocyclophotocoagulation can be performed using a fiberoptic probe passed through the pars plana during vitrectomy.

► Laser Suture Lysis

Trabeculectomy remains a popular method of glaucoma drainage surgery (see Chapter 11). In order to increase the degree of drainage and perhaps achieve greater long-term reduction in intraocular pressure—similar to that obtained with the older full-thickness drainage procedures—laser lysis of the partial-thickness scleral flap sutures can be performed in the early postoperative period. The black 10–0 nylon sutures are cut by focusing short-laser pulses upon them through the transparent conjunctiva, aided by compressing the overlying tissues with the Hoskins suture lens. The argon laser may be used, but if hemorrhage is present the krypton red or diode infrared laser is preferred to avoid flap perforation by hemoglobin absorption of argon blue-green laser wavelengths.

POSTERIOR & ANTERIOR CAPSULOTOMY AFTER CATARACT SURGERY

Modern cataract surgery uses phacoemulsification followed by posterior chamber intraocular lens implantation (see Chapter 8). If the posterior capsule supporting the intraocular lens later opacifies, vision can be restored by focusing Q-switched Nd:YAG laser pulses just posterior to the capsule to produce a central capsulotomy (thus avoiding further intraocular surgery). Careful focus through a condensing contact lens is necessary to avoid damage to the intraocular lens. There is a small increase in the risk of retinal holes and retinal detachment after capsulotomy, especially in high myopes. Opacification of the capsule is not preventable at present, although modern intraocular implants have a significantly lower rate.

Anterior capsular fibrosis may lead to contracture and occlusion of the visual axis. Radial incisions with the Q-switched Nd:YAG may obviate intraocular surgery.

► Anterior Vitreolysis

Incomplete clearance of vitreous from the anterior chamber during the management of vitreous loss secondary to trauma or surgery may result in pupillary distortion, chronic uveitis, and cystoid macular edema. The vitreous bands can be cut with the Q-switched Nd:YAG laser, using a condensing corneal contact lens. Topical pilocarpine constricts the pupil, thus tightening the vitreous strands to allow easier cutting. Multiple shots at minimal optical breakdown levels should be used to minimize concussion to cornea and iris. Although eyes with chronic cystoid macular edema have improved after cutting of vitreo-corneal bands, the bands should be cut as soon as they have been identified and before the development of these complications.

VAPORIZATION OF LID TUMORS

The carbon dioxide laser has been used to bloodlessly remove both benign and malignant lid tumors. However, because of scarring, lack of a histologic specimen, and inability to assess margins, laser treatment for this purpose appears inferior to surgery in most cases of malignant tumors.

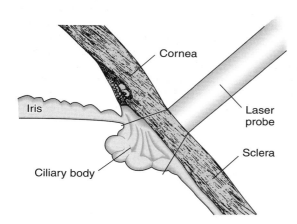

▲ **Figure 23–5.** Laser cyclophotocoagulation. The laser light passes through the conjunctiva and sclera and is absorbed by the pigment in the ciliary body, producing thermal coagulation of secreting epithelium.

CORNEAL REFRACTIVE SURGERY

The excimer lasers, particularly the 193-nm wavelength argon fluoride laser, can evaporate tissue very cleanly with almost no damage to cells adjacent to or under the cut. By using multiple pulses and progressively changing spot size to evaporate successive thin layers of the cornea, computer-controlled recontouring of the cornea (photorefractive keratectomy [PRK]) can precisely correct moderate myopic and astigmatic refractive errors (Figure 23–6). Hyperopic and highly myopic (over 6 diopters) errors respond less well. Although it quickly replaced radial keratotomy, in which radial incisions are made in the cornea with a blade and is less predictable, as well as being associated with complications—for example, deep scarring, ocular perforation, intraocular infection, and late hyperopic shift—PRK removes Bowman's membrane to which the corneal epithelium adheres, which can sometimes produce corneal haze. LASIK, in which a hinged lamellar flap of cornea is cut with a mechanical keratome, or with the femtosecond laser (IntraLASIK), the necessary laser ablation of the corneal bed is performed, and the flap replaced (Figure 23–7), preserves Bowman's membrane, and also provides faster visual recovery and less discomfort but with a slightly higher risk of long-term complications, especially in thin corneas. LASEK and epithelial LASIK (epi-LASIK), in which the flap is limited to the epithelium, potentially combine the benefits of both PRK and LASIK.

Modern excimer lasers have a smaller spot size, an eye-tracking system, and wavefront custom ablation. These improve accuracy of treatment and reduce the increase of spherical aberration induced by the corneal flap. Wavefront custom ablation is believed to cause fewer postoperative night-vision problems.

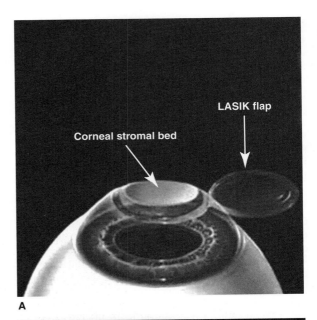

A

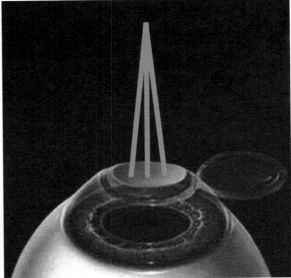

B

▲ **Figure 23–7.** LASIK. Diagrams of corneal flap **(A)** and multiple laser spots **(B)**.

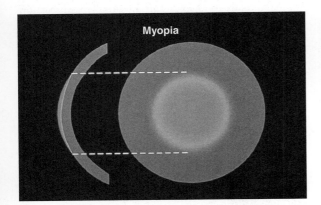

▲ **Figure 23–6.** Excimer laser photorefractive keratectomy. The laser cleanly photodecomposes corneal tissue in a controlled pattern to reshape the corneal curvature. (Photo courtesy of T Clapham, VISX Inc.)

Excimer lasers can also be used therapeutically (photo-therapeutic keratectomy—PTK) to remove superficial corneal opacities such as those associated with band keratopathy and to treat superficial corneal disease such as recurrent corneal erosions.

COSMETIC LASER EYELID SURGERY

Exposing wrinkled eyelid skin to repeated 1-ms pulses from the carbon dioxide laser—obtained by rapid pulsing of the laser tube or by computer-controlled rapid scanning of a continuous small laser beam—evaporates the epidermis and induces collagen contraction in the dermis. When the epithelium regenerates, the skin is tightened and small wrinkles and crow's feet are removed. The technique is more precise than older methods such as dermabrasion or chemical peels, but it still can sometimes be complicated by keloid scarring, hyperpigmentation, and herpesvirus infection. Surgeon experience is very important in obtaining good results. The erbium:YAG laser can be used in the same manner.

Green laser can also be used to remove xanthalesma. It is very effective but can cause depigmentation and should be avoided in darkly pigmented skin.

LASER DIAGNOSTIC IMAGING (ALSO SEE CHAPTER 2)

Confocal imaging is a video method that uses a rapidly scanning tiny laser spot whose reflected light is imaged through a pinhole upon a detector, thus suppressing all reflections except those from the focal plane. By scanning at multiple levels and then combining the images by computer processing, precise and reproducible 3-dimensional images of ocular structures can be produced. The principal use of these instruments is to evaluate and follow glaucoma-induced changes in the optic nerve head, but other uses include macular, lens, and corneal imaging. Laser interferometry is used to measure blood flow in the ciliary body and retinal blood vessels. Optical coherence tomography (OCT) can produce very high-resolution optical sections of the cornea, anterior segment, and retina to allow evaluation of diseases such as angle-closure glaucoma and macular edema.

REFERENCES

Blasi MA, Tiberti AC, Scupola A et al: Photodynamic therapy with verteporfin for symptomatic circumscribed choroidal hemangioma: five-year outcomes. Ophthalmology 2010 Apr 22. [Epub ahead of print] [PMID: 20417564]

Blumenkranz MS: Optimal current and future treatments for diabetic macular edema. Eye 2010;24:428. [PMID: 20075969]

Chan WM, Lim TH, Pece A, Silva R, Yoshimura N: Verteporfin PDT for non-standard indications – a review of current literature. Graefes Arch Clin Exp Ophthalmol 2010;248:613. [PMID: 20162298]

Lee JW, Lee JH, Lee KW: Prognostic factors for the success of laser iridotomy for acute primary angle-closure glaucoma. Korean J Ophthalmol 2009;23:286. [PMID: 20046690]

Lin SC: Endoscopic and transscleral cyclophotocoagulation for the treatment of refractory glaucoma. J Glaucoma 2008;17:238. [PMID: 18414112]

Li H, Sun T, Wang M, Shao J: Safety and effectiveness of thin-flap LASIK using a femtosecond laser and microkeratome in the correction of high myopia in Chinese patients. J Refract Surg 2010;26:99. [PMID: 20163074]

Muqit MM, Marcellino GR, Henson DB et al: Singe-session versus multiple-session pattern scanning laser panretinal photocoagulation in proliferative diabetic retinopathy: The Manchester Pascal Study. Arch Ophthalmol 2010;128:525. [PMID: 20457972]

O'Keefe M, Kirwan C: Laser epithelial keratomileusis in 2010 – a review. Clin Experiment Ophthalmol 2010;38:183. [PMID: 20398107]

Ramos JL, Li Y, Huang D: Clinical and research applications of anterior segment optical coherence tomography – a review. Clin Experiment Ophthalmol 2009;37:81. [PMID: 19016809]

Rapuano CJ: Phototherapeutic keratectomy: who are the best candidates and how do you treat them? Curr Opinion Ophthalmol 2010 May 12. [Epub ahead of print] [PMID: 20467315]

Ritch R, Tham CC, Lam DS: Argon laser peripheral iridoplasty (ALPI): an update. Surv Ophthalmol 2007;52:279. [PMID: 17472803]

Russo V, Barone A, Cosma A, Stella A, Delle Noci N: Selective laser trabeculoplasty versus argon laser trabeculoplasty in patients with uncontrolled open-angle glaucoma. Eur J Ophthalmol 2009;19:429. [PMID: 19396790]

Schmack I, Auffarth GU, Epstein D, Holzer MP: Refractive surgery trends and practice style changes in Germany over a 3-year period. J Refract Surg 2010;26:202. [PMID: 20229953]

Scanlon PH: Why do patients still require surgery for the late complications of proliferative diabetic retinopathy? Eye 2010;24:435. [PMID: 20057509]

Soong HK, Malta JB: Femtosecond lasers in ophthalmology. Am J Ophthalmol 2009;147:189. [PMID: 18930447]

Tan AM, Chockalingam M, Aquino MC et al: Micropulse transscleral diode laser cyclophotocoagulation in the treatment of refractory glaucoma. Clin Experiment Ophthalmol 2010;38:266. [PMID: 20447122]

Tanna M, Schallhorn SC, Hettinger KA: Femtosecond laser versus mechanical microkeratome: a retrospective comparison of visual outcomes at 3 months. J Refract Surg 2009;25:S668. [PMID: 19705541]

Wang D, Pekmezci M, Basham RP et al: Comparison of different modes in optical coherence tomography and ultrasound biomicroscopy in anterior chamber angle assessment. J Glaucoma 2009;18:472. [PMID:19680056]

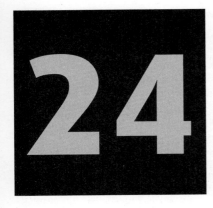

Low Vision

Gwen K. Sterns, MD, and Eleanor E. Faye, MD, FACS

In every subspecialty of ophthalmology, the patient with impaired vision represents a challenge in management. Whether reduced vision is temporary or permanent, it is the consequence of an eye disorder and, as such, is the responsibility of the ophthalmologist and optometrist. If the outcome of optimal medical and surgical intervention is diminished functional vision, the patient needs vision rehabilitation (also see Chapter 25). No person with low vision should have to search far and wide for low-vision care. Some level of care should be integrated into every ophthalmic practice, whether it is on-site or referral to a low-vision center.

Low-vision patients typically have impaired visual performance, that is, visual acuity not correctable with conventional glasses or contact lenses. They may have cloudy vision, constricted fields, or large scotomas. There may be additional functional complaints: glare sensitivity, abnormal color perception, or diminished contrast. Some patients have diplopia. A frequent complaint is confusion from overlapping but dissimilar images from each eye.

The term "low vision" covers a wide range. A person in the early stages of an eye disease may have near-normal vision. Others may have moderate to severe loss. All low-vision patients have some degree of useful vision even though the loss may be profound. They should not be considered "blind" unless they no longer have useful visual clues. Performance varies with each individual.

In the United States, over 6 million persons are visually impaired but not classified as legally blind.[1] Over 75% of patients seeking treatment are age 65 or older. Age-related macular degeneration accounts for an increasing number of cases. Other common causes of low vision are glaucoma, diabetic retinopathy, cataract, optic atrophy, corneal disease,

cerebral damage resulting in hemianopia, degenerative myopia, and retinitis pigmentosa. Approximately 9% of the low-vision population is pediatric, resulting from congenital eye disorders or trauma. (See Chapter 20 for discussion of the worldwide prevalence and causes of visual impairment.)

Effective low-vision intervention starts as soon as the patient experiences difficulty performing ordinary tasks. A treatment plan should consider the level of function, realistic goals for intervention, and the varieties of devices that could be helpful. Patients must face the fact that impaired vision is usually progressive. The sooner they adapt to low-vision devices, the sooner they can adjust to the new techniques of using their vision. Low-vision evaluation should never be delayed unless the person is in an active phase of medical or surgical treatment.

Visual performance can be improved by the use of optical and non-optical devices. The general term for corrective devices is "low-vision aids." In this chapter, the emphasis will be on assessment techniques, descriptions of useful devices, and a discussion of some of the functional aspects of common eye diseases.

MANAGEMENT OF THE PATIENT WITH LOW VISION

Comprehensive management includes (1) history of onset of the eye condition and the effect of the loss of vision on daily life; (2) examination for best corrected acuity, visual fields, contrast sensitivity, color perception (and glare sensitivity if it pertains to the patient's symptoms); (3) evaluation of near vision and reading skills; (4) selection and prescription (or lending) of aids that accomplish task objectives; (5) instruction in correct use and application of devices; and (6) follow-up to reinforce new patterns.

HISTORY TAKING

Specific features of the onset, treatments given, and current medications should be verified. Patients' responses indicate their understanding of their condition. Unrealistic or

---

[1]Legal blindness—defined as best corrected visual acuity of 20/200 or less in the better eye or a visual field of 20° or less—affects 1 000 000 individuals in the United States (see Chapter 20) It is an administrative definition that does not mean that the patient is unable to see anything.

Table 24–1. Common Activities That Are Adversely Affected by Visual Impairment Are Listed with Suggestions for Low- Vision Aids

Activity	Optical Aids	Non-Optical Aids
Shopping	Hand magnifier	Lighting, color cues
Fixing a snack	Spectacle magnifier	Color cues, consistent storage plan
Eating out	Hand magnifier	Flashlight, portable lamp
Identifying money	Spectacle, spectacle-mounted or hand magnifier	Arrange wallet in compartments, fold banknotes of different denominations differently
Reading print	Spectacle, spectacle-mounted, dome, hand, or stand magnifier Closed-circuit television	Lighting, high-contrast print, large print, reading slit
Writing	Hand magnifier	Lighting, bold-tip pen, black ink
Dialing a telephone	Telescope Hand magnifier	Large-print dial, hand-printed directory
Crossing streets	Telescope	Cane, ask directions
Finding taxis and bus signs	Telescope	
Reading medication labels	Hand magnifier	Color codes, large print
Reading stove dials	Hand magnifier	Color codes
Thermostat adjustment	Hand magnifier	Enlarged-print model
Using a computer	Intermediate add spectacles	High-contrast color, large-print program
Reading signs	Spectacle or spectacle-mounted magnifier Telescope Portable electronic magnifier	Move closer
Watching sporting event	Telescope	Sit in front rows

unreasonable attitudes need to be documented. Does the person understand the limitations of what can be achieved with low-vision rehabilitation? It is helpful to refer to a list of common daily activities the patient may not be able to perform efficiently (Table 24–1). From this list, it is possible to arrive at realistic treatment objectives for that person.

EXAMINATION

The patient should not have pupillary dilation before a low-vision evaluation. Refractive status should be confirmed to rule out a significant change, particularly after surgical intervention such as cataract or glaucoma surgery. A patient may have become myopic from a nuclear cataract or astigmatic from corneal warping after glaucoma drainage surgery. The most accurate acuity test is the Early Treatment Diabetic Retinopathy Study (ETDRS) chart (Figure 24–1), which has 14 five-letter lines of 0.1 log unit size difference with a LogMAR (logarithm of minimum angle of resolution) scale and a con-

venient metric or Snellen conversion. Masking of other lines may facilitate letter recognition. An integrated light box standardizes illumination. A 4-meter test distance is used when acuity is 20/20 to 20/200; a 2-meter distance for acuities less than 20/200 but 20/400 or better; and a 1-meter distance for acuities less than 20/400. The ETDRS chart makes obsolete the imprecise expression "finger counting." Alternatively, a Snellen chart can be used, either at the conventional testing distance of 20 feet (6 m) or less (see Chapter 2).

Projector charts are not recommended for testing subnormal vision because of low contrast and insufficient letter choice at low acuities.

The dominant eye and preferred eye should be noted.

The Amsler grid is the traditional test for evaluating the central field. Although it is relatively insensitive, it can be used to advantage in low vision, particularly to identify the dominant eye. At the test distance of 33 cm, the patient should first look at the chart *binocularly.* ("Can you see the dot?") Observe for eye or head turn. If the dot is seen, the

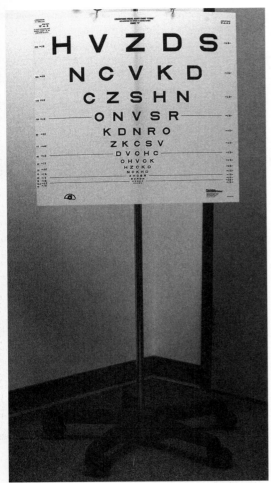

A

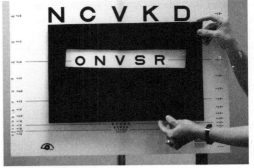

B

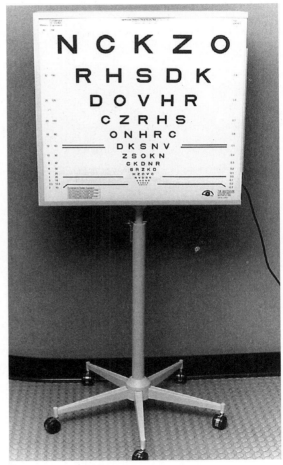

C

▲ **Figure 24–1.** **A:** Lighthouse modification of the Ferris–Bailey ETDRS chart. **B:** Masking of other lines to facilitate letter recognition. **C:** With integrated light box to standardize illumination.

patient is using either a viable macula or an eccentric viewing area. An eye turn or head tilt may confirm this. Ask the patient to report distortion or blank areas seen binocularly. Then check the grid *monocularly* and again ask the patient to report seeing the center fixation dot and any distortion or scotoma. If the grid is presented in this manner, the patient understands what is expected and the test can provide helpful data. For example, if a large scotoma in the dominant eye overrides the better nondominant eye, the patient probably will require occlusion of the dominant eye. If the dominant eye is the better eye, it will override the poorer nondominant eye and the patient can benefit from binocular correction.

Tests of contrast express the functional level of retinal sensitivity more accurately than any other test, including acuity. Of the available tests for contrast sensitivity, the recently developed Mars test using letters arranged on three 14×19 charts in 8 rows of 6 letters each has been evaluated favorably (Figure 24-2).[2] The contrast of each letter decreases by a constant factor of 0.04 log unit, which makes it the most sensitive of the clinical contrast tests. The test results identify the level of contrast loss: profound loss, severe loss, moderate loss, and normal adult contrast sensitivity. It is a rapid and accurate method of measuring an important visual function. Contrast sensitivity is a predictor of the retina's response to magnification. Regardless of acuity, if contrast is subthreshold or in the severe loss category, the patient is less likely to respond to optical magnification.

Simple color identification tests are done if the patient's complaints include difficulty with color cues.

NEAR VISION

Near vision may be evaluated with a combination of single-letter tests, such as with a reduced version of the ETDRS chart, and graded text, short sentences with simple vocabulary being helpful and non-threatening (Figure 24-3). Single letters and short words are presented first to establish near acuity. Graded text is then presented to establish reading skills with the selected optical devices.

SELECTION OF DEVICES & PATIENT INSTRUCTION

The dioptric range is selected from the outcome of acuity tests, modified by the results of the Amsler grid and contrast sensitivity tests. A rule of thumb for the starting power is to calculate the reciprocal of visual acuity—for example, an acuity of 20/160 suggests a starting lens of 8 diopters (160/20). Keep in mind that visual acuity is not a particularly sensitive measure of function. Scotomas within the reading field and the contrast sensitivity of the paramacular retina have a greater influence on ability to read magnified print through an optical lens.

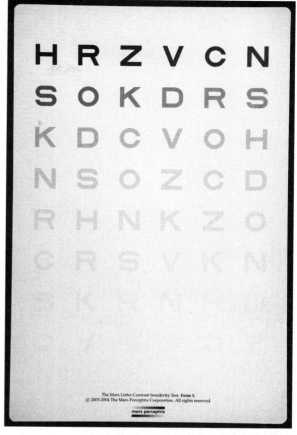

▲ **Figure 24–2.** Mars Letter-Contrast Sensitivity Test chart.

After the dioptric range has been agreed upon, the three major categories of devices are presented in sequence in the selected power. Lenses in a spectacle mounting are presented and evaluated first, followed by hand-held magnifiers and, third, stand-mounted magnifiers. Telescopes and television or computer-designed devices are increasingly prescribed as the population becomes more sophisticated in the use of advanced technology.

INSTRUCTION

Part of effective management of every low-vision patient is skilled instruction in using a device. Attention should be paid to daily living activities, which can be complemented by low-vision lenses but may also require referral to an agency for the visually impaired.

The patient uses the various devices under the supervision of an instructor until proficiency is achieved. During the instruction time, mechanics of the aids are reviewed, questions

[2]MARS Letter Contrast Sensitivity Test. Available from The Mars Perceptrix Corporation, 49 Valley View Road, Chappaqua, NY 10514-2523, www.marsperceptrix.com, Tel: 914-239-3526.

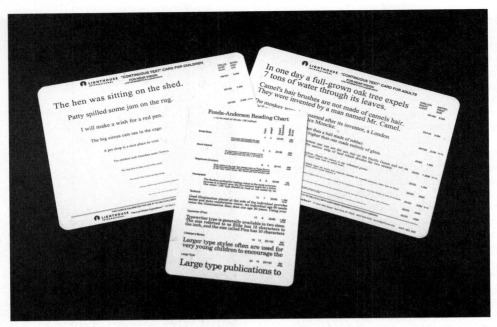

▲ **Figure 24–3.** Near-vision test charts, including the Lighthouse Continuous Text Cards for children and adults.

are answered, and goals reexamined. The patient is allowed ample time to learn correct techniques in one or more sessions, and possibly a loaner lens for home or job trial. Older patients usually need more adaptation time and reinforcement than younger or congenitally impaired persons.

Practitioners and staff benefit from training programs to learn how to manage a low-vision patient in the office. Basic setups for incorporating low vision into a practice are reviewed in a number of publications.

Instruction is the key to success in vision rehabilitation. Over 90% of patients succeed with instruction, whereas a 50% success rate (no better than chance) results from prescribing an aid without training.

FOLLOW-UP

In 2 to 3 weeks, the patient's progress is reviewed, adjustments are made, and prescriptions are finalized. If minor problems arise within the first few days after the appointment, they can usually be resolved by telephone.

▼ LOW-VISION AIDS

There are 5 types of low-vision aids: (1) convex-lens aids such as spectacle (including bifocal), spectacle-mounted, dome, hand-held, and stand-mounted magnifiers (Figure 24–4); (2) telescopes, either spectacle-mounted or hand-held

(Figure 24–5); (3) non-optical devices (adaptive aids) such as large print, reading stands, marking devices, reading, writing and signature guides, pill organizers, liquid level indicators, and large numeral and talking clocks, watches, timers, calculators, and scales (Figures 24–6); (4) tints and filters, including antireflective lenses (Figure 24–7), and illumination; and (5) electronic devices such as portable or desktop closed-circuit television (CCTV) reading machines (Figure 24–8), image scanners, and magnification, and voice synthesis and recognition computer software (Figure 24–9).

CONVEX-LENS AIDS (FIGURE 24–4)

Convex-lens aids, such as spectacle, spectacle-mounted, dome, hand and stand magnifiers are prescribed for over 90% of patients. The various mountings have inherent advantages and disadvantages.

The main advantage of spectacle and spectacle-mounted magnifiers is that both hands remain free to hold the reading material. They require the reading material to be held at the focal distance of the lens, for example, 10 cm for a 10-diopter lens. The stronger the lens, the shorter the reading distance, with increasing tendency to obstruct light (Figure 24–4 B). Lamps with flexible arms may be required for uniform lighting. Patients with binocular function may use spectacles in the 4- to 14-diopter range with base-in prism to aid convergence. Above 14 diopters, a monocular sphere must be used for the better eye.

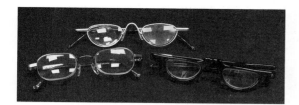

A

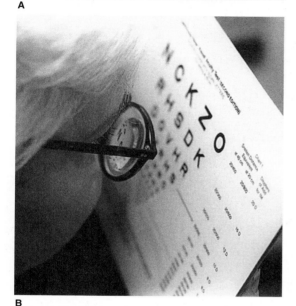

B

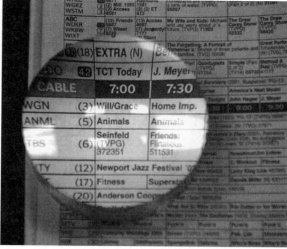

D

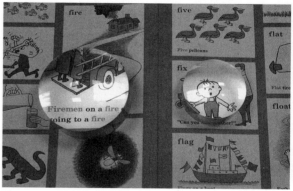

E

C

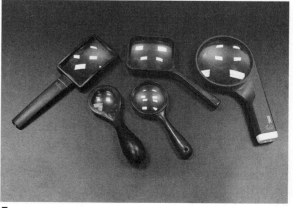

F

▲ **Figure 24–4.** Convex-lens aids. **A:** Spectacle magnifiers. **B:** Close reading distance with spectacle magnifier, both hands being free to hold reading material but light possibly being obstructed. **C:** Spectacle-mounted magnifiers. **D** and **E:** Dome magnifiers. **F:** Hand magnifiers of various strengths. **G:** Hand magnifier being used for kitchen task. **H:** Hand magnifiers suitable for carrying in a pocket or purse. **I:** Illuminated hand magnifiers of various strengths. **J:** Fixed focus stand magnifier, allowing writing on the material being read. **K:** A woman with macular degeneration uses a stand magnifier. Her hand tremor prevented her from using a hand magnifier.

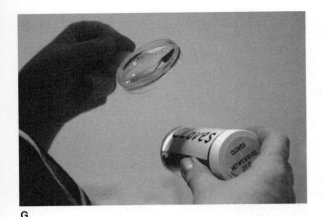

G

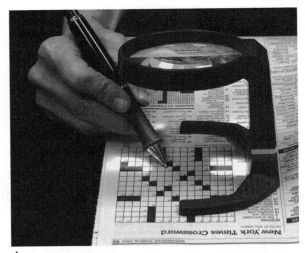

J

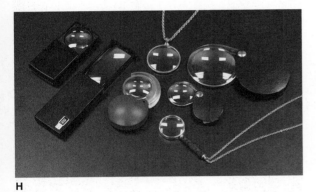

H

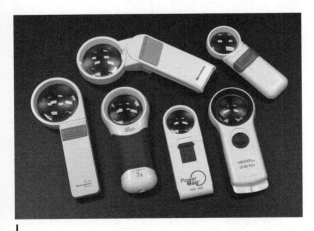

I

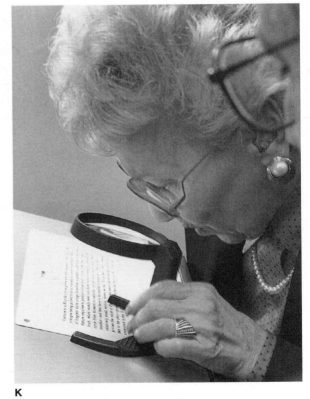

K

▲ **Figure 24–4.** (*Continued*)

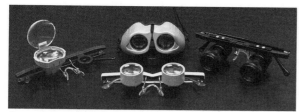

A

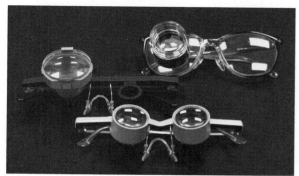

B

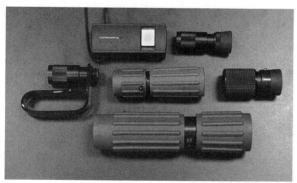

C

▲ **Figure 24–5.** Telescopes. **A:** Spectacle-mounted, including Galilean focusable (right). **B:** Spectacle-mounted for close tasks. **C:** Hand-held monocular.

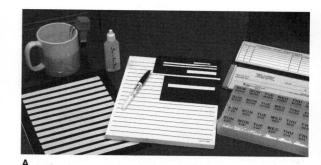

A

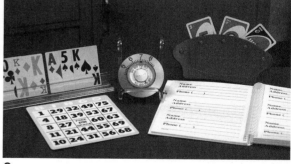

B

C

▲ **Figure 24–6.** Non-optical devices. **A:** Reading and writing guides, marking devices, pill organizer, and liquid level indicator. **B:** Large numeral and talking clocks, watches and timers. **C:** Large print address book, bingo card, playing cards, and thermostat.

Dome magnifiers, which are placed directly on the reading material, also allow both hands to be free, always provide a focused image, and maximize illumination, but the amount of magnification is limited and there may be problems with distortion and light reflection.

Hand magnifiers are convenient for shopping, reading dials and labels, identifying money, etc. They are often used by older people in conjunction with their reading glasses to enlarge print. The advantage of the hand-held lens is a greater working space between the eye and lens. Holding a lens, however, may be a disadvantage for a trembling hand or stiff joints. Hand magnifiers are available from 4 to 68 diopters.

Stand magnifiers are convex lenses mounted on a rigid base whose height is related to the power of the lens, for example, a 10-diopter lens is just under 10 cm from the

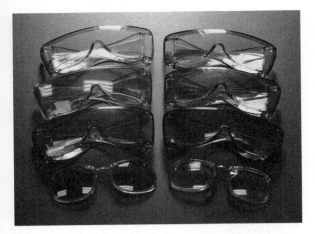

▲ **Figure 24-7.** Absorptive lenses to reduce glare and improve contrast. See color insert.

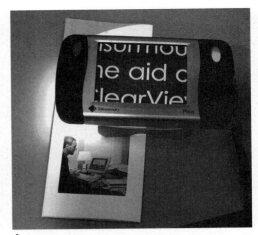

A

page, writing on the material being read being possible with the lower magnification devices. Because the lens mounting may block light, a lens with a battery-powered light may be the best choice. The most recent development in this device is the use of an LED light source, which allows for better illumination and longer battery life. Patients with corneal and lens pathology may not be able to tolerate the glare from an illuminated device.

TELESCOPES (FIGURE 24–5)

Telescopes are the only devices that can be focused from infinity to near. For low vision, the simplest device is the hand-held monocular for short-term viewing, particularly of signs. For patients with vocational or hobby interests, Galilean or Keplerian telescopes (internal prism systems) in a spectacle frame are practical. A recent development is a monocular autofocus telescope. The practical limit of power for hand-held units is 2–8×. Spectacle telescopes are difficult to use above 6×. All telescopes share the disadvantage of a small field diameter and shallow depth of field.

NON-OPTICAL DEVICES (ADAPTIVE AIDS) (FIGURE 24–6)

There are many practical items that augment or replace visual aids. They are traditionally called "non-optical devices," although "adaptive aids" is probably a better term. In daily life, difficulty in reading is not the only frustrating experience for the low-vision person. Cooking, setting thermostats and stove dials, measuring, reading a scale, putting on makeup, selecting the correct illumination, identifying banknotes and playing cards are only a few things that sighted people take for granted. Many devices are available for the visually impaired to assist in performing these tasks. The field is expanding rapidly and it is important to keep up to

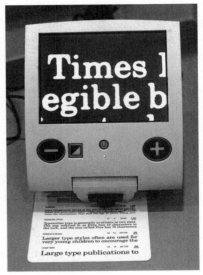

B

▲ **Figure 24-8. A** and **B:** Portable CCTV reading systems.

date with available aids and resources.

TINTS, COATINGS, AND ILLUMINATION

Many low-vision patients complain of poor contrast and glare, which particularly hinders traveling around on their own. A basic approach is to consider the effect sunlight has on cloudy media in causing glare and to remember that contrast is also affected by time of day, weather, and textures and colors in the surroundings. As a rule, light or medium gray lenses are prescribed to reduce light intensity. To improve contrast and reduce the effect of short-wave light rays, amber or yellow lenses are suggested (Figure 24–7). Companies,

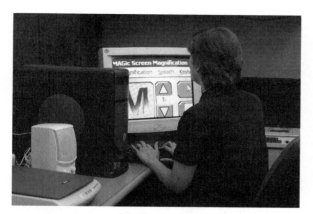

▲ **Figure 24–9.** Computer system with screen magnification software and image scanner.

device encourages a natural reading posture and is a good choice for school children to help them see their class work and view graphs, diagrams, or photos.

Portable video magnifiers allow the visually impaired to read medication labels, mail, price tags, and menus, or view videos. The devices have built in illumination and allow for contrast enhancement, color display, and variable magnification. Many are small enough to fit in a pocket or purse. Some have a built-in distance camera to allow viewing of signs, arrival and departure boards at airports, and classroom lectures. Electronic portable reading devices allow for downloading of printed material such as books and newspapers, with text to speech options. Some cellular phones can perform some of these tasks.

The rapid development of devices for the general population has benefited visually impaired patients by increasing choice and reducing cost, allowing them to regain their independence more easily.

such as Corning,NoIR, and Chadwick, design and manufacture lenses specifically for low-vision patients. Options include non-changeable filters and photochromic (variable tint) lenses. An additional antireflective coating should be considered for patients who are glare-sensitive. Because each patient responds differently to the various available tints and to the degree of light transmission that the lens provides, the use of trial lenses is advisable.

Adequate task and ambient lighting is essential for persons who depend principally on the macula for vision, enhancing contrast, reducing glare, and simulating natural lighting. Light that is too bright may cause strain, glare, and photophobia, which may be relieved by introducing amber to yellow filters that block ultraviolet and visible blue light below 527 nm. Patients with early cataracts, macular changes and corneal dystrophies may have difficulty reading with their current lighting. Older patients also notice difficulties with near tasks after changing to energy-saving light sources known as compact fluorescent light (CFL). Before changing the incandescent bulb to a CFL it is important to select the proper CFL bulb, one designated as "warm or soft light." Full-spectrum bulbs can improve lighting, eliminating glare and improving efficiency. Light that does not scatter and is aimed directly on the print or task is preferred. (Illumination is more fully discussed in Appendix II; Practical Factors in Illumination in the 17th edition.)

ELECTRONIC AND PORTABLE VIDEO MAGNIFIERS AND READING SYSTEMS (FIGURES 24-8 AND 24-9)

A closed-circuit television reading machine (CCTV) consists of a high-resolution monitor with a built-in camera with a zoom lens, if necessary an illumination system, and in the desk-top models an X-Y reading platform. Magnification from 1.5× to 45× is possible with adjustable font sizes, and the background can be reversed from white to dark gray. The

THE EFFECT OF THE EYE DISORDER

Treatment plans should take into account the effect of the eye disorder on both visual acuity and visual field. The type and strength of visual aid are influenced by the type and extent of the deficit.

Diseases resulting in low vision can be classified into 3 categories (Figure 24–10): (1) blurred or hazy vision throughout the visual field, characteristic of cloudy media; (2) central scotomas, characteristic of macular disorders and optic nerve disease; and (3) peripheral scotomas, such as the generalized constriction typical of retinitis pigmentosa and other peripheral retinal disorders, and advanced glaucoma, or homonymous hemianopia due to central nervous system disorders such as stroke.

BLURRED, HAZY VISION (FIGURE 24-10 B)

Generalized blurring and haziness of vision is the rule in any abnormality of the optical media. Glare and photophobia may also occur. Any corneal disease, cataract, capsular opacification, or vitreous opacity interferes with refraction of light rays entering the eye. Such random refraction causes reduced acuity, glare, and decreased contrast. Pupillary miosis further restricts the quantity of light reaching the retina. Patients have difficulty seeing stairs and steps and other low-contrast objects. Acuity varies with ambient light.

Useful parameters of visual function include visual acuity, glare, and contrast sensitivity. A potential acuity meter (PAM) used in conjunction with a glare test helps to differentiate retinal from media pathology.

▶ Management

Refraction should always be carefully done, including multiple pinholes, stenopeic slit, and keratometry. Modification of illumination and attention to details of room and task lighting are

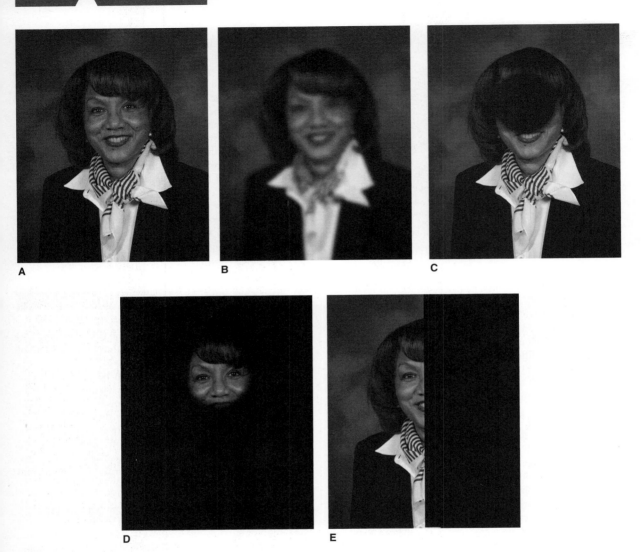

▲ **Figure 24–10. A:** Normal image. **B:** Blurred image. **C:** Central scotoma. **D:** Peripheral scotoma of peripheral retinal disorders or advanced glaucoma. **E:** Right homonymous hemianopia due to left cerebral hemisphere stroke.

most important. Antireflective lens coatings and neutral gray lenses reduce light intensity (and therefore glare). Yellow and amber lenses enhance contrast. Ultraviolet filters should be used particularly for pseudophakic patients. Large bold print provides the higher contrast the patient needs.

Magnification may or may not be effective depending on the patient's level of contrast sensitivity. A magnified image itself has low contrast. The glare from an illuminated stand magnifier may actually reduce reading acuity. Large bold print may be a better choice than a magnifier—or in case of surface glare from paper, a reading slit of matte black plastic

to reduce glare and outline the text. Contact lenses, keratoplasty, corneal laser refractive surgery, posterior capsulotomy, and cataract surgery may also be indicated.

If cataract seems to be interfering with optimal function, a combination of contrast sensitivity and glare tests may indicate the best time for surgery. The intraocular lens should contain an ultraviolet blocking agent. The surgeon may wish to discuss overcorrecting the power of the implant by a few diopters. The resulting myopia will provide clear intermediate distance vision without correction, which is more important for a visually impaired person than clear far-distance vision.

CENTRAL SCOTOMAS (FIGURE 24–10 C)

Central retinal (macular) function, predominantly utilizing cone photoreceptors, is essential for detailed, color, and daylight (photopic) vision. The two most common causes of macular disease are atrophic (dry) and neovascular (exudative, wet) age-related macular degeneration, both of which are increasingly prevalent in today's aging society. Other causes are macular holes, myopic macular degeneration, and congenital macular disorders. Optic nerve disease also predominantly affects central vision.

In the early stages of atrophic age-related macular degeneration, patients most often report blurred or distorted central vision. Peripheral vision is unaffected unless there is cataract. The loss of central vision interferes with reading and seeing details, including facial features. Dense scotomas are not present in atrophic macular degeneration and usually not in exudative disease unless there is retinal fibrosis following choroidal or subretinal hemorrhage. Contrast sensitivity decreases as the disease extends beyond the fovea. Macular degeneration generally does not hinder safe travel because the preserved peripheral vision is effective for orientation purposes. The efficacy of inhibitors of vascular endothelial growth factor (VEGF), such as bevacizumab and ranibizumab, in exudative age-related macular degeneration has increased the number of patients with macular degeneration who can benefit from low-vision rehabilitation.

Tests of visual function include visual acuity, Amsler grid, and contrast sensitivity. Reduced contrast indicates the need for higher magnification, more contrast, and more illumination than predicted from the visual acuity.

▶ Management

Patients with moderately advanced macular disease often spontaneously adopt an eccentric head tilt or eye turn to move images from nonseeing retina to a viable parafoveal area, known as a preferred retinal locus (PRL), of which there may be more than one in each eye. The ability to move the scotoma may be demonstrated to a patient during the Amsler grid test. Some patients respond to bilateral prisms in spectacles to relocate the image. Other patients may benefit from training to utilize a PRL, or to utilize another area of parafoveal retina, a trained retinal locus (TRL), that is more advantageous. Such training can be undertaken by occupational therapists or certified low-vision therapists, and can be facilitated with a scanning laser ophthalmoscope (SLO).

Magnifying lenses enlarge the retinal image, allowing use of eccentric fixation by compensating for lower retinal sensitivity in the parafoveal area. The power of the lens is related to the contrast sensitivity, as well as location and density of the scotoma. Patients may use different types of devices for various tasks: spectacles for reading, hand magnifier for shopping, CCTV for writing and typing. Most people learn to use low-vision aids successfully, particularly after instruction sessions to reinforce correct usage. Older people may require more time and repetition. All patients need to be reassured that complete loss of sight is only a remote possibility that should not be inferred by designation as legally blind, which is an administrative term.

PERIPHERAL SCOTOMA (FIGURES 24–10 D AND E)

Scotomas in the peripheral field are characteristic of end-stage glaucoma, retinitis pigmentosa, other peripheral retinal disorders including proliferative diabetic retinopathy treated with panretinal photocoagulation, and central nervous system disorders such as tumor, stroke, or trauma. The peripheral field is essential for orienting oneself in space, detecting motion, and awareness of potential hazards in the environment. The predominantly rod vision is most sensitive in twilight and at night. A person with a constricted field may be able to read small print yet need a cane or guide dog to get around.

▶ Management

If the central field diameter is less than 7°, magnification may not be advantageous. Telescopes and spectacle magnifiers may enlarge the image beyond the useful field. Hand magnifiers and closed-circuit television or computers may be the equipment of choice because the size of the image can be adjusted to match the size of the field.

Various training techniques have been advocated to expand the residual visual field in patients with homonymous hemianopia but their value has yet to be established. The reported benefits of the commercially available Vision Restoration Therapy (VRT), which involves twice-daily sessions for 6 months of responses to light stimuli projected on a video monitor, may be confounded by eye movements during visual field testing. Explorative Saccade Training (EST), which involves searching for numbers in the seeing and blind hemifields, has been reported to improve search response times in the blind hemifield and performance in social activities but is currently limited to research studies.

REFERENCES

Congdon N et al: Causes and prevalence of visual impairment among adults in the United States. Arch Ophthalmol 2004;122:477. [PMID: 15078664]

Crossland MD et al: Preferred retinal locus development in patients with macular disease. Ophthalmology 2005;112:1579. [PMID: 16087239]

Das A, Huxlin KR: New approaches to visual rehabilitation for cortical blindness: outcomes and putative mechanisms. Neuroscientist 2010 Jan 25. [Epub ahead of print[[PMID: 20103505]

Dougherty BE et al: An evaluation of the Mars Letter Contrast Sensitivity Test. Optom Vis Sci 2005;82:970. [PMID: 16317373]

Faye EE (editor): Clinical Low Vision, 2nd ed. Little, Brown, 1984.

Faye EE: Low vision aids. In: Clinical Ophthalmology, Vol 1: Refraction. Duane TD (editor). Harper & Row, 1990.

Faye EE: Pathology and visual function. In: *Functional Assessment of Low Vision*. Rosenthal BP, Cole RG (editors). Mosby, 1996.

Faye EE, Stuen CS: *The Aging Eye and Low Vision: A Study Guide*. The Lighthouse, 1995.

Forooghian F et al: Visual acuity outcomes after cataract surgery in patients with age-related macular degeneration: Age-Related Eye Disease Study Report No. 27. Ophthalmology 2009;116:2093. [PMID: 19700198]

Haymes SA et al: The letter contrast sensitivity test: clinical evaluation of a new design. Invest Ophthalmol Vis Sci 2006;47:2739. [PMID: 16723494]

Jobke S, Kasten E, Sabel BA: Vision restoration through extratriate stimulation in patients with visual field defects: a double-blind and randomized experimental study. Neurorehabil Neural Repair 2009;23:246. [PMID: 19240199]

Lighthouse Continuing Education. Annual catalog of courses, seminars and symposia. http://www.lighthouse.org/about/education/programs.htm, Fax: 212-821-9707; e-mail: education@lighthouse.org.

Lighthouse Information and Resource Service: Information and pamphlets about eye conditions, visual impairment, and blindness. http://www.lighthouse.org/services/rehab.htm, Tel: 800-829-0500.

Maberley DA et al: The prevalence of low vision and blindness in Canada. Eye 2006;20:341. [PMID: 15905873]

Markowitz SN, Aleykina N: The relationship between scotoma displacement and preferred retinal loci in low-vision patients with age-related macular degeneration. Can J Ophthalmol 2010;45:58. [PMID: 20130712]

Roth T et al: Comparing explorative saccade and flicker training in hemianopia: a randomized controlled study. Neurology 2009;72:324. [PMID: 19171828]

Shima N, Markowitz SN, Reyes SV: Concept of a functional retinal locus in age-related macular degeneration. Can J Ophtalmol 2010;45:62. [PMID: 20130713]

Smith HJ et al: A randomized controlled trial to determine the effectiveness of prism spectacles for patients with age-related macular degeneration. Arch Ophthalmol 2005;123:1042. [PMID: 16087836]

Watson GR et al: Effects of a preferred retinal locus placement on text navigation and development of advantageous trained retinal locus. J Rehabil Res Dev 2006;43:761. [PMID: 17310425]

Internet Resources

www.afb.org/seniorsitehome.asp

www.cdc.gov/visionhealth/

www.cdc.gov/visionhealth/pdf/improving_nations_vision_health.pdf

www.independentliving.com/products.asp?dept=30&deptname=Portable-Systems

www.lighthouse.org/

www.nei.nih.gov/nehep/programs/lowvision/index.asp

www.nei.nih.gov/nehep/newsletter/index.asp

http://one.aao.org/CE/EducationalContent/Smartsight.aspxhttp://www.spedex.com/napvi/

http://www.preventblindness.org/vpus/

Vision Rehabilitation

25

August Colenbrander, MD

Vision loss reduces the ability to cope with daily living activities, and affects the safety and quality of life. In developed countries, and increasingly in developing countries, the majority of irreversible vision loss occurs in the elderly and will represent an ever increasing part of ophthalmic practice (see Chapter 20). Unfortunately, many patients and caregivers still consider vision loss as an inevitable result of aging and often do not seek the help that is available. It is the task of the ophthalmologist to tell them that even if *"nothing can be done"* about many of the causes of vision loss, *"much can be done"* about its consequences. This chapter will deal with ways to alleviate the consequences of vision loss through comprehensive rehabilitation (also see Chapter 24).

STAGES OF VISUAL PROCESSING

Vision is a complex, multi-stage process. Dysfunction of the different stages causes different problems and requires different solutions.

The first stage is the *optical process* that puts an image of the outside world on the retina. This stage can be disrupted by refractive errors or media opacities, such as cataract. A good tool to evaluate this stage is visual (letter chart) acuity which measures the MAgnification Requirement (MAR) relative to the 20/20 reference standard. (MAR is usually known as minimum angle of resolution.) Magnification devices (see Chapter 24) are the natural choice to counteract this type of vision loss.

The second stage is the *receptor stage* that translates the optical image into neural impulses. If this stage is defective, vision is disrupted in a different way. A blind spot in the central retina (central scotoma) may necessitate shifting fixation to a less central retinal area (the preferred retinal locus, PRL) where the receptor mosaic is less dense. This causes reduced visual acuity, which can be counteracted by magnification (see Chapter 24). However, visual acuity tells only part of the story, since the condition at the PRL tells us nothing about the condition of the surrounding retina. Since normal vision involves constant eye movements, the object

of attention may move in and out of the scotoma. This *scotoma interference* is not quantified by visual acuity, although it may be apparent during testing, and cannot be remedied by magnification devices. The patient needs *training and practice* to improve fixation stability. This may be provided by occupational therapists or vision rehabilitation specialists, but it is up to ophthalmologists to recognize the need for this training and make the appropriate referral.

The third stage is that of *neural processing*. This process starts in the inner retina and proceeds via the visual cortex to higher cortical centers, where it eventually gives rise to visually guided behavior. This stage is undoubtedly the most complex and awareness of vision problems related to the processing of visual information is increasing, such as the perceptual consequences of traumatic brain injury (TBI) and cerebro-vascular accidents (CVAs), and in children the importance of the entity of cerebral (cortical) visual impairment (CVI). Relevant information needs to be brought to the attention of practicing ophthalmologists, and parents and educators need to be made more aware of compensatory techniques. Some cerebral defects produce obvious impairment of visual acuity and visual field. More subtle defects may exist in the presence of normal visual function on standard clinical testing. A patient with optical or retinal problems may stumble over a curb because of lack of contrast, whereas a patient with cerebral injury may be able to detect the change in contrast but unable to decide whether this is a line on the ground or the edge of a step. In this case, *vision enhancement* (better illumination, contrast) will not help and *vision substitution*, for example a cane to tactilely determine the step, may be more appropriate. Visual acuity is not a good measure of processing problems, and *training* is the main rehabilitative option. At the higher cerebral levels the information flow is no longer exclusively visual, but is integrated with information from other sources. Normally this integration is continuous and seamless. It only reaches our awareness if information from two sources is inconsistent and causes symptoms such as motion sickness.

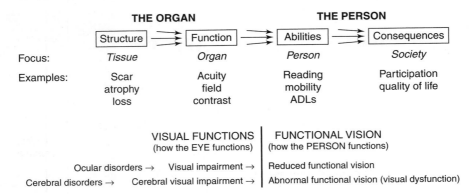

Figure 25-1. The aspects of visual functioning.

Full assessment of impaired cerebral visual processing may require neuropsychological testing but preliminary assessment by ophthalmologists or neurologists can be helpful, such as with the Cortical Vision Screening Test (CORVIST).

ASPECTS OF VISION LOSS

Since vision provides about one-half of all the input to the brain, it is no surprise that vision loss, whether minor or severe, can affect almost all aspects of life, and the complex phenomenon of vision cannot be captured from a single point of view. A convenient framework to discuss the various impacts of vision loss is by considering four aspects of visual functioning, *structure, function, abilities, and consequences* (Figure 25–1).

Structural changes, such as scarring, degeneration, and atrophy that are apparent on macroscopic and microscopic examination of tissue, do not necessarily indicate function, which is assessed by clinical tests, including visual acuity, visual field, and contrast sensitivity. In turn, this does not necessarily gauge the patient's ability to perform specific tasks, such as reading, getting around, recognizing faces, or undertaking activities of daily living. Occupational therapists and other rehabilitation professionals use all this information to work with patients and teach them how their residual vision can be used most effectively. In addition, the patient's participation in society and quality of life need to assessed.

Structure and function contribute to *visual functions*, which reflect the function of the visual system as an organ of the body, whereas how the person functions in vision-related activities reflects *functional vision*, which reflects how the patient functions as a person. Ophthalmology is well versed in analyzing the former, but the ultimate goal of all ophthalmic interventions should be to improve the quality of life, an aspect of the latter that often receives inadequate attention. Ophthalmic care, including in textbooks, traditionally prioritizes visual function, whereas for patients functional vision is more important, but the process is flexible and bi-directional such that intervention can be effective at all stages (Figure 25–2).

In medical practice, **treatment** is often overemphasized but comprehensive health care should include **prevention**, **treatment**, and **rehabilitation**, with social services also being involved in rehabilitation, particularly participation in society. The bi-directional nature of the process requires each aspect to be viewed and assessed from both sides, possibly needing different approaches even if they measure the

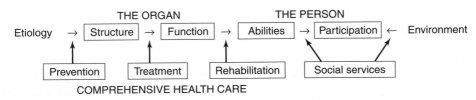

Figure 25-2. Interventions on flexible links.

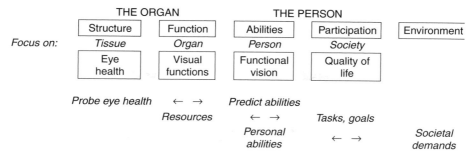

▲ **Figure 25–3.** Each aspect relates to adjacent aspects.

same parameter. For example, in ophthalmic practice visual acuity is measured to assess visual function, for which purpose best-corrected acuity for each eye separately is the best method. In rehabilitation, visual acuity is measured to estimate functional vision, for which purpose acuity with both eyes open is best, since this reflects the patient's normal situation. Similarly visual abilities can be assessed in terms of visual function, by measuring visual acuity, visual field, and color vision, but it needs to be undertaken with respect to the individual patient's activities, taking into account their difficulties and goals as well as their expectations and societal demands (Figure 25–3). Refractive surgeons have become very aware of individualizing treatment to the patient's needs. Also a single activity may require complex evaluation. Successful reading depends on being able to see the print, as well as reading speed, endurance, and enjoyment.

COMPREHENSIVE VISION REHABILITATION

Considering all of these aspects, it should be clear that comprehensive vision rehabilitation extends beyond the provision of low vision aids, although that is still vitally important (see Chapter 24). Any form of rehabilitation requires teamwork involving different professionals to deal with the various components. Since vision loss is the common denominator, the ophthalmologist should coordinate the team.

▶ History and Goal Setting

Before considering a rehabilitation plan, the patient's goals and needs are clarified. For the ophthalmologist this may involve only a general question, such as: *"How does your vision bother you?"* or *"Can you still read the newspaper?"* If the answer reveals a problem, clinicians should do the same as they do for retinal, glaucoma, or other problems and tell the patient: *"I understand your problem and I will refer you to someone who can help you."*

When future deterioration is a possibility, it is not necessary to wait until there is severe vision loss before recommending action. Early adaptations to minor loss can facilitate later adaptations to major loss. The possibility of deterioration of

vision is best made known from the beginning but accompanied with advice about the availability of skilled professionals and resources. Unfortunately, many practitioners are poorly trained in conveying bad news, a skill that should be taught and practiced in medical school. All ophthalmologists should master this skill, which includes informing the patient about options and knowing the appropriate referral sources.

The American Academy of Ophthalmology recognizes several levels of competence in vision rehabilitation. Some ophthalmology practices may employ professionals who can provide basic services in-house. Particularly for more complex cases, referral to specialized vision rehabilitation services is appropriate.

To determine the range of services that are appropriate, the American Academy of Ophthalmology recommends the following checklist:

- **Reading**—For many patients this is their foremost concern.
- **Activities of daily living (ADLs)**—Even though reading may be the most prominent complaint, most people spend the larger part of their day performing a variety of other activities.
- **Safety**—Are people at risk for falls? How do they cross the street?
- **Community participation**—Can they still participate at church or in community events?
- **Physical, cognitive, and psychosocial well being**—Since many patients with vision loss are elderly, this is an important aspect that should not be overlooked. If problems exist, it may affect the recommendations to be made.

Not all areas may have problems, but the checklist is important such that priorities can be set and specific rehabilitation goals formulated, reflecting the patient's needs and desires, not just the practitioner's expectations.

▶ Examination

The standard ophthalmic examination, including identification of any conditions amenable to specific treatment, needs to be adapted as discussed in Chapter 24.

Observation of visual performance is important in young children, where regular testing may not be possible. Reports from parents and teachers are often as informative as direct observation in the office. Even for adults, observation of the performance of daily living tasks can be helpful. It provides a baseline against which future progress can be measured. It can also give insight in the patient's problem-solving skills and motivation.

Questionnaires can assess the subjective difficulty of tasks, including those that cannot be assessed in the office. A disadvantage is that the responses are subjective, with some patients exaggerating their difficulties and others understating them.

Assessment of mobility, including identification of peripheral visual field loss, is very important and impaired mobility should trigger referral for assessment by an orientation and mobility (O+M) instructor. Mobility training may be crucial to reestablishing independence. Patients also need to be made aware of the importance of appropriate signaling of their visual impairment. Many feel that carrying a long cane or similar aid publicizes their vulnerability to individuals who might take advantage of it, but well-meaning individuals including drivers also need to be made aware of the patient's visual impairment.

▶ Comprehensive Rehabilitation Plans

A comprehensive vision rehabilitation plan requires attention to more than just how the eyes function. Figure 25–4 provides a summary of the possible interventions but not all will be needed in every case.

▶ Vision Enhancement (See Chapter 24)

Vision substitution refers to the use of senses other than vision. Common examples are talking books and voice-output devices (see Chapter 24), Braille, and long canes. Vision enhancement and vision substitution are not mutually exclusive but complementary. A patient may use a magnifier to read price tags and talking books for recreational reading.

A patient with retinitis pigmentosa with normal mobility in the day, may need a cane at night. Audio cassettes may have Braille labels.

Assistance is a form of vision substitution using the eyes of others. Family members, care givers, and office personnel should be familiar with sighted-guide techniques to effectively assist visually impaired patients with minimal embarrassment. Guide dogs are also a possibility but require training and care of the dog as well as training of the patient, who needs to be physically active and able to manage the dog.

Coping Skills: Vision loss often causes reactive depression, which renders the patient less receptive to rehabilitative suggestions. Conversely successful rehabilitation can be therapeutic and motivate the patient to further improvements. Dealing with depression may involve other professionals, but the authority of the ophthalmologist can play a major role in convincing patients that they can do far more than they may believe after the initial shock of vision loss.

Human Environment: As patients go through the stages of adaptation to vision loss, a supportive home environment is essential and it is important to include spouses, children, or significant others in the counseling process. The clinician should make sure that the significant others understand the underlying condition, what can be expected, and how to support the patient. Answering their questions directly is often better than leaving this to the patient, who initially may not have absorbed everything that was said. An overprotective environment that deprives patients of opportunities to do things themselves can be as detrimental as an over-demanding one that puts too much emphasis on the patient's shortcomings. The same applies to work, school, and social groups. Initially, patients often feel isolated and believe that they are the only ones experiencing these problems. This is where *peer support groups* can be helpful; in these groups they can experience how others are dealing with similar problems.

Physical environment: An uncluttered environment, where things have a defined, fixed place is helpful because it

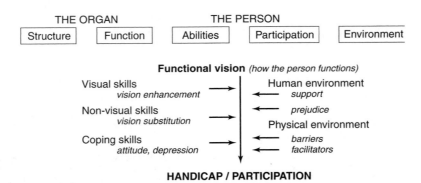

▲ Figure 25–4. Comprehensive rehabilitation.

eliminates the need for searching. Good general illumination and task lighting often help, because at higher illumination levels retinal cells that are damaged but not dead can still contribute. Good contrast is important, for instance milk should not be served in a white Styrofoam cup and edges of steps and stairs should be marked.

CONCLUSION

The patient's life does not end with the diagnosis of visual impairment. Similarly, the responsibility of the ophthalmologist does not end with the treatment of eye disease, but extends to counseling the patient and initiating rehabilitation, based upon knowledge of the available resources and referral pathways.

RESOURCES

Searching business telephone directories (yellow pages) and the internet under visual impairment, low vision, blindness, and rehabilitation can provide useful information on local rehabilitation resources.

General Information

The SmartSight initiative of the American Academy of Ophthalmology (www.AAO.org, search SmartSight) contains handouts for patients (including an extensive list of resources) as well as for practitioners.

The AFB Senior Site (www.AFB.org/seniorsitehome.asp) contains resources for seniors.

The MDsupport website (www.MDsupport.org) specializes in support and documentation for age-related macular degeneration.

The Lighthouse International in New York (www.lighthouse.org) offers extensive resources for all forms of vision loss.

These websites contain links to many more websites with additional information and often can provide information about local resources.

Personnel

Occupational Therapists (OT) (www.aota.org). This profession evolved in the health care field. They have broad rehabilitation training, but traditionally learned little about vision. This is changing as the demand for vision rehabilitation grows.

Another group includes Certified Low Vision Therapists (CLVT), Certified Orientation and Mobility Specialists (COMS), and Certified Vision Rehabilitation Therapists (CVRT). These professions evolved from the education field. Their training is vision-specific, but traditionally focused on students and younger age groups. They are certified by the ACVREP (www.acvrep.org).

For both groups their state chapters may provide information about available manpower.

Devices, Technology

Low-tech devices, such as magnifiers and telescopes, are available from many suppliers, who have their own websites. They are relatively low cost and can serve a large number of patients. Hi-tech devices, such as video-magnifiers, cost more and evolve more rapidly. For these, it is important to get up-to-date information from a specialist (see Chapter 24).

The Library of Congress provides an extensive library of free talking books.

Financial Support, Social Services

Financial support and social service programs may vary from state to state. All states have vocational rehabilitation programs. Special services are available for veterans through the VA Blind Rehabilitation Centers. Local agencies are often the best source of information.

APPENDIX
Functional Vision Score

August Colenbrander, MD

HISTORY

Vision loss is a complex phenomenon that cannot be fully understood unless many different aspects are considered (see Chapter 25). Yet, for certain applications it may be desirable to reduce this complex reality to a single number. Administrators prefer the oversimplification of the single number approach when they have to decide on eligibility for benefits or for worker's compensation cases, where the outcome also is a single number: the amount of compensation.

Formulas to calculate what was then called "Visual Economics" were first proposed in Germany in the late 1800s. In 1925 Snell proposed to the American Medical Association (AMA) a simpler formula for "Visual Efficiency." This formula, reflecting an 80% loss of employability for a visual acuity loss to 20/200, served until 2000. In its fifth (2001) and sixth (2008) editions the AMA *Guides to the Evaluation of Permanent Impairment* adopted the "Functional Vision Score" (FVS), which reflects an estimate of the ability to perform Activities of Daily Living (ADL).

On the new scale, 20/200 acuity is rated as an estimated 50% loss of ADL ability, rather than as an 80% loss of employability. Other changes include no longer considering the two eyes as separate organs, vision with both eyes open being the normal condition. The new scale has been shown to correlate well with other measures of ability.[1]

CALCULATING THE FUNCTIONAL VISION SCORE

Figure A–1 represents the steps in calculating the functional vision score and its use in calculating an AMA impairment rating.

▶ Functional Acuity Score

The first step is measuring the visual acuity. Use of an ETDRS type chart with a logarithmic progression of letter sizes and 5 letters on each line is preferred. The best corrected acuity is measured for each eye and with both eyes open.

According to the Weber–Fechner law, visual *ability* is proportional to the logarithm of the visual *acuity* value. This is reflected in the **visual acuity score (VAS)** (Table A–1). On an ETDRS type chart the VAS increases by 1 point for every letter read correctly; the scale is anchored at 20/20 = 100.

Next, the three VAS values—both eyes (OU), right eye (OD), left eye (OS)—are combined to provide a single **functional acuity score (FAS)**, 60% weighting being given to the acuity with both eyes open and 20% to each of the monocular values.

▶ Functional Field Score

In a similar way, a **visual field score (VFS)** and **functional field score (FFS)** are calculated. The VFS is determined with a grid (Figure A-2), which allocates 50 points to the central 10° area and 50 points to the remainder of the visual field. This division reflects that the representation of the central 10° of visual field occupies about 50% of the primary visual cortex. It also divides the score evenly between the central area, which is important for reading and detailed vision, and the outer area, which is important for orientation and mobility.

The points are allocated along two meridians in each of the upper quadrants and three meridians in each of the lower quadrants. On each meridian 5 points (2° apart) are assigned to the central area and 5 points (10° apart) to the outer area, their distribution being approximately logarithmic. The lower visual field is weighted 50% more than the upper visual field because of its greater importance in functional vision. The primary meridians are not used, to avoid the need for special rules for hemianopias.

The VFS is determined by counting the number of points seen within the visual field delineated by the Goldmann III4e (or equivalent, eg, Humphrey 10 dB) isopter.

The FFS is calculated from the three VFS values using the same weighted formula for calculating the FAS from the three VAS values (60% OU + 20% OD + 20% OS).

Finally, the FAS and FFS are combined into a single **functional vision score (FVS)**.

Thus far, the calculation follows strict mathematical rules. If there are other vision problems that are not reflected in a visual acuity or visual field loss, the examiner may apply an adjustment of maximally 15 points. Such an adjustment must be properly argued and documented.

[1]Fuhr PSW, Holmes LD, Fletcher DC et al. The AMA Guides Functional Vision Score is a better predictor of vision-targeted quality of life than traditional measures of visual acuity or visual field extent. Vis Impairment Res 2003;5:137–146 .

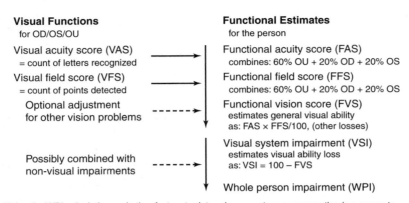

▲ **Figure A-1.** Steps in calculating the Functional Vision Score (FVS) and the AMA impairment ratings.

CALCULATING THE AMA IMPAIRMENT RATING

The FVS reflects visual function (20/20 = 100), whereas the AMA impairment rating reflects loss (20/20 = no loss = 0). Therefore, the AMA impairment rating is calculated by subtracting the FVS from 100.

Furthermore, a distinction is made between **visual system impairment (VSI)** and **whole person impairment (WPI)**. 100% VSI (total blindness) does not equal 100% WPI (death). Therefore, a gradual correction is made from VSI = 50% to VSI = 100%, so that 100% VSI = 85% WPI. This adjustment is justified by the increasing use of visual substitution skills (see Chapter 25) at lower visual acuity levels.

If there are impairments in other organ systems, these may be combined (through special tables) with the visual WPI percentage.

For a more detailed discussion with examples, the reader is referred to the AMA publication: Rondinelli RD (ed). *Guides to the Evaluation of Permanent Impairment,* 6th edition (2008), Chicago, IL: AMA Press, 2008:281–319.

Table A-1. Visual Acuity (VA) and corresponding Visual Acuity Score (VAS)

VA	VAS	VA	VAS
20/10	115	20/200	50
20/12.5	110	20/250	45
20/16	105	20/320	40
20/20	100	20/400	35
20/25	95	20/500	30
20/32	90	20/630	25
20/40	85	20/800	20
20/50	80	20/1000	15
20/63	75	20/1250	10
20/80	70	20/1600	5
20/100	65	20/2000	0
20/125	60		
20/160	55	CF < 2 ft	0
20/200	50	HM < 10 ft	0

Note that the VA columns list a geometric (logarithmic) sequence of visual *acuity* values. The VAS columns transform this to a linear sequence of visual *ability* estimates.
Also note that the VAS scale is not capped at 20/20, although AMA impairment ratings only reflect the loss relative to the 20/20 level.

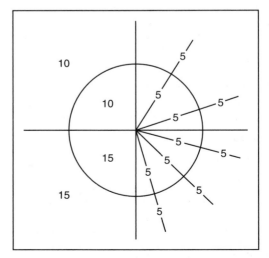

▲ **Figure A-2.** VFS grid, showing the total number of points in each region (left half) and how the points are allocated along the 5 meridians (right half). The radius of the circle is 10 degrees.

Glossary of Terms Relating to the Eye*

Accommodation: The adjustment of the eye for seeing at near distances, accomplished by changing the shape of the lens through action of the ciliary muscle, thus focusing a clear image on the retina.

Acquired: Contracted after birth.

Agnosia: Inability to recognize common objects despite an intact visual apparatus.

Albinism: A hereditary deficiency of melanin pigment in the retinal pigment epithelium, iris, and choroid.

Alternate cover test: Determination of the full extent of heterotropia and heterophoria by alternately covering one eye and then the other with an opaque object, thus eliminating fusion.

Amaurosis fugax: Transient loss of vision. Usually reserved for transient loss of vision due to retinal embolus.

Amblyopia: Reduced visual acuity in the absence of sufficient eye or visual pathway disease to explain the level of vision.

Ametropia: See Refractive error.

Amsler grid: A chart with vertical and horizontal lines used for testing the central visual field.

Angiography: A diagnostic test in which the vascular system is examined. The ocular circulation can be highlighted by intravenous injection of either fluorescein, which particularly demonstrates the retinal circulation, or indocyanine green, to demonstrate the choroidal circulation.

Aniridia: Congenital absence of the iris.

Aniseikonia: A condition in which the image seen by one eye differs in size or shape from that seen by the other.

Anisocoria: Unequal pupillary size.

Anisometropia: Difference in refractive error of the eyes.

Anophthalmos: Absence of a true eyeball.

Anterior chamber: Space filled with aqueous bounded anteriorly by the cornea and posteriorly by the iris.

Aphakia: Absence of the crystalline lens.

Aqueous: Clear, watery fluid that fills the anterior and posterior chambers.

Asthenopia: Eye fatigue from muscular, environmental, or psychological causes.

Astigmatism: Refractive error that prevents the light rays from coming to a point focus on the retina because of different degrees of refraction in the various meridians of the cornea or crystalline lens.

Axis: The meridian specifying the orientation of a cylindric lens.

Binocular vision: Ability of the eyes to focus on one object and then to fuse two images into one.

Biomicroscope: See Slitlamp.

Bitot's spots: Keratinization of the bulbar conjunctiva near the limbus, resulting in a raised spot—a feature of vitamin A deficiency.

Blepharitis: Inflammation of the eyelids.

Blepharoptosis (ptosis): Drooping of the eyelid.

Blepharospasm: Involuntary spasm of the lids.

Blind spot: "Blank" area in the visual field, corresponding to the light rays that come to a focus on the optic nerve.

Blindness: In the United States, the usual definition of blindness is corrected visual acuity of 20/200 or less in the better eye, or a visual field of no more than 20° in the better eye.

Botulinum toxin: Neurotoxin A of the bacterium *Clostridium botulinum* used in very small doses to produce temporary paralysis of the extraocular or facial muscles.

Buphthalmos: Large eyeball in infantile glaucoma.

Canal of Schlemm: A circular modified venous structure in the anterior chamber angle that drains aqueous to the aqueous veins.

Canaliculus: Small tear drainage tube in inner aspect of upper and lower lids leading from the punctum to the common canaliculus and then to the tear sac.

Canthotomy: Usually implies lateral canthotomy—cutting of the lateral canthal tendon for the purpose of widening the palpebral fissure.

Canthus: The angle at either end of the eyelid aperture; specified as outer (lateral) or inner (medial).

Cataract: An opacity of the crystalline lens.

Chalazion: Granulomatous inflammation of a meibomian gland.

---

*See also Definitions of Strabismus, Chapter 12.

Chemosis: Conjunctival edema.

Choroid: The vascular middle coat between the retina and sclera.

Ciliary body: Portion of the uveal tract between the iris and the choroid. It consists of ciliary processes and the ciliary muscle.

Coloboma: Congenital cleft due to the failure of some portion of the eye or ocular adnexa to complete growth.

Color blindness (deficiency): Diminished ability to perceive differences in color.

Concave lens: Lens having the power to diverge rays of light; also known as diverging, reducing, negative, or minus lens, denoted by the sign (−), and used to correct myopia.

Cones and rods: Two kinds of retinal photo receptor cells. Cones are primarily involved in fine visual discrimination (optimal visual acuity) and color vision; rods with peripheral vision and vision in decreased illumination.

Congenital: Existing at or before birth, not necessarily inherited (hereditary).

Conjunctiva: Mucous membrane that lines the posterior aspect of the eyelids and covers the anterior sclera.

Contact lenses: Thin lenses that fit directly on the eye, usually on the cornea but sometimes on the sclera.

Convergence: The process of directing the visual axes of the eyes to a near point.

Convex lens: Lens having power to converge rays of light and to bring them to a focus; also known as converging, magnifying, or plus lens, denoted by the sign (+), and used to correct hyperopia or presbyopia.

Cornea: Transparent portion of the outer coat of the eyeball forming the anterior wall of the anterior chamber.

Corneal graft (keratoplasty): Operation to replace a portion of the cornea, either involving the full thickness (penetrating keratoplasty), only a superficial layer (lamellar keratoplasty), or only the endothelium (endothelial keratoplasty), with donor cornea from the same human (autograft), or another human (homograft).

Cover test: Determination of the presence and degree of heterotropia by covering one eye with an opaque object and examining for any movement of the uncovered eye to fixate a target.

Cross cylinder: A specialized spherocylindrical lens used to measure astigmatism.

Crystalline lens: A transparent biconvex structure suspended in the eyeball between the aqueous and the vitreous. Its function is to bring rays of light to a focus on the retina. Accommodation is produced by variations in the magnitude of this effect. (Usually called simply the lens.)

Cyclodestructive procedures: Surgical techniques to reduce aqueous production by destroying portions of the ciliary body in the treatment of intractable glaucoma, using cryotherapy (cyclocryotherapy), lasers (cyclophotocoagulation), or diathermy.

Cycloplegic: A drug that relaxes the ciliary muscle, paralyzing accommodation.

Cylindrical lens: A segment of a cylinder, the refractive power of which varies in different meridians, used to correct astigmatism.

Dacryocystitis: Infection of the lacrimal sac.

Dacryocystorhinostomy: A procedure by which a communication is made between the nasolacrimal duct and the nasal cavity to relieve an obstruction in the nasolacrimal duct, or sac.

Dark adaptation: The ability to adjust to decreased illumination.

Diopter: Unit of measurement of refractive power of lenses.

Diplopia (double vision): Seeing one object as two.

"E" test: A system of testing visual acuity in illiterates, particularly preschool children.

Ectropion: Turning out of the eyelid.

Emmetropia: Absence of refractive error.

Endolaser: Application of laser from a probe inserted into the globe.

Endophthalmitis: Extensive intraocular infection.

Enophthalmos: Abnormal retrodisplacement of the eyeball.

Entropion: A turning inward of the eyelid.

Enucleation: Complete surgical removal of the eyeball.

Epicanthus: Congenital skin fold that overlies the inner canthus.

Epiphora: Tearing.

Esophoria: A tendency of the eyes to be convergent.

Esotropia: A manifest inward deviation of one eye.

Evisceration: Removal of the contents of the eyeball.

Exenteration: Removal of the entire contents of the orbit, including the eyeball and part or all of the lids.

Exophoria: A tendency of the eyes to be divergent.

Exophthalmos: Abnormal protrusion of the eyeball.

Exotropia: A manifest outward deviation of one eye.

Familial: Pertaining to traits, either hereditary or acquired, that tend to occur in families.

Far point: The point at which the eye is focused when accommodation is completely relaxed.

Farsightedness: See Hyperopia.

Field of vision: The entire area that can be seen without shifting gaze.

Floaters: Moving images in the visual field due to vitreous opacities.

Focus: A point to which rays of light are brought together to form an image; focal distance is the distance between a lens and its focal point.

Fornix: The junction of the palpebral and bulbar conjunctiva.

Fovea: 1.5-mm-diameter zone of the central retina, characterized histologically by thinning of the outer nuclear layer.

Foveola: 0.3-mm-diameter thinnest (0.25 mm) area of the central retina, clinically apparent as a depression, in which there are only cone photoreceptors and which provides optimal visual acuity. It corresponds to the retinal avascular zone on fluorescein angiography.

Fundus: The posterior portion of the eye visible through the pupil.

Fusion: Combining the images received by the two eyes into one image.

Glaucoma: Disease characterized by optic disc cupping and visual field loss, usually associated with elevated intraocular pressure.

Gonioscopy: A technique of examining the anterior chamber angle, utilizing a corneal contact lens.

Hemianopia: Blindness in one-half of the field of vision of one or both eyes.

Heterophoria (phoria): A tendency of the eyes to be misaligned that is overcome by fusion (latent deviation).

Heterotropia: See Strabismus.

Hippus: Exaggerated spontaneous rhythmic movements of the iris.

Hordeolum, external (sty): Infection of the glands of Moll or Zeis.

Hordeolum, internal: Meibomian gland infection.

Hyperopia, hypermetropia (farsightedness): A refractive error in which the focus of light rays from a distant object is behind the retina.

Hyperphoria: A tendency of one eye to deviate upward.

Hypertropia: Manifest upward deviation of one eye.

Hyphema: Blood in the anterior chamber.

Hypopyon: Pus in the anterior chamber.

Hypotony: Abnormally soft eye from any cause.

Inherited (hereditary): Transmitted from parents to offspring.

Injection: Congestion of blood vessels.

Iridectomy: Surgical excision of a sector of iris to form a direct communication between the anterior and posterior chambers.

Iridoplasty, peripheral (laser) iridoplasty: Procedure to contract the iris stroma by application of usually argon laser burns to the peripheral iris.

Iridotomy, peripheral (laser): Formation of a hole in the iris to form a direct communication between the anterior and posterior chambers, usually performed with the neodymium:YAG laser.

Iris: Colored, annular membrane, suspended behind the cornea and immediately in front of the lens.

Ishihara color plates: A test for color vision based on the ability to see numbers in a series of pseudoisochromatic multicolored charts.

Isopter: Boundary of the visual field to a particular target. Isopters to targets of different colors and sizes allow differentiation of relative from absolute visual field defects.

Jaeger test: A test for near vision using lines of various sizes of type.

Keratic precipitate (KP): Accumulation of inflammatory cells on the posterior cornea in uveitis.

Keratitis: Inflammation of the cornea.

Keratoconus: Cone-shaped deformity of the cornea.

Keratomalacia: Corneal softening, usually associated with vitamin A deficiency.

Keratometer: An instrument for measuring the curvature of the cornea, used in fitting contact lenses and determination of intraocular lens power prior to cataract surgery.

Keratopathy, bullous: Swelling of the cornea with painful blisters in the epithelium due to excessive corneal hydration.

Keratoplasty: See Corneal graft.

Keratoprosthesis: Plastic implant surgically placed in an opaque cornea to achieve an area of optical clarity.

Kerato-refractive surgery (refractive keratoplasty): Corneal surgery to correct refractive error.

Keratotomy: An incision in the cornea. In arcuate keratotomy, circumferential incisions are made to correct astigmatism.

Koeppe nodule: Accumulation of inflammatory cells on the iris in uveitis.

Lacrimal sac: The dilated area at the junction of the nasolacrimal duct and the canaliculi.

Laser in situ keratomileusis (LASIK): Corneal excimer laser ablation under a stromal flap to treat refractive error.

Laser subepithelial keratomileusis (LASEK): Corneal excimer laser ablation under an epithelial flap to treat refractive error.

Lens: A refractive medium having one or both surfaces curved. (See also Crystalline lens.)

Lensometer: An instrument for measuring the power of optical lenses.

Limbus: Junction of the cornea and sclera.

Macula: 5.5-6-mm-diameter area of central retina bounded by the temporal retinal vascular arcades. It is known to anatomists as the area centralis, to differentiate it from the macula lutea, and is defined as the part of the retina in which the ganglion cell layer is more than one cell thick.

Macula lutea: 3-mm-diameter area of the central retina defined anatomically by the presence of yellow xanthophyll pigment.

Maddox rod: A red lens composed of parallel series of strong cylinders through which a point of light is viewed as a red line—used to measure phorias.

Magnification: The ratio of the size of an image to the size of its object.

Megalocornea: Abnormally large cornea (> 13 mm in diameter).

Metamorphopsia: Wavy distortion of vision.

Microphthalmos: Abnormally small eye with abnormal function (see Nanophthalmos).

Miotic: A drug causing pupillary constriction.

Mydriatic: A drug causing pupillary dilation.

Myopia (nearsightedness): A refractive error in which the focus for light rays from a distant object is anterior to the retina.

Nanophthalmos: Abnormally small eye with normal function (see Microphthalmos).

Near point: The point at which the eye is focused when accommodation is fully active.

Nearsightedness: See Myopia.

Nystagmus: An involuntary rhythmic oscillation of the eyeball that may be horizontal, vertical, torsional, or mixed.

Ophthalmia neonatorum: Conjunctivitis in the newborn.

Ophthalmoscope: An instrument with a special illumination system for viewing the inner eye, particularly the retina and associated structures.

Optic atrophy: Optic nerve degeneration, manifesting clinically as pallor of the optic disk.

Optic disk: Ophthalmoscopically visible portion of the optic nerve.

Optic nerve: The nerve that carries visual impulses from the retina to the brain.

Orbital cellulitis: Inflammation of the orbital tissues surrounding the eye.

Orthoptics: The study and treatment of defects of binocular visual function or of the muscles controlling movement of the eyeballs.

Oscillopsia: The subjective illusion of movement of objects that occurs with nystagmus.

Palpebral: Pertaining to the eyelid.

Pannus: Infiltration of the cornea with blood vessels.

Panophthalmitis: Inflammation of the entire eyeball and orbital tissues.

Papilledema: Swelling of the optic disks due to raised intracranial pressure.

Papillitis: Inflammatory swelling of the optic nerve head.

Partially seeing child: For educational purposes, a partially seeing child is one who has a corrected visual acuity of 20/70 or less in the better eye.

Perimeter: An instrument for measuring the field of vision.

Peripheral vision: Ability to perceive the presence and movement of objects outside of the direct line of vision.

Phacoemulsification and phacofragmentation: Techniques of extracapsular cataract surgery in which the nucleus of the lens is disrupted into small fragments by ultrasonic vibrations, thus allowing aspiration of all the lens matter through a small wound.

Phakomatoses: A group of hereditary diseases characterized by the presence of spots, cysts, and tumors in various parts of the body—for example, neurofibromatosis, Von Hippel–Lindau disease, tuberous sclerosis.

Phlyctenule: Localized lymphocytic infiltration of the conjunctiva.

Phoria: See Heterophoria.

Photocoagulation: Thermal damage to tissues due to absorption of high levels of light (including laser) energy.

Photodecomposition: Tissue damage by direct separation of chemical bonds by absorption of very short-wavelength ultraviolet light (eg, from excimer lasers).

Photodisruption: Tissue damage produced by the breakdown of "plasma," which is a state of ionization created by spot focusing a high-energy laser source (eg, neodymium:YAG).

Photodynamic therapy (PDT): Retinal laser augmented by intravenous injection of a dye (verteporfin).

Photophobia: Abnormal sensitivity to light.

Photopsia: Appearance of sparks or flashes within the eye due to retinal irritation.

Photorefractive keratectomy (PRK): Surface corneal excimer laser ablation to treat refractive error.

Phototherapeutic keratectomy (PTK): Surface corneal excimer ablation to treat anterior corneal disorders, for example, recurrent corneal erosions.

Phthisis bulbi: Atrophy of the eyeball with blindness and decreased intraocular pressure, due to end-stage intraocular disease.

Placido's disk: A disk with concentric rings used to determine the regularity of the cornea by observing the ring's reflection on the corneal surface.

Poliosis: Depigmentation of the eyelashes.

Posterior chamber: Space filled with aqueous anterior to the lens and posterior to the iris.

Presbyopia ("old sight"): Physiologically blurred near vision, commonly evident soon after age 40, due to reduction in the power of accommodation.

Prism: A wedge of transparent material that deviates light rays without changing their focus.

Prism cover test: Extension of the alternate cover test using increasing strength prisms to quantify the total magnitude of ocular misalignment (heterophoria and heterotropia).

Prism diopter: The unit of prism power.

Pseudoisochromatic charts: Charts with colored dots of various hues and shades forming numbers, letters, or patterns, used for testing color discrimination (see Ishihara color plates).

Pseudophakia: Presence of an artificial intraocular lens implant following cataract extraction.

Pterygium: A triangular growth of tissue that extends from the conjunctiva over the cornea.

Ptosis: Drooping of the eyelid.

Puncta: External orifices of the upper and lower canaliculi.

Pupil: The round hole in the center of the iris that corresponds to the lens aperture in a camera.

Refraction: (1) Deviation in the course of rays of light in passing from one transparent medium into another of different density. (2) Determination of refractive errors of the eye and correction by lenses.

Refractive error (ametropia): An optical defect that prevents light rays from being brought to a single focus on the retina.

Refractive index: The ratio of the speed of light in a vacuum to the speed of light in a given material.

Refractive media: The transparent parts of the eye having refractive power, of which the cornea is most powerful but the (crystalline) lens is under voluntary control (see Accommodation).

Retina: Innermost coat of the eye, consisting of the sensory retina, which is composed of light-sensitive neural elements connecting to other neural cells, and the retinal pigment epithelium.

Retinal detachment: A separation of the neurosensory retina from the pigment epithelium and choroid.

Retinitis pigmentosa: A hereditary degeneration of the retina.

Retinoscope: An instrument for objective determination of the refractive error of an eye.

Rods: See Cones and rods.

Sclera: The white part of the eye—a tough covering that, with the cornea, forms the external protective coat of the eye.

Scleral spur: The protrusion of sclera into the anterior chamber angle.

Scotoma: A blind or partially blind area in the visual field.

Slitlamp biomicroscope: A combination light and microscope for examination of the eye, particularly allowing stereoscopic imaging.

Snellen chart: Used for testing central visual acuity. It consists of lines of letters or numbers, graded in size according to the distance at which they can be discriminated by a normal eye.

Sphincterotomy: A surgical incision of the iris sphincter muscle.

Staphyloma: A thinned part of the coat of the eye, causing protrusion.

Strabismus (heterotropia, tropia): Misalignment of the eyes (manifest deviation).

Sty: See Hordeolum, external.

Symblepharon: Adhesions between the bulbar and palpebral conjunctiva.

Sympathetic ophthalmia: Inflammation in both eyes following trauma.

Synechia: Adhesion of the iris to the cornea (anterior synechia) or lens (posterior synechia).

Syneresis: A degenerative process within a gel, involving drawing together of particles of the dispersed medium, separation of the medium, and shrinkage of the gel; specifically applied to the vitreous.

Tarsorrhaphy: A surgical procedure by which the upper and lower lid margins are united.

Tonometer: An instrument for measuring intraocular pressure.

Trabeculectomy: Surgical procedure for creating an additional aqueous drainage channel in the treatment of glaucoma.

Trabeculoplasty: Laser photocoagulation of the trabecular meshwork in the treatment of open-angle glaucoma.

Trachoma: A serious form of infectious keratoconjunctivitis due to chlamydial infection.

Transpupillary thermotherapy: Diffuse treatment of fundal lesions with low-energy diode laser.

Trichiasis: Inversion and rubbing of the eyelashes against the globe.

Tropia: See Strabismus.

Uncover test: Extension of the cover test to determine the presence of heterophoria by detection of corrective movement of the covered eye as it is uncovered.

Uvea (uveal tract): The iris, ciliary body, and choroid.

Uveitis: Inflammation of one or all portions of the uveal tract.

Visual acuity: Measure of the optical resolution of the eye.

Visual axis: An imaginary line that connects a point in space (point of fixation) with the foveola.

Vitiligo: Localized patchy decrease or absence of pigment on the skin.

Vitrectomy: Surgical removal of the vitreous to clear vitreous hemorrhage, allow treatment of retinal detachment or retinal vascular disease, or treat intraocular infection or inflammation.

Vitreous: Transparent, colorless mass of soft, gelatinous material filling the eyeball behind the crystalline lens.

Xerosis: Drying of tissues lining the anterior surface of the eye.

Zonule: The numerous fine tissue strands that stretch from the ciliary processes to the crystalline lens equator (360°) and hold the lens in place.

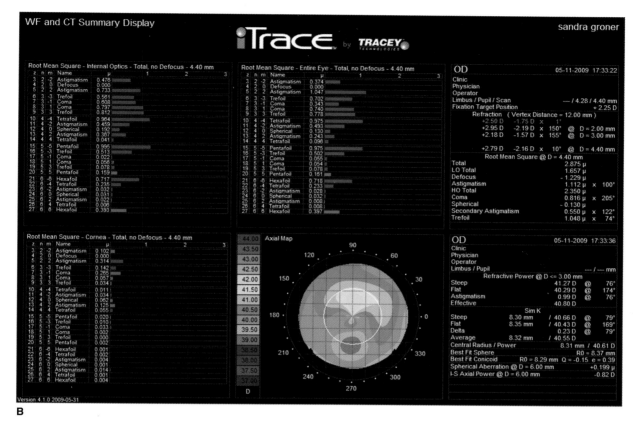

B

▲ **Figure 2–24. B:** Color-coded corneal topographic display of curvature across the entire corneal surface, combined with quantitative measurements of higher-order aberrations from the total eye (top right), lens (top left), and cornea (bottom left). (Photos courtesy of Tracey Technologies, Inc.)

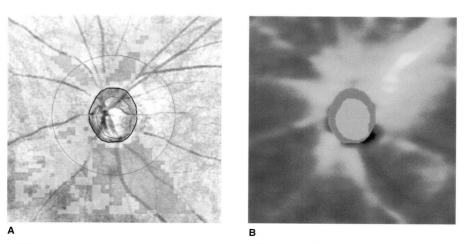

A   **B**

▲ **Figure 2–31.** OCT-derived color-coded maps of retinal nerve fiber layer thickness, with disc and cup masked **(A)** and indicating deviation from normal with cup and disc edges outlined **(B)**.

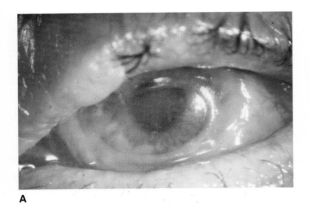

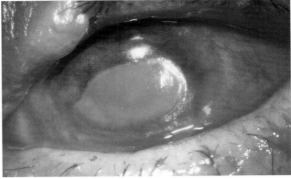

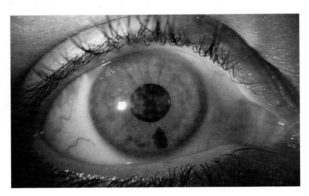

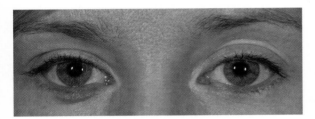

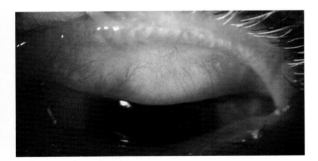

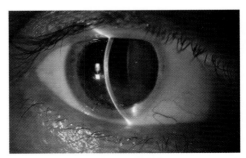

▲ **Figure 3–3.** Large corneal epithelial defect. **A:** Before instillation of fluorescein. **B:** After instillation of fluorescein.

▲ **Figure 4–2.** Severe anterior blepharitis.

▲ **Figure 5–6.** Corneal findings in EKC. Note the uniform, central round subepithelial opacities present in the cornea. (Courtesy of University of California, Davis, Cornea and External Diseases.)

▲ **Figure 5–2.** Conjunctival scarring secondary to trachoma. The superior tarsus is the classic site for subconjunctival scarring in association with trachoma.

▲ **Figure 5–22.** Demonstration with fluorescein staining of punctuate epithelial erosions found in dry eye syndrome due to Sjogren's syndrome, with greater distribution of epithelial lesions inferiorly. (Courtesy of University of California, Davis, Cornea and External Diseases.)

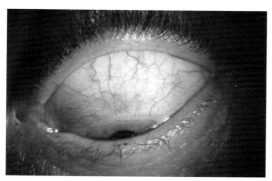

▲ **Figure 5–29.** Superior limbic keratoconjunctivitis with staining with rose bengal.

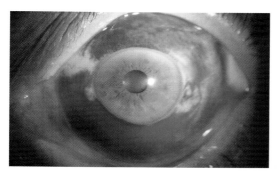

▲ **Figure 5–34.** Spontaneous subconjunctival hemorrhage while on warfarin. (Courtesy of University of California, Davis, Cornea and External Diseases.)

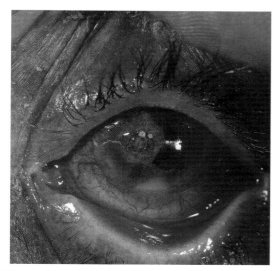

▲ **Figure 6–7.** Medical grade cyanoacrylate glue sealing small paracentral corneal perforation.

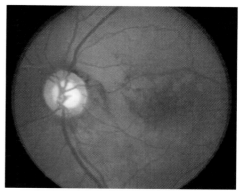

▲ **Figure 7–16.** Diffuse choroidal hemangioma surrounding the optic disc, with its cup appearing large and deep because of the pronounced circumpapillary choroidal vascular thickening. There is clumping of the retinal pigment epithelium in the central macula.

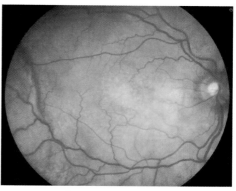

▲ **Figure 7–25.** Diffuse uveal lymphoid infiltration of primary uveal lymphoma, with focal accentuation temporally.

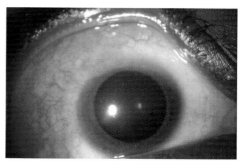

▲ **Figure 7–28.** Anterior diffuse scleritis. (Reproduced with permission from Pavesio C. Scleritis. In: Gupta A, Gupta V, Herbort CP, Khairallah M. *Uveitis Text and Imaging.* New Delhi, India: Jaypee Brothers Medical Publishers [P] Ltd: 2009.)

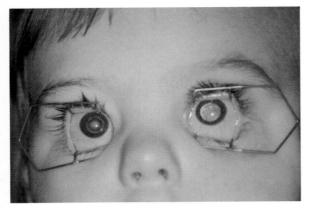

▲ **Figure 8–3.** Congenital cataract (right eye) with dilated pupils.

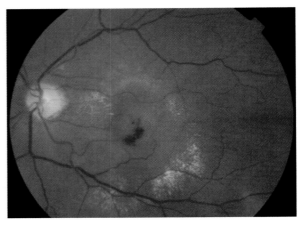

▲ **Figure 10–3.** RAP with superficial hemorrhage, retinal pigment epithelial detachment, and extensive exudation.

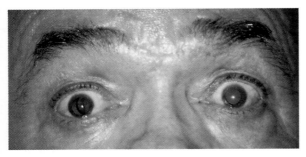

▲ **Figure 8–10.** Partially dislocated (subluxed) lens. (right eye) with dilated pupils.

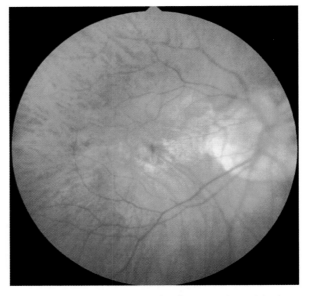

▲ **Figure 10–5.** Myopic macular degeneration with choroidal vessels visible through atrophic retinal pigment epithelium and peripapillary atrophy.

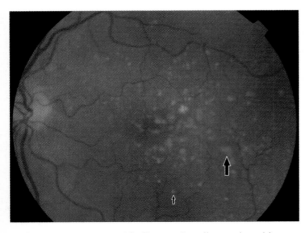

▲ **Figure 10–1.** AMD with discrete (small arrow) and large confluent (large arrow) macular drusen.

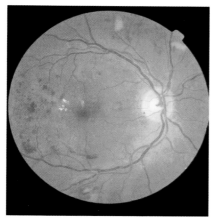

▲ **Figure 10–6.** Moderate nonproliferative diabetic retinopathy showing microaneurysms, deep hemorrhages, flame-shaped hemorrhage, exudates, and cotton-wool spots.

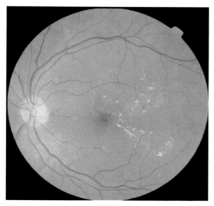

▲ **Figure 10–7.** Clinically significant macular edema with two circinate rings of exudates.

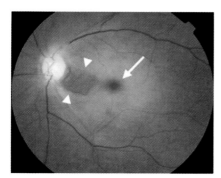

▲ **Figure 10–16.** Acute central retinal artery occlusion with cherry-red spot **(arrow)** and preserved retina due to cilioretinal arterial supply **(arrowheads)**. (Courtesy of Esther Posner.)

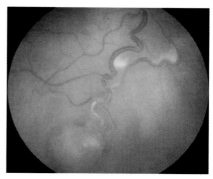

▲ **Figure 10–36.** Classic retinal capillary hemangioma inferiorly. The tumor is fed and drained by dilated tortuous retinal blood vessels. Note intraretinal and subretinal exudates along the blood vessels.

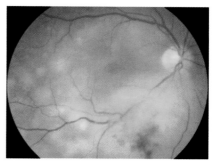

▲ **Figure 10–47.** Primary vitreo-retinal lymphoma in right eye. Fundus features include vitreous haze due to intravitreal cells, ill-defined retinal infiltrate of lymphoma cells inferotemporal to the optic disk, an associated patch of intraretinal blood, and scattered yellow subretinal retinal pigment epithelial infiltrates temporally and inferotemporally.

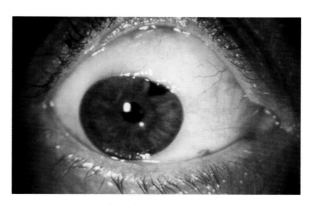

▲ **Figure 11–9.** Trabeculectomy showing an upper nasal "bleb" and peripheral iridectomy.

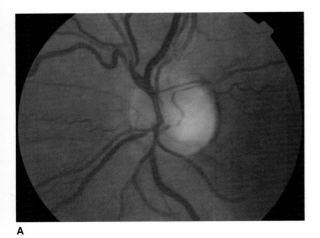

A

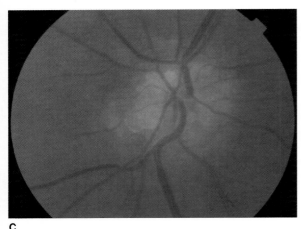

C

▲ **Figure 14–6.** Examples of optic atrophy. **A:** Primary optic atrophy due to nutritional amblyopia. **C:** Optic atrophy with optic disk drusen.

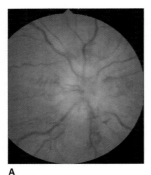

A

▲ **Figure 14–13.** Pseudo-Foster Kennedy syndrome due to sequential anterior ischemic optic neuropathy. **A:** Swollen right optic disk with hemorrhages due to current ischemic episode.

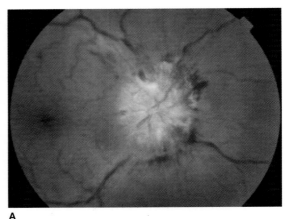

A

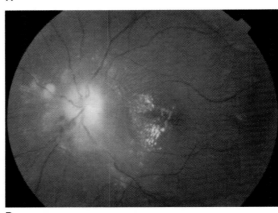

B

▲ **Figure 14–14.** Acute papilledema. **(A)** Optic disk swelling with cotton-wool spots and hemorrhages. **(B)** Retinal exudates.

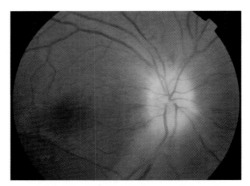

▲ **Figure 14–16.** Atrophic papilledema in idiopathic intracranial hypertension. The disk is pale and mildly elevated with blurred margins. The white areas surrounding the macula are reflected light from the vitreo-retinal interface.

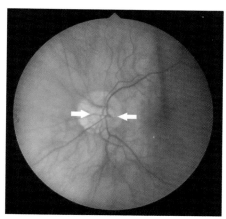

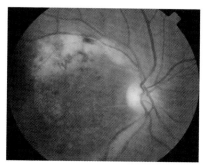

▲ **Figure 15–33.** Retinal changes in HIV infection—cytomegalovirus retinitis.

▲ **Figure 14–21.** Optic nerve hypoplasia. (Arrows indicate optic disk margins.)

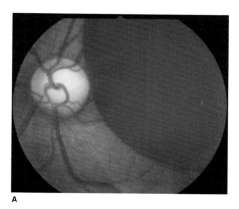

A

▲ **Figure 15–1. A:** Large preretinal hemorrhage due to severe straining.

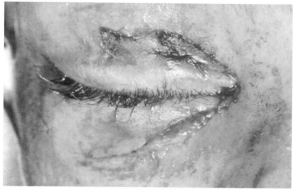

A

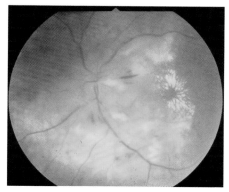

▲ **Figure 15–11.** Accelerated hypertension in a young woman manifesting as marked optic disk edema, macular star of hard exudates, serous retinal detachment, and retinal hemorrhages and cotton-wool spots.

B

▲ **Figure 19–1.** Eyelid laceration with concurrent open globe injury. **A:** Rather innocuous-appearing V-shaped eyelid laceration involving the upper and lower lids and medial canthal skin. **B:** Total dark red hyphema and hemorrhagic chemosis are evident when the lids are separated. Note also that laceration extends through both lacrimal canaliculi.

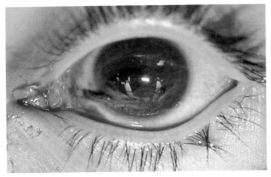

▲ **Figure 19–2.** Corneoscleral laceration inferonasally with pupil displaced toward the laceration and iris incarcerated in wound.

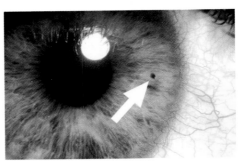

▲ **Figure 19–8.** Metallic corneal foreign body appearing as dark brown speck on the cornea (arrow).

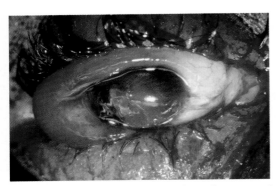

▲ **Figure 19–4.** Pellet gun injury to the right eye resulting in open globe injury. Note massive hemorrhagic chemosis, irregular corneal shape, distorted pupil, and dark brown iris tissue incarcerated into limbal wound.

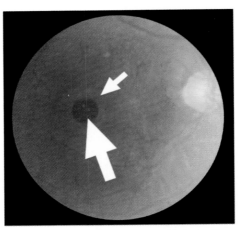

▲ **Figure 19–10.** Post-traumatic macular hole **(larger arrow)** with surrounding serous subretinal fluid **(smaller arrow).**

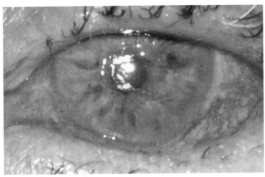

▲ **Figure 19–6.** Corneal abrasion stained with fluorescein.

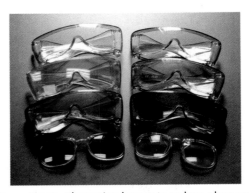

▲ **Figure 24–7.** Absorptive lenses to reduce glare and improve contrast.

INDEX

NOTE: Page numbers followed by *f* denote figures and *t* denotes table respectively.